Emergencies

Severe malaria	27
Sepsis	198
Cardiac arrest	263
Shock	272
Anaphylaxis	273
Acute severe asthma	296
The unconscious patient	406
Rising intracranial pressure	410
Bacterial meningitis	412
Extradural haematoma	436
Status epilepticus	444
Diabetic ketoacidosis	498
Acute poisoning	602
Snake bite	608

OXFORD MEDICAL PUBLICATIONS

Oxford Handbook of Tropical Medicine

Oxford Handbook of Tropical Medicine

Michael Eddleston
and
Stephen Pierini

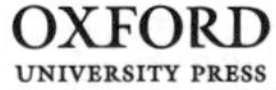

OXFORD
UNIVERSITY PRESS

Great Clarendon Street, Oxford OX2 6DP
Oxford University Press is a department of the University of Oxford.
It furthers the University's objective of excellence in research, scholarship, and education by publishing worldwide in

Oxford New York

Auckland Bangkok Buenos Aires Chennai
Cape town Dar es Salaam Delhi Hong Kong Istanbul Karachi
Kolkata Kuala Lumpur Madrid Melbourne Mexico City Mumbai Nairobi
São Paulo Shanghai Taipei Tokyo Toronto

Published in the United States
by Oxford University Press, Inc., New York

First published 1999
Reprinted 2002

British Library Cataloguing in Publication Data

Data available

Library of Congress Cataloging in Publication Data

Eddleston, Michael.
Oxford handbook of tropical medicine / Michael Eddleston and Stephen Pierini.
(Oxford medical publications)
Includes bibliographical references and index.
1. Tropical medicine—Handbooks, manuals, etc. I. Pierini, Stephen. II. Title. III. Title: Handbook of tropical medicine. IV. Series.
[DNLM: 1. Tropical Medicine handbooks. WC 39 E207o 1999]
RC961.6.E33 1999 616.9'883—dc21 98–50045

ISBN 019 262772 4

Typeset by author

Printed in Great Britain
on acid-free paper by
The Bath Press, Bath

Ideals – from the OHCM

Decisions and intervention are the essence of action; reflection and conjecture are the essence of thought; the essence of medicine is the combining of these realms of action and thought in the service of others. We offer the following ideals to stimulate both thoughts and action – these ideals are hard to reach – like the stars – but they can serve for navigation during the night.

- Do not blame the sick for being sick.
- If the patient's wishes are known, comply with them.
- Work for your patients, not your consultant.
- Use the ward rounds to boost the patient's morale, not your own.
- Treat the whole patient, not the disease – or the ward sister.
- Admit people, not strokes, infarcts, or crumble.
- Spend time with the bereaved; you can help them shed tears.
- Question your conscience – however strongly it tells you to act.
- The ward sister is usually right; respect her opinion.
- Be kind to yourself – you are not an inexhaustible resource.

Tony Hope and Murray Longmore

Dedicated to our parents, Katharine and Bobbie, Antonio and Thelma, for their endless support, encouragement, and love.

Contents

Foreword by David Heymann (Executive Director, Communicable Diseases, WHO) ix

List of abbreviations xiii

1. Introduction 1
2. The WHO/UNICEF approach to the Integrated Management of Childhood Illness 16
3. Major diseases
   - A. Malaria 18
   - B. HIV/STDs 46
   - C. Tuberculosis 110
   - D. Diarrhoeal diseases 128
   - E. Acute respiratory infections/pneumonia 178
4. Fevers/systemic signs 192
5. Cardiology 246
6. Chest medicine 284
7. Renal disease 314
8. Gastroenterology 344
9. Neurology 400
10. Dermatology/skin in systemic disease 458
11. Endocrinology 490
12. Haematology 508
13. Nutrition 550
14. Injuries/poisoning 598
15. Immunization 610
16. Laboratory investigations 626
17. Contact addresses 627
18. Index 629

"... we should not lose sight of the fact that the determinants of health are social and not pharmaceutical. Health is not primarily based on medicine, but on the circumstances under which we live."

Dr H. Grossman, Tanzania

"The world's biggest killer and the greatest cause of ill-health and suffering across the globe is listed almost at the end of the International Classification of Diseases. It is given the code Z59.5 – extreme poverty.

Poverty is the main reason why babies are not vaccinated, why clean water and sanitation are not provided, why curative drugs and other treatments are unavailable, and why mothers die in childbirth. It is the underlying cause of reduced life expectancy, handicap, disability, and starvation. Poverty is a major contributor to mental illness, stress, suicide, family disintegration and substance abuse. Every year in the developing world 12.2 million children under 5 years die, most of them from causes which could be prevented for just a few US cents per child. They die largely because of world indifference, but most of all they die because they are poor. . .

Beneath the heartening facts about decreased mortality and increasing life expectancy, and many other undoubted health advances, lie unacceptable disparities in health. The gaps between rich and poor, between one population group and another, between ages and between sexes, are widening. For most people in the world today every step of life, from infancy to old age, is taken under the twin shadows of poverty and inequity, and under the double burden of suffering and disease.

For many, the prospect of longer life may seem more like a punishment than a gift. Yet by the end of the century we could be living in a world without poliomyelitis, without new cases of leprosy, without deaths from neonatal tetanus and measles. But today the money that some developing countries have to spend per person on health care over an entire year is just US $4 – less than the amount of small change carried in the pockets and purses of many people in the developed world.

A person in one of the least developed countries in the world has a life expectancy of 43 years according to 1993 calculations. A person in one of the most developed countries has a life expectancy of 78 – a difference of more than a third of a century. This means that a rich, healthy man can live twice as long as a poor, sick man.

That inequity alone should stir the conscience of the world – but in some of the poorest countries the life expectancy picture is getting worse. In five countries life expectancy is expected to decrease by the year 2000, whereas everywhere else it is increasing. In the richest countries life expectancy in the year 2000 will reach 79 years. In some of the poorest it will go back to 42 years. Thus the gap continues to widen between rich and poor, and by the year 2000 at least 45 countries are expected to have a life expectancy at birth of under 60 years."

World Health Report 1995 – The state of world health. WHO: Geneva.

Foreword

The past century has brought tremendous advances in science and medicine, public health and sanitation, improving the health and extending the lives of millions of people worldwide. There have been many huge steps forward, from the research laboratory to the hospital bedside to the village health centre. But there have been huge setbacks too, and the challenges of tropical diseases – some of which have been with us for centuries – remain, especially among those who are economically underprivileged. The emergence of new diseases and the resurgence of old ones, together with the rise in antimicrobial resistance have placed an additional burden on clinicians battling these ancient diseases.

Public health measures, including vaccination, are a critical first step in disease prevention and control. When prevention has not been successful, rapid diagnosis and prompt treatment ensure successful control. Untreated, however, infectious diseases cause high levels of morbidity, mortality and in some instances long-term disability. The development of antimicrobial resistance is a particular concern and challenge in countries with limited access to second and third line drugs.

This book comes at a time when, because of international travel and trade, local health problems can rapidly become international health problems. More than ever, the ability of infections to spread quickly and disruptively underscores the need to ensure that local care is reliable and effective.

There have been many developments in the field of tropical medicine and public health over the years, and the World Health Organization continues to provide and update norms, standards and training materials for disease prevention, diagnosis and treatment. This vital information will of course only be useful if it reaches the places where it is most needed – that is health workers in the field, and particularly those in developing countries.

I am especially pleased therefore to have been asked to introduce this Handbook. Written following consultation with WHO staff, it addresses an important need for front-line health workers. It brings together a range of materials and advice for aiding in diagnosis, treatment and decision-making, providing a handy, compact reference for the tropical medicine practitioner in the field. A special feature of this book is its adaptability, with spaces throughout for health workers to add information relevant to their particular setting.

Tropical diseases promise to remain a challenge for many years to come. The success of programmes to fight these diseases starts first and foremost with people committed to prevention, care and cure, who need access to the best tools and information available. This Handbook is an additional step toward meeting that challenge.

David Heymann
Executive Director, Communicable Diseases, WHO

Introduction

This is a first attempt at producing a handbook which will be useful for junior doctors working in the developing world, often with few investigations and little senior support. We had been using the Oxford Handbook of Clinical Medicine for our studies in England but were unable to find anything similar which could have helped us discover clinical medicine in the tropics. Our work in Sri Lanka and Brazil showed us that there was clearly a great need for such a book amongst junior doctors.

We often came across technical guides produced by the WHO but were dismayed to see how rarely they found their way to the doctors working in district hospitals or peripheral clinics. All too often, because of logistic problems, the books arrived at the WHO office in the capital but then never left it. We have attempted to take these WHO management guidelines and put them into a concise form in a book which is cheap and small enough to find its way into the pocket of doctors far away from the capital. We hope that this will allow the most important recipients of this advice, the relatively inexperienced medical officer working in isolation, to be able to judge its value and benefit her patients. We must thank the WHO for their enthusiastic support of the handbook and their willingness to send us information to be included.

Making this book, specific to your local area – a request

Clinical medicine is very different in different countries. Even within a country, clinical practice high in the mountains will differ from that on the coast, or in the dry desert, or in the megacities. It is clearly not possible to write a handbook which will be specific for each and every place or hospital. However, we feel that there is enough in common across the tropics for a book such as this to be useful to junior doctors, supplying them with advice and guidance, often drawn up by the WHO. Readers will have to be critical and selective, deciding what is relevant for their own circumstances and facilities. The blank pages and lines have been left like this to allow each reader to adapt the book to his or her specific location.

We ask that readers send us back comments and criticisms so that we may improve the book in future editions. We hope to be able to offer free copies of future editions to those doctors who send us the best information – via a letter or an old annotated copy. Perhaps we will be able to publish the second edition in three versions – one for Africa, one for Latin America, and one for Asia.

Algorithms

We have taken most algorithms from one source – the WHO. We are not offering these algorithms as strict prescriptions but as hints, suggestions, of how to approach particular clinical situations. As we have emphasized throughout the book, the locally most common cause of any sign must be considered first while constructing a differential diagnosis. We expect readers to attack the algorithms with pencils, changing them to reflect their experience of local practice. We wish them to stimulate, not prescribe.

Acknowledgements

Many people have helped us get this idea off the ground. We particularly owe an immense debt to Robin Young for being our mentor early in the book's genesis, to Anne Prasad for reading through each page and giving us her editing and pharmaceutical skills, to Robin Bailey and Chris Whitty for reading multiple chapters and offering frequent criticism and encouragement, to Clare Sander and Gayathri Perera for writing the TB and haematology sections, and to Millie Davies for revising the book's drug doses.

From the time of our visit in 1995, we have been helped by many people from the WHO, in particular Pat Butler, David Bramley, Tore Godal, Gordon Stott, Jim Tulloch, Olivier Fontaine, Cathy Wolfheim, Mary Couper, Jono Quick, K. Behbehani, Peter Beales, Sergio Spinaci, David Heymann, Karin Esteves, Michael Ryan, John Clements, JW Lee, Bjorn Melgaard, Peter Piot, G. Vercautereng, Jim LeDuc and M. Thuriaux. Eileen Lloyd of the CDC helped us with the isolation guidelines. At the Wellcome Trust, we were welcomed by Robin Young, Chris Coyer, Denise Chew, Neil Packenham Walsh, and Simon Cathcart, and at the British National Formulary by Dinesh Mehta and James Reynolds.

Many people have read and commented on particular pages. We would like to thank Jean Alexander and the Department of Physiotherapy at the Radcliffe Infirmary, Oxford, William Howlett, Terence Ryan, Rob Davidson, Dunisha Samarasinghe, Chris Conlon, Steve Allen, Ariaranee Ariaratnam, Resvi Sheriff, David Mabey, Tony Bryceson, C Adams, Rustam Al-Shahi, Ra'ad Shakir, Dan Peckham, J Strang, Chris Tang, Bryan Angus, Philip Meyer, Michelle Murdoch, and Ali Khan. We also thank Anna Drage, Mike Pacey, and Charlotte Van Rooyen for their help for putting up with our constant interruptions. Thanks also to Wendy for her late night cups of tea and to Claire Schofield for being so patient.

Finally, we owe an immense debt to our long-suffering mentors David Warrell and David Theakston. May they continue to send fresh-faced medical students out to remote corners of the world in search of even more lethal poisons, venoms, and indigenous weapons.

Sources

We have used many sources for this book in addition to WHO publications. The most important are:

Weatherall D, Ledingham JGG, & Warrell DA, *Oxford Textbook of Medicine*, 3rd ed, OUP: Oxford 1996

Hope RA, Longmore M, Hodgetts T, Ramrakha P, *Oxford Handbook of Clinical Medicine*, 3rd ed, OUP: 1994

Cook GC, *Manson's Tropical Diseases*, 20th ed, Saunders: London 1996

Mandell G, *Principles and Practice of Infectious Disease*, 4th ed, Churchill Livingstone: New York 1995.

Evidence-based tropical medicine

At present, there is relatively little evidence-based tropical medicine. This will surely change and future editions will be able to incorporate this new information. Available resources are cited by Garner *et al.* 1998 *BMJ*, **317**, 531. This paper can be found on the web at <http://www.bmj.com/>

Note from the publishers

The publishers would like to thank the Editors of the *Oxford Textbook of Medicine*, 3rd edn., for permission to reproduce the figures on pages 21, 23, 41, 43, 45, 141, 155, 157, 187, 223, 227, 233, 245, 329, 355, 363, 375, 385, 393, 399, 421, 460, 461, 463, 483, 493, 563, 583, 597; the authors of the *Oxford Handbook of Clinical Medicine*, 3rd edn., for permission to reproduce the figures on pages 251, 253, 257, 263, 267, 283, 355, 359; the authors of *Nutrition for Developing Countries* for permission to reproduce the figures on pages 557, 559, 561, 575, 593; the World Health Organization for permission to reproduce the figures on pages 11, 31, 43, 83, 85, 86, 89, 90, 91, 93, 129, 145, 311, 321, 381, 383, 387, 397, 423, 517, 523; the Resuscitation Council UK Ltd for permission to reproduce the figures on page 263; Mr CBT Adams for permission to reproduce the figure on page 437; WB Saunders for permission to reproduce the figures on pages 227, 239, 243, 387, 415, 447, 489, 522, 525, 531; Edward Arnold for permission to reproduce the figures on pages 431, 433; the BMJ Publishing Group for permission to reproduce the figures on pages 204, 205, 295; the *New England Journal of Medicine* for permission to reproduce the figure on page 51; Tropical Health Technology (Teaching Aids at Low Cost, TALC) for permission to reproduce the figures on pages 213, 225, 227, 483, 485, 537, 539; Blackwell Science Ltd for permission to reproduce the figures on pages 34, 35; Antimicrobial Therapy Ltd for permission to reproduce the figures on pages 71, 77; Mandell for permission to reproduce the figure on page 371.

We would like to thank the following people who have informed us about corrections:

R Beharry
J Crawley
M Davies
N Gainsborough
J Hartley
J Keystone
L Marcus
D Warrell
Bridget Wills
V. Wuthiekanun

List of abbreviations

>	more than
<	less than
↑	raised
↓	lowered
→	leading to
%	per cent
~	approximately
+ve	positive
-ve	negative
1°	primary
2°	secondary

AII	aortic component of second heart sound
ABG	arterial blood gases
ACE	angiotensin-converting enzyme
ACS	acute confusional state
ACTH	adrenocorticotrophic hormone
AD	autosomal dominant (genetic inheritance)
AF	atrial fibrillation
AFB	acid-alcohol-fast bacilli
AFP	acute flaccid paralysis
AHA	autoimmune haemolytic anaemia
AHF	Argentinian haemorrhagic fever
AIDS	acquired immunodeficiency syndrome
ALL	acute lymphoblastic leukaemia
ALS	advanced life support
ALT	alanine transferase
AML	acute myeloblastic leukaemia
ANS	autonomic nervous system
AP	abdominal pain
APBA	allergic bronchopulmonary aspergillosis
AR	autosomal recessive (genetic inheritance)
ARF	acute renal failure
ARDS	acute respiratory distress syndrome
ARI	acute respiratory infection
ASO	antistreptolysin O
AST	aspartate transaminase
ATLS	advanced trauma life support
ATN	acute tubular necrosis
AV	atrioventricular
AXR	abdominal X-ray (plain)
Ba	barium
BAL	bronchoalveolar lavage
BCG	Bacille Calmette Guerin
Bd	bis die (twice a day)
BHF	Bolivian haemorrhagic fever
BL	Burkitt's lymphoma
BLS	basic life support
BMI	body mass index
BNF	British National Formulary

BOOP	bronchiolitis obliterans organizing pneumonia
BP	blood pressure
BPM	beats per minute
CA	carcinoma
CA^{2+}	calcium ions
CABG	coronary artery bypass graft
CAH	chronic active hepatitis
Cal	calorie
CAP	community-acquired pneumonia
CBD	common bile duct
CCF	congestive cardiac failure
CCHF	Crimean-Congo haemorrhagic fever
CDC	Centers for Disease Control and Prevention, Atlanta, USA
CDRI	Central Drug Research Institute
CF	cystic fibrosis
CID	*Clinical Infectious Diseases*
CK	creatinine kinase
CK-MB	creatinine kinase cardiac isoenzyme
Cl^-	chloride ions
CLL	chronic lymphocytic leukaemia
cm	centimetre
CMI	cell-mediated immunity
CML	chronic myeloid leukaemia
CMV	cytomegalovirus
CNS	central nervous system
COPD	chronic obstructive pulmonary disease
CPR	cardiopulmonary resuscitation
Cr	creatinine
CRF	chronic renal failure
CSD	catch scratch disease
CSF	cerebrospinal fluid
CT	computerized tomography
CVA	cerebrovascular accident (stroke)
CVI	Children's Vaccine Initiative
CVS	cardiovascular system
CXR	chest X-ray
D&V	diarrhoea and vomiting
DCL	disseminated cutaneous leishmaniasis
DCT	direct Coomb's test
DEC	diethylcarbamazine
DHF	dengue haemorrhagic fever
DIC	disseminated intravascular coagulation
dl	decilitre
DM	diabetes mellitus
DNA	deoxyribonucleic acid
DOTS	directly observed treatment strategy
DT	diphtheria toxoid
DTP	diphtheria toxoid, pertussis, and tetanus toxoid
DVT	deep vein thrombi
dxm	dexamethasone
EBV	Epstein-Barr virus
ECF	extracellular fluid
ECG	electrocardiogram

EEV	equine encephalitis virus
eg	for example
EHEC	enterohaemorrhagic *E. coli*
ELISA	enzyme linked immunosorbant assay
EPI	Expanded Programme on Immunization
ERCP	endoscopic retrograde cholangiopancreatography
ESR	erythrocyte sedimentation rate
ETEC	enterotoxigenic *E. coli*
ETT	exercise treadmill test
EUA	examination under anaesthesia
F	female
FBC	full blood count
FCPD	fibrocalculous pancreatic diabetes
FDP	fibrinogen degradation product
Fe	iron
FEV_1	forced expiratory volume in first second
FFP	fresh frozen plasma
Fhx	family history
FOB	faecal occult blood
Ft	feet (measurement)
g	gram
G^+	Gram-stain positive
GBS	Guillain-Barre syndrome
GCS	Glasgow coma scale
GFR	glomerular filtration rate
GH	growth hormone
GI	gastrointestinal
GN	glomerulonephritis
G6PD	glucose-6-phosphate dehydrogenase
GTN	glyceryl trinitrate
GTT	glucose tolerance test
GU	genitourinary
HA	haemaglutanin
HAV	hepatitis A virus
Hb	haemoglobin
HBeAg	hepatitis B virus e antigen
HBsAg	hepatitis B virus surface antigen
HBV	hepatitis B virus
HCC	hepatocellular carcinoma
HCV	hepatitis C virus
HDV	hepatitis D virus
HELLP	haemolysis, elevated liver enzymes and low platelet counts
HF	haemorrhagic fever
HHV-8	human herpes virus-8 (KSAV)
Hib	*Haemophilus influenzae* type b
HIV	human immunodeficiency virus
HL	Hodgkin's lymphoma
HLA	human lymphocyte antigen
HMMA	4-hydroxy-3-methoxymandelic acid
HMS	hyperreactive malarial splenomegaly
hrs	Hours
HSV	herpes simplex virus
HT	hypertension

HTLV	human T-cell lymphotrophic virus
HUS	haemolytic-uraemic syndrome
Hx	history
IBD	inflammatory bowel disease
ICP	intracranial pressure
ID	intradermal
IDD	iodine deficiency
IDDM	insulin-dependent diabetes mellitus
IHD	ischaemic heart disease
IMCI	WHO's Integrated Management of Childhood Illness
IM	intramuscular
INR	international normalized ratio
IPV	injected polio vaccine
ITP	idiopathic thrombocytopenic purpura
ITU	intensive therapy unit
IU	international unit
IUD	intrauterine contraceptive device
IV	intravenous
IVU	intravenous urography
J	joule
JE	Japanese encephalitis
JVP	jugular venous pressure
K^+	potassium ions
KCCT	kaolin cephalin clotting time
kg	kilogram
kJ	kilojoule
KOH	potassium hydroxide
kPa	kiloPascal
KS	Kaposi sarcoma
KSAV	Kaposi sarcoma associated virus
l	litre
LBBB	left bundle branch block
LBRF	louse borne relapsing fever
LD	lymphocyte depleted
LDH	lactate dehydrogenase
LFT	liver function test
Li^+	lithium ions
LIF	left iliac fossa
LN	lymph node
LOC	level of consciousness
LP	lymphocyte predominant
LP	lumbar puncture
LPS	lipopolysaccharide
LV	left ventricle
LVF	left ventricular failure
M	metre
M	male
MALT	mucosa-associated lymphoid tissue
max	maximum
MC	mixed cellularity
MC	mucosal leishmaniasis
MCH	mean cell haemoglobin
MCV	mean cell volume

mg	milligram
Mg^{2+}	magnesium ions
MI	myocardial infarction
mins	minutes
Ml	myocardial infarction
mm	millimetre
mmHg	millimetres of mercury
mmol	millimol
MMR	measles, mumps, and rubella vaccine
MND	motor neurone disease
MoH	Ministry of Health
Mosmol	milliosmol
MR	measles and rubella vaccine
MRDM	malnutrition-related diabetes mellitus
MST	morphine sulphate
mths	months
MU	megaunits (of benzylpenicillin = 0.6g)
MUAC	measuring the mid-upper arm circumference
N	north
NA	neuraminidase
Na^+	sodium ions
ND	notifiable disease (WHO)
NE	north east
NG	nasogastric
NGO	Non-governmental Organization
NGT	nasogastric tube
NHL	non-Hodgkin's lymphoma
NIDDM	non-insulin-dependent diabetes mellitus
NS	nodular sclerosing
NSAID	non-steroidal anti-inflammatory drug
N&V	nausea and/or vomiting
O_2	oxygen
OCP	oral contraceptive pill
Od	omni die (once daily)
OGS	oxygenic steroid
O/p	outpatient
OPV	oral polio vaccine
ORS	oral rehydration solution
OTM	Oxford Textbook of Medicine
$PaCO_2$	partial pressure of carbon dioxide in arterial blood
PAM	primary amoebic meningoencephalitis
PAN	polyarteritis nodosa
PCP	Pneumocystis carinii pneumonia
PCV	paced cell volume
PDPD	protein deficient pancreatic diabetes
PE	pulmonary embolism
PEFR	peak expiratory flow rate
pg	picogram
[illegible]	persistent generalized lymphadenopathy
[illegible]	portal hypertension
[illegible]	pelvic inflammatory disease
[illegible]	post-infective malabsorption
[illegible]	post kalar dermal leishmania

PML	progressive multifocal leukoencephalopathy
PMN	polymorphonuclear neutrophils
PNG	Papua New Guinea
PNS	peripheral nervous system
PO	per os (by mouth)
PO_4	phosphate
PR	per rectum (by the rectum)
PRV	polycythaemia rubra vera
PT	prothrombin time
PTB	pulmonary tuberculosis
PTH	parathyroid hormone
PTT	partial thromboplastin time
PV	per vaginam (by the vagina)
qds	quarter die sumendus (to be taken 4 times a day)
q2h	every 2 hours
q4h	every 4 hours, etc
RA	rheumatoid arthritis
RBBB	right bundle branch block
RBC	red blood cell
RDA	recommended daily allowances
RF	rheumatic fever
RHF	right heart failure
RIF	right iliac fossa
RIG	anti-rabies immunoglobulin
RMSF	Rocky Mountain spotted fever
RNA	ribonucleic acid
RR	respiratory rate
RSV	respiratory syncytial virus
RUQ	right upper quadrant
RV	right ventricular
RVF	Rift Valley fever
RVF	right ventricular failure
SAH	subarachnoid haemorrhage
SBE	subacute bacterial endocarditis
SC	subcutaneous
SCC	short course chemotherapy
SE	south east
SG	specific gravity
SIADH	syndrome of inappropriate ADH secretion
SLE	systemic lupus erythematosus
SOL	space-occupying lesion
SSPE	subacute sclerosing panencephalitis
STD	sexually transmitted disease
SVC	superior vena cava
TB	tuberculosis
TBRF	tick borne relapsing fever
Td	tetanus toxoid and low-dose diphtheria toxoid vaccine
tds	ter die sumendus (to be taken 3 times a day)
TFC	therapeutic feeding centre
TFT	thyroid function test
TIA	transient ischaemic attack
TIBC	total iron binding capacity
TMP/SMX	trimethoprim/sulfamethoxazole (co-trimoxazole)

TMR	Tropical Medicine Resource (The Wellcome Trust)
TSH	thyroid-stimulating hormone
TSS	tropical splenomegaly syndrome
TT	tetanus toxoid vaccine
TURP	transurethral resection of the prostate
UC	ulcerative colitis
U&E	urea and electrolytes – and creatinine
UK	United Kingdom
URT	upper respiratory tract
URTI	upper respiratory tract infection
USS	ultrasound scan
UTI	urinary tract infection
UV	ultraviolet
VEEV	Venezuelan equine encephalitis virus
VF	ventricular fibrillation
VHF	viral haemorrhagic fever
VMA	vanillyl mandelic acid
VSD	ventriculo-septal defect
VT	ventricular tachycardia
VZV	varicella-zoster virus
WCC	white cell count
WHO	World Health Organization
wks	weeks
yrs	Years
ZN	Ziehl-Neelson

1. Introduction

Traditional health care systems: a health resource of the majority 2
The Wellcome Trust's Tropical Medicine Resource (TMR) 3
The 1993 World Development Report – *Investing in Health* 4
The WHO's Essential Drugs Programme 6
Outbreaks 8
Universal precautions 12
Isolation precautions 15

Traditional health care systems: a health resource of the majority[1]

Gerard Bodeker, Global Initiative for Traditional Systems of Health, University of Oxford.

2

According to the World Health Organization (WHO), traditional health care systems constitute the main source of everyday health care for 60–80% of the population of most developing countries. The ratio of traditional health practitioners to population is substantially higher than that for trained medical personnel, representing an irreplaceable health care infrastructure. However, most traditional systems are outside the formal health sector or have marginal status within it.

Many traditional strategies are effective with such everyday conditions as wounds, skin disorders, respiratory conditions, and intestinal parasites. Some ineffective or unsafe practices also exist and underscore the need for training, research and policy development.

The cost of modern medicine influences traditional medicine utilization, as does limited availability of pharmaceutical drugs and drug resistance.[2] Villagers will often seek symptomatic relief from modern medicine, while using traditional medicine for what is perceived as the "true cause of the condition".

Training of traditional birth attendants is valuable, as with local healers who can disseminate health information, such as AIDS prevention. Some medical schools (e.g. Vietnam, and the University of Health Sciences in Moshi, Tanzania) provide training in traditional medicine to prepare students to understand the health care practices that the many patients use and to facilitate collaboration and cross-referral with traditional practitioners.

It is useful for the clinician to know that many herbal medicines can be effective and safe. An online database – NAPRALERT – accessible through Medline, gives pharmacological information on medicinal plants and herbal medicines. Herbal medicines can interact with pharmaceutical drugs to (i) potentiate the effects of pharmaceutical drugs or (ii) act antagonistically. The Central Drug Research Institute (CDRI) of India has patented a traditional Ayurvedic mixture of black pepper, long pepper and ginger, which allows for the dosage of the antibiotic rifampicin to be reduced by up to half in the treatment of tuberculosis and other mycobacterial infections. Many local plant-derived antimalarials appear to have antiplasmodial effects. However, certain antiplasmodial substances used in traditional medicines can interact antagonistically with pharmaceuticals.

Herbal drugs need not be assumed to be harmful or useless because no clinical trials have been conducted on them. Lack of research funding often underlies this deficiency. NAPRALERT and other databases, as well as national traditional medicine research centres, should be consulted in clarifying uncertainties regarding traditional medicine.

1. Bodeker G. *In* Hunter's Textbook on Tropical Medicine, 8th ed, W.B. Saunders Company 1998. Bodeker G, Parry E (eds) New approaches in traditional medicine, *Tropical Doctor*, 1997, **27**, Supplement 1.
2. Ong C-K, 1997, *Postgrad. Doctor Africa*, **19**, 52.

The Wellcome Trust's Tropical Medicine Resource (TMR)

Christopher Coyer, Head of the Tropical Medicine Resource, The Wellcome Trust, London

The Wellcome Trust has been actively involved in tropical medicine research for many years. Its founder, Sir Henry Wellcome, developed an interest in the subject through travelling the world and in 1902 established a tropical medicine research laboratory in Khartoum, Sudan.

Almost a century later many of the diseases that were of importance to researchers in 1902 are still having a devastating effect on human populations today. Malaria in particular has a hold on huge areas of the African continent, with current WHO estimates for global mortality being between 1.5 and 2.7 million people per year[1]. Growing parasite resistance to drug treatments and mosquito vector resistance to insecticides are both issues that need to be tackled by today's researchers. Tuberculosis is now a growing problem in many parts of the world and deaths through the effects of HIV/AIDs were estimated at 2.3 million people in 1997.

Today, Wellcome Trust funded units in Kenya, Thailand and Vietnam play a critical role in enabling high quality clinical and epidemiological field research and in providing training for local scientists. A new tool for tropical medicine training is the CD-ROM-based Topics in International Health series, which was first published by the Wellcome Trust in 1998.

The series consists of training materials for use by medical and life science students, their teachers and healthcare professionals worldwide. The following topics are already covered: malaria, trachoma, sexually transmitted diseases, sickle cell disease, leprosy, diarrhoeal diseases, schistosomiasis and tuberculosis; and disks on AIDS/HIV, nutrition and leishmaniasis are planned for the future. Each CD-ROM in the series contains tutorials, a complementary photographic image collection and an electronic glossary of terms. The series is intended for use within both the developed and the developing world, where the installation base of computers equipped with CD-drives is growing steadily.

The release of such materials is not something that has been done with the intention of replacing either textbooks or teachers, indeed quite the opposite is true. The intention is to broaden the range of materials that are available to teachers and their students, and to enrich the learning experience through the provision of interactive training materials. In any teaching model a balanced combination of teacher-directed time, printed resources, audio-visual media and individual student study, holds the key to successful learning. It is hoped that alongside the Oxford Handbook of Tropical Medicine, the Topics in International Health series will help support students and their teachers in schools and colleges of tropical medicine around the globe.

The Topics in International Health CD-ROMS are available from CABI Publishing. Email <publishing@cabi.org>, or write to CABI Publishing, CABI International, Walingford, Oxon, OX10 8DE, UK.

1. The World Health Report 1998, World Health Organization, Geneva, 1998

The 1993 World Development Report – *Investing in Health*[1]

In 1993, the World Bank published their annual World Development Report which was in that year dedicated to the issue of health. The report took as its starting point the disparity between the huge amount of money spent on health in the developing world (US $168 billion) and the lack of even basic health facilities for many of its poorest inhabitants.

These two pages give the key messages of the report. It has become one of the most influential health policy documents of recent years.[2] Its proposals, if put into effect, will have far-reaching consequences. We therefore feel that more doctors in the tropics should read the report and, whether in agreement or not, take part in the policy discussions which will influence the future of health policy and practice in their countries.

The report first discusses problems with health services which impede their supply of cost-effective health care to the majority of the population, especially the poor. Clearly not all are relevant for each and every country.

Problems with government health care provision

- ***Misallocation:*** public money is being spent on health interventions of low cost effectiveness (surgery for cancer) at the same time that critical and highly cost-effective interventions, such as treatment of TB and STDs, remain underfunded. In some countries, a single teaching hospital absorbs 20% of the MoH budget, even though almost all cost-effective interventions are best delivered at lower-level facilities.
- ***Inequity:*** the poor lack access to basic health care services and receive low-quality care. Government spending for health goes disproportionately to the rich in the form of free or below-cost care in sophisticated tertiary care hospitals and subsidies to private and public insurance.
- ***Inefficiency:*** much of the money spent on health is wasted – for example, brand name pharmaceuticals are purchased instead of cheap generic drugs and health workers are badly deployed and supervised.
- ***Exploding costs:*** in some middle-income developing countries health care expenditures are growing much faster than income. Increasing numbers of general physicians and specialists, the availability of new medical technologies, and expanding health insurance linked to fee-for-service payments together generate a rapidly growing demand for costly tests, procedures, and treatments.

The report then went on to propose solutions for the government.

1. Foster an environment that enables households to improve health

Household decisions shape health, but these decisions are constrained by the income and education of household members. In addition to promoting overall economic growth, governments can help to improve these decisions if they:

- pursue economic growth policies that will benefit the poor (this is fundamental; while child mortality fell everywhere during the 1980s, it fell twice as fast in countries where income increased by >1%/year);

- expand investment in schooling, particularly for girls, because the way that mothers use information and financial resources to shape their dietary, fertility, health care, and other lifestyle choices has a powerful influence on the health of other household members;
- promote the rights and status of women through political and economic empowerment and legal protection against abuse.

2. Improve government spending on health

The challenge for most governments is to concentrate resources on compensating for market failures and financing services that will particularly benefit the poor. Several directions for policy respond to this challenge:

- Reduce government expenditures on tertiary facilities, specialist training, and interventions that provide little health gain for the money spent. It is difficult to justify using government funds for such treatments when much more cost-effective services which benefit mainly the poor are not adequately financed.
- Finance and implement a package of public health interventions to deal with infectious disease control, prevention of AIDS, environmental pollution, and behaviours (such as drunk driving) that put others at risk. One potentially very effective intervention would be to use schools to deliver inexpensive treatment for schistosomiasis, intestinal worm infections, and nutrient deficiencies and to educate children about health and the risk of behaviours such as smoking & unsafe sex.
- Finance and ensure delivery of a package of essential clinical services. The comprehensiveness and composition of such a package can only be defined by each country taking into account epidemiological conditions, local preferences, and income. In most countries, public finance, or publicly mandated finance, of the essential clinical package would provide a politically acceptable way of distributing both welfare improvements and a productive asset – better health – to the poor.
- Improve management of government health services through such measures as decentralization of administrative and budgetary authority and contracting out of services.

3. Promote diversity and competition

There is not enough room to discuss the third set of proposals (relating to ways of organizing and financing health care) here. They have proven to be more controversial than the other proposals, with some authors questioning whether the developing world has the institutional capacity to carry out these reforms and regulate privately-financed health providers.[3]

Overall, the reforms proposed by the World Bank entail shifting new government spending for health away from specialized personnel, equipment, and facilities at the apex of health systems and "down the pyramid" toward the broad base of widely accessible care in community facilities and health centres.

1. World Development Report, *Investing in Health*, The International Bank for Reconstruction and Development/The World Bank. OUP: New York 1993
2. Buse K, 1998, *Lancet*, **351**, 665 3. Mills A, 1997, *TMIH*, **2**, 963

The WHO's Essential Drugs Programme

Mary Couper, DMP, WHO.

As far back as 1975, the World Health Assembly reviewed the main drug problems facing the developing world and outlined possible new drug policies. These policies were intended to extend the accessibility and rational use of the most necessary drugs to populations whose basic health needs could not be met by the existing supply system. The resulting essential drugs concept is basic to a National Drug Policy because it enables priorities to be set. It is intended to be adaptable to many different situations; exactly which drugs are regarded as essential remains a national responsibility. Its principle is that a limited number of drugs leads to better supply, more rational prescribing and lower costs, and easier quality assurance, procurement, storage, distribution and dispensing. Training and drug information can also be more focused and prescribers gain more experience with fewer drugs and recognize adverse reactions better. Essential drugs are usually cheaper and procurement of fewer items in larger quantities results in economies of scale.

At the heart of this work is the WHO model list of essential drugs. It is into its twentieth year and its success lies in the fact that it combines being a useful tool for effective drug supplies with a strong educational component. The list now contains 306 pharmaceutical products which "satisfy the health care needs of the majority of the population and should therefore be available at all times in adequate amounts and in the appropriate dosage form". The model list will also be the basis of a WHO model formulary which will include all the drugs on the model list together with prescribing information. WHO model prescribing information is currently being prepared. To date, five titles have been published on anaesthesia, parasitic diseases, mycobacterial diseases, STDs, HIV and associated infections, and skin diseases.

The concept of essential drugs has been disseminated and promoted extensively at the country level by the WHO's Action Programme on Essential Drugs, as well as by disease control programmes in the WHO, international and non-governmental organizations throughout the world, and bilateral agencies. The wide applicability of the concept is now evident from experience gained worldwide. Many countries have also successfully applied the concept to teaching hospitals and centres providing specialized care, and to the dissemination of drug information.

Antibiotic resistance and the rational use of antibiotics[1]

Particular emphasis has been placed on antimicrobial prescribing in recent years as a result of the ever-increasing problem of antimicrobial resistance. Resistance develops as soon as an antibiotic becomes widely used, particularly if it is used indiscriminately (such as being made available without prescription). Restriction in the use of particular antimicrobials is able to reduce the prevalence of resistant microorganisms since there is subsequently less drive to select for the resistant strains. This was recently reconfirmed in an excellent study from the USA where resistance against ceftazidime dropped from 24% to 8% among inpatients within 2 years of prescriptions requiring authorization by consultant microbiologists.[2]

The antimicrobial section of the WHO essential drugs list has been structured so as to promote the use of a number of well-established, widely available, relatively inexpensive drugs. Unfortunately, it is becoming increasingly common for important pathogens to emerge in a locality and be proved by susceptibility testing to have developed resistance to all these 'essential drugs'. In recognition of this problem, the WHO has now included a number of 'reserve antimicrobials' in the most recent version of the list. These are antibiotics which should be readily available but held in reserve and not used routinely. Examples of such drugs include the third-generation cephalosporins (eg ceftazidime), the fluoroquinolones, and vancomycin. While these antibiotics are useful for a wide variety of infections, because of the need to reduce the risk of the development of resistance and because of their relatively high cost, it is considered inappropriate to recommend their unrestricted use.

The importance of determining prevailing susceptibilities to important bacterial pathogens cannot be overemphasized since the selection of an antimicrobial is dependent upon this information. Prescribers also require access to independent information on essential antimicrobials. A further developing world problem relating to antimicrobials is the frequency with which patients are put at risk because of substandard drugs. A study in west Africa showed that 17 of some 450 drugs contained no detectable active ingredient. Most of these 17 products were antibiotics.

Each country needs to define its own list of 'essential' and 'reserve' antimicrobials. To promote their rational use and to prevent the development of resistance to them, each country must then develop a strategy for their use. The WHO and national drug regulatory authorities have recommended that countries should:

- make available independent authoritative information for prescribers and develop prescribing guidelines;
- monitor patterns of antibiotic resistance;
- ensure the quality of antimicrobial agents through regulation;
- encourage continuing education of both prescribers and the public;
- strengthen the control of antibiotic-related promotional activities;
- encourage research for innovative products.

1. Couper M, 1997, *CID*, 24, S154 2. White AC, 1997, *CID*, 25, 230

British National Formulary (BNF)

There is a lack of independent advice on drugs and prescribing in the developing world. Doctors need such help to combat the attempts of pharmaceutical industry representatives to promote their company's drugs with little objective proof of improved efficacy. We had hoped to put an essential drug formulary in this handbook but it has proved impossible to produce a good one with the space and resources available. We have decided therefore to push for more widespread availability of the BNF in the tropics. Although not written for these countries, the BNF offers truly authoritative advice and would usefully complement local formularies and the proposed WHO model formulary.

Outbreaks

Michael Ryan, EMC, WHO.

Clinicians usually deal with individual cases of an infectious disease. They diagnose and treat the case and where appropriate follow-up on the contacts of the case to prevent disease spreading further (eg TB). Occasionally, however, the physician notices something unusual. This may be in the form of a cluster of cases of either a specific disease or a collection of symptoms and signs (syndrome). This clustering of cases can occur:

- in time (eg a number of cases occurring in a short period)
- in place (eg a number of cases occurring in the same village)
- in person (eg a number of cases in the same age group).

The disease may be easily recognizable or the symptoms and signs may represent a disease that the clinicians have never seen before.

An outbreak is defined as the occurrence of two or more linked cases of a communicable disease. The response of the public health services to a suspected outbreak can only occur after the health services themselves become aware of the problem. The keys to outbreak control are early detection, reporting, and confirmation. This allows a coordinated response from the responsible agencies early in an epidemic.

Detection and reporting

Each country will have a number of infectious diseases that are considered to have epidemic potential (see opposite). These are usually under public health surveillance and it is the duty of a physician seeing a case of such a disease to report it to the public health service. However, outbreaks can occur of diseases which fall outside the regular list of epidemic-prone diseases or are even not known.

Early warning of a suspected outbreak may come from a variety of sources both official and non-official (see page 11). Health workers may routinely report individual cases of epidemic prone diseases to the public health services who are continually on the lookout for clusters of cases. They are also in the front line in the detection of outbreaks as in many cases it is the health workers themselves who notice a cluster of cases or something unusual. Other sources of information relating to suspected outbreaks include the media, NGOs, and the community themselves.

It is important that health workers report routinely what is required[1] and also that they report any suspected outbreaks to the next level so that investigation and confirmation may take place. It is useful to ask a number of questions before making a report such as this (see box opposite and figure on page 11). This will help one to collect all the relevant information. The answers will also aid in forming a hypothesis on the cause of the outbreak and be extremely useful in briefing the public health specialists who may investigate.

1. John J, 1998, *Lancet*, 352, 58

Notifiable diseases

These may well vary with locality. Check local guidelines.

- cholera
- AIDS
- diphtheria
- encephalitis
- measles
- tetanus
- viral hepatitis
- plague
- AFP
- dysentery
- leptospirosis
- human rabies
- tuberculosis
- whooping cough
- yellow fever
- haemorrhagic fever
- typhoid fever
- malaria
- food poisoning
- typhus fever
- simple continuous fever of >7 days duration
- any other disease occurring in large numbers

All cases of the above conditions should be reported ***on clinical suspicion alone***, without waiting for laboratory confirmation, by the doctor treating the case.

This may involve filling in a card and posting it to the Ministry of Health or local Health Directorate.

► Cases of cholera, plague, yellow fever, AFP (+/- AIDS) will require urgent notification - via telephone or telegram if possible.

Questions to be answered with any suspected outbreak

1. - Date of onset of symptoms and presentation of the first case
   - Number of cases/hospitalizations/deaths
   - Dates of onset, age, location, status (alive/dead) of all cases
2. - Symptoms and signs of this disease?
   - Suspected diagnosis?
   - Is the disease severe?
   - Is the disease spreading?
   - Are there secondary cases in any households?
3. - Have clinical specimens been collected?
   - Are any test results available (laboratory, X-ray)?
4. - Any suspicions about the pathogen, its source or route of transmission?

Confirmation

It is extremely important to confirm that an outbreak exists. This can be relatively straightforward if the disease is easily recognized clinically and there are laboratory tests that can be used to confirm the clinical diagnosis. The challenge in these situations is to properly document the cases, take the appropriate clinical specimens and get them to a recognized laboratory for testing. The difficulty arises when i) the symptoms and signs do not fit easily with a single disease entity or ii) where, although the disease is known, its source or transmission route are not known. In these situations the aetiology is unknown. It is very important to carefully document the cases to see if any information on the pathogen, its source, or transmission can be determined.

Multiple clinical specimens may need to be taken, concentrating on samples from the systems that are obviously involved. These samples will be of unknown biohazard and should be taken, transported, and processed with great care.

Response

The public health response in an outbreak can occur at any time from outbreak detection onward. The response may be general in the beginning and become more focused as the information on the disease and its transmission become clearer.

The clinician is an integral part of the response mechanism in outbreaks and is an important member of the outbreak response team that should coordinate all investigative and control activities.

Responses include:

- Treatment of cases
- Tracing of contact
- Isolation of cases
- Vaccination
- Vector control
- Safe burial of the dead
- Water warnings/treatment/orders/bans
- Food warnings/removals/bans
- Hospital infection control
- Epidemiological investigations to identify risk factors
- Health education on recognizing the disease, seeking care and preventing transmission

The responses are dependent on knowing about the pathogen, its source, and the route of transmission. In addition, the availability of an effective vaccine or treatment will affect decisions made about response.

At the end of an outbreak the response should be evaluated so that improvements can be made. Thorough evaluation and implementation of findings will lead to improvements in outbreak prediction, prevention and mitigation.

Prediction, prevention and preparedness

Prediction of the likely occurrence of epidemics can lead to effective preventive measures such as immunization or vector control. Diseases with epidemic potential in a given country should be subject to prevention and preparedness plans. The impact of an outbreak once started can be reduced by improving the rapidity and targeting of this response.

Figure: Steps in outbreak control

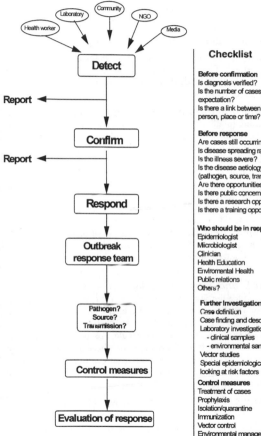

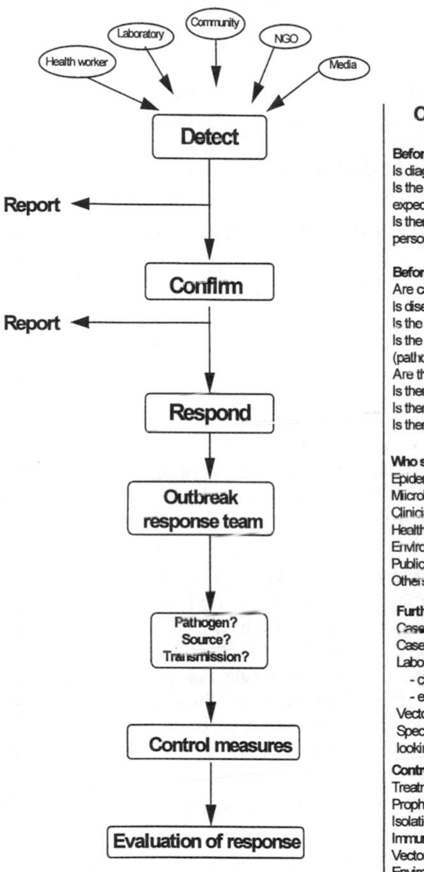

Checklist

Before confirmation
Is diagnosis verified?
Is the number of cases above expectation?
Is there a link between the cases in person, place or time?

Before response
Are cases still occurring?
Is disease spreading rapidly?
Is the illness severe?
Is the disease aetiology known (pathogen, source, transmission)?
Are there opportunities for control?
Is there public concern?
Is there a research opportunity
Is there a training opportunity

Who should be in response team
Epidemiologist
Microbiologist
Clinician
Health Education
Enviromental Health
Public relations
Others?

Further Investigation
Case definition
Case finding and description
Laboratory investigation
- clinical samples
- environmental samples
Vector studies
Special epidemiological studies looking at risk factors

Control measures
Treatment of cases
Prophylaxis
Isolation/quarantine
Immunization
Vector control
Environmental management
Health education

Universal precautions[1]

The purpose of these guidelines is to ensure that the accidental exposure of patients and health care workers to potentially infectious blood is reduced to an absolute minimum. They are based on the assumption that

► **ALL BODILY FLUIDS ARE POTENTIALLY INFECTIOUS**

- regardless of whether they are from a patient or a health worker, *and*
- regardless of whether laboratory tests are positive, negative, or not done.

Principles of infection control

- ***Handwashing*** – hands and other parts of the body that have been contaminated with blood or body fluids should be washed thoroughly with soap and water. Hands should also be washed immediately after removal of protective gloves.
- ***Gloves and other attire*** – health workers should wear gloves of suitable quality for all direct contact with blood and body fluids. When gloves are not available, other methods should be used to prevent direct contact with blood; for example, forceps, a towel, gauze or, if these are unavailable, even a leaf may be employed to hold a blood-stained needle or syringe. If gloves are not disposable they should be changed, washed, and disinfected or sterilized after contact with each patient. When injuries from sharp instruments are possible (eg when they are being cleaned), extra-heavy-duty gloves are recommended and the instruments should be handled with extreme caution. During procedures in which there may be splashing or suspensions of blood (eg during surgery or childbirth), the eyes, nose, and mouth should be protected with a face shield or mask and glasses, and gowns or aprons worn.
- ***Needlestick and other sharp injuries*** – methods should be devised to reduce the risk of needlestick and other injuries from sharp instruments, which should always be handled with extreme care. The handling of anything sharp should be reduced to a minimum. To prevent needlestick injuries, needles should not be recapped, bent, broken, removed from disposable syringes, or otherwise manipulated by hand. After use, needles and other sharp instruments should be placed in puncture-proof containers located as close as possible to where they are used and then handled as infected material.
- ***Mouth-to-mouth resuscitation*** – although HIV has been recovered from saliva, there is no conclusive evidence that saliva is involved in HIV transmission. Nevertheless, to reduce occupational exposure to HIV, mouthpieces, resuscitation bags, or other ventilation devices should be used if available when resuscitation is necessary. Resuscitation equipment should be used once only and discarded, or be thoroughly cleansed and disinfected. Mouth-to-mouth mucus extractors should be replaced, if possible, by electrical hand-operated or foot-operated suction machines.

Injections and skin-piercing

- Injections and other procedures in which the skin or mucous membranes are pierced for preventative, diagnostic, cosmetic or therapeutic purposes play an important role in both traditional and modern care.
- It is important to restrict injections and other skin-piercing procedures to situations in which the indications are clearly and appropriately defined. In many situations drugs given by injection would be equally effective if given orally. Reducing the number of unnecessary injections and procedures, such as episiotomies, is therefore important in protecting both the health worker and the patient.
- To avoid person-to person transmission of HIV, single-use (disposable) instruments should be used once only. To prevent reuse, they should then be destroyed under careful supervision. Multiple-use (reusable) instruments should always be washed and appropriately sterilized (or disinfected) according to existing guidelines. Chemical disinfection must not be used, however, for needles and syringes. If these procedures are always strictly observed, the risk of HIV transmission through injections and other skin-piercing procedures can be eliminated.

Invasive procedures

- An invasive procedure may be defined as a surgical entry into tissues, cavities, or organs, whether for an operation or for repair of injury. Strict precautions for infection control should be observed in relation to blood and other body fluids.

In addition:

- Health workers who perform or assist in vaginal or Caesarean deliveries should wear gloves and gown or apron when handling the placenta and until the blood has been removed from the infant's skin and post-delivery care of the umbilical cord is complete.
- If a glove is torn or a needlestick or other injury occurs, the glove should be changed and the hands washed carefully as soon as the safety of the patient permits. The needle or instrument involved in the accident should be removed from the sterile field.

Postmortem procedures

- Health workers performing postmortem procedures should follow the precautions outlined above and the standard guidelines for the health care setting involved.

1. Piot P, *AIDS in Africa – A Manual for Physicians*, WHO, Geneva 1992

Disposal of infected wastes

- Needles and other sharp instruments or materials should be placed in a puncture-proof container immediately after use and should preferably be incinerated.
- Liquid wastes such as bulk blood, suctions fluids, excretions and secretions should be carefully poured down a drain connected to an adequately treated sewer system, or disposed of in a pit latrine.
- Solid wastes, such as dressings and laboratory and pathology wastes, should be considered as infectious and treated by incineration, burning or autoclaving. Other solid wastes, such as excreta, may be disposed of in a hygienically controlled sanitary landfill or pit latrine.
- Solid waste materials in the home (dressings, diapers, menstrual pads) should be considered infectious. They should preferably be burned; if this is not possible, they should be deposited in a domestic or public hygienically-controlled sanitary landfill or pit latrine.

Laundry

- Soiled linen should be bagged where used and not sorted or rinsed where patients are being cared for. Linen soiled with blood or other body fluids should be placed and transported in leakproof bags. If leakproof bags are not available, the linen should be folded with the soiled parts inside. When handling soiled linen, gloves and protective apron should be worn.
- Linen should be washed with detergent and water at a temperature of at least 71°C (160°F) for 25 minutes. If low-temperature laundry cycles are used (less than 70°C [158°F]), chemicals suitable for low-temperature washing should be used at the appropriate concentration as recommended by the manufacturer.

Laboratory specimens

- Gloves should be worn by anyone handling and processing specimens of blood.
- All open wounds on hands and arms should be covered with a watertight dressing. Hands should always be washed with soap immediately after exposure to specimens.
- Specimens should be placed in containers with a secure lid to prevent leakage during transport. Care should be taken to avoid contamination of the outside of the container. When samples are mailed or otherwise transported, they should be placed inside unbreakable plastic containers.
- Working surfaces should be covered with a non-penetrative material that is easy to clean thoroughly, eg plastic film. Any spillage of blood or other body fluid should immediately be decontaminated with a disinfectant such as sodium hypochlorite 0.5% before cleaning.
- Specimens should be carefully disposed of by pouring them down a drain connected to a sewer. If this is not possible, blood and body fluids should be decontaminated with an appropriate disinfectant such as sodium hypochlorite 0.5% before disposal. Gloves should preferably be worn during disposal.
- Hands must be carefully washed after laboratory activities.

Isolation precautions[1,2]

Ethleen Lloyd, Special Pathogens Branch, Centers for Disease Control and Prevention USA.

These guidelines have been developed by the CDC and WHO following their experience with viral haemorrhagic fevers (VHF) in central Africa. Isolation precautions are based on the principle of establishing a physical barrier to prevent the transmission of disease from an infectious patient. Protection of skin and mucous membranes from fomites and droplets is a major consideration. The barrier can be in many forms, from wearing protective clothing to the use of isolation rooms. As in earlier outbreaks, patient isolation was critical in the management of the Ebola haemorrhagic fever outbreak in Kikwit during 1996 and it is therefore advised in the management of all suspected VHF patients (see chapter 4). The guidelines replace universal precautions.

- Reinforce and ensure the use of universal precautions in non-isolation areas of the health facility.
- Isolate the patient.
- Wear protective clothing (enhanced by use of two sets of gloves, two sets of clothing, plastic apron, boots, eyewear, bonnet, and mask) in the isolation area, cleaning and laundry area, laboratory, or when in contact with the patient.
  [Because of experimental infection of primates by aerosols, the observed high mortality among health care workers, and the desire to provide the maximum protection, masks which meet the US HEPA or N series standards are recommended.]
- Handle needles and other sharp instruments safely. Do not recap needles. Dispose of non-reusable needles, syringes, and other sharp patient-care instruments in puncture-resistant containers.
- Avoid sharing equipment between patients. Designate equipment for each patient, if supplies allow. If sharing equipment is unavoidable, make sure it is not reused by another patient until it has been cleaned, disinfected, and sterilized properly.
- Disinfect all spills, equipment, and supplies safely (this is enhanced by using disinfectant sprayers and 0.05% hypochlorite solutions).
- Dispose of all contaminated waste by incineration or burial (including safe disposal of corpses).
- Appropriate information should be provided to the families and community about the prevention of VHF and the care of infected patients.

1. CDC and WHO, *VHF Isolation Precautions: Infection Control of Viral Hemorrhagic Fevers in the African Health Care Setting*, WHO: Geneva 1997.
2. Public Health Service, US Department of Health and Human Services, Centers for Disease Control and Prevention, Atlanta, Georgia. Garner JS, Hospital Infection Control Advisory Committee, *Guidelines for isolation precautions in hospitals*, January 1996.

2. The WHO/UNICEF approach to the Integrated Management of Childhood Illness

Seven out of every ten deaths of children less than 5yrs in the developing world are due to acute respiratory infections (ARI), diarrhoea, measles, malaria, or malnutrition – and often to a combination of these conditions (see below). Every day, millions of parents seek health care for their children, taking them to hospitals, health centres, pharmacists, community health care providers, and traditional healers. At least three out of four of these children are suffering from one of these five conditions.

Deaths among children <5yrs in the developing world

• ARI	(in association with malnutrition)	19%
• diarrhoea	" " " "	19%
• measles	" " " "	7%
• malaria	" " " "	5%
• malnutrition (as a direct cause)		21%
• one or more of these 5 conditions		71%

Because there is considerable overlap in the signs and symptoms of several of these major childhood diseases, a single diagnosis for a sick child is often inappropriate. ► Focusing on the most apparent problem may lead to an associated, and potentially life-threatening, condition being overlooked. Treating the child may be complicated too by the need to combine therapy for several conditions.

Recognizing this overlap, the Division of Child Health and Development (CHD) and Special Programme for Research and Training in Tropical Diseases (TDR) of the WHO, together with UNICEF and other WHO divisions, have developed the *Integrated Management of Childhood Illness* strategy. IMCI aims to improve the management and prevention of illness in children from one week to 5 years of age via three main components: improving health worker skills, improving aspects of the health system, and improving family and community practices, all based on standard guidelines that have been adapted to the local epidemiology and other factors. The strategy ensures effective combined treatment of the five major childhood illnesses, speeds referral of seriously ill children, and empowers parents to care for their sick children at home, whenever possible. It emphasizes the prevention of disease through immunization, improved nutrition including breastfeeding, and the use of bednets to protect against malaria.

Since potentially fatal child illnesses are often brought to the attention of health workers at first-level facilities, IMCI aims to improve their performance through training and support. Health workers are trained to manage childhood illness effectively in an integrated fashion. They are also trained in communication skills, so that they may help mothers understand how best to ensure the health of their children.

- ► The full guidelines for the integrated management of childhood illness are not given here since they do not fit into the format of this handbook. Booklets detailing the approach can be obtained from the national WHO or UNICEF office in each country or directly from the WHO (see chapter 17 for the address).
- The guidelines were fully field tested and are now being introduced in more than 50 countries worldwide. ► They need to be adapted to country-specific policies and guidelines in all countries.

Summary of case management:

The training course developed by the WHO and UNICEF teaches the following case management process:

1. First assess the child, asking questions of the mother, examining the child, and checking immunization status.
2. Classify the child's illness, and decide whether to i) refer urgently, ii) give specific medical treatment and advice, or iii) give simple advice on home management.
3. Identify specific treaments – only give urgent treatments to children who are being referred.
4. Give practical treatment instructions. Teach the mother how to give oral drugs, how to increase fluids during diarrhoea, and how to treat simple infections at home. Advise the mother on the signs which indicate the child should immediately be brought back to the clinic, and when to return for follow-up.
5. Assess feeding in children <2yrs and those with low weight for age. Record any feeding problems, and provide counselling on feeding problems.
6. Organize follow-up.

Summary of patient assessment

1. Check for general danger signs which indicate that the child is severely ill.
2. Check for cough or difficulty in breathing which might indicate pneumonia.
3. Check for diarrhoea – whether acute watery diarrhoea, dysentery, or persistent diarrhoea – and dehydration.
4. Check for fever and presence of stiff neck. Management then depends on whether the locality is a high malaria risk area or not.
5. Check for evidence of measles.
6. Check for ear problems or mastoiditis.
7. Assess nutritional status in all children, identifying severely malnourished children who need referral to hospital.
8. Assess for severe pallor suggestive of significant anaemia.
9. Check the child's immunization status and give vaccines as required.

3A. Malaria[1]

Malaria 20
Epidemiology 22
Falciparum malaria 24
Severe malaria 26
Diagnosis 30
Key to identification of malaria parasites on blood films 32
Management 36
Chemotherapy 38
Chemoprophylaxis 42
Multidrug-resistant malaria and treatment failure 44
The future of malaria 44

1. Warrell DA, 1990, Severe and complicated malaria. *Trans RSTMH*, **84**, suppl. 2 pp. 1–65.
   WHO, *WHO Manual for Diagnosis and Treatment of Malaria in Africa*, WHO, Geneva

WHO revised guidelines

The new WHO guidelines for severe falciparum malaria have just been published. They have been extensively revised (we have not been able to reflect these changes fully in this corrected reprint). Their citation is: WHO 2000. Severe falciparum malaria. *Transactions of the Royal Society of Tropical Medicine and Hygiene* **94**, supplement 1, 1–90. They will hopefully soon become available on the web at either the Society's website <www.rstmh.org> or the WHO's website <www.who.int>.

Combination chemotherapy

The rapid spread of drug resistance amongst malaria parasites has meant that chloroquine is no longer effective in much of the world. Single therapy with pyrimethamine-sulphadoxine (PSD) is following the same path. Antimalarials effective against resistant parasites are at least 10× more expensive and probably unaffordable in Africa. The success of combination chemotherapy in treating TB and HIV has resulted in the call for treatment of malaria with chloroquine, PSD, or malarone together with an artemesin derivative in an attempt to slow resistance to the first drug. This is discussed in White NJ 1999, *Lancet* 353, 1965.

Malaria

Malaria is a disease caused by four species of protozoan parasites of the genus *Plasmodium*: *P. falciparum*, *P. vivax*, *P. ovale* and *P. malariae*.

Malaria is best thought of as a collective name for different diseases, since the epidemiology of transmission and severity of the disease vary greatly from region to region, village to village and even from person to person. These differences are due to mosquito biting/breeding habits, parasite species, compliance with drug treatment regimens, patterns of resistance and an individual's immunity, to name but a few.

At present about 40% of the world's population is exposed to malaria (~2000 million people) with over 1 million deaths occurring per year.

Falciparum malaria versus benign malaria; severe versus uncomplicated malaria

P. falciparum infection can follow a relatively mild or uncomplicated course. However, in some patients, particularly young children and non-immune adults, it may become a severe life-threatening disease. *P. falciparum* is responsible for most severe manifestations of malaria.

The benign malarias are *P. ovale*, *P. malariae* and *P. vivax*. Nearly all infections are uncomplicated and patients rarely die during acute infection with these species. However, chronic infection or infection of pregnant women may cause marked morbidity. The benign malarias may recur after treatment and after long intervals because of latent hypnozoite infection of the liver.

Life cycle and transmission

The parasite matures and reproduces sexually in a mosquito of the *Anopheles* genus. Transmission occurs via the bite of the female mosquito, which requires a blood meal for the development of her eggs. The parasite sporozoites (see opposite) enter the human bloodstream with the saliva of the biting mosquito and invade the liver cells, where they develop and multiply. Merozoites, released into the blood from the liver, invade red blood cells and initiate the cycle of development and multiplication that brings about the clinical symptoms of the disease due to haemolysis, blood cell sequestration and widespread immune effects.

Incubation periods: *P. falciparum* 7–14 days (but highly variable, especially in the semi-immune or after prophylaxis); *P. vivax* 12–17 days; *P. ovale* 15–18 days; *P. malariae* 18–40 days (but 5–10% >1 year after initial infection).

Malaria parasite life cycle

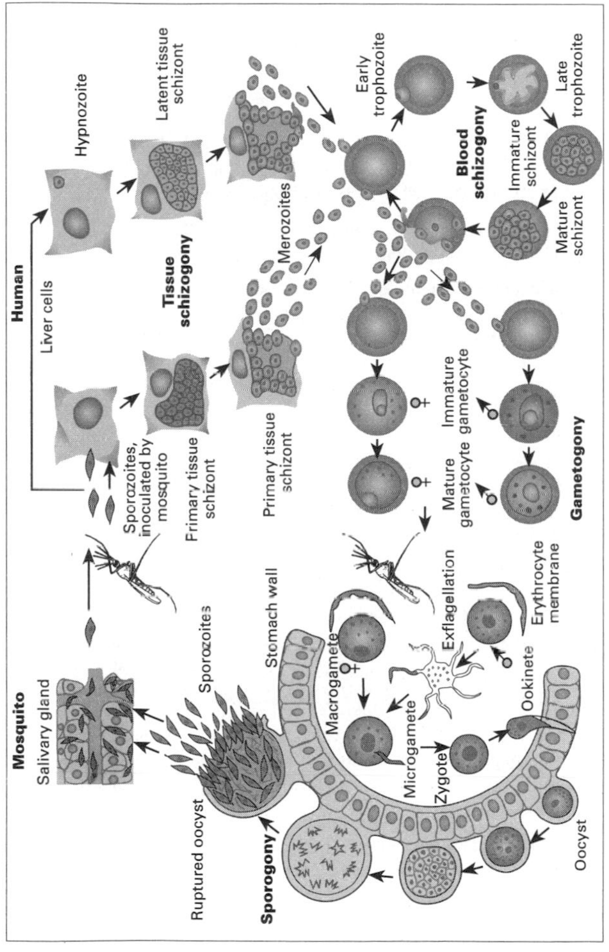

Epidemiology

Malarial transmission depends upon i) mosquito longevity, ii) density of both mosquito and humans and iii) the mosquitos' man-biting habit. Clinically the host's immune response is also important. Transmission may be measured using either the parasite rate (% of blood films which are +ve) or the spleen rate (% of population with splenomegaly), although the latter is less reliable since splenomegaly may be a result of other diseases. Neither method, however, attempts to record the clinical impact of the disease on a given population.

Two distinct types of transmission emerge, although it should be stressed that these represent extremes:

- ***stable malaria*** wherein disease predominantly affects children and pregnant women with little yearly variation in incidence;
- ***unstable malaria*** which affects all ages equally.

The old classification of hypoendemic, mesoendemic, holoendemic, and hyperendemic areas is no longer used.

► Malaria control in stable areas is problematic, since interventions which reduce transmission, but do not eradicate the disease, may impair the development of naturally acquired immunity in the population resulting in a pattern of unstable disease.

Protection against malaria

The worldwide distribution of the various forms of malaria is affected by two protective mechanisms – the development of partial immunity in persons continually exposed to infection and the presence of certain red blood cell polymorphisms which affect the parasite's ability to infect and survive in red blood cells.

Partial immunity **–** requires 4–10yrs of repeated malarial infection, possibly with differing genetic variants. In areas of stable transmission, neonates are usually protected by maternal antibodies for 6 months, following which there is a period of increased susceptibility. Repeated exposure results in the development of clinical immunity, usually by the age of 5yrs in those who survive the repeated infections. Depending upon the level of transmission, antiparasite immunity appears later, at around 10yrs of age, at which time the prevalence of parasitaemia may reach 50%. Adults tend to get less severe bouts of disease with lower parasite densities. Partial immunity wanes after ~5yrs without reinfection. It is also decreased by pregnancy, severe illness, and surgery.

Non-immune protection **–** certain haematological disorders, notably sickle cell trait but also G6PD deficiency, β thalassaemia trait, and ovalocytosis, partially protect against severe disease. The lack of Duffy antigen on RBCs in some west Africans accounts for their immunity to *P. vivax* infection, since these antigens act as receptors for merozoite entry into RBCs.

Distribution of malaria

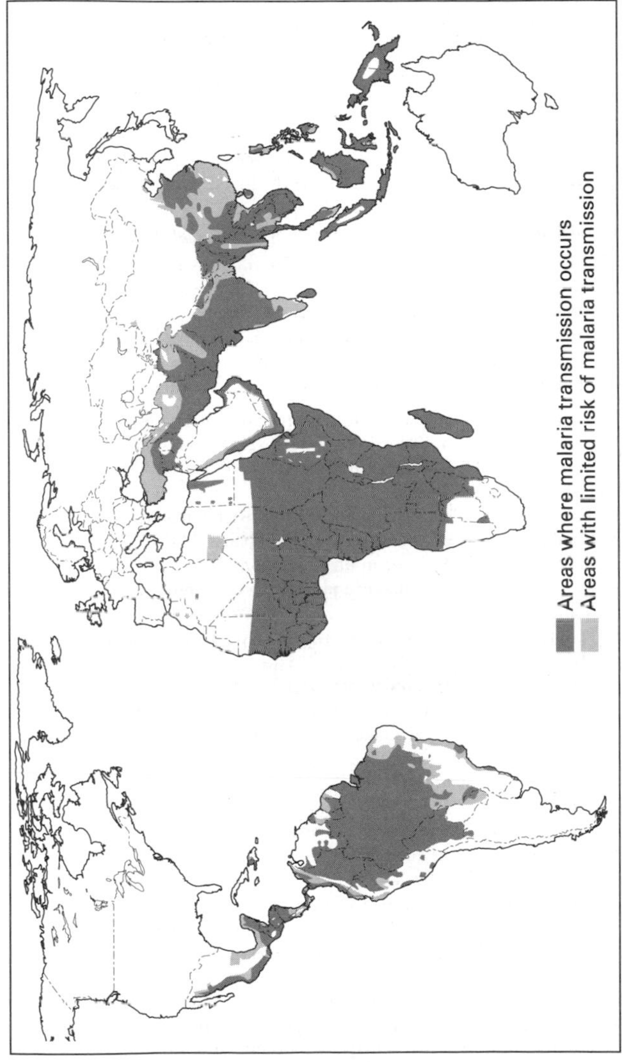

Falciparum malaria

Clinical features: Acute symptoms are often preceded by a prodromal illness consisting of malaise, headache, myalgia and anorexia. ► The symptoms of uncomplicated malaria are often very non-specific and the patient thinks she has flu.

Adults: typical symptoms and signs include:

- **Fever:** changing from cold (shivers, rigors, vomiting) → hot (temp. up to 41°C, flushing, tachycardia) → sweating or drenching → sleep. ► Daily fever is common, but patients may be afebrile in severe *P. falciparum* infection.
- **Anaemia:** (due to a variety of factors) may be severe in *P. falciparum* malaria. Reticulocytosis is often absent due to marrow suppression.
- **Splenomegaly:** usually occurs early in an acute attack. Repeated infections may result in hypersplenism.
- **Jaundice:** commonly mild. May be severe in *P. falciparum* malaria.

Children: Most malarial deaths occur in children aged 1–5yrs therefore ► observe children carefully.

Common features include: fever, early cough, vomiting, diarrhoea, anaemia, hypoglycaemia. Jaundice, pulmonary oedema, and renal failure are rarer in children than adults, although progression to other severe complications is usually faster (1–2 days) in children.[1]

Pregnant women: Malaria during pregnancy increases the risk of miscarriage, stillbirth, prematurity, low birthweight, and neonatal death, as well as maternal morbidity and mortality. High fever is thought to contribute to foetal distress.

- The risk is greatest in primigravidae in unstable malarial areas.
- Cerebral malaria is more common – in Thailand 50% of mortality due to cerebral malaria occurs in pregnant women.
- Parasitaemia is usually higher and anaemia more profound and this may result in heart failure.

► Pregnant women are at greater risk of hypoglycaemia and pulmonary oedema.

- Congenital transmission is rare and usually occurs in non-immune individuals infected with *P. vivax* or *P. malariae*. Neonatal illness presents with fever, haemolytic anaemia, and failure to thrive in the first days/weeks of life.

Complications

Falciparum malaria may progress to severe (malignant) malaria and death, or resolve leaving some residual immunity. Persistent anaemia is common and further attacks, due to recrudescence of blood forms which may persist between attacks, can occur up to 1yr after initial infection. In Thailand, 30% of patients with *P. falciparum* malaria develop symptomatic *P. vivax* infection within 2 mths <u>without</u> re-exposure to parasites, implying an initial dual infection.

- Malaria is not altered by simultaneous HIV infection.
- Malnutrition does not appear to increase susceptibility to disease, although if present it will increase mortality and morbidity.

The benign malarias

- ***P. vivax*** and ***P. ovale*** **–** may relapse up to 5yrs after initial infection despite treatment which eliminates all blood forms. This is due to latent liver hypnozoites undergoing schizogony and re-entering the blood stream.
- ***P. malariae*** **–** persistent parasites may cause recurrent fevers even decades after 1° infection. The fevers decrease in frequency and severity over time. Anaemia and splenomegaly may, however, be persistent.
- ***P. malariae*** **–** may cause glomerulonephritis and nephrotic syndrome.
- ***P. vivax*** **–** a rare complication is splenic rupture (mortality 80%). It is more common following infection and results from acute enlargement +/– trauma. It presents with sudden and persistent abdominal pain, guarding, fever, shock, and lowered haemocrit.

Chronic malaria

Symptoms include recurrent acute attacks of malaria, anaemia, hepatosplenomegaly, diarrhoea, weight loss, and increased incidence of other infections (especially bacterial gastroenteritis). It may resolve, with the onset of partial immunity, or progress, with 2° complications. Chronic malaria is associated with an increased incidence of Burkitt's lymphoma due to impaired T-cell immunity.

Hyperreactive malarial splenomegaly (formerly called tropical splenomegaly syndrome) may develop with recurrent infections. It is characterized by splenic pain, profound anaemia, 2° infection, fever, and jaundice.

Management: should be aimed at eradicating current malarial infection and improving the anaemia with iron and folic acid supplements – a process which usually takes ~2 years.

1. Marsh K, 1995, *NEJM*, **332**, 1399

Severe malaria

See WHO criteria for severe malaria opposite.

Severe malaria is caused by *P.falciparum* and is characterized by multi-system involvement due to i) RBC sequestration in the microvasculature, ii) RBC destruction and iii) immune activation. Onset can be rapid, with death (particularly in children) occurring in a matter of hours. Beware late diagnosis or misdiagnosis in travellers from endemic regions.

- **Cerebral malaria** is the most important complication (20% mortality). It most often occurs in non-immunes and children. It is defined as unrousable coma not attributable to other causes. Neck rigidity and photophobia are not usually seen and Kernig's sign is –ve. There may be one or more of: diffuse cerebral dysfunction, convulsions (~50% are generalized), focal neurological signs, coma, brainstem failure. Retinal haemorrhages occur in 15% of African and SE Asian cases. Neurological sequelae are found in at least 5% of survivors (10% in children) and include hemiparesis, cerebellar ataxia, cortical blindness, hypotonia and mental retardation. ***In children*** cerebral malaria carries a 10–40% mortality, most deaths occurring within the first 24hrs.[1]
  ► Reduced consciousness may follow a febrile convulsion in a child, but if cerebral malaria is suspected do not wait to see if the level of consciousness improves – the patient may die if treatment is delayed. Malarial convulsions can occur at any temperature and post-ictal coma may last >1/2 hr. In deep coma, abnormalities of posture and muscle tone are frequently seen. For young children use the Blantyre Coma Scale (shown opposite) to grade the coma.
- **Anaemia:** a normocytic anaemia with haemocrit <15% (or Hb <5g /dl) in the presence of parasitaemia >10,000/ml is a common presentation in African children. Look for pallor, breathlessness, gallop rhythm, respiratory distress, pulmonary oedema, and neurological signs. Anaemia is made worse by 2° bacterial infections, haemorrhage, and pregnancy. Hyperparasitaemia or G6PD deficiency can result in massive IV haemolysis. In children, repeated episodes of otherwise uncomplicated malaria may lead to chronic normochromic anaemia with dyserythropoeitic changes in the bone marrow. ► Children are prone to developing rapid, severe, anaemia following *P.falciparum* infection, which may contribute to both neurological and cardiopulmonary signs.
- **Jaundice:** is common in adult patients and has haemolytic, hepatic, and/or cholestatic components. Unconjugated and conjugated bilirubin may all be raised to >50μmol/l (3.0mg/dl). Clinical signs of liver failure are not seen unless there is concomitant viral hepatitis.
- **Renal impairment:** usually occurs in adults and is characterized by a raised serum Cr (>265μmol/l, or 30mg/dl) and urea, with oliguria or anuria (<400ml urine/24 hrs in an adult) due to acute tubular necrosis. In some cases there is polyuria. It has a poor prognosis (45% die).

1. Molyneux ME, 1989, *QJM*, 71, 441

WHO criteria for severe malaria

One or more of:

- cerebral malaria
- severe normocytic anaemia
- renal failure
- hyperparasitaemia
- pulmonary oedema
- hypoglycaemia
- circulatory collapse
- spontaneous bleeding/DIC
- repeated generalized convulsions
- acidaemia/acidosis
- malarial haemoglobinuria

Other manifestations include:

- impaired consciouness, but rousable
- prostration, severe weakness
- jaundice
- hyperpyrexia

Blantyre Coma Scale[1]

	Score
Best motor response	
• Localizes painful stimulus *	2
• Withdraws limb from painful stimulus **	1
• No response or inappropriate response	0
Best verbal response	
• Cries appropriately with painful stimulus, or if verbal speaks	2
• Moan or abnormal cry with painful stimulus	1
• No vocal response to painful stimulus	0
Eye movements	
• Watches or follows (eg mother's face)	1
• Fails to watch or follow	0

To obtain "coma score" add the scores from each section.

* Pressure with blunt end of pencil on sternum/supraorbital ridge.
** Pressure with horizontal pencil on nailbed of finger or toe.

- **Blackwater fever** is massive haemoglobinuria (urine becomes very dark), often following treatment or prophylaxis with oxidant drugs such as primaquine. It is more common in patients with G6PD or other RBC enzyme deficiencies.

- **Hypoglycaemia** (whole blood glucose <2.2 mmol/l, 40mg/dl) may be due to reduced hepatic function or quinine/quinidine-induced hyperinsulinaemia (pregnant women are particularly prone). It presents with anxiety, sweating, breathlessness, dilated pupils, oliguria, hypothermia, tachycardia, and light-headedness, eventually leading to decreased consciousness, convulsions, and coma. In a fasting adult hepatic glycogen stores last ~2 days, those of a child maybe as little as 12 hrs. Hence, hypoglycaemia is common in 1–3yr olds (especially those with cerebral malaria, hyperparasitaemia, or convulsions). It indicates a poor prognosis. It is not associated with signs of malnutrition. In Malawi 37% of hypoglycaemic children died and 42% of survivors had neurological sequelae compared with 4% and 7% respectively of normoglycaemic controls.[1]

- **Lactic acidosis:** pH <7.3 or raised plasma and CSF lactate levels (plasma >15mmol/l) and a low plasma HCO_3^- carry a poor prognosis,[2] especially in children with cerebral malaria. Lactate levels >5mmol/l frequently exceed the buffering capacity of the body and result in metabolic acidosis. Watch for abnormally slow & deep ventilation.

- **Fluid and electrolyte disturbances:** such as hypovolaemia and dehydration are common. Low Na^+, Cl^-, PO_4^-, and Ca^{2+}, and endocrine dysfunction are common, although rarely severe.

- **Pulmonary oedema:** carries a 50% mortality and may occur at a time when the patient is otherwise improving. Excess fluid replacement is a common cause – look for a raised RR (excluding aspiration or acidosis). Predisposing causes include hyperparasitaemia, renal failure, and pregnancy (occurs suddenly after delivery). Hypoxia may cause convulsions and death within a few hours.

- **Shock (algid malaria):** cold, clammy cyanotic skin (core : skin temp difference >10°C; weak rapid pulses; supine systolic BP <70mmHg (50 in children) suggests circulatory collapse. Commonly due to 2° infection, or metabolic acidosis, pulmonary oedema, dehydration, GI bleed.

- **DIC:** is due to pathological activation of coagulation mechanisms. Look for bleeding gums, epistaxis, petechiae, haematemesis, and/or melaena with significant blood loss. Occurs in <10% of patients, but is more common in non-immunes (especially travellers). Blood film shows thrombocytopaenia and schistocytes (broken RBCs). ↑ PT, PTT and FDPs.

- **Hyperpyrexia:** (rectal temperature >40°C) is more common in children. It is associated with convulsions, delirium, and coma and may result in permanent neurological sequelae or death.

1. Taylor T, 1988, *NEJM*, **319**, 1040 2. Taylor T, 1993, *QJM*, **86**, 99

- **Hyperparasitaemia** is a parasite density >10^6 ring stage forms/ml, although in highly endemic areas patients may tolerate greater densities, without clinical features.
- **Gastrointestinal symptoms** are common in children. Nausea, vomiting, abdominal pain and diarrhoea without blood or pus are frequently seen. There may also be ulceration of the stomach and duodenum, malabsorption and increased bacterial infections. Persistent vomiting is a major cause of treatment failure and needs urgent parenteral drug administration.
- **2° infection** of lungs (e.g. following aspiration), urinary tract (following catheterization) and post-partum sepsis are common complications. Gram –ve septicaemia may occur without any focus of infection.

Respiratory distress and lactic acidosis

The majority of respiratory distress in children with malaria is due to metabolic acidosis. It predominantly presents as deep breathing with an increased amplitude of chest excursion. Severe metabolic acidosis (BE >–12) is associated with an 8× increased risk of death in Kenyan children. Deep breathing is an accurate clinical indicator of acidosis – it is not due to congestive failure secondary to severe anaemia – and requires rapid intervention.

Indicators of a poor prognosis

- hyperlactataemia (>6mmol/l or arterial pH <7.3)
- hyperventilation
- bleeding
- convulsions
- hyperparasitaemia (>10^6 ring stage forms/ml)
- decerebrate posturing
- hypothermia (<36.5°C)
- sustained hyperthermia (>39°C)
- severe anaemia (PCV <15% or Hb <5 g/dl)
- deep coma (3–5 on GCS)
- age <3yrs
- jaundice
- uraemia (>21.4mmol/l)
- shock
- hypoglycaemia (plasma glucose <2.2mmol/l)
- peripheral leucocytosis (>12,000/ml)
- ALT and AST raised three-fold above normal limits

Diagnosis

Blood films: specific diagnosis requires identification of parasites in smears of the patient's blood. See blood film diagrams and thick/thin film methodology.

► Keep a high index of suspicion and carry out multiple blood films. Do not forget infection via transfusion, needlestick injuries, and brief airport stopovers in travellers. Unlike the benign malarias, *P. falciparum* schizogony occurs in capillaries and, therefore, the presence of schizonts in peripheral blood samples indicates severe infection.

Pitfalls in diagnosis

- A negative film does not exclude disease. Repeat ×3 at intervals (taking the blood at the height of fever). The patient may have been partially treated – **ASK** – since it is unlikely that schizogony is so highly synchronized that it would give totally negative peripheral blood films.
- In endemic areas a positive film does not prove that malaria is responsible for the current symptoms.
- Cross-contamination of slides is possible in bulk-staining.
- Correlation between parasite density and disease severity is weak.

Other tests which may be useful include: FBC (anaemia, ↓WCC, although often ↑ in severe disease, thrombocytopenia); glucose; bilirubin; U&E (hyponatraemia, uraemia); pH (HCO_3); urinalysis; blood culture.

- A useful negative finding is the absence of rash and lymphadenopathy.

Other methods of diagnosis currently available include serodiagnosis, monocytic malarial pigment, quantitative buffy coat method, dipstick, and PCR.

Differential diagnosis: any febrile illness, septicaemia, influenza, hepatitis, leptospirosis, relapsing fevers, haemorrhagic fevers, scrub typhus, gastroenteritis, trypanosomiasis, UTI, mastitis, meningitis, babesiosis, typhoid fever, ascending cholangitis, puerperal sepsis, heat stroke.

Cerebral malaria

► This complication of falciparum malaria is diagnosed clinically.
Check the retinae for haemorrhages +/– papilloedema. It is essential to do a lumbar puncture to distinguish meningitis from cerebral malaria. However, some argue that it should be delayed until there is an improvement in conscious level. If this practice is followed, then antibiotics must be given empirically for meningitis as soon as possible.[1]

In all cases, signs of raised ICP should be sought. CSF is clear with ↑ lactic acid and protein and <10 leukocytes/ml. CT is usually normal although there may be EEG disturbances. Abdominal reflexes are usually absent in cerebral malaria.

Differential diagnosis: meningitis; encephalitis; febrile convulsion in children (post-ictal coma lasts <1/2 hr); eclampsia; diabetic, hepatic, uraemic, or hypoglycaemic coma; trauma; psychosis; favism; poisoning.

1. Newton CRJC, 1991, *Lancet*, **337**, 573; Waller D, 1991, *Trans RSTMH*, **85**, 362; Wright PW, 1993, *Paed Inf Dis J*, **12**, 37

How to prepare a thick and thin film on the same slide

1. Clean the tip of the patient's left index finger.
2. Pierce the pulp of the fingertip with a sterile lancet or needle.
3. Squeeze the finger until a droplet of blood forms and place it onto the middle of a clean slide (holding the slide by the edges). This is for the thin film.
4. Place a further 3 droplets of blood onto the slide at a point to one side of the first droplet. These are for the thick film.
5. Using a second clean slide as a spreader, touch the first, small drop with the edge and allow the blood to run along its edge. With the spreading slide at 45°, push the spreader forwards slowly, ensuring even contact, so that the blood is spread as a thin film over the surface of the slide. See picture below.
6. Using the corner of the spreading slide, amalgamate the three drops of blood on the other half of the slide in to a single small, denser film about 1cm in diameter.
7. Label the slide with a pencil and allow to dry horizontally.

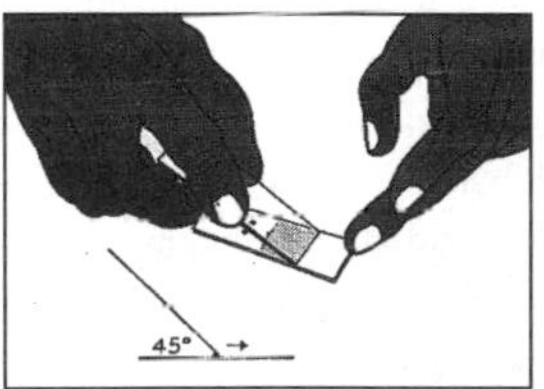

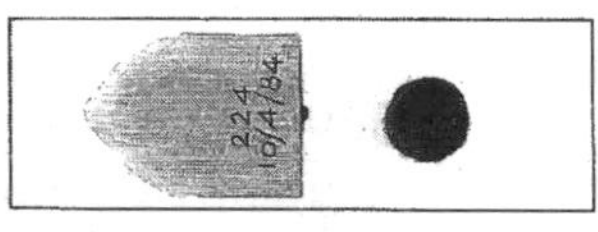

Correctly prepared slide

Problems: Badly positioned blood droplets, too much or too little blood, using a greasy slide, a chipped edge of the spreader slide.

Staining (consult a laboratory manual for more details)
Giemsa stain may be used for both films but is costly and more difficult to do. Thin films must first be fixed in methanol then dipped in 10% Giemsa for 20–30mins, thick films in 5% solution for 30mins. Field's stain uses 2 solutions, A and B which are cheaper and more suited to rapid bulk staining. For thick films dip dried slides into solution A for 5secs, avoiding agitation. Wash in tap water (preferably neutral pH) for 5secs then dip into solution B for 3secs. Wash again in water for 5secs then allow to dry vertically. The centre of the film may not be stained, but optimal parasite staining occurs at the edges of the film. For thin films use solution B before solution A.
Leishman's stain may be used for thin films. 0.5ml stain is added to each horizontal film, left for 30secs then 1.5ml of buffered water added and left for 8min. The slide is then washed in tap water.

Key to identification of malaria parasites on blood films[1]

1. Are there one or more red-stained chromatin dots and blue cytoplasm? YES – go to 2. NO – what you see is not a parasite.

2. Are the size and shape correct for a malaria parasite? YES – go to 3. NO – what you see is not a malaria parasite.

3. Is there malaria pigment in the cell? YES – go to 7. NO – go to 4.

4. Does the parasite have one chromatin dot attached to blue cytoplasm in the form of a regular ring in the cytoplasm? YES – this is a trophozoite. NO – go to 5.

5. Does the parasite have one chromatin dot attached to blue cytoplasm in the form of a small solid or regular ring or with a vacuole? YES – this is a trophozoite. NO – go to 6.

6. Is the parasite with one chromatin dot irregular or fragmented? YES – this is a trophozoite. NO – go to 8.

7. Does the parasite with malaria pigment have one chromatin dot? YES – go to 8. NO – go to 9.

8. Does the parasite have a vacuole or is it fragmented in some way? YES – this is probably a late trophozoite stage. NO – go to 11.

9. Does the parasite have 2 chromatin dots attached to a ring and also have a vacuole? YES – this is a trophozoite. NO – go to 10.

10. Does the parasite have between 2 and 32 chromatin dots and pigment? YES – this is a schizont.

11. Is the parasite rounded or 'banana-shaped'? Rounded – go to 12, 'banana-shaped' – go to 14.

12. Does the rounded parasite have clearly stained chromatin and a deep blue cytoplasm? YES – this is a female gametocyte. NO – go to 13.

13. Does the rounded parasite have a reddish overall colour, so that the chromatin is indistinct? YES – this is a male gametocyte.

14. Does the 'banana-shaped' parasite have densely stained blue cytoplasm and bright red chromatin? YES – this is a female gametocyte. NO – go to 15.

15. Does the 'banana-shaped' parasite have a reddish overall colour, so that the chromatin is indistinct? YES – this is a male gametocyte.

1. *Basic Malaria Microscopy – Learner's guide*. WHO, Geneva, 1991.
The diagrams of malarial blood cells are taken from BJ Bain, *Blood Cells, a Practical Guide*. Blackwell Science, Oxford, 1995, with permission.

	Early trophozoite (ring form)	Mature trophozoite
Plasmodium vivax	Thick rings, $\frac{1}{3}$–$\frac{1}{2}$ the diameter of the red cell 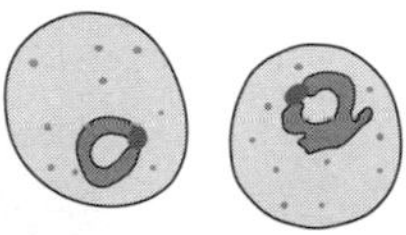 A few Schnuffner's dots Accolé (shoulder) forms and double dots less common than with *P. falciparum*	Ameboid rings, $\frac{1}{2}$–$\frac{2}{3}$ the diameter of the red cell Pale blue or lilac parasite with prominent central valuole 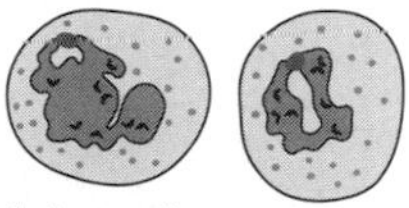 Indistinct outline Scattered fine yellowish-brown pigment granules or rods
Plasmodium ovale	Thick, compact rings, $\frac{1}{3}$–$\frac{1}{2}$ the diameter of the red cell 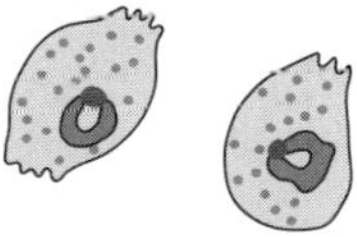 Numerous Schuffner's dots but paler than with *P. vivax*	Thick rings, less irregular than those of *P. vivax*, $\frac{1}{3}$–$\frac{1}{2}$ the diameter of the red cell 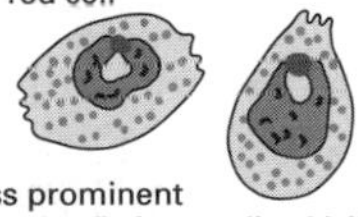 Less prominent vacuole, distinct outline Yellowish-brown pigment which is coarser and darker than that of *P. vivax* Schuffner's dots prominent
Plasmodium falciparum	Dellcate rings, $\frac{1}{6}$–$\frac{1}{4}$ the diameter of the red cell 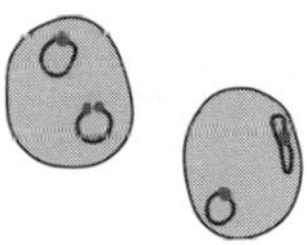 Double dots and accolé forms common	Fairly delicate rings, $\frac{1}{3}$–$\frac{1}{2}$ the diameter of the red cell 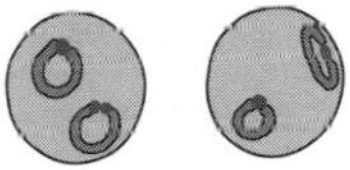 Red-mauve stippling (Maurer's dots or clefts) may be present Mature trophozoites are less often present in peripheral blood than ring forms
Plasmodium malariae	Small, thick, compact rings Small chromatin dot which may be inside the ring 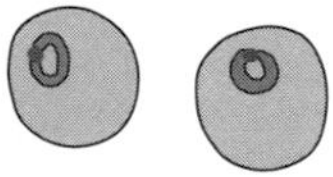 Double dots and accolé forms rare	Ameboid form more compact than *P. vivax* Sometimes angular or band forms 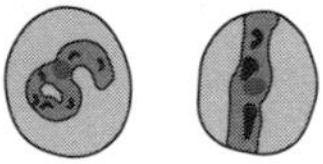 Heavy, dark-yellow-brown pigment No stippling unless ovestained

	Early schizont	Late schizont
Plasmodium vivax	Rounded or irregular Ameboid Loose central mass of fine yellowish-brown pigment 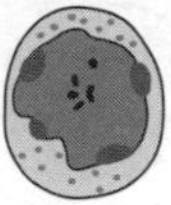 Schizont almost fills cell Schuffner's dots	12–24 (usually 16–24) medium-sized merozoites 1–2 clumps of peripheral pigment 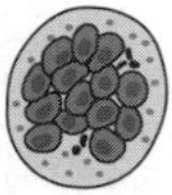 Schizont almost fills cell Schuffner's dots
Plasmodium ovale	Round, compact Darkish brown pigment, heavier and coarser than that of *P. vivax* 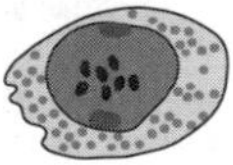 Schuffner's dots	6–12 (usually 8) large merozoites arranged irregularly like a bunch of grapes 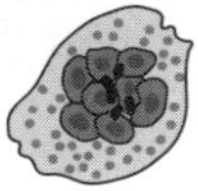 Central pigment Schuffner's dots
Plasmodium falciparum	Not usually seen in blood Very small, ameboid Scattered light-brown to black pigment	Not usually seen in blood 8–32 (usually few) very small merozoites; grouped irregularly Peripheral clump of coarse dark brown pigment
Plasmodium malariae	Compact, round, fills red cell 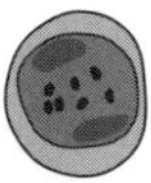 Coarse dark yellow-brown pigment	6–12 (usually 8–10) large merozoites, arranged symmetrically, often in a rosette or daisy head formation 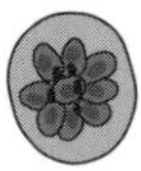 Central coarse dark yellowish-brown pigment

	Gametocyte	
	Macrogametocyte	Microgametocyte
Plasmodium vivax	Round or ovoid, almost fills enlarged cell Blue cytoplasm 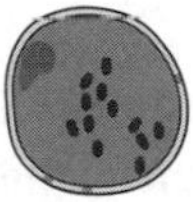 Eccentric compact red nucleus Scattered pigment	Round or ovoid, as large as a normal red cell but does not fill the enlarged red cell 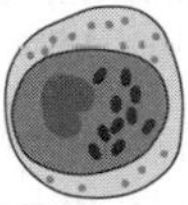 Faintly staining Larger, lighter red central or eccentric nucleus Fine, scattered pigment
Plasmodium ovale	Similar to *P. vivax* but somewhat smaller 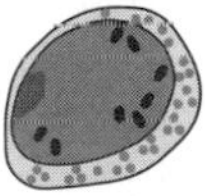 Pigment coarser and blacker, scattered but mainly near the periphery	Similar to *P. vivax* but smaller 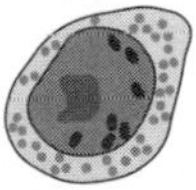
Plasmodium falciparum	Sickle or crescent shaped Deforms cell which often appears empty of haemoglobin 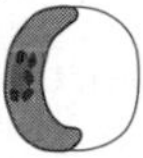 Blue cytoplasm Compact central nucleus with pigment aggregated around it	Oval or crescentic with blunted ends Pale blue or pink 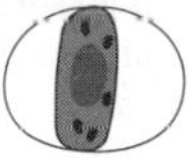 Large pale nucleus with pigment more scattered than in macrogametocyte
Plasmodium malariae	Similar to *P. vivax* but smaller, round or oval, almost fills cell, blue with a dark nucleus 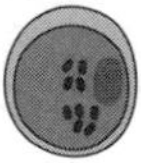 Prominent pigment concentrated at centre and periphery	Similar to *P. vivax* but smaller, pink or paler blue than macrogametocyte with a larger, paler nucleus 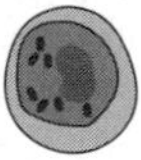 Prominent pigment

Management

►► Decide whether you are dealing with a *P. falciparum* infection. If there are signs of severe infection, do not wait for laboratory confirmation. Weigh the patient and start treatment immediately

Basic rules:

- In most instances, uncomplicated malaria can be treated on an out-patient basis.
- Await blood film results for uncomplicated malaria.
- Advise patients to return promptly if symptoms get worse or do not get better within 48hrs.
- Be wary of sending home children who have mild symptoms but high levels of parasitaemia since they may deteriorate rapidly.

All patients will need antimalarial chemotherapy

Antimalarial treatment with an appropriate agent should be started immediately. Choose the drug bearing in mind likely compliance, side-effects, local resistance, and costs – see next page. What is the locally recommended chemotherapy?

Most patients will need antipyretics and analgesics

If fever causes distress or the child is prone to febrile convulsions, give paracetamol. Avoid aspirin in children.

► In hyperpyrexia, quickly begin tepid sponging and fanning to rapidly reduce temperature. Consider giving IM antipyretics.

Consider the following for patients with severe disease:

1. ***50% dextrose*** – 50ml (children: 1.0ml/kg) given by IV bolus for hypoglycaemia. Follow this with 10% dextrose IV with electrolytes (beware hyponatraemia). Monitor blood glucose levels regularly.
2. ***Rehydration*** – particularly if D&V is present. Adults with severe *P. falciparum* malaria usually require 1–3l of isotonic saline over the 1st 24 hrs – aim to maintain the JVP between 0 and 4 cm in the patient lying at 45°. Avoid overhydration. Monitor renal output, BP, JVP every hour. Be careful to take into account volumes of fluids given with any IV drugs. If the patient remains oliguric, peritoneal dialysis or haemodialysis may be indicated.
3. ***Blood transfusion*** – with pathogen-free, compatible fresh blood or packed cells.

   ►► This is urgent, particularly in children, if the haematocrit falls below 15% (Hb <5g/dl) and is accompanied by acidosis or respiratory distress. Give blood 10mg/kg over 30mins, then a further 10mg/kg over 2–3hrs without diuretics in children with respiratory distress and severe anaemia. In DIC, fresh blood, clotting factors, or platelets should be transfused as required.

   ► The overall clinical condition of the patient must be weighed against the risks incurred by transfusion.

4. ***Oxygen and mechanical ventilation*** – may be required in respiratory distress. Ensure that the airway is clear and the head of the bed is raised if the distress is due to pulmonay oedema. If due to overhydration, stop all IV fluids and give IV frusemide. Haemofiltration may be used, if available. If these interventions fail, withdraw 250ml of blood into a sterile transfusion bag so that it may be given back to the patient at a later time, if required.
5. ***Diuretics*** – such as frusemide 20–80mg IV. Should be given in pulmonary oedema – if there is no response, the dose can be increased up to 200mg – and haemoglobinuria.
6. ***Broad spectrum antibiotics*** should be started immediately after taking blood cultures if 2° bacterial infection is suspected. Continue until specific sensitivities are known from the blood cultures. Bacteraemia occurs in ~8% of children with severe anaemia, rising to ~12% in those under 30 months.
7. ***Dopamine*** may be given in shock through a central line if the BP or JVP are not maintained following the use of plasma expanders.
8. ***Vitamin K*** 10mg IV by slow injection may help normalize the PT and PTT. Heparin should be avoided.

Cerebral malaria

Treat as above with the following additional specific measures:

- Nurse the patient on her side to avoid aspiration of vomit. Turn every two hours.
- Unless anuric, the patient should be catheterized and have temperature, heart and respiratory rates, BP, and fluid balance measured regularly.
- Consciousness must be assessed regularly with the Glasgow or Blantyre Coma Scores.
  ► If convulsions arise – be alert since they may be subtle – treat with diazepam 0.15mg/kg (up to a maximum of 10mg in adults) by slow IV injection. [An alternative is diazepam 0.5mg/kg rectally.]
- Avoid corticosteroids or other ancillary agents for cerebral oedema since they are of no proven benefit.

Chemotherapy

- Aim to reduce the parasitaemia as quickly as possible, using oral agents if they are tolerated. ► Beware local patterns of resistance. ►► If the species is unknown or there is mixed infection, treat as *P.falciparum.*
- If the parasite count has not fallen by at least 75% 48hrs after starting therapy, the count should be rechecked and, if confirmed, a different antimalarial drug used.
- During pregnancy, quinine is still the treatment of choice for *P.falciparum*/severe disease despite the remote possibility of induced abortion since preservation of the mother's life is paramount. Avoid mefloquine in the first trimester of pregnancy.

Antimalarial preparations and their recommended doses[1]

1. Quinine – used in the treatment of *P.falciparum* malaria and in emergency IV treatment of benign malaria where oral drugs are not tolerated.

For uncomplicated disease, give 10mg/kg quinine salt PO tds, *together with* tetracycline 4mg/kg PO qds, *or* doxycycline 3mg/kg PO daily, *or* clindamycin 10mg/kg PO bd, each for one week.

For severe disease, give 20mg/kg of the dihydrochloride salt IV over 4hrs, followed by 10mg/kg infused over 2–8hrs every 8hrs until oral therapy is tolerated.

- Oral doses which are vomited out within 1hr of adminstration should be repeated immediately.
- Doses should be reduced by one-third in patients with renal failure.
- Compliance with 7 days of oral quinine is poor because it tastes bitter.
- IV doses should be given in 500ml of 0.9% sodium chloride solution into a large vein. ► **Check** if the patient has already received chloroquine, quinine, or mefloquine – if yes, omit the loading dose – and that cardiac monitoring is available. ► Watch for hypoglycaemia (particularly in pregnant women) and ↓ the rate of infusion if arrhythmias occur. Switch to oral drugs when possible.
- Where IV access is unavailable, quinine may be given IM (20mg/kg loading dose followed by 10mg/kg tds) but beware of tissue damage and risk of heart block. Dilute the preparation 5-fold and give in divided doses by deep IM injection into the anterior thigh.

2. Mefloquine – related to quinine, this is a newer preparation which is useful for multidrug resistant forms of *P.falciparum.* It is available as a hydrochloride (Larium). Temporary adverse psychiatric effects have been reported in people using this drug for prophylaxis (severe in 1:1500 cases). The benefit of treating potentially life-threatening multidrug resistant malaria outweighs this risk. The adverse effects may respond to chlorpromazine. ► Do not administer within 12hrs of the last quinine dose. ► Do not use in early pregnancy. Warn women to avoid conception within 3 months of taking mefloquine. ► Avoid in severe disease because of the risk of neurological syndromes. ► Do not use if taken as prophylaxis.

Give 15mg/kg base PO stat (+/– 2nd dose of 10mg/kg 8–24hrs later)
[In the USA, 1 tablet = 228mg base; elsewhere 1 tablet = 250mg base.]

3. Chloroquine – its use against *P. falciparum* infection is now no longer recommended due to widespread resistance. It should also not be used if it has previously been taken as prophylaxis. In these situations, treat with quinine unless absolutely certain of sensitivity.

However, chloroquine is still the drug of choice for benign malaria in most parts of the world, although resistant strains are emerging (see below). It is safe during pregnancy at the recommended doses. Use oral preparations whenever possible.

For uncomplicated disease, give 10mg/kg base PO followed by *either* 10mg/kg base at 24hrs and 5mg/kg base at 48hrs, *or* 5mg/kg base at 12, 24, and 36hrs (each regimen gives 25mg/kg total dose)

For *P. vivax* or *P. ovale*, add primaquine 0.25mg base/kg daily for 14 days to obtain a radical cure (see below). If the patient is known to have G6PD deficiency, use a reduced dose to avoid haemolysis. Watch out for black urine; reduce the dose if this occurs.

IV route should be considered when a patient cannot swallow, has D&V, or if IV quinine/quinidine is not available. ► Excessively rapid administration may result in fatal cardiovascular collapse.

Give10mg/kg base at a constant rate by IV infusion over 8hrs, followed by 15mg/kg base over 24hrs. If IV route is not available, give 3.5mg/kg base IM/SC q6h (up to a total dose 25mg/kg base).

Radical cures and primaquine in benign malaria

- Treatment with a blood schizontocidal drug, such as quinine, will not eliminate parasites from the liver. Therefore patients infected with *P. vivax* or *P. ovale* are also given primaquine to kill the liver hypnozoites and prevent recrudescence at a later timepoint.
- Since primaquine is also gametocidal, it is sometimes given to patients infected with *P. falciparum* in non-endemic regions. This prevents the blood gametocytes being taken up by local mosquitos and possibly initiating local foci of infections.
- A major drawback is primaquine's ability to cause severe intravascular haemolysis in patients with G6PD deficiency. Weekly doses of 45mg are better tolerated than daily doses of 15mg.
- Relatively primaquine resistant strains of *P. vivax* have been reported in the Pacific region which require at least 6mg/kg total dose (~twice normal dose).

1. White N, 1996, *NEJM*, **335**, 801, British National Formulary, and WHO, 2000, *Trans RSTMH* **94**, suppl 1, 1–90

4. Tetracycline/doxycycline – used in conjunction with quinine in the treatment of quinine-resistant *P. falciparum* and in patients hypersensitive to sulfadoxine-pyrimethamine. See quinine text for doses. Do not give in pregnancy, ↓ dose in renal failure.

5. Sulfadoxine-pyrimethamine – there is now widespread resistance to this drug combination. It is used in combination with 1–3 days of quinine, particularly for the severely ill patients and patients without immunity, but is no longer recommended.

Give: • 20mg/kg sulfadoxine *plus* 1mg/kg pyrimethamine as a single dose. (2–3 tablets of Fansidar is usual adult dose.)

6. Quinidine – if quinine is unavailable, this related compound may be given. It is important to have cardiac monitoring available during IV infusion of this drug.

Give: • 7.5mg/kg base IV at a constant rate over 1hr, *followed by* 0.02mg base/kg/min.

7. Halofantrine – used in the treatment of uncomplicated chloroquine-resistant *P. falciparum* malaria as a last alternative to quinine or mefloquine. ► Side-effects include Q–T interval prolongation and ventricular arrhythmias, particularly in patients with coronary heart disease, cardiomyopathy, and congenital heart disease. Do not take in combination with arrhythmogenic drugs or drugs which cause electrolyte disturbances. ► Do not use to treat recrudescent infections within 28 days of 1° mefloquine therapy.

Give: • 8mg/kg PO repeated at 6 and 12hrs on an empty stomach.
• Repeat 1 week later in those without immunity.
► Needs ECG monitoring due to cardiotoxicity.

8. Artemisinins – are highly effective in clearing multidrug resistant *P. falciparum* parasites. IM artemether is as effective as IM quinine (although recrudescence rates may be higher). Artesunate suppositories are quick, easy, and free of the risks associated with IV injections. In uncomplicated disease, artesunate is used in combination with mefloquine.

Artenusate: • 10–12mg/kg PO in divided doses over 3–7 days, *plus*
• a total of 25mg/kg mefloquine.

If used alone, the total dose is given over 7 days [usually 4mg/kg on day 1, 2mg/kg on days 2 & 3, and 1mg/kg on days 4–7]. 1 tablet is 50mg.

For severe disease, give 2.4mg/kg IV or IM initially, followed by 1.2mg/kg at 12 and 24 hrs, then 1.2mg/kg daily. [60mg of artenusic acid is dissolved in 0.6ml of 5% $NaHCO_3$, diluted to 3–5ml with 5% dextrose and given IV or IM. 1 ampule = 80mg.]

Artemether: • same regimens as for artesunate in uncomplicated disease. 1 capsule = 40mg.

For severe disease, give 3.2mg/kg IM initially, followed by 1.6mg/kg daily. ► Do not give IV. 1 ampoule = 80mg.

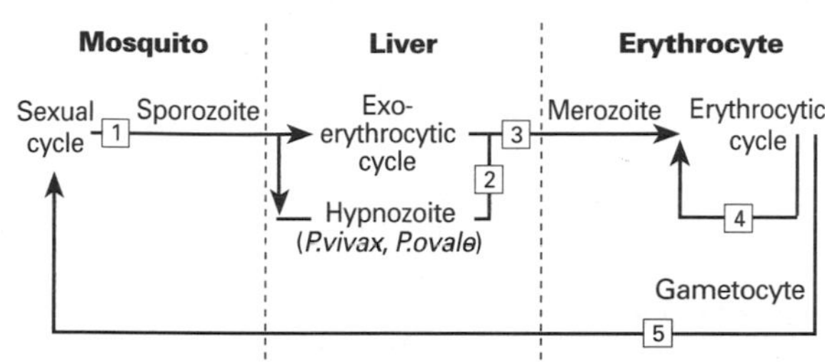

Stage specificity of antimalarial drugs:

1. sporontocidal (eg proguanil, pyrimethamine, atovaquone);
2. hypnozoitocidal (eg primaquine);
3. tissue schizontocidal (eg proguanil, pyrimethamine);
4. blood schizontocidal (eg chloroquine, quinine, artemesin);
5. gametocytocidal (eg primaquine; chloroquine in benign malarias)

9. Atovaquone/proguanil (malarone) – a new drug that is now licensed in some countries for the treatment of uncomplicated falciparum malaria where resistance to other drugs is suspected. Each tablet contains proguanil hydrochloride 100mg and atovaquone 250mg. Doses: adult and child >40kgs, 4 tablets daily for 3 days; child 11–20kg, 1 tablet; 21–30kg, 2 tablets; 31–40kg, 3 tablets, all daily for 3 days.

10. Atovaquone/tetracycline combinations – a new drug that requires clinical trials before its role in treatment is known.

11. Amodiaquine – can be effective against R1, R2, and R3 chloroquine-resistant *P.falciparum* (see section on drug resistance). IV preparations are not available, although the related amopyroquin is administered IM.

Chemoprophylaxis

► **Prophylaxis never affords full protection and measures should be taken at all times to reduce insect bites.** Also always be aware of the possible onset of malarial symptoms and present early for blood film investigation.

Travellers to malarial areas should preferably begin prophylaxis 1 week (2–3 in the case of mefloquine) before arrival and must continue for 4 weeks after departure. ► Any febrile illness occurring within 1 year of travel could be malaria. For long-term non-immune residents in malarial areas a balance must be reached between risks of infection and drug side-effects. It may be possible to target prophylaxis to transmission seasons alone.

Drugs used in prophylaxis

1. Proguanil – used for prophylaxis in pregnant women and non-immune individuals in areas of low risk only. It is more commonly used in combination with chloroquine (see below).
Dose: 200mg PO daily in adults, including pregnant women. Children <1yr 25mg/day; 1–4yrs 50mg/day; 5–8yrs 100mg/day, and 9–14yrs 150mg/day. A folic acid supplement should be taken during pregnancy.

2. Chloroquine – used with proguanil in low risk areas, for pregnant women and non-immunes only.
Dose: 300mg (as base) PO weekly in adults, including pregnant women. Children require 5mg/kg weekly.

Chloroquine binds to melanin, including that of the retina, causing concern that long-term prophylaxis may lead to visual impairment and blindness. For this reason, total lifetime exposure should not exceed 100g. Twice-yearly retinal screenings should be performed in anyone who has taken 300mg of chloroquine weekly for >5yrs. However, retinopathy was usually reported following the high doses that were formerly used in the treatment of rheumatoid arthritis and other similar diseases.

3. Mefloquine – now the drug of choice for prophylaxis in many areas due to chloroquine resistance.
Dose: 250mg PO weekly in adults and children >45kg (60mg weekly in children 3 months–5yrs; 125mg for 6–8yrs, 180mg for 9–14yrs). It is not recommended in neonates.

4. Doxycycline – useful in areas where chloroquine and mefloquine resistance is prevalent.
Dose: 1.5mg/kg PO daily, up to a max of 100mg. Do not use in children <12yrs, pregnant, or lactating women. Conception should be avoided for >1 week after its use.

5. Pyrimethamine-dapsone (Maloprim) – used in areas of chloroquine resistance (with chloroquine to cover *P. vivax*) when mefloquine or doxycycline are contraindicated.
► Pyrimethamine-sulfadoxine (Fansidar) **is not used for prophylaxis** due to the risk of Stevens–Johnson syndrome and bone marrow toxicity.
Dose: 12.5mg pyrimethamine plus 100mg dapsone (1 tablet of Maloprim) PO weekly for adults. Children: 1–5yrs 1/4 dose, 6–11yrs 1/2 dose, >11yrs full adult dose.

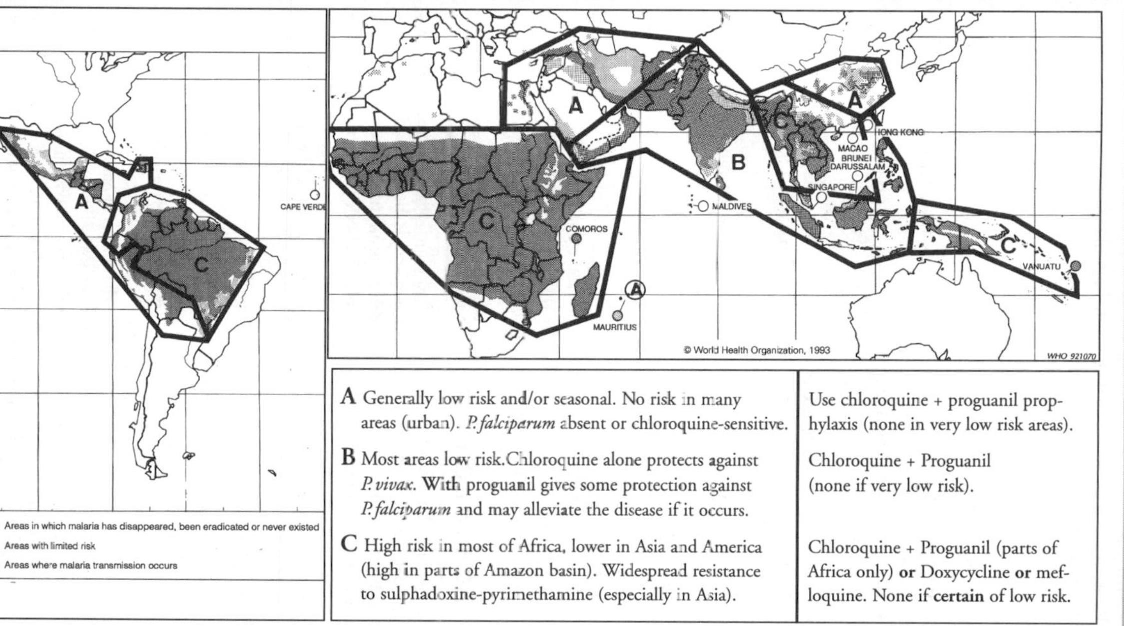

A Generally low risk and/or seasonal. No risk in many areas (urban). *P. falciparum* absent or chloroquine-sensitive.	Use chloroquine + proguanil prophylaxis (none in very low risk areas).
B Most areas low risk. Chloroquine alone protects against *P. vivax*. With proguanil gives some protection against *P. falciparum* and may alleviate the disease if it occurs.	Chloroquine + Proguanil (none if very low risk).
C High risk in most of Africa, lower in Asia and America (high in parts of Amazon basin). Widespread resistance to sulphadoxine-pyrimethamine (especially in Asia).	Chloroquine + Proguanil (parts of Africa only) **or** Doxycycline **or** mefloquine. None if **certain** of low risk.

Multidrug-resistant malaria and treatment failure

Resistance is a growing problem throughout the world (see map opposite), particularly with *P. falciparum* malaria. In certain areas, prophylaxis with chloroquine and pyrimethamine-sulfadoxine, and treatment with mefloquine or pyrimethamine-sulfadoxine are no longer recommended. *P. vivax* resistance has been reported in areas of SE Asia.

Chloroquine resistance is classified as follows:

- **R1:** Recrudescence occurs within 4 weeks of apparently successful treatment.
- **R2:** Despite improvement with treatment, parasitaemia persists and increases soon afterwards, heralding a clinical deterioration in the patient.
- **R3:** Complete resistance in which the patient continues to deteriorate (and the parasitaemia increases) despite treatment until chloroquine is replaced by an effective drug.

Treatment failure is defined as a failure of either symptoms to begin to improve or the parasite count to have fallen by 75% within 48hrs. It is possible with any drug and may result from:

- inadequate treatment (patient non-compliance or oral drug vomited)
- parasite resistance to drug
- poor drug quality
- a non-malarial cause for the symptoms.

Reassess the patient and if malaria is still thought to be the cause, change to a different treatment and ensure that the patient is taking it.

The future of malaria

It was once believed that by a combined effort of treatment, prophylaxis and particularly control measures, malaria could be eradicated. This view has been abandoned, largely because the assumptions that were made at the time of planning were not applicable practically. The current aims are to reduce morbidity, prevent mortality and reduce socioeconomic losses. Efforts continue around the world to produce an effective vaccine, an elusive goal, although several are currently being tested.

Role of education

1. To promote prompt and effective diagnosis and treatment, educating the population as to when to seek treatment, when prophylaxis is required and the importance of completing the treatment.
2. To reduce contact between mosquito and humans.
3. To control mosquito breeding by draining stagnant water, removing litter and debris which may hold water, using larvicides and larvivorous fish in mosquito breeding pools or polystyrene balls in wells and water tanks (these practices will also reduce breeding oportunities for the mosquito vectors of other diseases such as dengue fever). DDT spraying is still widely used but may eventually be replaced by new methods.

Areas of multidrug-resistant malaria

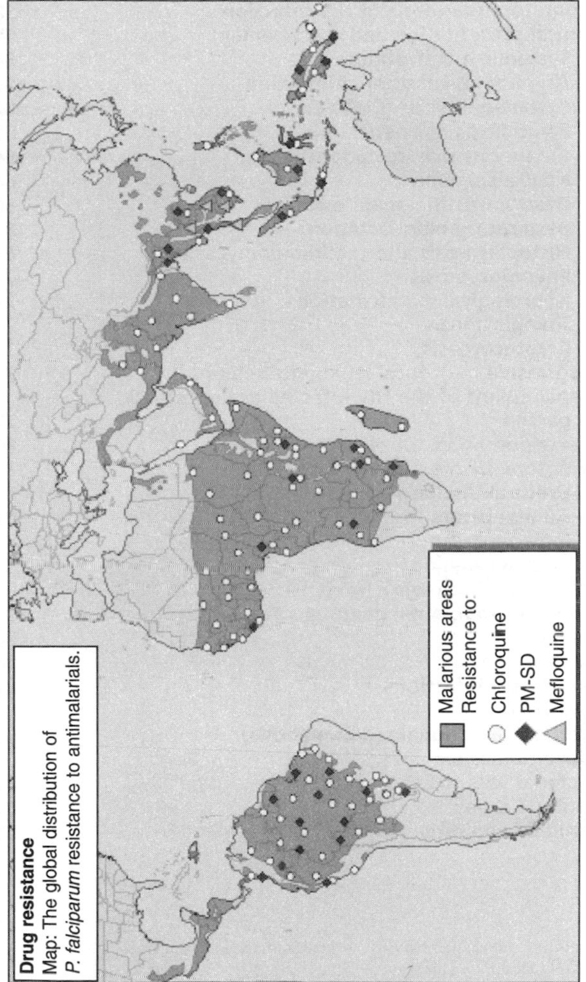

3B. HIV/STDs[1]

Sexually transmitted diseases 48
HIV infection/AIDS 50
Clinical features 52
Diagnosis 54
Laboratory diagnosis of HIV infection 56
Clinical presentation and management 58
A. Systemic manifestations 58
Atypical mycobacterial infection 62
Cytomegalovirus (CMV) 62
Penicilliosis marneffei 62
B. Cutaneous manifestations 64
Kaposi sarcoma 64
C. Gastrointestinal manifestations 66
D. Respiratory manifestations 68
Histoplasmosis and coccidioidomycosis 68
Pneumocystosis 70
E. Neurological manifestations 72
Toxoplasmosis 74
Cryptococcosis 76
Progressive multifocal leukoencephalopathy 76
Management of the HIV-infected asymptomatic person 78
Prevention and control 80
Symptomatic management of STDs 82
A. Urethral discharge 82
B. Genital ulcers 84
C. Inguinal bubo 84
D. Scrotal swelling 86
E. Vaginal discharge 88
F. Lower abdominal pain 92
Syphilis 96
Gonorrhoea 100
Chlamydial infections 102
Chancroid 104
Granuloma inguinale (donovanosis) 104
Trichomoniasis 106
Bacterial vaginosis 106
Genital herpes 108
Canidida vaginitis 108

1. Much of this chapter has been adapted from the following publications of the World Health Organization:
WHO Model Prescribing Information – Drugs Used in Sexually Transmitted Diseases and HIV Infection, WHO: Geneva 1995
Management of Sexually Transmitted Diseases, Global Program on AIDS, WHO: Geneva 1994.

HIV/STDs

Sexually transmitted diseases (STDs)

The recent demonstration that treatment of STDs reduces the transmission of HIV has re-emphasized the importance of these diseases.[1] STDs are also responsible, directly or indirectly, for much sterility, stillbirth, miscarriage, blindness, brain disease, disfigurement, cancer, and death throughout the world. The burden on the medical services is immense – several hundred million new cases are treated each year.

► Only two means of decreasing HIV transmission have thus far been proven to work:
- syndromic treatment of STDs (Tanzania)
- government promotion of condom use (Uganda and Thailand).

Their control requires a multidisciplinary approach:

1. correct diagnosis
2. effective early treatment
3. education on avoidance of contact and prevention of transmission
4. promotion and provision of condoms
5. tracing, treating, and counselling of sexual partners
6. appropriate clinical follow-up.

► It is essential that persons are treated when first seen and counselled to modify their sexual behaviour.

Syndromic approach to diagnosis and treatment

Where diagnostic facilities and effective therapies are available, all persons attending a STD clinic should be screened using laboratory tests for HIV, syphilis, chlamydia, and gonorrhoea infection. However, many cases will be treated in primary health centres where these laboratory facilities are unavailable. As a result, the WHO has developed a syndromic approach to empirical treatment that is based on the commonly seen clinical signs and symptoms. This approach is presented in the second half of this section.

> These charts have been designed to provide a framework for evaluation and treatment, but they should not replace clinical judgement based on local knowledge. They need to be trialled in, and adapted for, local circumstances.

Single-dose antibiotics should be used whenever possible. Where repeated oral doses are prescribed for ambulatory patients, drug administration should be supervised if at all possible.

► Particular attention must be made to local patterns of antibiotic resistance when these are known, particularly for gonococcal infection and to a lesser extent chancroid.

1. Gosskurth H, 1995, *Lancet*, **346**, 530

STDs and reproductive tract infections are caused by:

Microbe		*Condition*
• Bacteria		
Neisseria gonorrhoeae	→	gonorrhoea
Gardnerella vaginalis plus anerobic bacteria	→	bacterial vaginosis
Haemophilus ducreyi	→	chancroid
Calymmatobacterium granulomatis	→	donovanosis
Treponema pallidum	→	syphilis
Chlamydia trachomatis	→	urethritis/cervicitis
	→	lymphogranuloma venereum
• Fungi		
Candida albicans	→	candidiasis
• Protozoa		
Trichomonas vaginalis	→	trichomoniasis
• Viruses		
human immunodeficiency virus	→	AIDS
herpes simplex virus	→	genital herpes
human papillomavirus	→	genital warts
• Arthropods		
Phthirus pubis	→	pubic lice
Sarcoptes scabiei	→	scabies

Other microbes can be passed sexually, for example hepatitis B and CMV, but are not considered STDs. Gastrointestinal microbes such as hepatitis A can also be transmitted through anal sexual intercourse.

HIV infection/AIDS

The human immunodeficiency viruses have infected over 30 million people and are the cause of the acquired immunodeficiency syndrome (AIDS) pandemic that is currently sweeping through the world. Most disease is caused by HIV-1 – it is more virulent and widespread than HIV-2 which mostly occurs in west Africa. The viruses attach to and enter T lymphocytes that bear the CD4 protein on their surface. These '$CD4^+$' lymphocytes coordinate the body's immune response and as their numbers fall during the late stages of AIDS, profound immunosuppression occurs. This lays the patient open to a variety of infections that would not normally cause disease in an immunocompetent person – so-called opportunistic infections. The specific opportunistic infections that occur will depend on both • the area of the world and • the patient's degree of immunosuppression. Certain tumours, caused by viruses, are more common in AIDS patients: lymphomas (EBV) and Kaposi sarcoma (a novel herpesvirus KSAV or HHV-8).

There is currently no vaccine and no cure for the viral infection itself. Good therapies have been developed, however, for many of the opportunistic infections, and antiretrovirals appear to at least temporarily slow the pace of the viral infection. Unfortunately, these drugs are expensive and therefore not universally available.

There are three stages to the disease:

1. ***an acute retroviral illness***, similar to mononucleosis, that occurs in ~50% of patients 2–5 weeks post-infection,
2. ***an asymptomatic stage*** during which the body's immune system attempts to control the virus [NB that the virus is not latent at this stage but is instead in balance with the immune system. Billions of virus particles are both produced and destroyed each day],
3. ***a symptomatic stage*** as the immune system's function becomes compromised and the patient suffers from multiple opportunistic infections as well as the direct effects of HIV itself.

Transmission is via:

- unprotected intercourse (both heterosexual and homosexual)
- from the mother to fetus or infant before, during, or after birth (virus is passed from an infected mother to her child in milk)
- receipt of infected blood products
- injections or treatments with unsterile needles, syringes, or skin-piercing instruments.

Sexually transmitted diseases, particularly those that cause genital ulceration, increase the risk of sexual transmission. In the developing world, heterosexual intercourse appears to be the major mode of transmission for adults, followed by blood transfusion and unsterile needles. Children are at risk of infection perinatally and from blood transfusion.

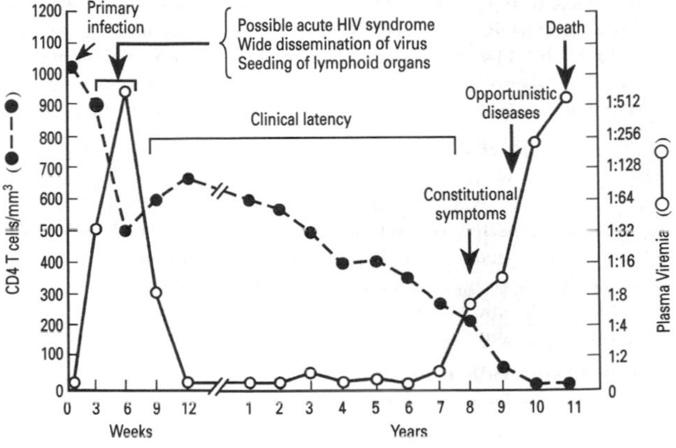

The natural history of HIV infection. In many parts of the world, the period of clinical latency may be shorter than represented here and symptoms may appear at higher CD4 levels. (Reproduced with permission from reference 1)

Chemotherapy of an acute infection rarely completely removes the causative agent from the body. Normally, the host's immune response continues to control and suppress the infection. Since the immune system is impaired in AIDS patients, the infection will recur once treatment is stopped. Therefore, AIDS patients need to recei[illegible] therapy for the rest of their lives after an acute infection – t[illegible] is termed ***2° chemotherapy***.

Trials now indicate that treatment of HIV+ people [illegible]an prevent infections with microbes such as TB – ***1° chemopr[illegible]phylaxis***.

1. Pantaleo G, 1993, *NEJM*, **328**, 327

Clinical features

Acute retroviral illness: this occurs in some patients 10–30 days post-exposure and lasts 3–21 days. It is similar to infectious mononucleosis with a variety of signs and symptoms – malaise, fever, sore throat, myalgia, anorexia, anthralgia, headache, diarrhoea, nausea, generalized lymphadenopathy, macular eruption involving trunk and arms, thrombocytopenia. Rare complications include aseptic meningoencephalitis and mono/polyneuritis. Atypical lymphocytes may be seen in the blood film.

Asymptomatic HIV infection: lasts for a variable period of time before immune system dysfunction produces symptoms. In the USA, ~50% of HIV-infected individuals develop symptoms by 10 years; most of the others are expected to develop AIDS in the future. The length of the asymptomatic period in the developing world is unclear – it may be shorter, reflecting the generally lower level of health compared to the USA. The only sign of infection during this period may be generalized lymphadenopathy, probably due to HIV itself.

Symptomatic HIV infection: weight loss and weakness are the commonest manifestations. Opportunistic infections attack multiple systems (see following pages). Certain opportunistic infections become more common as the CD4 count falls – this is reflected in the WHO's proposals for staging HIV infection and disease by clinical signs and symptoms.

WHO clinical staging system for HIV infection and disease

The following staging system has been developed for epidemiological purposes. It may also prove useful for both estimating a patient's prognosis and following the development of AIDS. The system can be adapted for each locality using the blank spaces. The presence of any of these manifestations in a previously healthy adult should suggest HIV infection. Any suspicion of HIV infection should be confirmed by laboratory tests after discussion with and consent of the patient.

A performance scale: has been developed by the WHO for the staging of HIV infection and AIDS that is compatible with the clinical staging system opposite.

Performance level

1. asymptomatic, normal activity
2. symptomatic, normal activity
3. bedridden <50% of the day during the last month
4. bedridden >50% of the day during the last month

HIV encephalopathy = clinical findings of disabling cognitive and/or motor dysfunction interfering with activities of daily living, progressing over weeks to months, in the absence of a concurrent illness or condition other than HIV infection that could explain the findings.

HIV wasting syndrome = weight loss >10% of body weight, plus either unexplained chronic diarrhoea (>1 month) or chronic weakness and unexplained prolonged fever (>1 month).

Clinical stage 1

- Asymptomatic
- Persistent generalized lymphadenopathy (PGL)

Clinical stage 2

- Weight loss <10% of body weight
- Minor mucocutaneous lesions (seborrhoeic dermatitis, prurigo, fungal nail infections, recurrent oral ulcerations, angular cheilitis)
- Zoster within the last five years
- Recurrent upper respiratory tract infections (incl. bacteria sinusitis)
-

Clinical stage 3

- Weight loss >10% of body weight
- Unexplained chronic diarrhoea for >1 month
- Unexplained prolonged fever (intermittent/constant) for >1 month
- Oral candidiasis (thrush)
- Oral hairy leukoplakia
- Pulmonary tuberculosis within the past year
- Severe bacterial infections (pneumonia, pyomyositis)
-

Clinical stage 4

- HIV wasting syndrome
- *Pneumocystis carinii* pneumonia (PCP)
- Toxoplasmosis of the brain
- Cryptosporidiosis with diarrhoea, for >1 month
- Cryptococcosis, extrapulmonary
- Cytomegalovirus (CMV) disease of an organ other than liver, spleen, or lymph nodes
- Herpesvirus infection, mucocutaneous for >1 month, or visceral of any duration
- Progressive multifocal leukoencephalopathy (PML)
- Any disseminated endemic mycosis
- Candidiasis of the oesophagus, trachea, bronchi, or lungs
- Atypical mycobacteriosis, disseminated
- Nontyphoid salmonella septicaemia
- Extrapulmonary tuberculosis
- Lymphoma
- Kaposi sarcoma
- HIV encephalopathy
- Invasive cervical cancer

Diagnosis

Almost all HIV-infected individuals have detectable levels of anti-HIV antibodies by three months post-infection (three weeks for the new, third-generation ELISAs). Patients who have AIDS can also be diagnosed by the presence of particular conditions that are characteristic of this disease. Some conditions are so typical that, if present, AIDS can be diagnosed, for epidemiological purposes only, in the absence of laboratory tests for either anti-HIV antibodies or declining CD4 count. This is recognized in the following algorithm:

WHO algorithm to aid recognition of *symptomatic* HIV infection

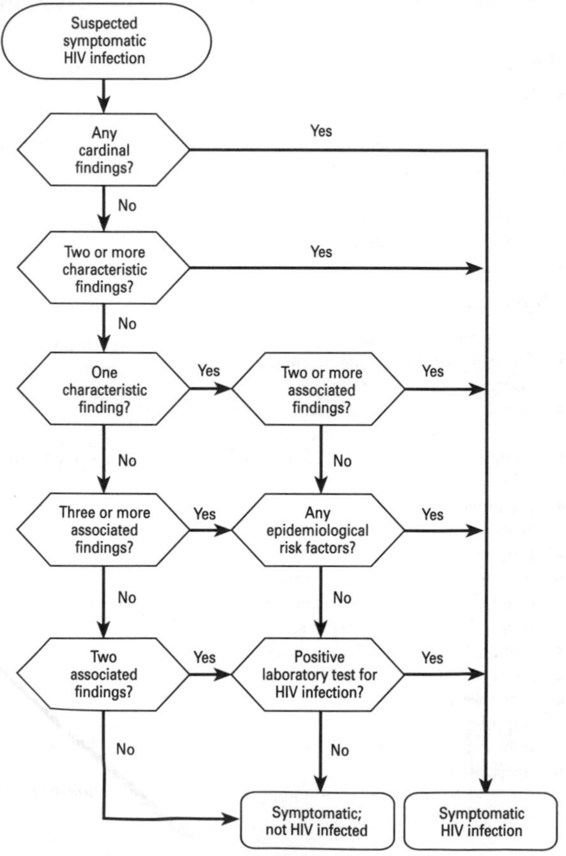

Cardinal findings:

- Kaposi sarcoma (intraoral, generalized, or rapidly progressive/invasive lesions)
- *Pneumocytis carinii* pneumonia
- *Toxoplasma* encephalitis
- oesophageal candidiasis
- CMV retinitis

Characteristic findings in the absence of obvious causes of immunosuppression:

- oral candidiasis (in a patient not taking antibiotics)
- hairy leukoplakia
- cryptococcal meningitis
- tuberculosis (miliary, extrapulmonary, noncavitary pulmonary disease)
- herpes zoster (past or present; particularly >1 dermatome; age <50 yrs)
- severe pruritis
- Kaposi sarcoma (other than as a cardinal finding)
- high-grade B-cell extranodal lymphoma

Associated findings in the absence of obvious causes of immunosuppression:

- weight loss – recent, unexplained; >10% of baseline body weight
- fever – continuous or intermittent; for >1 month
- diarrhoea – continuous or intermittent; for >1 month
- ulcers – genital or perianal; for >1 month
- cough – for >1 month
- neurological complaints or findings – particularly (focal) seizures; peripheral neuropathy (sensory or motor); focal central motor or sensory deficit; dementia; progressively worsening headache
- generalized lymphadenopathy – extrainguinal
- drug reactions – previously not seen eg to thiacetazone, sulfonamides
- skin infections – severe/recurrent; eg warts, dermatophytes, folliculitis

Epidemiological risk factors:

1. ***Present or past high-risk behaviour:***
    - drug injecting
    - multiple sex partners
    - sex partner(s) with known AIDS or HIV infection
    - sex partner(s) with known epidemiological risk factor or from an area with high prevalence of HIV infection
    - males having penetrative sexual intercourse with males
2. ***Recent history of genital ulcer disease***
3. ***History of transfusion after 1975*** of unscreened blood, plasma, or clotting factor; or (even if screened) from an area with a high prevalence of HIV infection
4. ***History of scarification, tattooing, ear piercing, or circumcision*** using non-sterile instruments

Laboratory diagnosis of HIV infection[1]

There are 3 main purposes for which HIV antibody testing is performed:

- ***transfusion/transplant safety*** – screening of donated blood and organs to prevent HIV transmission.
- ***surveillance*** – unlinked and anonymous testing for monitoring the prevalence of, and trends in, HIV infection over time in a given population.
- ***diagnosis of HIV infection*** – voluntary testing of serum from asymptomatic persons or from persons with clinical signs and symptoms suggestive of HIV infection or AIDS.

The first objective requires extremely sensitive tests that will pick up all contaminated blood/organs and thus prevent them from entering the blood/organ supply. The third objective requires very specific tests so that there are few false positives – ie HIV-uninfected people are not told that they are infected. The second objective requires tests that are sensitive and specific but not to the same degree as the other two objectives.

UNAIDS/WHO have developed three testing strategies that maximize accuracy in these different settings while minimizing cost. They are described in reference 1. Guidelines laid down by the national Health Ministry will determine which test is used for the above objectives.

An HIV test kit bulk-purchase programme has been established by WHO and UNAIDS in order to provide national AIDS control programmes with accurate tests at the lowest possible cost.

Clinical diagnosis

Before carrying out a test to diagnose HIV infection, ask yourself:

- What is the purpose of carrying out this test?
- Will this person gain from being diagnosed as HIV positive?

In many parts of the world, there is no antiretroviral therapy that would make an early diagnosis clinically useful. In addition, most patients are treated symptomatically whether they are HIV infected or not. Newly diagnosed patients have received hostility from their community; there are also reports of newly diagnosed women being assaulted.

However, as experience accrues with prophylaxis or vaccination to combat common infections such as TB or pneumococcal pneumonia, and as the value of antiretroviral therapy in preventing mother-to-child transmission becomes more defined, an early diagnosis will become of use to more patients.

- Overall, therefore, diagnostic testing for HIV should be carried out only after careful thought.
- Diagnostic tests for HIV infection should never be considered as positive, and the patient informed, until they have been confirmed by a second assay.

1. UNAIDS/WHO – Revised recommendations for the selection and use of HIV antibody tests, 1997 *Weekly Epidemiol. Rec*, 72, 81.

Counselling

If you decide to offer an HIV test, counselling is essential. Studies indicate that a patient who knows him or herself to be infected will practise safer sexual practices if the HIV testing is accompanied by counselling and if future psychological support is provided.

- *Pre-test counselling* – ensures that the patient understands the purpose of the test and the consequences of a positive result.
- *Post-test counselling* – helps the patient come to terms with a positive result or to encourage HIV negative individuals to practise low risk behaviour.

A physician should be able to discuss the diagnosis of HIV infection, the transmission of the virus and its prevention, and the best ways of staying healthy with HIV and of taking care of common HIV/AIDS-related problems.

Clinical presentation and management

A list of the main causes for each manifestation of AIDS, in order of significance, should be established for each country, in light of the available information. We currently know too little about the causes of many of the common manifestations of AIDS in many parts of the world. This information is essential if better treatment protocols for particular manifestations are to be developed. While opportunistic infections are important causes of disease in patients with AIDS, the infections that are common in HIV-negative patients in the same area also tend to be common in HIV infected patients. They are often simply more severe and life-threatening.

The infections and conditions that are characteristic of patients with AIDS in a certain locality will also occur in other immunosuppressed patients – such as those with haematological malignancies.

A. Systemic manifestations

► Always consider TB (and in relevant geographical regions, fungal infection such as penicilliosis, coccidioidomycosis) as a cause of systemic illness in HIV-infected persons. The manifestations of TB in such a person are extremely diverse – see chapter 3C.

1. Weight loss – is often the first sign of HIV infection. After treatment for an intercurrent infection, some patients gain weight again but normally only for a short time. Accelerated weight loss is a sign of disease progression (some lose up to 40% of their weight and die in extreme cachexia). No specific cause is identified in most patients.

2. Weakness and anorexia – are frequently present, but may be absent even at times of great weight loss.

3. Fever – Hx and Ex first to look for localizing signs (chapter 4). If these are absent, the fever may be an '*HIV-associated fever*'. This is defined as a fever with a duration of >2 weeks as the only clinical presentation in a patient with a prior history of symptomatic HIV infection, or in a known HIV-positive patient with an asymptomatic prior history. The fever is often intermittent and accompanied by night sweats and chills.

However, when resources are limited, the identification of non-HIV aetiologies for fever may sometimes be impossible. Fever due to HIV itself should only be considered after other treatable causes – a diagnosis of last resort.

***Aetiology*:**

- Infections – mycobacterial (TB, atypical mycobacteria), fungal (cryptococcosis, histoplasmosis), bacterial (bacteraemia due to *Salmonella* spp, *S. pneumoniae*, *H. influenzae*), viral (disseminated CMV, EBV), protozoal (*P. carinii*, *T. gondii*, visceral leishmaniasis).
- HIV infection itself.
- Malignancy – lymphoma.
- Drugs – many possibilities.

► When no alternative cause for the fever can be found, try discontinuing the patient's drugs one at a time.

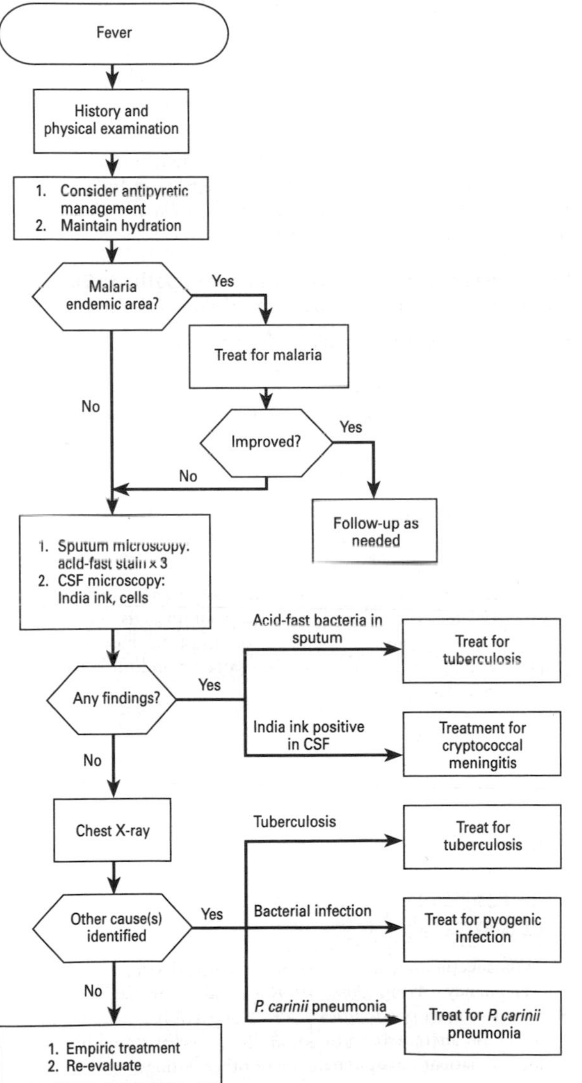
Fever
History and physical examination
1. Consider antipyretic management
2. Maintain hydration
Malaria endemic area?
Yes
Treat for malaria
Improved?
Yes
Follow-up as needed
No
No
1. Sputum microscopy: acid-fast stain × 3
2. CSF microscopy: India ink, cells
Any findings?
Yes
Acid-fast bacteria in sputum
Treat for tuberculosis
India ink positive in CSF
Treatment for cryptococcal meningitis
No
Chest X-ray
Other cause(s) identified
Yes
Tuberculosis
Treat for tuberculosis
Bacterial infection
Treat for pyogenic infection
P. carinii pneumonia
Treat for P. carinii pneumonia
No
1. Empiric treatment
2. Re-evaluate

4A. Lymphadenopathy: defined as lymph node enlargement in a patient with symptomatic HIV infection.

Aetiology:

- HIV infection itself
- Infections – bacterial (TB, syphilis), fungal (histoplasmosis) or viral (CMV)
- Malignancies – lymphadenopathic Kaposi sarcoma (not necessarily associated with cutaneous Kaposi sarcoma), lymphoma
- Dermatological conditions – seborrhoeic dermatitis, chronic pyoderma.

A careful physical examination should identify any local or contiguous infection that might explain the lymphadenopathy. ► Infections prevalent in the region concerned, eg trypanosomiasis or *Paracoccidioides brasiliensis* infection, should also be considered.

4B. Persistent generalized lymphadenopathy (PGL) is common in HIV$^+$ patients and is often due to HIV alone. It is defined as follows:

- More than 3 separate lymph node groups affected
- At least 2 nodes >1.5 cm in diameter at each site
- Duration of >1 month
- No local or contiguous infection that might explain the lymphadenopathy

It is important to exclude the following treatable causes:

- **syphilis:** (papulosquamous rash +/– evidence of recent genital ulcer)
- **tuberculosis:** (suggestive clinical signs → CXR and/or node aspiration for AFB)

If excluded, asymptomatic patients do not need further investigation. However, if nodes are rapidly enlarging, or there is nodal asymmetry or systemic symptoms, a lymph node must be biopsied to exclude lymphoma, lymphadenopathic Kaposi sarcoma and infiltrative fungal or mycobacterial disease.

GPA/WHO flowcharts

The flowcharts presented in this section were developed by the Global Programme on AIDS of the WHO to aid the management of HIV-infected persons in resource-poor settings with a high incidence of both malaria and tuberculosis. Similar flowcharts may be useful for the management of these patients in other settings.

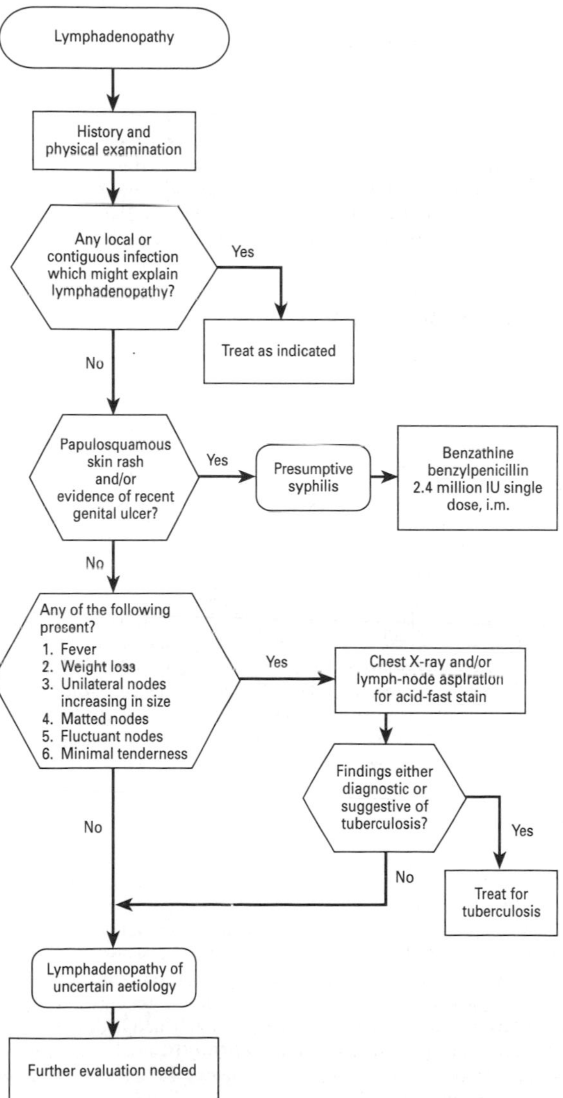
Lymphadenopathy
History and physical examination
Any local or contiguous infection which might explain lymphadenopathy?
Yes
Treat as indicated
No
Papulosquamous skin rash and/or evidence of recent genital ulcer?
Yes
Presumptive syphilis
Benzathine benzylpenicillin 2.4 million IU single dose, i.m.
No
Any of the following present?
1. Fever
2. Weight loss
3. Unilateral nodes increasing in size
4. Matted nodes
5. Fluctuant nodes
6. Minimal tenderness
Yes
Chest X-ray and/or lymph-node aspiration for acid-fast stain
Findings either diagnostic or suggestive of tuberculosis?
Yes
Treat for tuberculosis
No
No
Lymphadenopathy of uncertain aetiology
Further evaluation needed

Atypical mycobacterial infection

Non-tuberous mycobacteria have long been known to cause disseminated infection or pneumonia in patients with underlying illnesses. However, the prevalence of these diseases has increased markedly since the emergence of AIDS. They are environmental pathogens worldwide, but do appear to occur less commonly among HIV-infected persons in Africa compared to other parts of the world. Any of the known pathogenic mycobacteria can cause a febrile illness with weight loss, malaise, and night sweats. Other signs: anaemia, hepatosplenomegaly, lymphadenopathy, and widespread organ involvement particularly the GI tract. ***Diagnosis*** is by Ziehl-Neelsen staining of intracellular AFB in biopsies (also sputum but not necessarily indicative of disease); specialized blood culture – allows differentiation from TB. ***Management:*** clarithromycin 250–500mg PO bd *plus* rifabutin 450–600mg PO daily *plus* ethambutol 15mg/kg PO daily. Therapy improves symptoms; it is not clear if it improves survival.

Cytomegalovirus (CMV)

Most people have been infected by this herpesvirus by the age of 40. In nearly all cases infection is asymptomatic; <10% have a self-resolving mononucleosis-like illness. In the immunocompromised host, however, it may cause a severe febrile illness with protean manifestations involving multiple organs. Chorioretinitis is the most common manifestation. GI involvement may include colon, oesophagus and liver; CNS infection is rare. Other organs that may rarely be involved include lungs and adrenal glands. Both lung and bowel involvement can be fatal – the former presents similarly to pneumocystosis; intense inflammation in the latter can result in perforation and peritonitis or haemorrhage. Untreated infection of the retina rapidly produces blindness.

CMV may be isolated from urine, and blood from both symptomatic and asymptomatic persons. However, the ***diagnosis*** of CMV disease is often based on identification of typical inclusion bodies on histopathological examination, presence of IgM antibody, or seroconversion. The disease in most AIDS patients is a reactivation of a chronic/latent infection. ***Treatment*** with antiviral agents, such as ganciclovir or foscarnet, is able to treat disease and prevent reactivation but it is extremely expensive.

Penicilliosis marneffei

A disseminated and progressive fungal infection that is becoming increasingly recognized in immunosuppressed patients in SE Asia and S China. It may be misdiagnosed as tuberculosis or another disseminated fungal infection (histoplasmosis, cryptococcosis) due to its common mode of presentation: fever, anaemia, weight loss, skin lesions, sepsis and/or lymphadenopathy.[1] Other sites include lungs (painful, non-productive cough; CXR may show abscesses, cavities), liver, spleen, (rarely bones, joints). ***Diagnosis*** is via Giemsa stain of bone marrow, lymph node or skin scraping for yeast-like organisms; serology. ***Treatment:*** amphotericin B IV for 2 weeks followed by itraconazole for 6 weeks. Relapses are common – retreat with amphotericin B or fluconazole.

1. Duong TA, 1996, *Clin Infect Dis*, **23**, 125

B. Cutaneous manifestations

Many people with HIV have cutaneous manifestations (see opposite), some of which are fairly specific for AIDS. Others are very non-specific and may be signs of systemic disease – biopsy and scraping are required for a diagnosis. The skin of AIDS patients often becomes dry and atrophic and the hair becomes thinner, losing its colour.

A generalized papular pruritic reaction is found in many African HIV$^+$ patients, often as a 1° lesion. In certain high risk groups, it is quite specific for HIV infection. The cause is not known. Papules, scratch marks, and hyperpigmented macules are symmetrically distributed over the body, but particularly the extensor arm surface, back of the hands, ankles, and dorsum of the feet. They last throughout the patient's illness.

Kaposi sarcoma (KS)

This is a tumour of endothelial cells, probably caused by a recently identified sexually-transmitted herpesvirus, called Kaposi sarcoma associated virus (KSAV or HHV-8), that presents with lesions of the skin and in many cases the viscera. It is common in Africa. Two other forms are recognized: classic KS in equatorial Africa that is slowly progressive in adults (aggressive in children/adolescents) and limited to one anatomical region, particularly the feet, and an indolent skin tumour of elderly men in the US and elsewhere.

Clinical features: the multiple lesions are nodular and pigmented, appearing black on black skin and purple on pale skin. Early lesions, being small, macular and erythematous, are often difficult to recognize. While mostly asymptomatic, especially at first, the lesions may become infiltrated or ulcerate. They occur on all parts of the body, not just the skin, and are rarely limited to one anatomical region. Lesions on the face, soles, and in the oral cavity are common. Visceral disease may occur without skin involvement – the only visible lesion may be in the oral cavity. Oral lesions are 1) often not raised, and 2) may result in bleeding, pain, and dysphagia. KS commonly involves lymph nodes (→ lymphoedema), GI tract (mostly stomach, duodenum, rectum; it rarely → intestinal obstruction, bleeding) and lungs (dyspnoea, cough, chest tightness, bronchoconstriction, rarely fever). However, any organ may be involved.

Diagnosis: can be made clinically in most cases; a punch biopsy otherwise shows characteristic histology (biopsy very rarely → haemorrhage); (as KSAV becomes characterized, ? → importance of serology).

Management: the clinical course of KS is often indolent, patients normally dying from intercurrent infections. However, pulmonary KS can be rapidly fatal. The lesions may respond to chemotherapy; relapse is common. Local treatment such as surgical excision, radiation, or topical liquid nitrogen can be used for individual lesions on the face or in the mouth.

Cutaneous manifestations of AIDS

Neoplasia	Kaposi sarcoma	non-Hodgkins lymphoma
	squamous cell CA	basal cell CA
Infections	herpes zoster	herpesvirus infections
	superficial fungal infections	angular cheilitis
	chancroid	cryptococcosis
	histoplasmosis	human papillomavirus
	impetigo	lymphogranuloma venereum
	molluscum contagiosum	mycobacterial infection
	syphilis	furunculosis
	folliculitis	pyomyositis
Others	pruritic papular dermatitis	seborrhoeic dermatitis
	drug eruptions	vasculitis
	xeroderma	psoriasis
	granuloma annulare	thrombocytic purpura
	telengiectasia	hyperpigmentation
	dry atrophic skin	hair changes

C. Gastrointestinal manifestations

Studies of AIDS patients in different parts of the world have begun to identify the most common causes of GI disease. It is becoming clear that these differ between regions, eg *Cryptosporidium* spp and CMV are the commonest gut pathogens in parts of Africa and in India, respectively. Further studies should help define the most common causes of the GI signs and symptoms in each region with clear advantages for treatment when diagnostic workup is limited.

1. Chronic diarrhoea – defined as 'liquid stools 3 or more times per day, continuously or episodically for >1 month, in a patient with symptomatic HIV infection'.

Aetiology: although the cause is often not identified, possibilities include:

- Infections – cryptosporidiosis, *Isospora belli*, *Giardia lamblia*, *Salmonella* spp, *Shigella flexneri*, *Campylobacter* spp., *Entamoeba histolytica*, CMV, *Strongyloides stercoralis*, atypical mycobacteria.
- Malignancies – Kaposi sarcoma, lymphoma.
- Idiopathic (possibly HIV infection).

2. Colitis – may present with severe abdominal cramps and distension, rebound tenderness and megacolon. Watery diarrhoea (+/– blood) is common. The cause is often not identified; possibilities include CMV and ulcerative Kaposi sarcoma.

3. Dysphagia – the commonest cause is treatable oesophageal candidiasis; other causes include CMV and herpes virus.

Oesophageal candidiasis

Anyone with weight-loss and dysphagia due to oral candidiasis requires treatment with fluconazole (50–100mg PO daily for 14–30 days or, if required, 400mg IV on day 1, then 200mg IV until clinical response). Recurrence is common after stopping antifungals. Diagnosis is by barium swallow, fine-needle aspiration of enlarged lymph nodes, or oesophagoscopy.

4. Perianal discomfort – anogenital ulcerations are caused by herpes viruses, *T. pallidum* and *H. ducreyi*. Perianal warts are caused by human papillomavirus.

5. Hepatic disease – intrahepatic opportunistic infections or malignancies have been found commonly on postmortem in AIDS patients, although the liver lesions appear to be part of widespread disseminated disease.

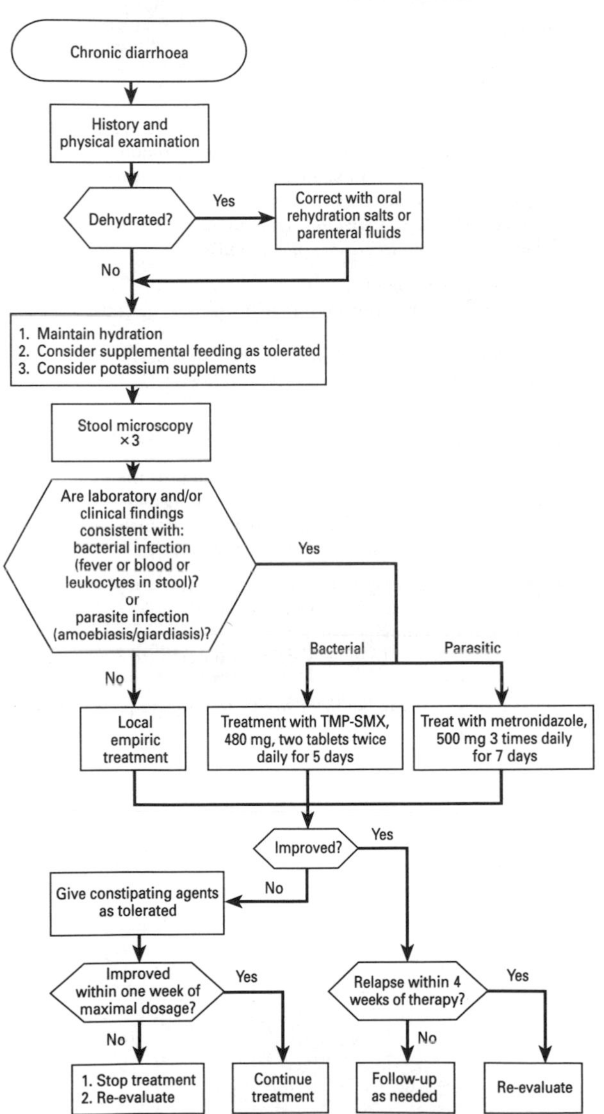
Chronic diarrhoea
History and physical examination
Dehydrated?
Yes
Correct with oral rehydration salts or parenteral fluids
No
1. Maintain hydration
2. Consider supplemental feeding as tolerated
3. Consider potassium supplements
Stool microscopy ×3
Are laboratory and/or clinical findings consistent with: bacterial infection (fever or blood or leukocytes in stool)? or parasite infection (amoebiasis/giardiasis)?
Yes
Bacterial
Parasitic
No
Local empiric treatment
Treatment with TMP-SMX, 480 mg, two tablets twice daily for 5 days
Treat with metronidazole, 500 mg 3 times daily for 7 days
Improved?
Yes
No
Give constipating agents as tolerated
Improved within one week of maximal dosage?
Yes
No
1. Stop treatment
2. Re-evaluate
Continue treatment
Relapse within 4 weeks of therapy?
Yes
No
Follow-up as needed
Re-evaluate

D. Respiratory manifestations

Persistent or worsening cough, chest pain, dyspnoea, cyanosis, or tachypnoea

Aetiology:

- Infections –
- ► Particularly: • TB in Africa
  • PCP in Asia and the Americas

  Otherwise, bacterial pneumonia (*S. pneumoniae*, *H. influenzae*), fungal infection (cryptococcus, histoplasmosis, coccidioidomycosis), atypical mycobacteria, CMV, toxoplasmosis, *Nocardia asteroides*, *Candida albicans*, *Legionella pneumophila*
- Malignancies – Kaposi sarcoma, lymphoma
- Others – lymphoid interstitial pneumonitis

These may be exacerbated by

- ***pleural effusion/empyema*** (associated with TB, bacterial infection or cancer)
- ***pneumothorax*** (associated with TB, PCP or cancer)
- ***pericardial effusion*** (often associated with TB)

Histoplasmosis and coccidioidomycosis

Although these fungi are normally local infections of the lung, they may cause disseminated disease in AIDS patients – see chapter 6. Early signs are non-specific or pulmonary, including: cough, fever, malaise, weight loss, and interstitial infiltrates on CXR. D&V may occur.

Management: haematogenous spread may result in rapid deterioration so therapy should be started in severe cases on clinical suspicion (+/– the presence of serum antibody). Give:

1. amphotericin B 0.5–1mg/kg IV daily for 6 weeks (to a maximum total of 3g) *then*
2. amphotericin B 0.5mg/kg IV at weekly intervals to prevent relapse.

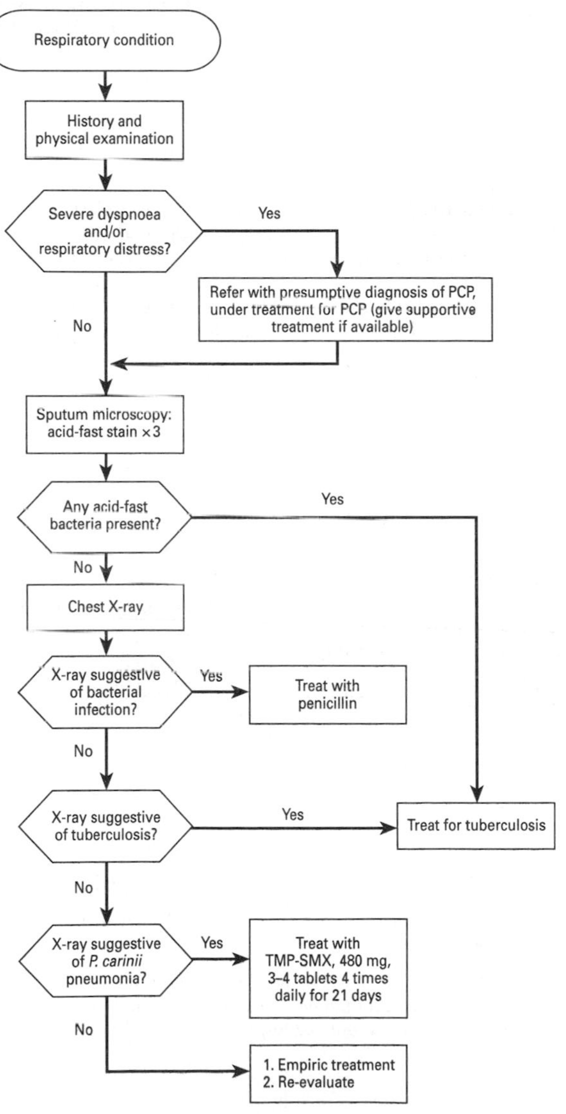
Respiratory condition
History and physical examination
Severe dyspnoea and/or respiratory distress?
Yes
Refer with presumptive diagnosis of PCP, under treatment for PCP (give supportive treatment if available)
No
Sputum microscopy: acid-fast stain ×3
Any acid-fast bacteria present?
Yes
No
Chest X-ray
X-ray suggestive of bacterial infection?
Yes
Treat with penicillin
No
X-ray suggestive of tuberculosis?
Yes
Treat for tuberculosis
No
X-ray suggestive of P. carinii pneumonia?
Yes
Treat with TMP-SMX, 480 mg, 3–4 tablets 4 times daily for 21 days
No
1. Empiric treatment
2. Re-evaluate

Pneumocystosis

The causative protozoa, *Pneumocystis carinii*, is a ubiquitous microbe that does not cause disease in the immunocompetent. It is a common cause of pneumonia (*P. carinii* pneumonia – PCP) in adult AIDS patients except in Africa – where it has been reported in HIV^+ infants. Its rarity in African adults may be due to the high prevalence of more virulent respiratory pathogens such as TB. In contrast, in Brazilian and Thai AIDS patients, *P. carinii* is as common a respiratory pathogen as TB.

Respiratory failure results from an irreversible fibrotic reaction caused by protozoal multiplication in the alveolar septal walls throughout the lungs.

Clinical features: are initially insidious and easily missed (minority → fulminant infection). They include dyspnoea and non-productive cough, rarely mild pleuritic chest pain. Auscultation reveals rales and rhonchi only in an advanced stage. Similarly, early CXR may be normal; later they show bilateral interstitial and alveolar infiltrates in middle and lower zones, usually with peripheral sparing. Cavities may form. Severe clinical symptoms in the absence of findings on examination or CXR is highly suggestive of PCP. Extrapulmonary infection has been reported.

Diagnosis: Pneumocystosis is strongly suspected in a patient who does not have TB but has bilateral pulmonary infiltrates resistant to antimicrobials. Examination of Gram-Wright stained lavage from bronchoscopy is the ideal investigation. When bronchoscopy is not available, non-invasive induced sputum method has proved sensitive – stain sputum after inhalation of 3% nebulized saline.

Management:

1.
- co-trimoxazole 100–120mg/kg/day IV/PO in 2–4 divided doses, *or*
- pentamidine isethionate 4mg/kg IV daily,
  both regimens for 21 days.

2. ► If the patient is cyanosed, the simultaneous administration of corticosteroid decreases risk of death. Give:
- prednisolone 40mg bd for 5 days, *followed by*
- 40mg daily for 5 days *then*
- 20mg daily for 10 days
- [alternatively, give methylprednisolone IV].

3. Maintenance dose:
- co-trimoxazole 960mg PO bd, *or*
- dapsone 100mg PO twice weekly, *or*
- pentamidine isethionate 300mg by aerosol every 4wks,
  all regimens for life.

Prevention: in regions where PCP is a significant clinical problem, prophylactic treatment should be started for all patients with symptomatic HIV infection or CD4 counts <200/μl.

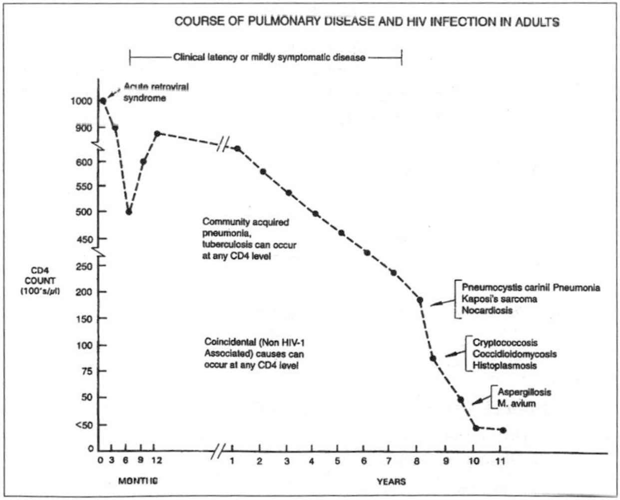

This represents the situation in the USA. Infections may occur at higher CD4 counts in the developing world.

E. Neurological manifestations

1. Headache – defined as a headache in a patient with symptomatic HIV infection, often persistent or severe and rapidly increasing or not responding to common drugs used for pain relief. It can be with or without fever.

Aetiology:

- Infections – chronic meningitis due to tuberculosis, cryptococcus or chronic HIV infection; meningoencephalitis due to *Toxoplasma* or viruses (eg CMV); neurosyphilis, progressive multifocal leukoencephalopathy
- Malignancies – lymphoma
- Drug side-effect – zidovudine

Causes of headache (chapter 9) not related to HIV infection, particularly malaria, should be identified and treated. Infectious diseases prevalent in the region concerned that can lead to headache should also be considered and treated, if possible.

2. Progressive behaviour changes and dementia – (subacute AIDS encephalopathy) – cognitive dysfunction may be common in AIDS patients. It has an insidious onset; signs/symptoms include:

- loss of concentration and recent memory
- mental slowing
- motor signs such as tremor and slowness
- apathy
- social withdrawal
- uncoordination

In time, it progresses to:

- severe dementia • mutism • incontinence • paraplegia.

This condition appears to be due to direct HIV infection of the CNS – no association has been found between this condition and opportunistic infections. However, progressive multifocal leukoencephalopathy (see page 76) can cause similar signs.

3. Meningism – acute HIV infection may cause signs of meningism. If chronic, they are likely to be due to cryptococcus or tuberculosis.

4. Visual impairment – commonly due to CMV infection or toxoplasmosis.

5. Focal neurological signs including seizures – are most commonly due to *T. gondii* or B-cell lymphoma. Candida, cryptococcus, and mycobacteria also cause space occupying lesions in the CNS.

6. Peripheral neuropathy (chapter 9) – due to HIV; other viruses; vasculitis; compression by a lymphoma; alcohol, and increasingly by drug therapy (isoniazid, antiretrovirals).

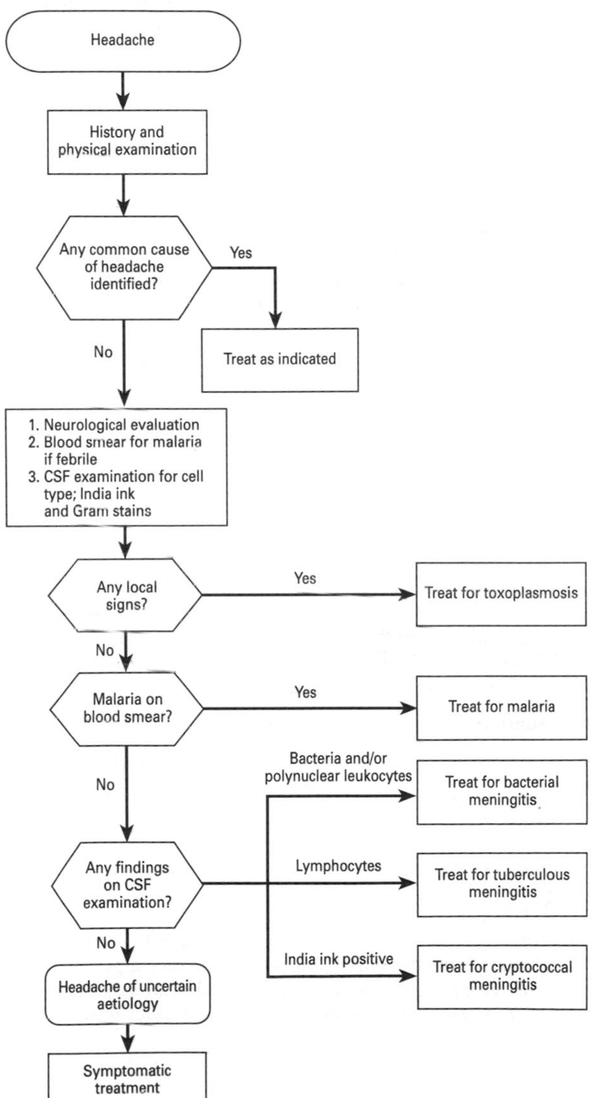
Headache
History and physical examination
Any common cause of headache identified?
Yes
Treat as indicated
No
1. Neurological evaluation
2. Blood smear for malaria if febrile
3. CSF examination for cell type; India ink and Gram stains
Any local signs?
Yes
Treat for toxoplasmosis
No
Malaria on blood smear?
Yes
Treat for malaria
No
Bacteria and/or polynuclear leukocytes
Treat for bacterial meningitis
Any findings on CSF examination?
Lymphocytes
Treat for tuberculous meningitis
India ink positive
Treat for cryptococcal meningitis
No
Headache of uncertain aetiology
Symptomatic treatment

Toxoplasmosis

Infection by *Toxoplasma gondii*, an obligate intracellular parasite, is a common asymptomatic infection of normal adults that very rarely results in a mononucleosis-like syndrome. Primary infection of women in the early stages of pregnancy results in fetal infection and serious congenital malformations.

Following acute infection, a latent infection ensues that may become reactivated in immunocompromised patients. In this situation, toxoplasmosis is a serious disease primarily of the brain, but also involving lungs, heart, and chorioretina. Focal *Toxoplasma* encephalitis with brain abscesses is a common manifestation of AIDS; a rarer diffuse form is rapidly fatal.

Transmission: via • licking fingers or eating food (incl. vegetables) contaminated with oocytes from cat faeces or • ingesting tissue cysts in undercooked meat from domesticated animals. Infection occurs in multiple animal species but the cat appears to be the definitive host. Mother to fetus transmission occurs in humans but there is little evidence of other human-to-human transmission.

Clinical features: if symptomatic, a 1° infection presents as a mononucleosis with discrete, non-tender lymphadenopathy without suppuration. After reactivation in an immunosuppressed patient, subacute CNS disease may occur, presenting with focal brain signs: commonly hemiparesis, speech abnormalities, cranial nerve lesions, altered higher function, coma. Diffuse cerebral involvement presents with generalized CNS dysfunction without focal signs. Pneumonitis manifests as fever with cough and dyspnoea; chorioretinitis is rare.

Diagnosis: isolation of toxoplasma from blood/body fluids during acute infection; demonstration of tissue cysts in Giemsa-stained tissue sections or centrifuged body fluids; characteristic lymph node histology (reactive follicular hyperplasia, epithelioid histocytes blurring germinal centre margins, focal cellular distension of sinuses); serology.

Management:

- pyrimethamine 75mg PO (first day, then 25–50mg PO daily) *plus*
- sulfadiazine 4–6g PO weekly *plus*
- Ca^{2+} folinate 15mg PO (or IV) three times weekly

all for at least four weeks.

Maintenance therapy = pyrimethamine 25mg PO and sulfadiazine 2g PO, both 3–5 times per week for life.

Prevention: pregnant women and the immunocompromised should be warned not to eat undercooked meat and to take care of personal hygiene close to domestic cats; vaccines. Chemical prophylaxis may be of value in preventing toxoplasmosis in immunocompromised individuals.

HIV/STDs

Cryptococcosis

This fungal infection often presents in AIDS patients as a subtle chronic meningitis. Rarely it manifests as a fulminant disease with extraneural involvement. It is ubiquitous in the environment and therefore presumed exposure is common; overt infection is rare in the immunocompetent.

Early clinical features include low grade fever, headache, weight loss; neck stiffness occurs later with N&V +/– photophobia. If untreated → confusion and coma. Focal signs are rare. CSF is clear; WBC may be absent or a few PMN. Other sites: lungs (if → pneumonia, high mortality), skin (non-specific lesions often painless on face/scalp; may be first sign), bone, GI tract. Blood WCC is generally unchanged.

Diagnosis: add 1 drop of sediment from >3 ml CSF to 1 drop India ink, mix and smear onto a slide under a coverslip (if correctly made, newsprint should be readable through it). Search the whole slide for cryptococci: double refractile cell wall, distinctly outlined capsule, refractile intracytoplasmic inclusions. Others: antigen in serum/CSF; fungal culture.

Management: suggested regimens:

- amphotericin B 0.3mg/kg IV daily
  plus
  flucytosine 150mg/kg/day PO in 4 divided doses for >42 days, *or*
- amphotericin B 0.5–0.6mg/kg IV daily for >42 days, *or*
- amphotericin B 0.5–0.6mg/kg IV daily for 14 days
  followed by
  fluconazole 200–400mg/day PO for >28 days

Maintenance therapy:

- amphotericin B 1mg/kg IV weekly *or*
- fluconazole 200mg PO daily, both for life.

Progressive multifocal leukoencephalopathy

This is caused by the JC polyomavirus and presents with altered mental status and/or limb weakness. Autopsy shows patchy areas of demyelination and necrosis, which show up as pale areas on a CT scan. ***Diagnosis:*** immunohistochemistry on brain biopsies but, since there is no specific treatment and taking a biopsy can ↑ morbidity, this is rarely indicated. The clinical course is often indolent; patients normally die of other infections.

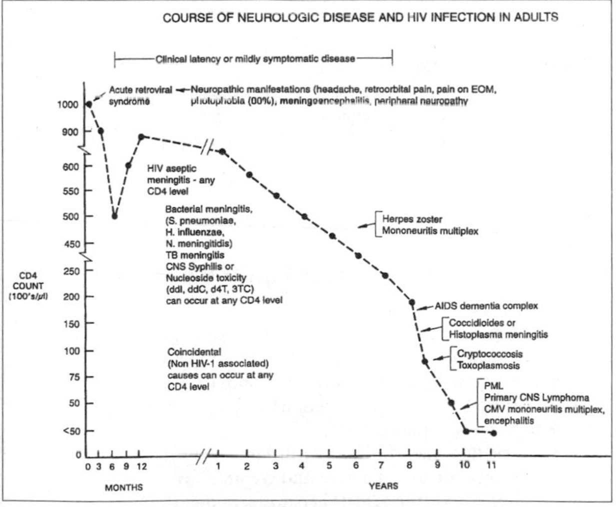

This represents the situation in the USA. Infections may occur at higher CD4 counts in the developing world.

Management of the HIV-infected asymptomatic person

This involves both • counselling and • medical care.

Counselling

Its general purpose is to promote and maintain the maximum possible level of psychological and physical health among infected people, their partners and relatives, their caregivers, and others who see themselves at risk of HIV infection. It has two particular aims:

1. to support the ability of infected persons and those who care for them to cope with the stresses of HIV/AIDS
2. to prevent the transmission of HIV to others

Medical management

of HIV$^+$ asymptomatic persons has the following aims:

1. early detection of HIV-associated disease and treatment
2. primary prophylaxis when indicated
3. determination of the appropriate time to start retroviral therapy

Where the facilities exist, knowledge of the degree of immune deficiency by CD4 count assists in i) interpretation of symptoms, and determining when to initiate ii) 1° prophylaxis eg for PCP and iii) retroviral therapy. The frequency of visits should ↑ as the CD4 count falls. Where this is not practical due to scarce resources, priority should be given to regular follow-up in clinic (eg every 6 months) with only minimal laboratory investigations (eg Hb and total WCC). Total lymphocyte count fluctuates greatly due to concurrent infection – it is only a crude guide to CD4 status and degree of immune deficiency

A. History – check for

- fever
- night sweats
- weight loss
- anorexia
- dysphagia
- diarrhoea
- cough
- odynophagia
- worsening headache
- pruritus
- seizures
- visual symptoms
- diffuse lymphadenopathy
- skin rash

Ask specifically about current medication.

B. Physical examination – should cover the following:

1. ***general:*** weight loss, fever
2. ***neurological system:*** peripheral neuropathy, cognitive disorders
3. ***skin changes:*** herpes zoster, herpes simplex, folliculitis, tinea, Kaposi sarcoma, pruritis, seborrhoeic dermatitis, severe psoriasis
4. ***oral cavity:*** thrush, hairy leukoplakia, gingivitis, KS, lymphoma
5. ***eyes:*** perform a fundoscopy
6. ***lymph nodes:*** look for focal or diffuse enlargement
7. ***lungs:*** check for consolidation and crepitations
8. ***abdominal examination:*** hepatosplenomegaly
9. ***genitalia:*** chancre, ulcers
10. ***anus:*** ulcers, warts

C. Laboratory investigations and X-ray – as stated above, in areas with limited resources, these can be limited to Hb and total WCC. However, the following investigations may be considered:

1 Tests to assess degree of immunodeficiency

- total lymphocyte count *(poor marker)*
- CD4 lymphocyte count and percentage
- viral RNA (use best available test)

2 Tests to assess potential infection

- serology: toxoplasmosis, CMV, syphilis, hepatitis B
- tuberculin skin test (becomes suppressed with ↑ immunosuppression)
- complete blood count
- liver function tests
- chest X-ray

D. Drug therapy – primary prophylaxis and the administration of vaccines may be of value. Local prevalence of the following infections will determine whether primary prophylaxis or vaccination should be offered

- tuberculosis
- *P. carinii* pneumonia
- toxoplasmosis
- pneumococcal pneumonia
  (either via vaccine or prophylactic antibiotics)

Antiretroviral chemotherapy

Triple therapy is currently unaffordable to all but the richest sections of the developing world. However, recent clinical trials of short-course antiretroviral chemotherapy (zidovudine, nevirapine) in pregnant women in the developing world have shown reductions in perinatal transmission. There is currently an intense debate about the benefits and economics of supplying such drugs in the developing world (see *Lancet* 355; 2095). As a consequence, these drugs are being considered for inclusion in the WHO's Essential Drug List.

Prevention and control

In the absence of either effective widely available anti-retroviral drugs or a vaccine, primary prevention is the only method of attempting to control the AIDS pandemic. Strategies to control HIV infection should be aimed at the main methods of transmission: sexual, parenteral, and vertical.

Note that the only two strategies which have been proven to work are syndromic treatment of STDs and government promotion of condom use.

Sexual – changing high-risk sexual behaviour through health education would have a major effect on sexual HIV transmission. It would also have a marked effect on STD transmission. Creative educational approaches, respecting cultural traditions, are necessary to make the population aware of the dangers of HIV infection and AIDS and to encourage protective measures. Several governments have now initiated such health education programmes. However, these programmes will have to be accompanied by approaches that influence the social and environmental determinants of risk to enable those vulnerable to infection to protect themselves.[1]

Blood transfusion – screening of blood donations for HIV antibody may result in high benefit-to-cost ratio for the prevention of AIDS in populations with a high infection rate. Drawbacks are cost, logistics and the lack of detectable HIV antibodies for 3–6 months (reduced to 3–6 weeks with new 3rd generation ELISAs) after infection in some persons. Efforts to identify and exclude high risk donors have proven to be difficult, but they may be important in decreasing the risk of HIV^+ seronegative persons donating blood.

Injections – prevention of infection through contaminated needles is feasible through the use of universal precautions (p 12). However, the use of disposable needles and syringes may be prohibitively expensive for some countries and health workers should be trained to give as few injections as possible and to sterilize reusable equipment. The risk from infected needlestick injuries to health workers appears to be very low – about 0.5% of persons receiving needlestick injuries with body fluids from an HIV-infected person become infected.

Vertical – most importantly this involves the prevention of HIV infection in women of childbearing age, and advice on contraception to HIV^+ women. The WHO recommends that breastfeeding should remain the standard advice to pregnant women, including those known to be HIV^+, where the primary causes of infant deaths are infectious disease and malnutrition. Where this is not the case, HIV^+ women are advised not to breastfeed but to use a safe feeding alternative for their babies.

Occupational exposure – it appears to be relatively difficult to become infected following occupational exposure to the virus in the hospital. Careful adherence to barrier precautions (see p 12) should decrease potential exposure.

1. d'Cruz-Grote D, 1996, *Lancet*, **348**, 1071

HIV/STDs

Symptomatic management of STDs[1]

A. Urethral discharge

Male patients complaining of urethral discharge and/or dysuria should be examined for evidence of discharge. If none is seen, the urethra should be gently massaged from the ventral part of the penis towards the meatus. If microscopy is available, a urethral specimen should be collected – a Gram-stained urethral smear showing more than 5 PMNs per field (×1000) in areas of maximal cellular concentration is indicative of urethritis.

The major pathogens causing urethral discharge are

- ***Neisseria gonorrhoeae***
- ***Chlamydia trachomatis***

Unless a diagnosis of gonorrhoea can be definitively excluded by laboratory tests, the treatment of the patient with urethral discharge should provide adequate coverage of these two organisms.

Recommended treatment regimens:

- therapy for uncomplicated gonorrhoea (p 100) ***plus***
- doxycycline 100mg PO bd ***or*** tetracycline 500mg PO qds, both for 7 days.

Alternative regimen when tetracyclines are contraindicated or not tolerated:

- therapy for uncomplicated gonorrhoea (p 100) ***plus***
- erythromycin 500mg PO qds

Alternative regimen where single-dose therapy for gonorrhoea is not available:

- co-trimoxazole 480mg 10 tablets PO daily for 3 days ***plus***
- doxycycline 100mg PO bd ***or*** tetracycline 500mg PO qds, both for 7 days.

This can only be used in areas where co-trimoxazole has been shown to be effective against uncomplicated gonorrhoea.

Follow-up

Patients should be advised to return if symptoms persist 7 days after start of therapy. Persistent or recurrent symptoms may be due to • poor compliance, • reinfection, • infection with a resistant strain of *N. gonorrhoeae*, or • infection with *T. vaginalis*. Where symptoms persist or recur after adequate treatment of the index patient and partner(s), both (or all) should be referred for laboratory investigation. The investigation should include a Gram stain to confirm the presence of urethritis and to look for *N. gonorrhoeae*. *T. vaginalis* may be identified by microscopic investigation of a first voided urine sample, although this test has a fairly low sensitivity as compared to culture. If the presence of *T. vaginalis* is confirmed, treat as per p 106.

1. This syndromic approach to the management of STDs is taken directly from the WHO publication: *Management of Sexually Transmitted Diseases*, GPA, WHO: Geneva 1994.

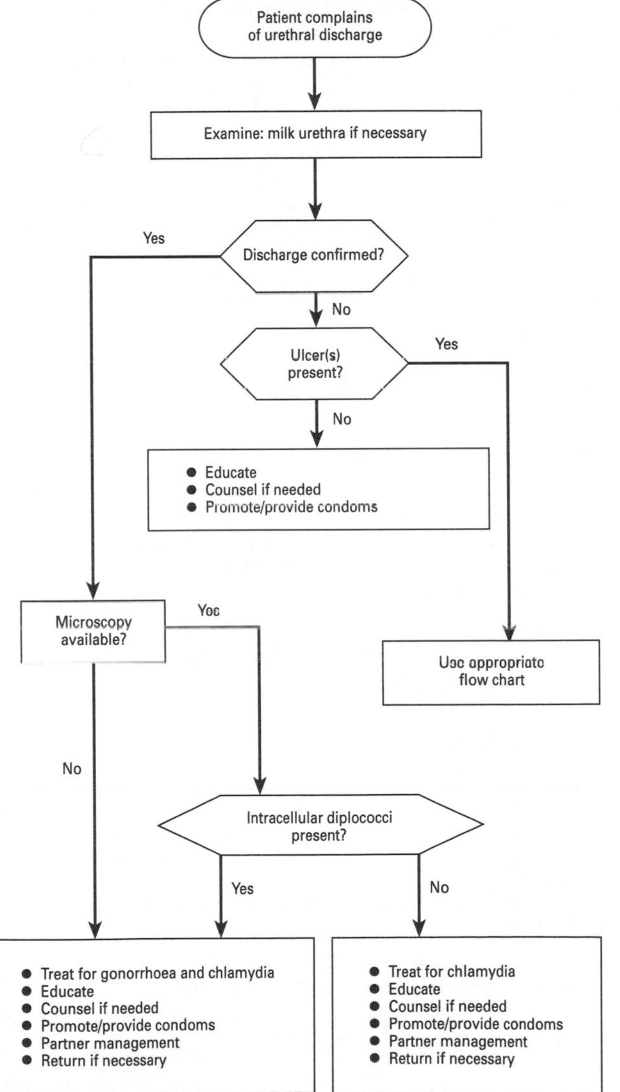
Patient complains of urethral discharge
Examine: milk urethra if necessary
Discharge confirmed?
Yes
No
Ulcer(s) present?
Yes
No
● Educate
● Counsel if needed
● Promote/provide condoms
Microscopy available?
Yoc
Uoc appropriato flow chart
No
Intracellular diplococci present?
Yes
No
● Treat for gonorrhoea and chlamydia
● Educate
● Counsel if needed
● Promote/provide condoms
● Partner management
● Return if necessary
● Treat for chlamydia
● Educate
● Counsel if needed
● Promote/provide condoms
● Partner management
● Return if necessary

B. Genital ulcers

The frequency with which genital ulcers are caused by specific organisms varies dramatically in different parts of the world. Clinical differential diagnosis of genital ulcers is inaccurate, particularly in settings where several aetiologies are common. Clinical manifestations may be further altered in the presence of HIV infection.

After examination to confirm the presence of genital ulceration, treatment appropriate to local aetiologies and antibiotic sensitivity patterns should be given. For example, in areas where both syphilis and chancroid are prevalent, patients with genital ulcers should be treated for both conditions at the time of their initial presentation to ensure adequate treatment in case of loss to follow-up. In areas where granuloma inguinale is also prevalent, treatment for this condition should be included.

Laboratory-assisted differential diagnosis is rarely helpful at the initial visit, and mixed infections are common. For instance, in areas of high syphilis incidence, a reactive serological test may reflect a previous infection and give a misleading picture of the patient's present condition.

Recommended regimen:

- therapy for syphilis (p 98) ***plus***
- therapy for chancroid (p 104) ***and/or***
- therapy for granuloma inguinale (p 104)

Genital ulcer and HIV infection

In HIV-infected patients, prolonged courses of treatment may be necessary for chancroid. Moreover, where HIV infection is prevalent, an increasing proportion of cases of genital ulcer is likely to harbour herpes simplex virus. Herpetic ulcers may be atypical and persist for long periods in HIV-infected patients.

Follow-up

Patients with genital ulcers should be followed up weekly until the ulceration shows signs of healing.

C. Inguinal bubo

Inguinal bubo, an enlargement of the lymph nodes in the groin area, is rarely the sole manifestation of an STD and is usually found together with other genital ulcer diseases. Non-sexually transmitted local and systemic infections (eg infections of the lower limb) can cause swelling of the inguinal lymph nodes.

In the presence of enlarged and/or painful lymph nodes, look for genital ulcers:

- If present, follow the genital ulcer flowchart.
- If absent, treat for lymphogranuloma venereum.

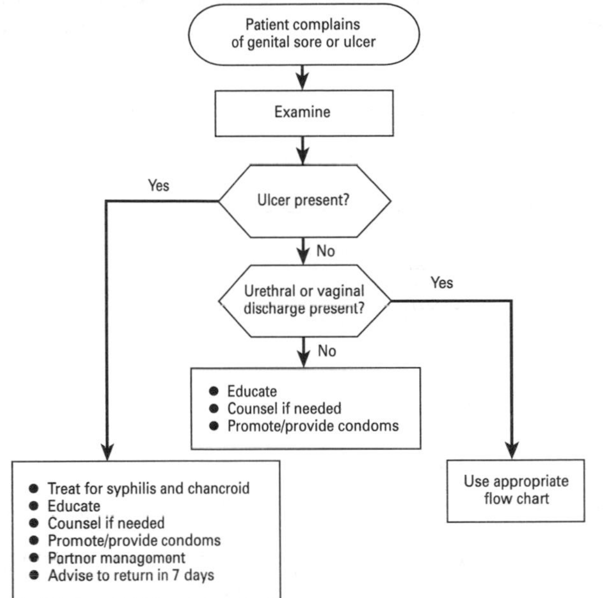

Causes of genital ulcers: syphilis, chancroid, granuloma inguinale, HSV, scabies, aphthosis, drug reactions, Behçet's disease, carcinoma

D. Scrotal swelling

Scrotal swelling can be caused by trauma, tumour, torsion of the testis, or epididymitis. Inflammation of the epididymis is usually accompanied by pain, oedema and erythema and sometimes by urethral discharge, dysuria, and/or frequency. The adjacent testis is often also inflamed (orchitis), producing epididymo-orchitis.

► Sudden onset of unilateral swollen scrotum may be due to trauma or testicular torsion and requires immediate referral. The testis will be irreversibly damaged within 6hrs – see opposite.

When not treated effectively, STD-related epididymitis may lead to infertility.

The most important causative agents are:
- *Neisseria gonorrhoeae*
- *Chlamydia trachomatis*

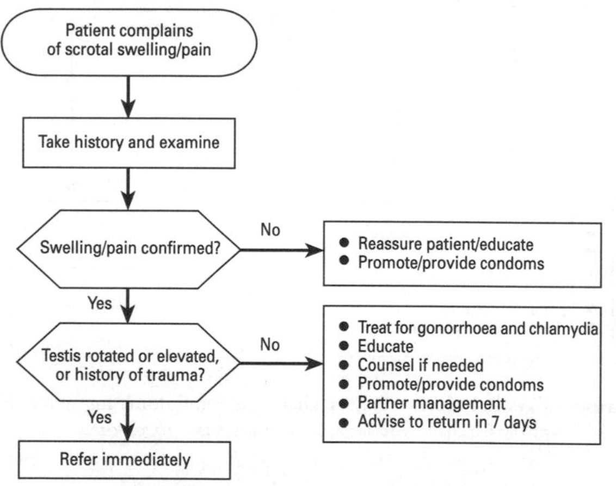

Recommended regimen:

- therapy for uncomplicated gonorrhoea (p 100) ***plus***
- doxycycline 100mg PO bd ***or*** tetracycline 500mg qds, both for 7 days.

For alternative regimens when tetracyclines are contraindicated or not tolerated, or where single-dose therapy for gonorrhoea is not available, see p82.

Adjuvants to therapy:

Bed rest and scrotal elevation until local inflammation and fever subside.

Torsion of the testicle

► The aim is to recognize this condition before the cardinal signs and symptoms are fully manifest, as a torted testis will survive for about 6hrs. If in any doubt, surgical exploration is required. It is more common in 15–30yr olds, but may occur at any age.

Clinical features: sudden onset of pain in one testis, making walking very uncomfortable. Abdominal pain, nausea and vomiting are common. Lifting or supporting the testis does not ease the pain (as it classically does in epididymitis). The testis is hot, swollen and tender. ***Differential diagnosis:*** includes epididymitis (tends to occur in older patients, with slower onset and symptoms of UTI), tumour, trauma, acute hydrocele.

Treatment: ask for consent for a possible orchidectomy (removal of the testis) and *bilateral* fixation (orchidopexy) before surgery to untwist the testis.

E. Vaginal discharge

Vaginal discharge is most commonly caused by vaginitis, but may also be the result of cervicitis.

◆ **Cervicitis** is caused by
- *Neisseria gonorrhoeae*
- *Chlamydia trachomatis*

◆ **Vaginitis** is caused by
- *Trichomonas vaginalis*
- *Candida albicans*
- *Gardnerella* spp plus anaerobic bacterial infection

Non-infectious causes of vaginal discharge (eg neoplasia, oestrogen deficiency, foreign body) often have a slower onset. Any form of immunosuppression, such as diabetes or AIDS, will predispose to *C. albicans* infection.

► Effective management of cervicitis is more important from a public health point of view. However, it is often difficult to clinically distinguish between vaginitis and cervicitis. The symptom of vaginal discharge is neither sensitive nor specific for either condition. Recent studies suggest that an assessment of the woman's risk status helps greatly in making a diagnosis of cervicitis, but further evaluation of the following three flowcharts is needed, particularly with regard to risk factors, which will vary from country to country. The risk factors listed below need to be adapted to the local situation.

► Where it is not possible to differentiate between cervicitis and vaginitis, and risk assessment is positive, patients should be treated for both.

1. Cervicitis – recommended regimen:

- therapy for uncomplicated gonorrhoea (p 100) ***plus***
- doxycycline 100mg PO bd ***or*** tetracycline 500mg qds, both for 7 days.

For alternative regimens when tetracyclines are contraindicated or not tolerated, or where single-dose therapy for gonorrhoea is not available, see p82.

2. Vaginitis – recommended regimen:

- metronidazole 2g PO stat, ***or***
- metronidazole 400–500mg PO bd for 7 days

plus either

- nystatin 100 000 IU intravaginally daily for 14 days, ***or***
- miconazole ***or*** clotrimazole 200mg intravaginally daily for 3 days, ***or***
- clotrimazole 500mg intravaginally stat.

WHO suggested risk factors:

Risk factors: either
◆ partner is symptomatic, or
◆ two of:
1. age <21
2. single
3. >1 partner
4. new partner in last 3 months

Vaginal discharge without use of speculum or microscope

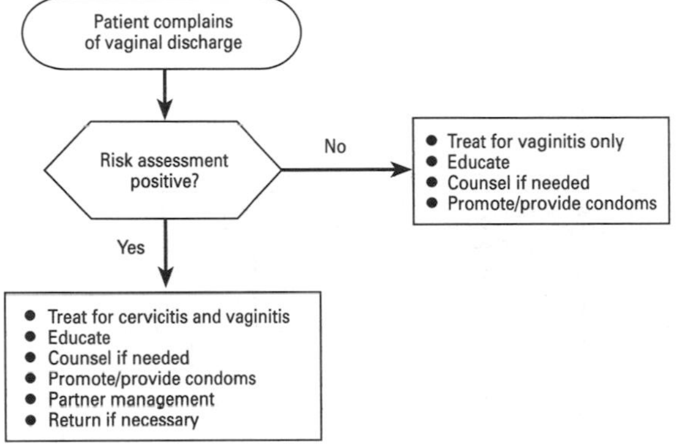

Locally derived risk factors:

Risk factors: either
- ◆ partner is symptomatic, or
- ◆ two of: 1.
  2.
  3.
  4.

Vaginal discharge with use of speculum only

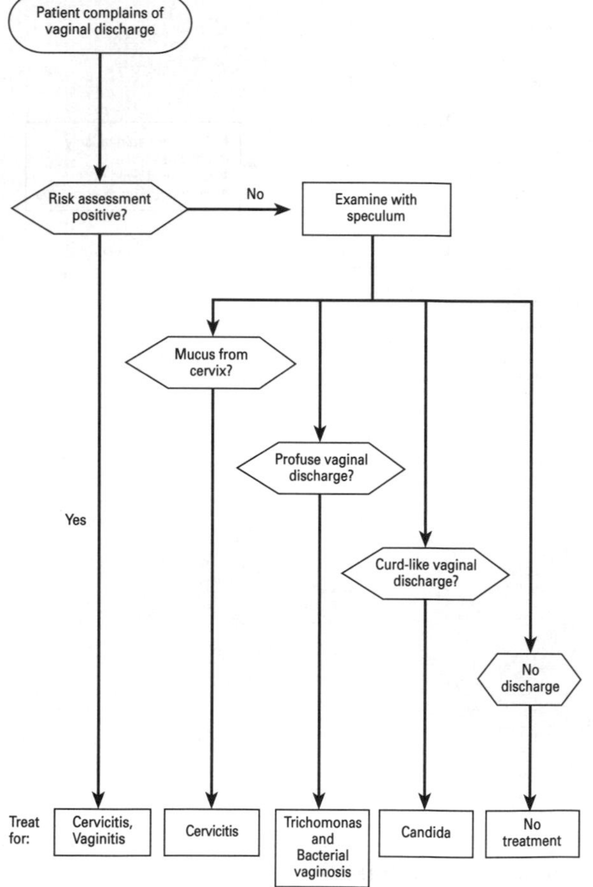

For all patients:
- Educate
- Promote/provide condoms
- Counsel

For all infected patients:
- Manage partners
- Organize follow-up

Vaginal discharge with use of speculum and microscope

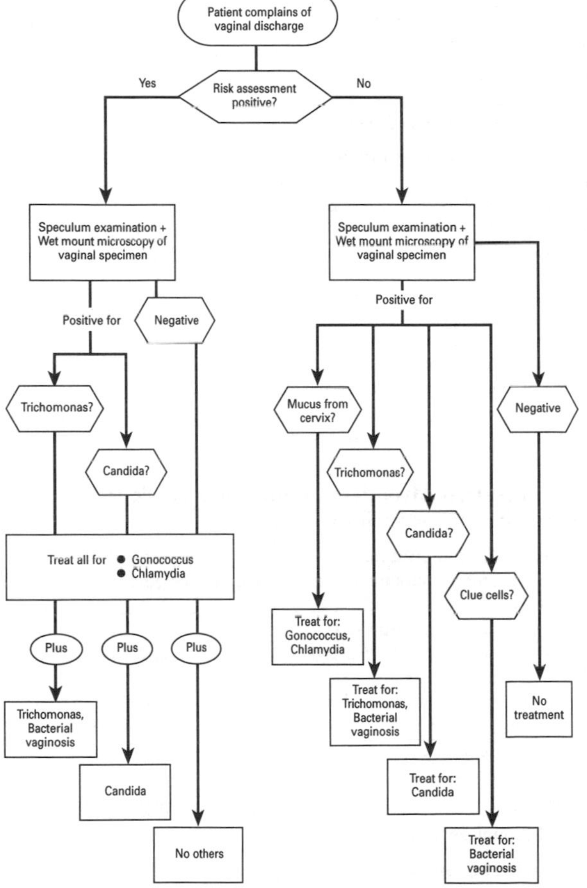

For all patients:
- Educate
- Promote/provide condoms
- Counsel

For all infected patients:
- Manage partners
- Organize follow-up

F. Lower abdominal pain

All sexually active women presenting with lower abdominal pain should be carefully evaluated for the presence of salpingitis (pelvic inflammatory disease [PID]) and/or endometriosis. In addition, routine bimanual and abdominal examinations should be carried out on all women with a presumptive STD since some women with PID or endometriosis will not complain of lower abdominal pain.

Women with endometriosis may present with complaints of:
- vaginal discharge
- bleeding
- uterine tenderness on pelvic examination.

Symptoms suggestive of PID include
- abdominal pain
- vaginal discharge
- dysuria
- fever
- dyspareunia,
- menorrhagia,
- pain associated with menses,
- nausea and vomiting

PID is difficult to diagnose because clinical manifestations are varied. PID becomes highly probable when one or more of the above symptoms are manifested in a woman with adnexal tenderness, evidence of lower genital tract infection, and cervical motion tenderness. Enlargement or induration of one or both Fallopian tubes, tender pelvic mass, and direct or rebound tenderness may also be present. The patient's temperature may be elevated but is normal in most cases. In general, clinicians should err on the side of overdiagnosing and treating milder cases.

Hospitalization of patients with acute pelvic inflammatory disease should be seriously considered when:

- the diagnosis is uncertain
- surgical emergencies such as appendicitis and ectopic pregnancies have to be excluded
- a pelvic abscess is suspected
- severe illness precludes management on an outpatient basis
- the patient is pregnant
- the patient is unable to follow or tolerate an outpatient regimen
- the patient has failed to respond to an outpatient regimen
- clinical follow-up 72 hours after the start of antibiotic therapy cannot be guaranteed.

► Many experts recommend that all patients with PID should be admitted to hospital for treatment

PID is caused by:
- *N. gonorrhoeae*
- *C. trachomatis*
- anaerobic bacteria (*Bacteriodes* spp, G$^+$ cocci)
- (• Gram-negative rods)
- (• *Mycoplasma hominis*)

Since it is difficult to clinically differentiate between these organisms, therapy should be effective against all.

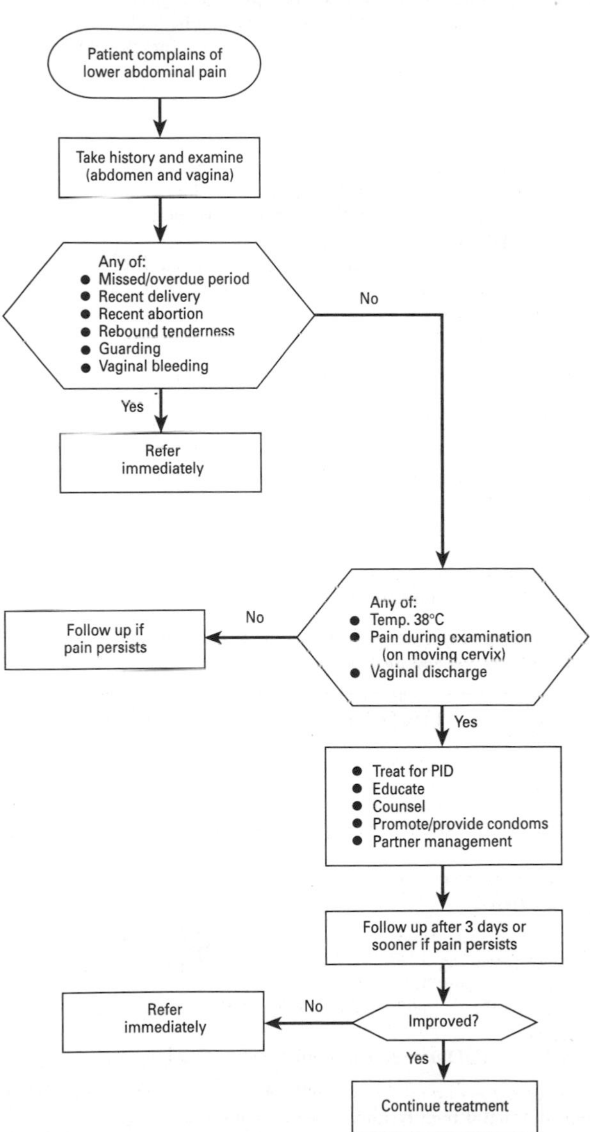
Patient complains of lower abdominal pain
Take history and examine (abdomen and vagina)
Any of:
Missed/overdue period
Recent delivery
Recent abortion
Rebound tenderness
Guarding
Vaginal bleeding
No
Yes
Refer immediately
Any of:
Temp. 38°C
Pain during examination (on moving cervix)
Vaginal discharge
No
Follow up if pain persists
Yes
Treat for PID
Educate
Counsel
Promote/provide condoms
Partner management
Follow up after 3 days or sooner if pain persists
Improved?
No
Refer immediately
Yes
Continue treatment

Inpatient therapy

Recommended regimens – use one of:

1. • ceftriaxone 500mg IM once daily ***plus***
• doxycycline 100mg PO/IV bd ***or*** tetracycline 500mg PO qds ***plus***
• metronidazole 400–500mg PO/IV bd ***or*** chloramphenicol 500mg PO/IV qds

2. • clindamycin 900mg IV q8h ***plus***
• gentamicin 1.5mg/kg IV q8h

3. • ciprofloxacin 500mg PO bd ***or*** spectinomycin 1g IM qds ***plus***
• doxycycline 100mg PO/IV bd ***or*** tetracycline 500mg PO qds ***plus***
• metronidazole 400–500mg PO/IV bd ***or*** chloramphenicol 500mg PO/IV qds

For all three regimens, therapy should be continued until at least 2 days after the patient has improved and should then be followed with either:

- doxycycline 100mg PO bd or
- tetracycline 500mg PO qds, both for 14 days.

► Tetracyclines are contraindicated in pregnancy.

Outpatient therapy

Recommended regimen:

- single-dose therapy for uncomplicated gonorrhoea (p 100 – only ceftriaxone has been shown to be effective for PID; other single-dose regimens have not been formally evaluated) ***plus***
- doxycycline 100mg PO/IV bd ***or*** tetracycline 500mg PO qds, for 14 days, ***plus***
- metronidazole 400–500mg PO/IV bd for 14 days

Alternative regimen where single-dose therapy for gonorrhoea is not available:

- co-trimoxazole 480mg 10 tablets PO daily for 3 days ***plus***
- doxycycline 100mg PO bd ***or*** tetracycline 500mg PO qds, both for 14 days, ***plus***
- metronidazole 400–500mg PO/IV bd for 14 days

► This can only be used in areas where co-trimoxazole has been shown to be effective against uncomplicated gonorrhoea.

Adjuncts to therapy: removal of intrauterine contraceptive device (IUD)

The IUD is a risk factor for the development of PID. Although the exact effect of removing an IUD on the response of acute salpingitis to antimicrobial therapy and on the risk of recurrent salpingitis is unknown, removal of IUD is recommended soon after microbial therapy has been initiated.

► When an IUD is removed, contraceptive counselling is essential.

Follow-up – outpatients with PID should be followed up at 72 hours and admitted if their condition has not improved.

HIV/STDs

Syphilis

A worldwide disease caused by the spirochaete *Treponema pallidum* that has greatly increased in incidence over the last few decades, coincident with an increase in its resistance to common antibiotics. The disease can be divided into four phases:

1. local 1° infection,
2. dissemination associated with 2° syphilis,
3. a latent period during which infectivity is low (however, relapses into 2° syphilis may occur during the 1st four years after contact – the early latent period)
4. late syphilis. This occurs after many years with the widespread production of *gummas* – agranulomatous lesions with a necrotic centre and surrounding obliterative endarteritis. Other late manifestations result from long term damage to the cardiovascular and central nervous systems.

Transmission: is almost exclusively through abraded skin at sites of sexual contact with infected persons. Other modes include congenital transmission (which produces severe disease in the infant) and infection by blood transfusion.

Clinical features:

1° syphilis: 9–90 days after infection, a primary ulcer or chancre forms on the genitalia (p 104). It is typically solitary, 'punched out', indurated and painless with a clear exudate and resolves over a few weeks. Atypical lesions occur and there may be multiple ulcers in HIV^+ patients. There is regional lymphadenopathy. The lesions are highly infective.

2° syphilis: coincides with the greatest number of treponemes in the body and blood, 1–6 months after contact. Specific features include: • a transient, variable (not vesicular) rash particularly on trunk, soles and palms; • in warm, moist areas where 2 skin surfaces are in contact, the papules enlarge and coalesce to form highly infectious plaques called *condylmata lata*; • silver grey lesions with red periphery on mucosal surfaces called *mucous patches* (eg snail track ulcers in the mouth). • There is also low grade fever, malaise, generalized lymphadenopathy, arthralgias, and occasionally focal involvement of eyes, meninges, parotid glands, or viscera (kidney, liver, GI tract).

Late syphilis: the commonest manifestations are areas of local tissue destruction in skin, bones, liver and spleen due to gumma formation. Others:

1. *Cardiovascular system* – ascending aorta aneurysm +/– aortic regurgitation & coronary artery stenosis.

2. *CNS*

- chronic meningitis – cranial nerve defects, hemiparesis, seizures
- parenchymal disease (general paralysis of the insane) – psychoses, dementia, hyperactive reflexes, tremor, speech and pupillary (Argyll Robertson) disturbances
- tabes dorsalis – shooting pains in limbs, peripheral neuropathy, ataxia, Charcot's joints, a positive Romberg's sign.

HIV/STDs

Diagnosis: during 1° and 2° disease, repeated dark field microscopy for motile spirochaetes in lesion exudates; later – serology, either treponeme specific (FTA, TPHA) for exposure or non-specific (VDRL, RPR) for active disease. ► All patients with syphilis should be encouraged to have an HIV test because of the high frequency of dual infection and its implications for clinical assessment and management.

Management:

Early syphilis (1°, 2° or latent syphilis of <2 years duration):

1. • benzathine penicillin G 1.5g, IM stat as two injections into separate sites, *or*

• procaine penicillin G 1.2g daily IM for 10 days.

2. Some experts recommend treating 2° and latent disease with extended regimens:

• benzathine penicillin G once weekly for 3 weeks, *or*

• procaine penicillin daily for 15 days.

The 10 day course of procaine penicillin has been recommended for HIV⁺ patients.

3. For penicillin-allergic patients, alternatives include

• tetracycline[1] 500mg PO qds *or*

• doxycycline[1] 100mg PO bd, both for 15 days.

Late syphilis (not neurosyphilis) (includes latent syphilis of >2 years or indeterminate duration):

1. • benzathine penicillin G 1.5g IM, as two injections into separate sites, weekly for 3 weeks *or*

• procaine penicillin G 1.2g IM daily for 21 days.

2. Alternatives for penicillin-allergic patients include:

• tetracycline[1] 500mg PO qds (probably better) *or*

• doxycycline[1] 100mg PO bd, both for 30 days.

However, penicillin is the preferred therapy and should be given whenever possible.

3. Some experts recommend examination of CSF in these patients for asymptomatic neurosyphilis.

Neurosyphilis

1. • benzathine penicillin G 14.4g, administered IV daily for 14 days, in four hourly doses of 2.4g, *or*

• procaine penicillin G 1.2g IM daily *plus* probenecid 500mg PO qds, for14 days – ensure patient's outpatient compliance for this regimen.

2. Alternative regimen for penicillin allergic patients:

• tetracycline[1] 500mg PO qds *or*

• doxycycline[1] 200mg PO bd, both for 30 days.

Third generation cephalosporins may also be useful.

3. Consult a neurologist if possible and follow up carefully.

Follow-up early syphilis at 3, 6 and 12 months to assess treatment and possible reinfection.

1. Tetracyclines are contraindicated in pregnant women

Management of pregnant women

Pregnant women should be treated with penicillin whenever possible. Alternatives include erythromycin 500mg PO qds for 15 days (early syphilis) or 30 days (other forms of syphilis). NB The effectiveness of erythromycin is highly questionable, particularly for neurosyphilis, and many failures have been reported. The baby should be evaluated and treated soon after birth. An extended course of a 3rd generation cephalosporin should probably be given to pregnant women whose allergy is not manifested by anaphylaxis.

Gonorrhoea

Gonorrhoea results from infection with the Gram-negative coccus, *Neisseria gonorrhoea*. Primary infection through sexual contact usually involves the mucosal surfaces of the urethra, cervix, rectum, and oropharynx.

► Without early effective treatment, both local and disseminated complications can occur. Although sensitive to penicillin for many years, recent decades have seen the rise in strains resistant to penicillin, tetracycline and doxycycline. ► Conjunctival infection of neonates during vaginal delivery is a serious condition that may cause blindness if not treated early.

Clinical features: in ***men***, urethral discharge and dysuria occur 2–5 days after infection. The discharge is initially mucoid, but rapidly becomes profuse and purulent (in contrast to non-gonococcal urethritis, p 102). Local complications include acute epididymitis or prostatis, periurethral abscess and urethral stricture. In ***women***, after an incubation period of around 10 days, infection produces signs of cervicitis (sometimes with urethritis) – vaginal discharge, dysuria and intermenstrual bleeding. Unlike men, many women are asymptomatic or have insufficient symptoms for presentation to medical facilities. Local complications include pelvic inflammatory disease and perihepatitis. Frequency and urgency are uncommon in both men and women.

Hematogenous dissemination is a rare complication in untreated patients. It may result in meningitis, endocarditis, osteomyelitis, sepsis or acute destructive monoarthritis with synovial effusion. Reactive polyarthropathy and papular/pustular dermatitis are recognized complications.

Diagnosis: gram-negative intracellular diplococci in smears – urethra in men (>90%), endocervix in women (less reliable); culture.

Management: ► all patients with gonococcal infection should also be treated for chlamydia since they often coexist, unless facilities are available to exclude specifically chlamydial infection. Sexual partners should be treated at the same time.

1. ***In uncomplicated genital and anal infection*** use ceftriaxone 250mg or spectinomycin 2g, both IM stat, unless local antibiotic resistance data indicate that the strain should be sensitive to a less expensive microbial. [Alternatives include: ciprofloxacin 500mg PO stat (***not during pregnancy***) and cefixime 400mg PO stat.] ► Always use locally recommended regimen.
2. ***For pharyngeal infection*** use ceftriaxone 250mg IM stat, or cotrimoxazole 480mg 10 tablets once daily for three days.
3. ***In disseminated infection*** use ceftriaxone 1g IV/IM daily or spectinomycin 2g IM bd for
   - 7 days in local infection and arthritis
   - 14 days in meningitis
   - 28 days in endocarditis.
4. ***Gonococcal conjunctivitis*** is highly contagious and should be treated by barrier nursing (p 12), in addition to frequent saline irrigation and antibiotics: ceftriaxone 1g IM, spectinomycin 2g IM, ciprofloxacin 500mg PO [or kanamycin 2g IM], all stat.

Locally recommended regimens:

1. uncomplicated infection:

2. pharyngeal infection:

3. disseminated infection:

4. gonococcal conjunctivitis:

Pregnant patients:

Chlamydial infections

Chlamydia trachomatis is an obligate intracellular bacteria that causes two STDs in adults, depending on the strain –1) an infection of urethra, endocervix (may → infertility) or rectum and 2) lymphogranuloma venereum. It is also the cause of ocular trachoma which is a major cause of blindness worldwide.

1. Urethritis/endocervicitis/proctitis

The D-K serotypes of chlamydiae have become the most common STD in the developed world. They are prevalent throughout the world, frequently coexisting with gonococcal infections, and are the commonest cause of non-gonococcal urethritis (NGU) in ***men***. Complications in men include epididymitis and, in homosexual men, chronic proctitis. Infection in ***women*** is often subclinical or non-specific. However, it is associated with cervicitis, salpingitis and endometriosis and is a major cause of female subfertility worldwide. ► Screening women through culture or serology and treating them for asymptomatic chlamydial infection appears to be of value in reducing complications.

2. Lymphogranuloma venereum

A chronic STD caused by L1, 2 & 3 strains of *C. trachomatis*. The 1° lesion is a painless genital ulcer (rarely visible in women) that heals in a few days. After a latent period of days or months, an acute, fluctuant inguinal lymphadenopathy (buboes) develops. With time, the buboes may spread locally and ulcerate → sinuses/fistulae. Subsequent chronic blockage of lymphatic drainage produces genital lymphoedema which is often quite severe in women.

Diagnosis: by microscopy although this is difficult – intracellular bacteria may be seen on smears of material from lesions or bubo aspirate (immunofluorescence is helpful if available – ? refer); otherwise culture.

Management

- ***Uncomplicated urethritis*** – doxycycline[1] 100mg PO bd or tetracycline[1] 500mg PO qds [alternatives: erythromycin 500mg PO, qds or sulfadiazine 1g PO, qds] for 7 days (except sulfadiazine = 10 days). The addition of trimethoprim to a sulphonamide does not increase its activity against *C. trachomatis*. Treatment >7 days does not appear to improve the cure rate in uncomplicated infection. ► Compliance with the 7-day regimens is critical. Because resistance to these regimens has not been observed, it is unnecessary to undertake a cure evaluation on completion of treatment. Patients should be asked to return if symptoms persist. ► Partners must be treated at the same time.
- ***lymphogranuloma venereum*** – as above but for 14 days (or longer if clinically indicated). Fluctuant lymph nodes should be aspirated through healthy skin. ► Incision and drainage, or excision, of nodes will delay healing and are contraindicated. (Late sequelae such as stricture/fistula, however, may require surgical intervention.)

1. Tetracyclines are contraindicated in pregnant women

HIV/STDs

Chancroid

An acute STD caused by the bacterium *Haemophilus ducreyi* that is characterized by painful ulceration and frequent bubo formation. It is highly infectious and the commonest cause of genital ulcers in Africa and SE Asia. Chancroid is much more common in males, suggesting a female carrier state.

Clinical features: 3–7 days post-infection, *painful* vesicular papules form which rapidly develop into soft ulcers with undermined, ragged edges. Ulcers are haemorrhagic and sticky (often secondarily infected); if multiple, they may become confluent; and they occur at sites of trauma during intercourse (extragenital is rare). Commonly 7–14 days later, inguinal nodes become involved: painful, matted, tethered to erythematous skin = *bubo*. A discharging sinus may develop, in time becoming a spreading ulcer. The lesions heal slowly and commonly relapse.

Diagnosis: clean the ulcer with saline, then remove material from the undermined edge; or aspirate pus from bubo. Gram stain the smear – *H. ducreyi* are Gram –ve rods (fine, short, round-ended) often seen in shoal-of-fish or railroad track formation. Beware contaminating 2° organisms. Culture is difficult.

Granuloma inguinale (donovanosis)

The bacterium *Calymmatobacterium granulomatis* causes chronic ulceration of the genitalia and surrounding tissues. Males are more frequently infected than females; patients' sexual partners are often uninfected.

Clinical features: 1–6 weeks following infection, an indurated painless papule forms which slowly develops into a 'beefy' granulomatous ulcer with characteristic rolled edges. The lesion is elevated, well defined and bleeds easily with trauma. The usual sites are in the anogenital region, thighs and perineum; rare intravaginal (or rectal) lesions may present with PV (PR) bleeding. Healing is uncommon without treatment – 2° infection can follow → painful, destructive lesions, as can squamous cell carcinoma. Inguinal nodes are not involved unless there is 2° infection. Subcutaneous granulomas form which may be mistaken for enlarged lymph nodes (hence their name 'pseudobubo') – they may also become an abscess, discharging via a sinus, or an infected ulcer. Elephantoid enlargement of genitalia may occur during healing.

Diagnosis: crush a piece of granulation tissue from the active edge of the lesion between 2 slides, air-dry and stain with Giemsa or Gram stains. Large mononuclear cells are filled with the cytoplasmic Gram –ve rods (Donovan bodies – look like closed safety pins due to bipolar staining).

Management: no controlled trials have been published. Recommended regimen:

- co-trimoxazole 960mg PO bd for >14 days, until the lesions have healed. Alternatives:
  - tetracycline[1] 500mg PO qds *or*
  - doxycycline[1] 100mg PO bd, both for 7 days.

Management of chancroid:

- erythromycin 500mg PO tds for 7 days
  alternatives:
  - ciprofloxacin 500mg PO stat, *or*
  - ceftriaxone 250mg IM stat, *or*
  - spectinomycin 2g IM stat, *or*
  - co-trimoxazole 960mg PO bd for 7 days.

Erythromycin should be used wherever possible – there is evidence that single-dose regimens are associated with an unacceptably high failure rate in some parts of the world and in HIV$^+$ patients, and that co-trimoxazole is less effective in some parts of Africa and Asia.

► Treatment outcome and the development of antibiotic resistance should be carefully monitored when the alternative regimens are used.

1. Tetracyclines are contraindicated in pregnant women

Trichomoniasis

Vaginal infection with *Trichomonas vaginalis* produces an irritating, pruritic (rarely bad smelling) discharge, 5–28 days post-infection. Dyspareunia, dysuria and urethral infection occur in some patients; lower abdominal pain is rare. The discharge is copious, sometimes yellow or green, and pools in the posterior fornix. The vagina and exocervix become inflamed; colposcopy reveals cervical hemorrhages in 50% of symptomatic cases. However, the infection is frequently asymptomatic in women (? up to 50%) and in most men. It occasionally causes urethritis.

Diagnosis: is by light microscopy. The parasite can readily be seen in a wet film of a posterior fornix smear as a motile, pear-shaped flagellate, particularly when the lighting is reduced.

Management:

1. Metronidazole 2g PO stat or 400–500mg PO bd for 7 days for both symptomatic and asymptomatic women.
2. Notify and treat all sexual partners. Infection is most often asymptomatic in men, sometimes → NGU. The 7 day regimen works well, efficacy of the single dose is less clear.
3. Patients should return after 7 days if symptoms persist. Failure can be due to • resistance or • reinfection. Patients often respond well to retreatment with the 7 day regimen.
4. Refractory infections should be treated with metronidazole 2g PO daily plus 500mg applied intravaginally each night for 3–7 days.
5. ► *During pregnancy*, metronidazole may only be used at the minimum effective dose during the 2nd and 3rd trimesters.

Bacterial vaginosis

Bacterial vaginosis is a common form of vulvovaginitis that is often milder than either candidiasis or trichomoniasis. It is caused by coinfection with *Gardnerella vaginalis* and anaerobic bacteria such as *Bacteroides* and *Prevotella* spp. *G. vaginalis* alone appears to be insufficient to cause bacterial vaginosis.

Most women have a grey/white, homogenous discharge with bubbles and a pungent odour, that adheres to the vaginal wall; it is usually not present in large quantities. Dysuria, dysparaeunia and abdominal pain are uncommon – marked abdominal pain should raise the suspicion of concurrent conditions. Erythema and oedema are uncommon. The cervix is not involved; a cervical discharge suggests concurrent infection.

Diagnosis: is by microscopic examination of a wet smear for 'clue cells' – vaginal epithelial cells that are covered with tiny coccobacilli – and the presence of large clumps of coccobacilli in Gram-stained smears. The discharge has few neutrophils.

Management:

1. Metronidazole 400–500mg PO bd for 7 days.
2. ♂ partners are not routinely treated (although this may result in ♀ recolonization; if infection recurs in ♀, treat partner). However, he should be assessed for other STDs.

HIV/STDs

Genital herpes

A condition that is caused by herpes simplex viruses, predominantly HSV-2 (70–95%). Recurrent infection occurs frequently with reactivation of the latent virus from the dorsal root ganglia. Asymptomatic shedding is common and may be an important cause of reinfection. Infections are often prolonged and severe in the immunocompromised.

Transmission occurs by direct contact with infected genital secretions. After an incubation period of 2–7 days, local infection and inflammation result in multiple vesicular lesions that rapidly ulcerate. The ulcers are greyish and extremely painful; they occur on the penis in ♂ and the vagina, cervix, vulva, and perineum in ♀, often accompanied by a vaginal discharge (also found in anus). 1° infection is accompanied by fever, malaise, and inguinal lymphadenopathy; extragenital involvement occurs in up to 20% of cases. Encephalitis is a recognized complication of genital herpes.

Diagnosis: culture, serology in 1° infection; rarely multinucleated giant cells in scrapings from suspected lesions (also found in VZV infection).

Management:

1. ***First clinical episode (take a careful history)*** – aciclovir 200mg PO 5× daily for 7 days will reduce formation of new lesions, duration of pain, time required for healing and viral shedding but probably not the incidence of recurrence.
2. ***Recurrences*** – aciclovir 200mg PO 5× daily for 5 days or, if recurs >6 times/year, aciclovir 200mg PO tds continuously. Recurrences become more common after >1 year of treatment, so some experts recommend stopping aciclovir after 1 year so that recurrence rates can be reassessed. The minimum continuous dose that will suppress recurrence should be determined empirically. However, aciclovir does not stop viral shedding and transmission to sexual partners may be increased with asymptomatic infection. ► Recommend the use of condoms.
3. ***HIV⁺ patients*** – HSV infection may become destructive in immunocompromised persons. Treat with aciclovir 400mg PO 3–5× daily. Persistence and recurrences are common.

Candida vaginitis

This is not normally a STD – it results from the overgrowth of a commensal vaginal fungus, *Candida albicans*. Antibiotic therapy, pregnancy and immunosuppression are predisposing factors. The woman shows a thick, curd-like white discharge (rarely, a scanty discharge) with Gram +ve fungal hyphae but no neutrophils. Visualization of the hyphae is made easier by the addition of 10% KOH to clear the epithelial cells. Intense vulval pruritis and erythema are characteristic. The perineum may also become involved; endometritis is rare but it can be followed by 2° bacterial infection. Occasionally a woman can infect her partner → balanitis.

Management: nystatin 100 000 IU intravaginally daily for 14 days, [alternatives include: miconazole or clotrimoxazole 200mg intravaginally daily for 3 days, or clotrimoxazole 500mg intravaginally stat].

3C. Tuberculosis (TB)[1]

Clare Sander

Tuberculosis 112
Disease and pathogenesis 114
Clinical features 116
Diagnosis 120
Treatment 122
Tuberculosis and HIV 126

1. Most of the information presented in this chapter comes from two recently published books:
Treatment of tuberculosis: Guidelines for national programmes, WHO: Geneva
Crofton J, *Clinical Tuberculosis*, Macmillan 1997

Staining for acid-alcohol-fast bacilli (AFB)

1. Wear a mask, as samples are potentially infective. Keep sputum handling to a minimum. Smear a sample of sputum onto a clean slide, spreading it over an area roughly 2cm by 2cm. Try to get the more greenish, purulent sputum from your sample if possible.
2. Heat-fix the sample over a bunsen flame, avoiding over-heating and burning.
3. Flood the slide with Carbol Fuchsin and heat by flaming a lit alcohol swab beneath the slide until steam rises. Leave for 5mins.
4. Wash with 3% acid alcohol and leave for 3–5mins.
5. Rinse under tap water.
6. Counter-stain with Malachite Green and leave for 5mins.
7. Wash with tap water.
8. Drain to dry (do not blot dry).

Staining for bacteria

1. Prepare the sputum smear on a slide as above and heat-fix over a flame.
2. Place on a rack and flood with Gram stain for 1min.
3. Wash the stain from the slide with clean water.
4. Flood the slide with Lugol's iodine for 1min.
5. Tilt the slide and pour on acetone or alcohol for 5–10s max. to decolourize, before washing with water.
6. Flood the slide with the neutral red counter-stain for 30s.
7. Wash the stain from the slide and allow to dry vertically.

Tuberculosis (TB)

Tuberculosis is curable, yet it kills more people than any other infectious disease. Approximately 1/3 of the world population is infected with *Mycobacterium tuberculosis,* with 8–10 million developing overt disease and ~3 million dying each year. About 95% of cases occur in the developing world and 75% of these in the 15 to 50 age group. As a result, it greatly hinders productivity and economic development in countries with a high disease burden.

Control of this global emergency is achievable but it requires commitment to:

- the organization of services at both national and local level
- effective diagnosis and treatment of those who present for health care
- implementation of the directly observed treatment strategy for chemotherapy (DOTS)
- raise international funding to assist with the implementation of DOTS and to research new pharmaceuticals and vaccines.

These measures are required soon so as to prevent an increase in the number of TB cases, deaths, and the development of multi-drug resistance. The epidemic needs stopping before it becomes untreatable.

Microbiology

The genus *Mycobacterium* has about 50 members which are classified into two broad groups:

- **Typical:** *M. tuberculosis* (causes the most morbidity and mortality), *M. bovis, M. africanum*
- **Atypical:** *M. avium complex, M. kansasii, M. scrofulaceum, M. fortuitum, M. ulcerans, M. marinum* (cause opportunistic infections, and disease in animals).

These bacteria are slender, curved rods distinguished by their cell wall which renders them acid-fast (retains carbolfuschin dye when decolourized with acid ethanol) – the Ziehl-Neelsen (ZN) test. They multiply slowly so 4–6 weeks are required for culture. Infections tend to run an insidious and chronic course.

Transmission

- ***M. tuberculosis*** is spread by the inhalation of droplets coughed up by sputum-positive individuals (NB isoniazid + rifampicin have a high early bactericidal activity and render sputum non-infectious by about 2 weeks). Bacilli are susceptible to UV light, so daytime outdoor transmission is rare. Overcrowded, poorly ventilated housing increases the risk of transmission. Other infected body fluids are more of a theoretical than real risk.
- ***M. bovis*** spreads by the ingestion of bacilli from non-pasteurised dairy products. Domesticated and wild animals are the usual host.
- **Atypical mycobacteria** are saprophytes in soil and water which can be inhaled or introduced through skin abrasions. There is no patient–patient transmission.

Reasons for global TB burden

The main reasons for the increasing global TB burden are:

- poverty
- neglect (inadequate case detection, diagnosis, and cure)
- changing demography (increasing world population and changing age structure)
- the impact of the HIV pandemic
- poor patient compliance with the long treatment courses
- ease of international travel
- long-term warfare in some parts of the world

Directly observed treatment strategy (DOTS)

The thrust of the WHO Global Tuberculosis Control programme is to diagnose and treat infectious patients effectively and thereby interrupt the chain of transmission. The DOTS scheme uses trained health care workers to watch patients take their anti-TB medication either daily or 3× weekly for six to eight months, ensuring good compliance. It is being expanded throughout the world and consistently produces 85% or higher cure rates. It has been shown to be one of the most cost-effective of all health interventions. Use of community members such as shop-owners to supervise treatment will enable this strategy to be extended further.

Disease and pathogenesis

Primary TB

Aerosolized droplets of *M. tuberculosis* enter alveoli and initiate a non-specific acute inflammatory response at the periphery of the lung. The bacilli are ingested by macrophages and transported to hilar lymph nodes. The bacilli may either be contained here or spread via the lymphatics or bloodstream to the rest of the body. With the development of cell-mediated immunity (CMI), lymphocytes enter infected areas. Their secretion of cytokines recruits and activates macrophages, transforming them into specialized histiocytes which organize into granulomas surrounded by lymphocytes.

In an immunocompetent host, most granulomas heal and calcify. They can sometimes be seen on CXR as a 1° complex: calcified peripheral lung lesion (Ghon focus) and hilar lymph nodes. However, although the lesions become calcified, bacilli persist intracellularly in macrophages in a quiescent state and may become activated at a later time.

Post-primary TB

In a minority of cases, predominantly infants and children, primary infection is not contained and disseminated disease (miliary TB and meningitis) develops at the same time as primary infection.

Post-primary TB also occurs as a reactivation of latent infection. It involves exponential multiplication of bacilli at sites of dissemination, which are either pulmonary or extrapulmonary. In high prevalence countries, only ~10 % of adults infected with *M. tuberculosis* develop secondary disease and this usually occurs many years after primary infection. Infants are at increased risk of developing overt disease, with some studies showing up to 43% of infected babies going on to develop clinical disease.

Risk factors for disease progression

- Age (weakened immunity at the extremes of age)
- Malnutrition
- Intercurrent infection eg malaria, worms, measles, whooping cough
- Toxic factors eg alcohol & smoking
- Poverty (overcrowding; increased exposure to tubercle bacilli)
- Immune suppression eg HIV, steroids
- Host genetic factors eg HLA type has a weak influence

Non-*Mycobacterium tuberculosis* disease

M. bovis causes a spectrum of disease similar to *M. tuberculosis* but with a predilection for cervical lymphadenitis and gastrointestinal disease.

Atypical mycobacteria are associated with a wide range of clinical conditions in the immunosuppressed host (see chapter 3B). In the immunocompetent host, they principally cause localised disease of the:

- lungs (similar process to pulmonary *M. tuberculosis*)
- lymphadenitis (predominantly in children)
- skin and soft tissue

Tuberculin test

These tests (Mantoux and Heaf) rely on the fact that cell-mediated hypersensitivity develops 4–6 weeks after infection. They involve intradermal injection of PPD (purified protein derivative), a crude mixture of antigens, using a needle and syringe for the Mantoux and a six-pronged gun for the Heaf. An assessment of skin induration takes place 48hrs (Mantoux), or 2–7days (Heaf) later. A positive test indicates exposure, not immunity, to mycobacteria. A negative test does not exclude TB since many factors eg HIV, malnutrition, severe illness may suppress the test.

BCG vaccination

The Bacille Calmette Guerin (BCG) is a live attenuated vaccine derived from serially culturing an isolate of *Mycobacterium bovis*. Although its mode of action is unknown, a widely accepted theory states that by inducing a form of immune responsiveness characteristic of post-primary TB, BCG vaccination prevents dissemination of bacilli from initial sites of infection, thereby preventing the serious manifestations of primary TB, namely meningitis and miliary TB.

Clinical features

Primary TB

The initial infection is usually asymptomatic, but there may be fever, malaise, cough (+/– sputum), or erythema nodosum. The diagnosis is made by tuberculin test conversion, occasionally by the detection of acid fast bacilli (AFB) in sputum specimens. A CXR may show segmental consolidation (any lobe) +/– enlarged lymph nodes. The 1° complex is only seen months–years later.

Post-primary TB

Is usually symptomatic. ***Non-specific symptoms*** are common and include:

- weight loss
- anorexia
- fever
- night sweats
- malaise.

► **TB may affect any organ in the body** resulting in organ specific symptoms and signs. In adults, pulmonary TB is the commonest manifestation. Extrapulmonary disease is more common in children than adults.

1. **Pulmonary TB** involves the lung parenchyma. It may cause a productive cough, haemoptysis, chest pain, breathlessness. Examination may be unremarkable or the patient may look ill and wasted with a fever and tachycardia. Chest examination may reveal fine crepitations in the lung apices, bronchial breathing, localized wheeze, or signs of a pleural effusion. Differential diagnoses include pneumonia, COPD, lung cancer, lung abscess, and bronchiectasis.
   Diagnosis: ~65% of pulmonary TB cases are sputum smear +ve (AFB detectable on direct microscopy of three sputum samples).
   ► It is essential that direct smears of sputum are made if a patient has had a cough for >3wks. See opposite.
   Complications include: pleural effusion and empyema (consider pleural biopsy when tapping fluid), pleurisy, pneumothorax, cor pulmonale, TB bronchiectasis, aspergillomata in cavities, and dissemination to other organs.

2. **Miliary TB** most commonly affects infants and the immunosuppressed. It classically presents with a few weeks' history of gradual onset fever, malaise and weight loss. There may be evidence of tuberculous lesions in the lungs, hepatomegaly, splenomegaly, choroidal tubercles, and neck stiffness (meningitis often complicates miliary TB). Death occurs within weeks in the absence of therapy.
   Diagnosis: CXR characteristically shows diffuse, small, nodular opacities. Sputum and tuberculin tests are often negative, biopsy of liver, bone marrow, lymph nodes, or lung parenchyma may yield AFBs or granulomata.

Case definitions

Smear-positive pulmonary tuberculosis (PTB)

1. >1 sputum specimen positive for AFB
or

2. 1 sputum specimen positive for AFB, *plus*
CXR consistent with PTB, *plus*
a decision by the physician to treat with a full curative course of anti-TB chemotherapy
or

3. 1 sputum specimen positive for AFB which is also found to be culture-positive

Smear-negative PTB - (requires CXR or culture)

1. 2 sets (>1 sputum specimen 2 wks apart) negative for AFB, *plus*
CXR consistent with PTB, *plus*
lack of any clinical response to 1 week of antibiotic therapy
or

2. if severely ill – as above but requiring only 1 set of specimens negative for AFB
or

3. sputum specimens which are negative for AFB but culture positive.

3. **TB adenitis** can involve any lymph nodes, although cervical nodes are the most frequent site (known as *scrofula*). Nodes are initially rubbery and non-tender, becoming harder and matted with time. The condition is usually indolent; rarely the nodes suppurate to form sinuses and fistulae. TB nodes may enlarge during anti-TB therapy – this responds to increased corticosteroid cover.
   Diagnosis: is by surgical biopsy and culture. Usually a single node is involved and excision is curative. Needle aspiration and ZN stain may be positive in AIDS patients

4. **Skeletal TB** usually affects the spine (Pott's disease). Vertebral collapse causes gibbus deformity and paraplegia may develop. Paravertebral cold abscesses are frequently seen but do not require drainage.
   Diagnosis: is by X-ray and biopsy. Treat medically unless the patient is neurologically compromised, or the spine is unstable. ► Such patients require urgent referral. Hip and knee joint TB respond well to immobilization and chemotherapy.

5. **TB meningitis** is most commonly seen in children. The diagnosis should be considered in a child with headache, irritability, vomiting, decreased consciousness, or any unusual progressive neurological syndrome. Seizures are the most common presentation in adults. Meningeal signs are common as are cranial nerve findings (III, IV, VI & VIII particularly), reflecting basilar distribution of the disease. Seizures may also occur.
   Diagnosis: examine the CSF. There is typically a lymphocytosis with raised protein & decreased glucose. Send (preferably) >10ml CSF for culture (this takes time). ZN stain of CSF has a poor return.

6. **Gastrointestinal TB** may present during primary TB with complications of mesenteric adenitis including obstruction, ascites, and fistula formation. Organisms swallowed from extensive cavitating pulmonary disease can cause disease at terminal ileum and caecum. The patient presents with diarrhoea, pain, or ascites. Consider the diagnosis if diarrhoea does not respond to treatment for typical causes.
   Diagnosis: ZN stain and culture of ascitic tap and needle biopsy of the peritoneum. Laparotomy may be necessary. Treat with chemotherapy. Surgery may be necessary for obstruction and fistulae.

7. **Pericardial TB** presents with fever, pericardial pain, and occasionally tamponade. A friction rub may be heard. Exudative effusion and chronic constriction are late sequelae, but frequently respond to prednisolone. Increasingly diagnosed in HIV^{+} patients.
   Diagnosis: is via ZN stain of a pericardial tap. Pericardial calcification may be seen on CXR years later (although this is uncommon). Echocardiography is helpful for identifying an effusion.

8. **Genitourinary TB** can involve any part of male or female GU tract. Presentation is insidious. Renal TB presents with symptoms of UTI with microscopic pyuria and haematuria but sterile urine culture. TB salpingitis presents either as infertility or lower abdominal pain. Painful epididymal swelling is the most common presentation of GU TB in males.

Scheme to aid diagnosis of TB in children[1]

1. Score chart for child with suspected TB

Score	0	1	3
Length of illness	Less than 2 weeks	2–4 weeks	More than 4 weeks
Nutrition (weight)	Above 80% for age	60 – 80%	Less than 60%
Family TB past or present	None	Reported by family	Proved sputum positive

2. Score for other features if present:

- positive tuberculin test **3**
- large painless lymph nodes: firm, soft, sinus in neck, axilla and groin **3**
- unexplained fever, night sweats, no response to malaria treatment **2**
- malnutrition, not improving after 4 weeks **3**
- angle deformity of the spine **4**
- joint swelling, bone swelling, or sinuses **3**
- unexplained abdominal mass or ascites **3**
- CNS: change in temperament, convulsions, or coma (admit to hospital) **3**

3. If the TOTAL score is 7 or more – treat for TB

Treat children with a score less than 7 if

- a CXR is characteristic of TB infection, *or*
- the child does not respond to two 7-day courses of two different antibiotics.

1. Adapted from *Clinical tuberculosis*, courtesy of Dr Keith Edwards

Diagnosis

Diagnostic algorithms will depend on the facilities available. ▶ Microscopy for tubercle bacilli is the "gold-standard" diagnostic method.

- **To diagnose pulmonary TB**, see the flowchart opposite. Sputum should always be examined if a productive cough has been present for > 3wks. 3 specimens are required – ideally collected at 1st presentation, a subsequent morning, and the morning the patient returns for follow up. Some patients, particularly children, have no sputum or are unable to produce it, but nebulization with 3% hypertonic saline may aid collection. Gastric lavage, or laryngeal swabs may also be used. Since there is no "gold-standard" diagnostic test for smear –ve PTB, it is important to follow recommended guidelines as closely as possible. See table at start of chapter for staining guidelines.
- **To diagnose extrapulmonary TB**, the possibility of TB infection must first be recognized. The relevant body fluid or tissue then requires microscopic examination and culture. See p. 111.

Microscopy: involves examining Ziehl-Neelsen stained smears or tissue with a light microscope under oil immersion.

Culture: is more sensitive than microscopy but will rarely be available for routine use. Many media are available but Lowenstein-Jensen is the most commonly used. A Reference Laboratory can assess drug sensitivities and investigate individuals with treatment failure.

Radiology is very useful but ▶ a suspicious X-ray should never be treated without sputum examination.

- Certain features seen on CXR are strongly suggestive of TB: upper zone patchy/nodular shadows (unilateral or bilateral), cavitation especially >1, calcified shadows, diffuse small nodular opacities (miliary TB).
- Features on CXR that may suggest TB include: an oval or round solitary shadow (coin lesion), hilar and paratracheal nodes, mycetoma (fungus ball, complication of old TB), halo shadow.
- A normal radiograph can rarely be seen in 2° endobronchial TB.

Tuberculin test exists in 2 forms. It is useful as an epidemiological tool, but its use is limited in the diagnosis of individuals. It measures exposure to TB (plus BCG), not active disease. Co-existing disease and malnutrition can result in false negative results.

- ***Mantoux*** – inject 5IU of PPDRT23 (read label carefully before choosing dose) intradermally between mid and upper 1/3 of dorsal surface of clean dry forearm. Use a tuberculin syringe and 26 gauge 10mm long intradermal needle. Read after 48–72hrs by measuring diameter of induration (NOT erythema). The bigger the reaction, the more +ve the test. Induration >10mm strongly suggests disease.
- ***Heaf*** – place a drop of undiluted PPD on clean dry skin at the junction of mid and upper 1/3 of the anterior surface of the forearm. Adjust the needle length on the Heaf gun (2mm for adults, 1mm for young children), dip the needles and end-plate in spirit and ignite briefly, cooling for >10 secs. Depress handle of gun – the needles will pierce the skin. Grade response at 2–7 days (see opposite).

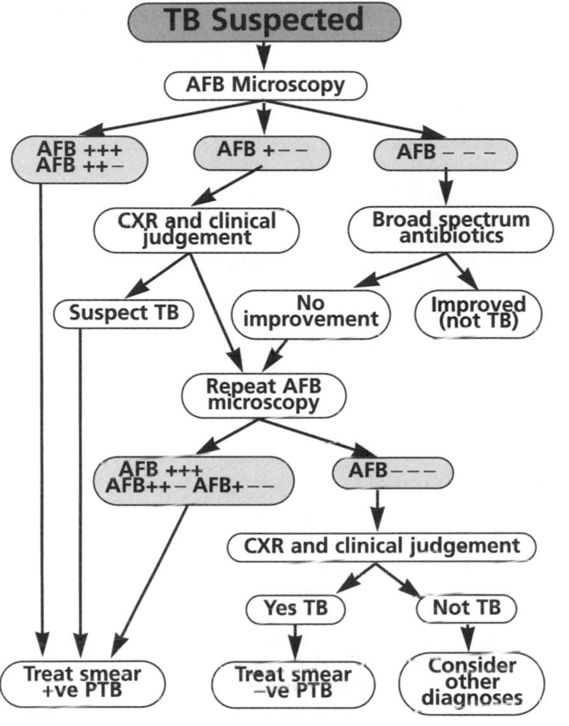

Grading of Heaf test response

- *Grade I* 4 or more discrete patches
- *Grade II* Confluent patches forming a ring
- *Grade III* Disc of induration
- *Grade IV* Disc of induration >10mm diameter, or vesiculation of disc

Treatment

► TB is a curable disease. Effective treatment is an important form of prevention.

Aims of treatment: • to cure patients with least interference to their lives • to prevent death in the seriously ill • to prevent extensive damage to the lungs • to avoid disease relapse (ie obtain sterilization) • to prevent development of resistant bacilli • to protect the patient's family and community from infection.

General management: recommended treatment regimens are similar irrespective of the site of disease, although some advise a prolonged consolidation phase for TB meningitis and bony disease. Short course chemotherapy (SCC) containing rifampicin & lasting 6–8 months has been shown to be more cost-effective than "standard regimens" which use 12 months of thiacetazone, isoniazid & 2 months of streptomycin. SCC consists of two phases:

- ***intensive phase*** which lasts 2 months, uses at least 3 drugs, and aims to decrease the population of viable bacteria as rapidly as possible and prevent the emergence of resistance.
- ***consolidation (continuation) phase*** which lasts 4–6 months, uses at least 2 drugs, and aims to eliminate the remaining bacilli.

Criteria used for selecting a drug regimen

Case definitions, used to determine treatment categories, depend on:

1. **Site –** pulmonary or extra-pulmonary
2. **Severity –** which depends on
   - bacillary load • extent of disease
   - anatomical site (meningitis, miliary, pericarditis, bilateral pleural effusions, spinal, intestinal & GU are severe; lymphadenopathy, unilateral pleural effusion, bone, peripheral joint & skin are less severe).
3. **Bacteriology –** sputum smear +ve or –ve
4. **History of previous treatment –**
   - new case
   - relapse – previously been declared cured, now sputum +ve
   - treatment failure – smear +ve despite >5months treatment
   - treatment after interruption of >2months
   - chronic case – remained smear +ve after a full treatment course

See table on the next page for treatment regimens

From the public health perspective, the highest treatment priority should be given to infectious cases, ie prioritized from category I (highest priority) to IV (lowest priority).

Monitoring treatment

- Sputum-positive patients should be monitored by sputum smear examination after 2 months of treatment. All other patients should be monitored clinically.
- Monitoring for adverse drug reactions is essential.

The essential anti-TB drugs

anti-TB drug (abbreviation)	*Mode of action*	*Recommended dose (mg/kg)*	
		Daily	*3×/week*
Isoniazid (H)	bactericidal	5	10
Rifampicin (R)	bactericidal	10	10
Pyrazinamide (Z)	bactericidal	25	35
Streptomycin (S)	bactericidal	15	15
Ethambutol (E)	bacteristatic	15	30
Thiacetazone (T)	bacteristatic	2.5	N/A

Special groups

- Give pyridoxine to diabetic, malnourished, alcoholic, and pregnant individuals treated with isoniazid to prevent peripheral neuropathy.
- Avoid ethambutol in young children as they are unable to report changes in visual acuity – a recognized side-effect of this drug.
- Women of child-bearing age on oral contraceptives must receive an alternative or additional form of contraception (eg an IUD) during, and for 4–8 weeks after stopping, rifampicin therapy. Rifampicin is such a potent inducer of liver enzymes that even a high-dose oral contraceptive may not be sufficient protection.
- Corticosteroids have an adjunct role in pericarditis, pleural effusion and severe meningitis, decreasing mortality & late complications.

Pregnancy

- Authorities suggest that rifampicin is safe in pregnant women.[1] A large case series concluded that it did not increase the risk of congenital malformations.
- Avoid streptomycin – it is ototoxic to the fetus.
- There is no need to restrict breastfeeding.

1. *Martindale: the Extra Pharmacopoeia*, p. 269

Compliance: is central to both achieving cure and preventing the development of resistance. Patients begin to feel better just a few weeks after commencing treatment so the importance of a full course of treatment must be explained clearly to both patient and family. The DOTS scheme will increase compliance and is less expensive and disruptive than hospitalization. Fixed proportion combination pills decrease the chance of accidental monotherapy.

Resistance: small numbers of naturally resistant organisms exist in all populations. Secondary resistance mainly results from poor prescribing and poor compliance. ► Prevent resistance by never using monotherapy and never adding a single drug to a failing regimen. Multidrug resistance is becoming increasingly important, especially in HIV+ patients.

Treatment failure: can result from either poor compliance or resistance. Manage in a stepwise fashion:

1. Check compliance and take drug history.
2. Repeat treatment in a supervised fashion.
3. If possible send specimen to a reference lab for culture and sensitivity.
4. Treat with all 1st line drugs for 6mths (longer if resistant to rifampicin).
5. If treatment fails again (incurable infection) stop treatment & consider isoniazid monotherapy. The need for long term isolation needs to be addressed by the community.

Control programmes will typically involve some or all of:

- ***Socioeconomic development*** – critically important for long-term control. Includes improved housing, ventilation, and nutrition.
- ***Health education and promotion*** – to increase awareness of the disease and therefore increase numbers presenting for diagnosis. Additionally to discourage spitting, smoking, and excess alcohol.
- ***BCG vaccination of newborns*** – safe, cheap, thought to prevent life-threatening disseminated TB in children. Trials demonstrate variable efficacies in different countries. Protection is of limited duration, so vaccinaton causes shifts in age-specific TB rates. WHO recommends its use in asymptomatic HIV^+ infants but not in children with AIDS.
- ***Chemoprophylaxis*** – use isoniazid for 6mths. Indications depend on resources of country and local risk of TB but include:
    - healthy contacts of new cases with a positive tuberculin test
    - recent tuberculin test conversion (not due to BCG)
    - infants of sputum positive mothers
    - close contacts aged <5yrs with a strongly +ve tuberculin test
    - HIV^+ people with a positive tuberculin test

    ► Lifelong chemoprophylaxis in HIV is controversial.

    ► Isoniazid has been shown to protect against the development of TB and slow the rate of progression to AIDS.
- ***Chemotherapy*** – using DOTS and case finding.
- ***Contacts*** – examine sputum of all household members. In adult contacts, if sputum is negative, re-examine and check sputum in 1mth. In children, use a tuberculin test if possible. If positive and the child is unwell (having excluded other diagnoses), treat for TB; if the child is well, use prophylactic isoniazid.

► Familiarize yourself with the local National Control Programme.

Treatment of TB: Guidelines for national programmes (see page 123 for drug abbreviations)

TB treatment category	*TB patients*	*Alternative TB treatment regimens* *Initial phase*	*Continuation phase*
I	• New smear-positive PTB • New smear-negative PTB with extensive parenchymal involvement • New cases of severe forms of extrapulmonary TB	2 months of: daily EHRZ (*or* daily SHRZ)	6 months of daily HE, *or* 4 months of daily HR, *or* 4 months of 3×/week HR
II	• Sputum-positive - relapse • Sputum-positive - treatment failure • Sputum-positive after an interruption in treatment of >2 months	2 months of daily SHRZE	5 months of daily HRE, *or* 5 months of 3×/week HRE
III	• New smear-negative PTB (other than those in category I • New less severe forms of extra-pulmonary TB	2 months of daily HRZ	6 months of daily HE, *or* 4 months of daily HR, *or* 4 months of 3×/week HR
IV	• Chronic case (still sputum-positive after supervised retreatment)	Not applicable (Refer to WHO guidelines for use of second-line drugs in specialized centres)	

Tuberculosis and HIV

TB is a common, serious, but very treatable complication of AIDS. It is estimated that 5–6 million people are dually infected with *M. tuberculosis* and HIV worldwide and that 30–50% of those with AIDS in the developing world also develop clinical TB. Currently, 70% of cases of dual infection occur in Sub-Saharan Africa and 20% in Asia. However, as the HIV epidemic spreads in Asia even larger numbers are predicted to occur because of the pre-existing high prevalence of latent TB amongst young adults in this population.

► Importantly, the increased burden of TB caused by the HIV epidemic is causing the TB services in poor communities to collapse under the pressure of rising demands.

Differences in management of TB in HIV$^+$ patients – the 'new tuberculosis'

Presentation: extrapulmonary disease is seen more frequently, particularly lymphadenopathy, pleural effusions, pericardial disease, miliary disease and meningitis. However, PTB is still the commonest form. The development of TB may be the 1st sign of HIV infection, so counselling and HIV testing may be appropriate for patients presenting with TB.

Diagnosis: can be harder because

- more sputum smears are –ve & +ve smears tend to contain fewer AFBs
- tuberculin tests are often falsely –ve
- CXRs are often atypical. Hilar lymphadenopathy, bi-basal pneumonia, and pleural effusions are seen more often and cavitation less often.

Differentiating PTB from other HIV-related pulmonary diseases can be difficult. However, rapid diagnosis and implemention of therapy is crucial. When clinical suspicion is high and other diagnoses have been excluded as far as possible a trial of anti-TB chemotherapy may be appropriate. Failure to respond within 2–4 wks suggests that the diagnosis is unlikely and that the patient should be re-evaluated.

Treatment: use the same criteria to determine treatment categories and the same drug regimens as for HIV negative individuals.

However, be aware that:

- Drugs tend to be more toxic, particularly thiacetazone (associated with severe, sometimes fatal skin reactions). Use ethambutol instead.
- Streptomycin requires IM injection and should probably be best avoided in areas of high HIV prevalence, unless sterile needles/syringes are in good supply.
- There are many common drug interactions eg rifampicin and ketoconazole in combination decrease serum levels of rifampicin..
- Case-fatality rates are greater in coinfected individuals than in HIV-ve TB patients. However, treatment with short-course chemotherapy still offers the best chance of clearing the infection.

Reciprocal interaction between *M. tuberculosis* & HIV

The relationship between HIV and TB is not simply that they commonly coexist in the same individual. In addition, each infection worsens the progression and prognosis of the other.

Effect of HIV on TB: the risk of developing active TB is 6–100 fold greater in HIV-infected individuals compared to non-infected individuals. It is not clear whether this increased risk is due to increased susceptibility to exogenous infection or due to increased reactivation of latent infection. Both mechanisms may play a role.

Effect of TB on HIV: active TB accelerates the progression of HIV. HIV^+ patients with TB have a decreased survival compared to HIV^+ patients with matched CD4 counts who do not have TB.

Consequences of HIV for TB control include:

- overdiagnosis of sputum smear –ve PTB
- underdiagnsosis of sputum smear +ve PTB
- inadequate supervision of anti-TB chemotherapy
- low cure rates
- high case fatality rates during treatment
- high default rates because of adverse drug reactions
- high rates of TB recurrence and therefore increased emergence of drug resistance

3D. Diarrhoeal diseases

Faecal staining 129
Diarrhoeal diseases 130
Classification of diarrhoea 130
Antimicrobial drugs 131
Acute diarrhoea with blood 132
Bacillary dysentery (shigellosis) 132
Enterohaemorrhagic *E. coli* (EHEC) 132
Balantidium enterocolitis 134
Campylobacter enterocolitis 134
Yersinia enterocolitis 134
Amoebic dysentery 136
Salmonella entercolitis 138
Trichuriasis (whipworm) 140
Antibiotic-associated colitis 140
Acute diarrhoea without blood 142
Rotavirus 142
Enterotoxigenic *E. coli* (ETEC) 142
Enterotoxin-producing *S. aureus* 142
Giardiasis 144
Cholera 146
The cholera outbreak 148
Clostridium perfringens 150
Cryptosporidiosis 150
Chronic diarrhoea 152
Malabsorption and steatorrhoea 152
Post-infective malabsorption (PIM or tropical sprue) 154
Other causes of malabsorption 156
Other causes of chronic diarrhoea 156
Strongyloidiasis 158
Intestinal flukes 160
Dehydration 162
Estimation of fluid defect 164
Oral rehydration solution (ORS) 164
Treatment plan A 166
Treatment plan B 167
Treatment plan C 170
Management of persistent diarrhoea 172
Complications of diarrhoea 174
Antidiarrhoeal drugs 175
Prevention of diarrhoea 176
Some difficulties encountered in home therapy for diarrhoea 177

How to make a direct faecal smear

1. Write the patient's name on a clean slide.
2. Place a drop of sterile saline in the centre of the left hand side of the slide and place a drop of iodine in the centre of the right hand side of the slide. Fig 1.

3. With a match or applicator, pick up a small portion of faeces (~2mg – or about the size of a match head) and add it to the drop of saline. Repeat and add to the iodine. Mix the faeces with the drops to form suspensions. Fig 2.

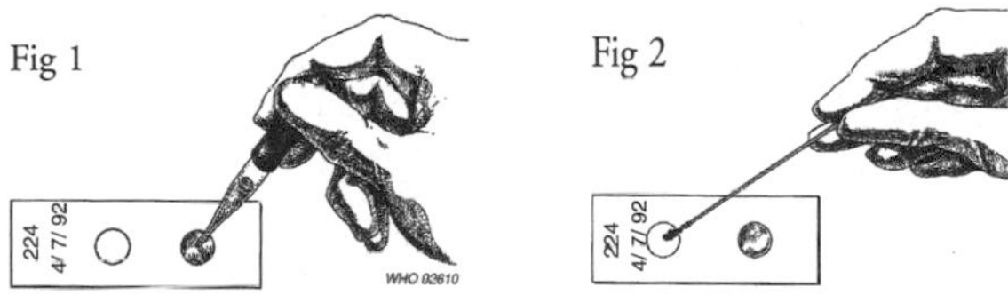

Fig 1 Fig 2

4. Cover each drop with a coverslip. Fig 3.

5. Examine each drop with the ×10 objective, or, for identification, with the higher power objectives, searching in a systematic manner. When organisms are seen, switch to higher power for more detail. Fig 4.

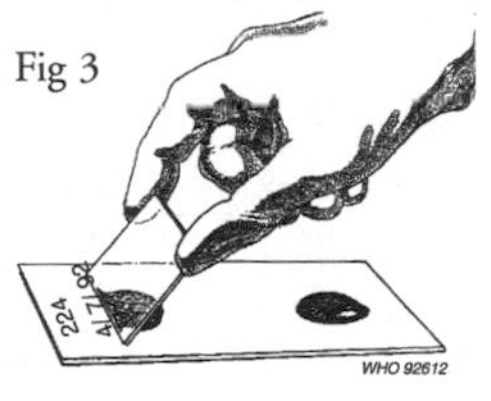

Fig 3

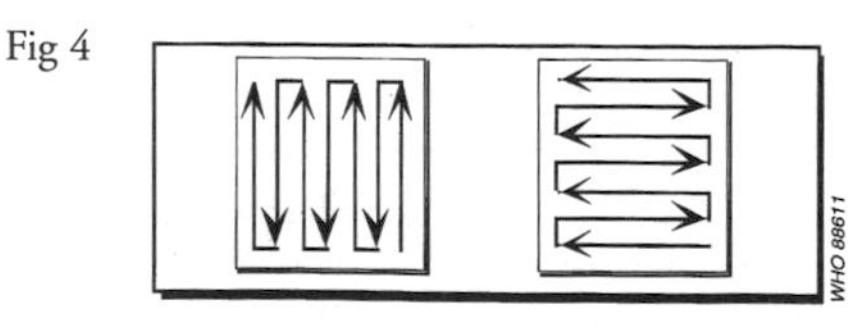

Fig 4

Diarrhoeal diseases

Diarrhoea is defined as the passage of abnormally loose or fluid stools more frequently than normal. Normal bowel habit varies greatly from person to person, but above 12 months of age, more than 3 loose stools per day is considered abnormal.

Infective diarrhoea is the second highest cause of death due to infection in the world, with ~3–4 million fatalities each year. 80% of deaths are in children under 2yrs, specifically during and shortly after weaning, since breastfeeding confers significant protection against intestinal infections. Repeated attacks of diarrhoea initiate a vicious cycle of malnutrition, reduced immunity and more intestinal infections.

An accurate history is vital for all cases of diarrhoea, since it will give clues to the aetiology and severity of disease. Include in the past medical history any similar episodes and also any current medication.

► A diagnosis based upon the clinical history and signs present is often sufficiently accurate, since treatment will usually focus on maintaining hydration. Antimicrobials will only be needed in severe disease.

Some key questions to be asked:

1. How long has the diarrhoea been present?
2. Is (or was) there fever?
3. What is the stool like – specifically is there blood (bright red or dark) and/or mucus?
4. How frequent are the motions?
5. Is there any abdominal pain – where?
6. Is there a sense of tenesmus (incomplete emptying following defaecation)?
7. Has the patient vomited – how much, when, what?
8. Has the patient been in contact with anyone with similar symptoms?
9. Have they eaten or drunk anything unusual prior to the onset of symptoms?
10. Is anyone else in the family ill?

► In examining the patient, one should look for signs of dehydration and malnutrition, as well as for clues to determine the disease aetiology.

Investigations: for general assessment include Hb, FBC, U&E, and glucose. Usually stool culture & microscopy is required for definitive diagnosis. Specific tests may be indicated, but the results will often come back too late to influence management. ► Do a blood film for malaria.

Classification of diarrhoea

It is useful to subdivide diarrhoeal diseases according to duration and presence of blood in the stool, since the causative agents are largely different in each group. Here we shall divide the diseases into acute diarrhoea with blood (dysentery), acute diarrhoea without blood, and chronic diarrhoea.

▸ Antimicrobial drugs

In the majority of cases, symptoms of diarrhoea improve with treatment of dehydration alone, without the need for antibiotics.

In certain circumstances, however, antimicrobial drugs may be beneficial. These include:

1. ***Bloody diarrhoea (dysentery) which does not improve after 3 days of rehydration treatment.*** If a specific cause is found it should be treated appropriately (see relevant section below). If no cause can be found, an antimicrobial effective against *Shigella* should be used in the first instance.
2. ***Cholera with severe dehydration:*** any suspected case of cholera should be treated with an effective antimicrobial and control agencies notified.
3. ***Laboratory-proven, symptomatic cases of* G. intestinalis *infection*** which do not improve after 3 days of ORS therapy should be treated with an antimicrobial.

Acute diarrhoea with blood

The presence of blood in diarrhoea (dysentery) usually signifies ulceration of the large bowel. By far the commonest cause in the tropics is shigellosis (bacillary dysentery) which is unfortunately also more likely to progress to complications and death.

Bacillary dysentery (shigellosis)

Shigella dysenteriae, Sh. flexneri, Sh. boydii and *Sh. sonneii* cause the disease known as bacillary dysentery, with the former two species responsible for most morbidity and mortality (which may reach 20%). The disease may occur both endemically and epidemically, with children most frequently affected. The incubation period in humans (the only natural host) is 1–5 days following direct person to person contact (from cases of asymptomatic excreters) or ingestion of contaminated water and food.

Clinical features: range from mild disease in which there is intermittent watery diarrhoea alone, to severe systemic complications. In severe cases, onset is usually rapid, with tenesmus, fever and passage of frequent (up to 100/day) bloody mucoid stools. Intestinal complications include: toxic megacolon, perforation, and protein-losing enteropathy. Systemic complications include: dehydration, hypoglycaemia and electrolyte imbalance (particularly hyponatraemia), haemolytic-uraemic syndrome, convulsions (particularly in children, often before the onset of diarrhoea), Reiter's syndrome, thrombotic thrombocytopenic purpura, pneumonia. Invasive disease may give '*rose spots*' – crops of 2–4mm papules which fade on pressure, usually appearing on the upper abdomen and lower chest.

Diagnosis: the clinical distinction between bacillary and amoebic dysentery is usually impossible. Stool microscopy may show leukocytes, but for confirmation, culture of stool samples and rectal swabs is needed.

Management

1. Oral rehydration is sufficient for mild disease.
2. In severe disease, ampicillin or trimethoprim (or co-trimoxazole) should be given, although due to resistance, quinolones such as ciprofloxacin may be the most appropriate agent. Antimicrobial sensitivities should be sought from individual cultures wherever possible.

Prevention: no vaccine is currently available.

Enterohaemorrhagic *E. coli* (EHEC)

Although rare, these verotoxin-producing bacteria have been associated with a number of outbreaks of inflammatory, haemorrhagic colitis, with features similar to disease caused by *Sh. dysenteriae.* It is commonly implicated in the haemolytic-uraemic syndrome.

Management

1. Careful rehydration and symptomatic relief is usually sufficient.

Causes of acute diarrhoea with blood

1. Bacillary dysentery (shigellosis).
2. *Balantidium coli* enterocolitis.
3. *Campylobacter* enterocolitis.
4. Enterohaemorrhagic *E. coli.*
5. *Yersinia* enterocolitis.
6. Amoebic dysentery.
7. *Salmonella* enterocolitis
8. Massive *Trichuris* infection.
9. Antibiotic-associated colitis (pseudomembranous colitis).
10. *S. mansoni* or *S. japonicum* infection.

Balantidium enterocolitis

Balantidium coli is a rare protozoal pathogen of humans. It exists in cyst and trophozoite forms, the former being responsible for transmission. Trophozoites invade the intestinal mucosa producing inflammation and ulceration.

Clinical features: infection closely resembles amoebic colitis and may take one of three forms:

- Asymptomatic carrier state (80%).
- Acute dysentery which may be associated with nausea, abdominal pain, and weight loss. This is potentially fatal.
- Chronic diarrhoea, frequently without blood.

Diagnosis: rests upon identification of the trophozoite in the faeces

Management: tetracycline 500mg PO tds for 10 days in severe disease. The parasite is also sensitive to ampicillin and metronidazole.

Campylobacter enterocolitis

C. jejuni, C. coli or *C. laridis* cause frequent epidemics in nurseries or paediatric wards. Infective bacteria may continue to be excreted in the faeces up to 3 weeks after the cessation of diarrhoea.

Clinical features: the disease is normally self-limiting in 5–7 days. Severe, disseminated infection can occur with concurrent malnutrition, hepatic dysfunction, malignancy, diabetes mellitus, renal failure and immunosuppression. Complications include bacteraemia, meningitis, deep abscesses, cholecystitis, and reactive arthritis.

Diagnosis: Gram stain or dark field microscopy of faecal smears +/–culture. In severe disease, colonoscopic biopsy may be needed.

Management

1. Careful rehydration and symptomatic relief is usually sufficient.
2. In severe disease, use erythromycin. Resistant strains (especially *C. coli*) may need trimethoprim (or co-trimoxazole) or ciprofloxacin.

Yersinia enterocolitis

Yersinia enterocolitica is a rare cause of diarrhoea in the tropics. There may be low-grade fever, bloody diarrhoea and abdominal pain affecting mainly children <5yrs, plus nausea, vomiting, headache or pharyngitis. Infection may spread to cause: septicaemia; peritonitis; hepatic, renal and splenic abscesses; pyomyositis, and osteomyelitis, although such complications are more common in immunocompromised adults or in patients who are iron overloaded (e.g. haemochromatosis).

Diagnosis: culture from stool or other focal sites of infection.

Management:

1. Careful rehydration and symptomatic relief is usually sufficient.
2. In complicated disease, use trimethoprim (or co-trimoxazole), tetracycline or chloramphenicol.

Diarrhoeal diseases

Amoebic dysentery

Around 480 million people world-wide are infected by the protozoite *Entamoeba histolytica* and although only about 10% are symptomatic, it is the third leading parasitic cause of death after malaria and schistosomiasis, with an annual mortality of ~100,000. Severe infection occurs in pregnant women, very young children, the malnourished, and people on steroids.

Transmission: occurs via the faeco-oral route, usually through food and drink becoming contaminated with human faeces. Prevalence is highest in areas where human faeces are used as fertilizer. Sexual transmission also occurs. Cysts are ingested and pass into the small and large intestine, dividing to form metacysts and trophozoites which produce further cysts. These are evacuated in the stool and remain viable and infective for several days (up to 2 months in cool, damp conditions). *E. histolytica* has the capacity to destroy almost any tissue in the body, with amoebic liver abscess being the most common extra-intestinal manifestation.

Clinical features: range from the asymptomatic carrier state to fulminant colitis with perforation and multi-organ involvement. Intestinal amoebiasis usually has an insidious onset with abdominal discomfort and diarrhoea becoming increasingly bloody and mucoid as severity increases. Tenesmus occurs in half the patients and is always associated with recto-sigmoid involvement. On palpation, there is frequently tenderness over the caecum, transverse and sigmoid colon and the liver may be enlarged and tender. Colonoscopy may reveal hyperaemic, necrotic ulcers covered with a yellowish exudate, particularly in the region of the flexures. Following repeated amoebic infection, an amoebal granuloma (amoeboma) may develop (most frequently at the caecum) where it may be palpable and mistaken for a malignant mass.

Extra-intestinal amoebiasis: the commonest form is liver abscesses. These may in turn give rise to pericardial, pleuropulmonary, cerebral, genitourinary, or cutaneous disease. It may occur without dysentery.

Diagnosis: is often difficult. Examine at least 3 stool samples using concentration and permanent stain techniques, preferably before administration of medications or contrast media since these interfere with amoebae recovery. The presence of *E. histolytica* trophozoites containing ingested erythrocytes is diagnostic of amoebiasis. However, the demonstration of cysts in a patient with GI symptoms does not necessarily indicate that amoebiasis is causing these symtoms. Culture of amoebae is a more sensitive method of diagnosis, but is impractical for most clinical laboratories. Monoclonal antibodies, DNA probes and ELISAs are being developed.

Management:

1. Metronidazole 400 mg PO tds for 10 days *followed by*
2. Diloxanide furonate 500 mg tds for 10 days.
3. If there are signs of peritonism, add a broad spectrum antibiotic.
   (Metronidazole is effective against the trophozoite, but because it has little effect on the cysts treatment should be followed by a luminal amoebicide such as diloxanide).

Prevention: improved hygiene; no vaccine is yet available.

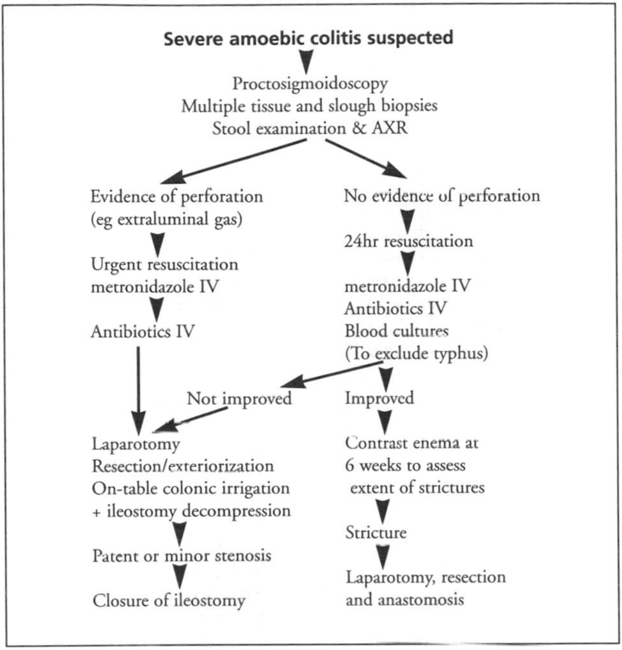

Severe amoebic colitis suspected

↓

Proctosigmoidoscopy
Multiple tissue and slough biopsies
Stool examination & AXR

→ Evidence of perforation (eg extraluminal gas)
↓ Urgent resuscitation metronidazole IV
↓ Antibiotics IV
↓ Laparotomy
Resection/exteriorization
On-table colonic irrigation
+ ileostomy decompression
↓ Patent or minor stenosis
↓ Closure of ileostomy

→ No evidence of perforation
↓ 24hr resuscitation
↓ metronidazole IV
Antibiotics IV
Blood cultures
(To exclude typhus)
→ Not improved → Laparotomy
↓ Improved
↓ Contrast enema at 6 weeks to assess extent of strictures
↓ Stricture
↓ Laparotomy, resection and anastomosis

E. histolytica trophozoite in faecal smear size 15–60µm

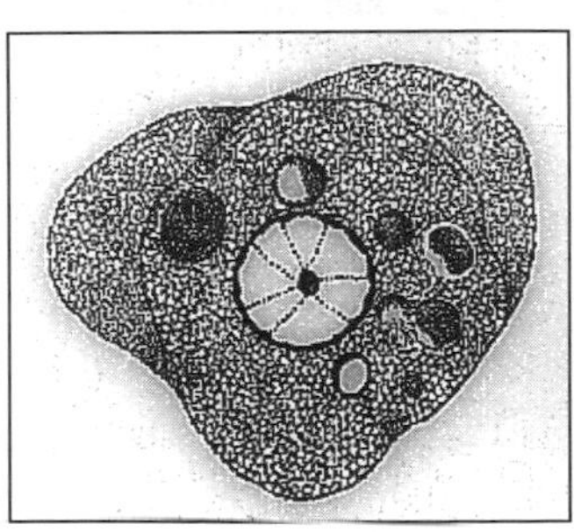

Salmonella enterocolitis

Salmonella typhimurium and *S. enteritidis* enterocolitis has become an important public health problem in the developing world. Transmission is faeco-oral, usually by ingestion of contaminated food (they survive freezing at −20°C). The organisms are widely distributed among wild and domestic animals. The incubation period is 24–48hrs (up to 72hrs); bacteria are then excreted in the faeces for up to 8 weeks following infection. There are associations with both malaria and HIV infection.

Clinical features: range in severity according to the serotype involved. Two (often overlapping) clinical syndromes are seen.

- ***Acute enterocolitis:*** nausea and vomiting, headache, fever, and malaise, rapidly progressing to diarrhoea with cramping abdominal pains. Initially voluminous and watery, the stool changes to 'colitic stool' with blood and mucus as the disease progresses. There may be LIF pain and rebound tenderness. Infrequently, ileal involvement is dominant with symptoms mimicking appendicitis. ► Severe colitis may be complicated by toxic megacolon.
- ***Invasive salmonellosis:*** bacteraemia rates of 8% have been recorded, with higher rates for certain serotypes. Predisposing factors are: extremes of age, immunosuppression, malignancy, gastric hypoacidity (eg antacid use), concurrent severe disease, bartonellosis, and sickle cell disease. Systemic illness is characterized by swinging fevers, rigors, and general toxicity accompanying the diarrhoea, or a typhoid-like illness characterized by sustained fever, splenomegaly, rose spots and minimal diarrhoea. There may be metastatic spread to meninges (almost exclusively in children <2yrs old), bones and joints, lungs, endocardium and arteries, liver, spleen, ovaries or kidneys. A reactive arthritis is infrequently seen. Patients with chronic schistosomiasis are prone to salmonella bacteraemia since the bacteria live within the helminth and are protected from antibiotics.

Diagnosis: requires isolation of the bacteria from faecal samples or blood cultures. Sigmoidoscopy may be used in severely ill patients.

Management

1. Careful rehydration and symptomatic relief is usually sufficient.
2. Most antibiotics do not influence the clinical course and may prolong bacterial carriage.
3. To patients with severe colitis and/or invasive disease *plus* those in whom the risk of developing severe disease is high, give ciprofloxacin 500 mg PO bd for 5 days.

   Chloramphenicol, amoxicillin or trimethoprim (or co-trimoxazole) may be effective in systemic disease, but local resistance is increasing. Cefotaxime is highly effective, where available.

Diarrhoeal diseases

Trichuriasis (whipworm)

Thought to infect up to 25% of the world's population, *Trichuris trichiura* are 3–4cm long and colonize the colon and rectum after ingestion of faecally contaminated soil.

Life cycle: ingested eggs hatch in the small intestine releasing larvae which mature in the villi for ~1 week before colonizing the caecum and colorectum. Released eggs pass out in the stool and can resist low temperatures, but not desiccation. The time from ingestion to appearance of eggs in the faeces is ~60 days. The perianal area is covered with eggs and auto-infection occurs by the eggs being carried from the anal margin directly to the mouth.

Clinical features: are often absent in mild infections. However, co-infection with *Ascaris lumbricoides* or hookworms (which is common) may result in RIF pain, vomiting, distension, flatulence, and weight loss. Heavy worm burden can result in lower GI haemorrhage, mucopurulent stool and dysentery with rectal prolapse. 2° infection with *E. histolytica* or *B. coli* can aggravate mucosal ulceration and exacerbate dysentery. In such cases there may be finger clubbing and growth retardation in children.

Diagnosis: is by detection of eggs in the stool. An egg count may be done and indicates the degree of infection (>30,000/g stool is heavy infection, implying the presence of several hundred adult worms). There may be anaemia and hypoalbuminaemia, though eosinophilia usually indicates concomitant *Toxocara* infection. Proctoscopy may reveal worms attached to a reddened, ulcerated rectal mucosa. AXR can show changes similar to those seen in Crohns disease.

Management

1. Mebendazole 600mg or albendazole 400mg, both PO once, are equally effective, although there may be regional differences in albendazole sensitivity.

Prevention: control is as for other soil-transmitted helminths.

Antibiotic-associated colitis

This condition was previously called pseudomembranous colitis or *Clostridium difficile* colitis. It is caused by overgrowth of *C. difficile* following broad-spectrum oral or IV antibiotic therapy, particularly clindamycin (see opposite). It is rare in the tropics.

Clinical features: vary from the asymptomatic to toxic megacolon and are due to the production of toxins. Sigmoidoscopy shows characteristic yellow plaques (pseudomembranes) on the mucosa.

Management

1. Metronidazole 400mg PO tds for 5 days.
   Vancomycin is an expensive alternative.

Prevention: careful use of broad-spectrum antibiotics.

Life cycle of *T. trichiura*

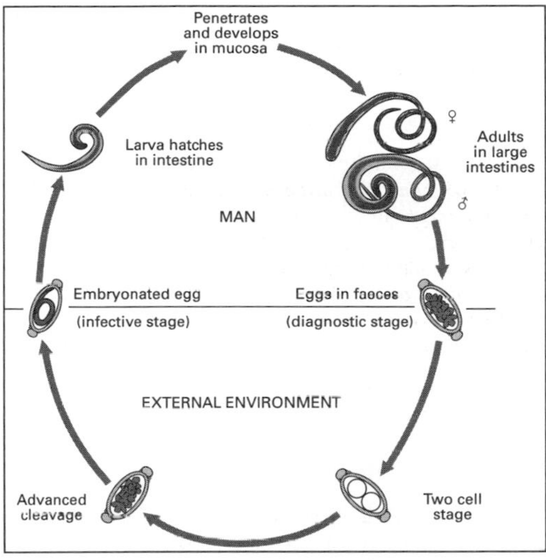

Faecal smear of *T. trichiura* egg ~50μm long

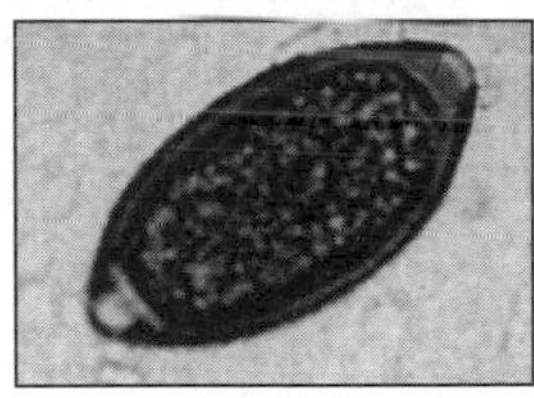

Clindamycin

Because it may cause potentially fatal antibiotic-associated colitis, clindamycin has few primary indications (staphylococcal joint and bone infections; intra-abdominal sepsis). However, the WHO considers clindamycin to be a valuable drug which should be used when other antibiotics are known to be ineffective or inappropriate for a given individual. It should be stopped immediately that diarrhoea occurs.

Acute diarrhoea without blood

See opposite for causes.

Rotavirus

In developed countries, viral infections account for up to 60% of all gastroenteritis in children under 5yrs. In contrast, rotavirus cause <5% of all episodes of diarrhoea in developing countries, but of these 40–50% require hospitalization. Nearly all children in the tropics have been infected with rotavirus at least once before the age of 2yrs.

Clinical features: vomiting is an early feature; the diarrhoea may be so liquid that it is confused with urine. Colicky abdominal pains, ill-defined tenderness, and exaggerated bowel sounds are common. The stool has a characteristic smell.

Management: is supportive, aiming to prevent dehydration. Continue breast feeding, but stop bottled milk and solids until the child improves or is hungry. Beware confusion with surgical causes of diarrhoea in the neonate such as Hirschsprung's disease, intussusception, bowel atresia.

Other viruses such as Norwalk agent and enteric adenoviruses may be responsible for producing acute diarrhoea without blood or fever.

Enterotoxigenic *E. coli* (ETEC)

ETEC accounts for 20% of diarrhoeal cases, second only to rotavirus as a cause of in-patient gastroenteritis in developing countries. Transmission is by the faeco-oral route either directly or via contaminated food or water. It may account for up to 80% of **"traveller's diarrhoea"** which is said to affect between 20–50% of the estimated 12 million travellers from industrialized countries to the tropics/subtropics annually. Other causes of traveller's diarrhoea are listed opposite.

Clinical features: toxins stimulate Cl^-, Na^+ and water efflux into the intestinal lumen, resulting in voluminous, watery diarrhoea after an incubation period of 1–2 days. Vomiting and abdominal cramps are frequently a feature and up to 10 motions per day may be passed.

Diagnosis: depends upon culture of *E. coli* from the faeces, though usually by the time this is done symptoms have subsided.

Management: is for dehydration. Trimethoprim or ciprofloxacin are most likely to be effective in severe disease.

Enterotoxin-producing *S. aureus*

Commonly spread from the milk of cows with staphylococcal mastitis, but may also grow in prepared foods. The incubation time is short; 2–6hrs. (since the enterotoxin is preformed).

Clinical features: vomiting rapidly followed by diarrhoea which may be very severe, though usually short-lived.

Management: is supportive; antibiotics are useless.

Causes of acute diarrhoea without blood:

1. Almost any infection in a child or neonate, notably rotavirus in infants.
2. Malaria, especially *P. falciparum* (see chapter 3A).
3. Mild shigellosis, salmonella enterocolitis, or *Campylobacter* infections.
4. Enterotoxigenic *E. coli* (commonly causing traveller's diarrhoea).
5. Enterotoxin-producing strains of *Staphylococcus aureus*.
6. Giardiasis.
7. Cholera.
8. Food poisoning by *Clostridium* spp.
9. Cryptosporidiosis.
10. Strongyloidiasis
11. Food toxins.

Causes of traveller's diarrhoea:

Enterotoxigenic *E.coli*	30–80%
Campylobacter jejuni	~20%
Shigella spp.	5–15%
Salmonella spp.	3–15%
Giardia intestinalis	0–3%
Unknown	15–20%

Giardiasis

Giardia intestinalis (also known as *G. lamblia, G. duodenalis*) is the most common human protozoan GI pathogen, having a world-wide distribution. Its prevalence rates can reach ~30% in the tropics, with infection being highest in infants and children. It causes 3% of traveller's diarrhoea.

Transmission: the cysts can survive for long periods outside the host in suitable environments eg. surface water. They are notably NOT killed by chlorination. Infection follows ingestion of cysts in faecally contaminated water (rarely food) or through direct person to person contact. Partial immunity may be acquired through repeated infections.

Clinical features: in endemic areas, the asymptomatic carrier state is common. Symptoms of acute disease usually begin within 3–20 days of infection; most patients recover within 2–4 weeks, although in 25% of travellers symptoms persist for up to 7 weeks. Diarrhoea is the major symptom; it is watery initially, becoming steatorrhoeic and often associated with nausea, abdominal discomfort, bloating, weight loss, and sometimes sulphurous, offensive burps.

Some patients develop a chronic diarrhoea associated with weight losses of up to 20% of ideal body weight, fat malabsorption, deficiencies (particularly of vitamins A and B_{12}), and in some cases 2° hypolactasia.

Complications: growth and development may be retarded in severely affected infants and children, in whom malabsorption exacerbates malnutrition. Chronic giardiasis is associated with allergic and inflammatory conditions such as lymphoid nodular hyperplasia. Protein-losing enteropathy, lactose intolerance, and irritable bowel syndrome have been reported in W African children.

Diagnosis: detection of cysts (and occasionally trophozoites) in faecal samples by light microscopy. Examine 3 separate samples, since cysts are excreted only intermittently. Trophozoites may be detected in biopsies of small intestine mucosa. ELISA tests now exist for faecal *Giardia* antigens. Serology is not useful because of cross-reactivity in non-infected individuals in endemic areas.

Management

1. Careful rehydration and symptomatic relief is usually sufficient.
2. If symptoms persist, an antigiardial drug will decrease the severity and duration of symptoms. It is not clear whether asymptomatic carriers in endemic areas should be treated.
   Drug failure due to resistance is increasing. Recommended drugs include metronidazole, mepacrine and furazolidone.

Prevention: attention to personal hygiene, appropriate treatment of water supplies, encouraging breast feeding (shown to partially protect against infection). Research continues into possible vaccines.

Trophozoites of *Giardia* spp in stool isolates

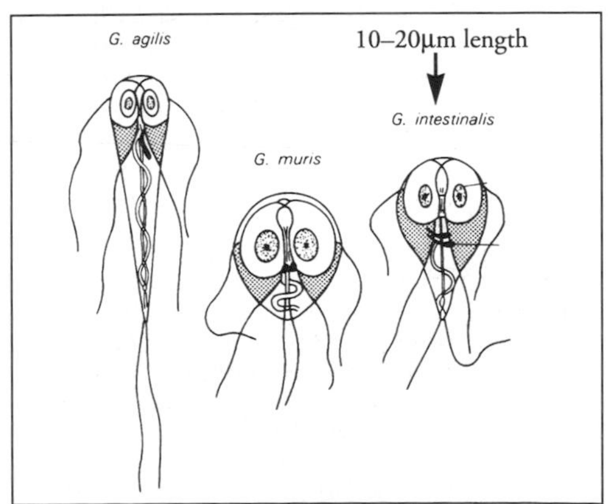

Cholera

The enterotoxic *Vibrio cholerae* produces a characteristically watery diarrhoea, often described as a rice-water stool, which if untreated may be fatal in up to 80% of cases. Vibrios are Gram-negative, aerobic, comma-shaped rods which are oxidase positive, ferment both sucrose and glucose but not lactose and can be divided into several serovars with *V. cholerae* 01 causing cholera.

V. cholerae is killed by heating at 55°C for 15 mins and by most disinfectants yet it can survive in saline conditions for up to two weeks at ambient temperatures. In most cases the bacteria survive for only limited periods on foodstuffs, with the notable exception of chitinous shellfish upon which they may survive for 14 days if refrigerated.

Transmission: humans are the only known natural host. Infection usually requires a large infective dose and occurs via contaminated food or water. The incubation period ranges from a few hours to 5 days. Only a minority of infected people develop symptoms – studies suggest that there are ~40 asymptomatic carriers of El Tor to every symptomatic case (~5:1 for classical biotype). This is true both in endemic areas and during outbreaks, hence the need for meticulous hygiene.

Clinical features: symptomatic infection varies between mild self-limiting diarrhoea and severe watery diarrhoea of up to 30 litres per day. Even severe diarrhoea is painless; it leads to electrolyte imbalances, metabolic acidosis, prostration, and death from dehydration within hours. Vomiting commences shortly after the onset of diarrhoea in 80% of cases. Shock typically follows ~12hrs later, with impaired consciousness due to hypovolaemia and hypoglycaemia. This is particularly bad in children who, unlike adults, may have a mild fever. Renal failure, ileus, and cardiac arrhythmias accelerate death, which may occur in untreated cases within 12hrs. Muscular and abdominal cramps occur owing to loss of Ca^{2+} and Cl^- ions.

Diagnosis: in epidemics, the diagnosis may be made on clinical grounds alone. In non-epidemic periods or places, acute watery diarrhoea resulting in severe dehydration or the death of a patient over 5yrs should suggest cholera. Dark-field microscopy of faecal material shows comma-shaped bacteria darting about; this is quickly halted upon addition of diluted 01 antisera. Transportation of samples should be in alkaline peptone water and kept cool. Culture requires selective media such as TCBS agar. If possible, specimens should be sent to a reference laboratory for bio- and serotyping.

Management of cholera

1. In all but a few cases treatment consists solely of meticulous attention to rehydration, usually with oral preparations. This will reduce mortality to less than 1%. See below for rehydration management. In some emergency cases where ORS was not available, sucrose and rice-water-based solutions have been given with success.

Epidemiology of *V. cholerae*

V. cholerae serovar 01 is the causative agent of cholera. There are two biotypes of the 01 serovar: classical and El Tor; each of these biotypes is further divided into three serotypes: Ogawa, Inaba and Hikojima.

The classical biotype caused the first six cholera pandemics in south Asia during the 19th and early 20th centuries. The El Tor biotype was first recognized in 1906 but until 1963 was restricted to Sulawesi. During the 1960s, the seventh pandemic started with spread of the El Tor biotype, Inaba serotype, out of Indonesia into South Asia, Africa and, since 1991, Latin America. This biotype has now replaced the classical biotype throughout much of the world, except Bangladesh.

Other *V. cholerae* serovars cause a cholera-like illness. The 0139 serotype first appeared in southern India in 1992. Unlike other non-01 strains, it caused cholera with similar epidemiological and clinical pictures to 01 cholera. The major difference noted in Bangladesh is that it tends to affect adults. Previous exposure to the 01 serovar does not confer protection.

2. Antibiotics should be given to only the most severe cases, where they have been shown to reduce both the volume and duration of diarrhoea.
   • doxycycline is the drug of choice for adults (except pregnant women) in whom a single dose of 300mg is sufficient.
   • tetracycline 500mg PO qds for 3 days can be given to adults, although resistance has been reported in central Asia and Africa.
   ►Follow local guidelines based on susceptibilities.
   • give children or pregnant women co-trimoxazole 30mg/kg PO daily. This may also be used for adults: 960mg PO bd for 3 days.

Prevention: public health measures aimed at improving food and water hygiene and sanitation are the most important factors. Currently, killed whole cell vaccines are available and although they offer some individual protection (50–60%), their use in outbreaks is not recommended.

Health education: plays a major role in both preventing outbreaks and limiting the spread of infection once one occurs. This should not only concentrate upon ensuring food and water hygiene, but also such additional measures as disinfecting patients' clothing by boiling for 5 mins, drying out bedding in the sun, burying stools, etc. In larger health centres, patient excreta may be mixed with disinfectant (eg. cresol) or acid before disposal in pit latrines. Semi-solid waste should be incinerated. Funerals should be held quickly and near to the place of death, discouraging the arrival of mourners from uninfected areas, ritual washing of the dead, and funeral feasts (if this is culturally possible).

The cholera outbreak

Under the terms of the International Health Regulations of 1969, it is obligatory to notify the WHO of all cholera cases. Suspected cases should be reported immediately by national health authorities and laboratory confirmation sent as soon as it is obtained. This should be followed by weekly reports containing the number of new cases and deaths since the last report, the cumulative totals for the year, and if possible the age distribution and number of patients admitted to hospital, all preferably recorded by region or other geographical division (see chapter 1 for more information). This data should be sent to WHO headquarters as well as to the appropriate regional office.

Usually there is a national coordinating committee to implement and regulate control and prevention measures, though often it is up to the front-line doctors to initiate the process and frequently they remain in close collaboration with national and international bodies. Mobile control teams may be needed in inaccessible areas or in countries with no national co-ordination and these are responsible for: establishing and operating temporary treatment centres, training local staff, educating the public, carrying out epidemiological studies, collecting stool, food and water samples for laboratory analysis, and providing emergency logistical support to health posts and laboratories. Emergency treatment centres may be needed if appropriate facilities do not exist or are swamped with patients. These should aim for simple, rapid treatment. Strict isolation or quarantine measures are not needed.

Estimated minimum supplies needed to treat 100 patients during a cholera outbreak[1]

- 650 packets of ORS solution (1 litre)
- 120 bags of 1 litre Ringer's lactate solution,[2] with giving sets
- 10 scalp vein sets
- 3 NG tubes, 5.3mm outside diameter (16 French), 50cm long for adults
- 3 NG tubes; 2.7mm outside diameter (8 French), 38cm long for children.

For adults:

- 60 capsules of doxycycline 100mg (3 caps per severely dehydrated adult patient)
  or
- 480 capsules of tetracycline 250mg (24 capsules per severely dehydrated patient).

For children:

- 300 tablets of trimethoprim-sulphamethoxazole 120mg (15 tablets per severely dehydrated child).

***If selective chemoprophylaxis is planned*:**
the additional requirements for 4 close contacts per severely dehydrated patient (c. 80 people) are:

- 240 capsules of doxycycline 100mg (3 capsules per person)
  or
- 1920 capsules of tetracycline 250mg (24 capsules per person).

Other necessary supplies:

- 2 large water dispensers with tap for bulk ORS manufacture
- 20 1litre bottles, 20 half-litre bottles for ORS dispensing
- 40 200ml cups
- 20 teaspoons
- 5kg cotton wool
- 3 reels of adhesive tape.

1. The supplies listed are sufficient for IV fluid followed by oral rehydration salts for 20 severely dehydrated patients and for ORS alone for 80 patients
2. If Ringer's lactate solution is unavailable, physiological saline may be substituted.

Clostridium perfringens

Clostridium perfringens produces two forms of gastrointestinal disease: simple food poisoning (caused by type A) and necrotic enterocolitis (type C).

1. Food poisoning – see opposite.

2. Necrotic enterocolitis (pigbel)

This is common in Uganda, SE Asia, China, and the highlands of Papua New Guinea. It occurs when *C. perfringens* type C is eaten, normally in meat, by people who are malnourished, heavily infected with *Ascaris lumbricoides*, or have a diet rich in sweet potatoes. The latter two are associated with high levels of heat-stable trypsin inhibitors which inhibit the luminal proteases, preventing them inactivating the toxin.

Clinical features: symptoms usually begin 48 hrs following ingestion but may start up to one week later. It is classified into 4 types:

- Type I (***acute toxic***) presents with fulminant toxaemia and shock. It usually occurs in young children and carries an 85% mortality rate.
- Type II (***acute surgical***) presents as mechanical or paralytic ileus, acute strangulation, perforation, or peritonitis. It has a 40% mortality.
- Type III (***subacute surgical***) presents later, with features similar to type II. Mortality is also ~40%.
- Type IV is of ***mild diarrhoea*** only, though it may progress to type III.

In types II–III a thickened segment of bowel is sometimes palpable. Blood and pus are passed with the stool in severe disease.

Diagnosis: isolation of *C. perfringens* from stool or peritoneal fluid culture. Serological diagnosis is also possible.

Management: type I and II disease require urgent surgery after appropriate resuscitation. Give IV chloramphenicol or benzylpenicillin and *C. perfringens* type C antiserum, where available. Milder cases may require glucose and electrolyte infusions, with IV broad-spectrum antibiotics if there are signs of extraintestinal spread. Give an antihelminthic effective against *Ascaris*. Oral food intake should commence after 24hrs.

Prevention: immunization with type C toxoid has greatly reduced the incidence and severity of the disease in Papua New Guinea.

Cryptosporidiosis

The protozoan *Cryptosporidium parvum* is a common opportunistic infection in HIV$^+$ patients. It also causes outbreaks of diarrhoea in the immunocompetent after drinking lamb or calf faeces-contaminated water. It accounts for up to 17% of childhood diarrhoea in the developing world, with a mortality during the first year of life of ~3%.

Clinical features: non-specific chronic diarrhoeal illness, often present for >5 months. It may be severe, mimicking cholera, in AIDS patients.
Diagnosis: faecal detection of the oocysts (red spheres in ZN stain).
Management: rehydration with symptomatic relief; as yet, no drug has been shown to be effective against this organism.

Food poisoning from bacteria or their toxins

Organism/toxin	*Principal foods*	*Time after food*	*Clinical features*
Staph. aureus	Meat, poultry, dairy produce	1–6hrs	D, V & AP
B. cereus	Fried rice, sauces, vegetables	1–5hrs 6–16hrs	V D, AP
Red bean toxin		1–6hrs	D, V
Zinc		1–6hrs	V, AP
Scombrotoxin	Fish	1–6hrs	D, flushing, sweating mouth pain
Mushroom toxin		1–6hrs	D, V, AP
Ciguatera	Fish	1–6hrs	fits, coma, renal/liver failure
Salmonella spp	Meat, poultry, dairy produce	8–72hrs (mean 12–36hrs)	D, V, AP, fever
Campylobacter spp	Poultry, raw milk, eggs	1–10 days (mean 2–5 days)	D, AP
C. perfringens A	Cooked meat	8–24hrs (mean 8–15hrs)	D, AP, V
Vibrio parahaemoliticus	Seafood	4–96hrs (mean 12hrs)	D, V, AP, cramp, headache
Shigella spp	Faecal contamination	1–7 days (mean 1–3 days)	D(bloody), V, fever
C. botulinum	Poorly canned food, smoked meats	2hrs–8 days (mean 12–36hrs)	diplopia, paralysis
L.monocytogenes	Dairy produce, meat, vegetables, seafood	1–7 weeks	septicaemia, septic abortion
E. coli	Dirty water	8–44hrs	D, V, cramps
Y. enterocolitica	Pork and beef	24–36hrs	fever, AP, D

V = vomiting, D = diarrhoea, AP = abdominal pain.

Chronic diarrhoea

Defined as diarrhoea lasting >2 weeks. Causes are listed opposite.

Malabsorption and steatorrhoea

May be due to a wide range of causes. The key signs and symptoms are:

1. Diarrhoea: stool is typically loose, bulky, offensive, greasy, light coloured and difficult to flush away.
2. Abdominal symptoms: discomfort, distension, flatulence.
3. Nutritional deficiencies: eg glossitis, pallor, muscle pain bruising, hyperpigmentation, CNS or PNS signs, skeletal deformity.
4. General ill health: anorexia, weight loss, lethargy, dyspnoea, fatigue.
5. Features related to underlying cause: surgical scars, systemic disease.

Investigating malabsorption

Do FBC, U&Es ESR, LFTs, stool culture and microscopy. Others include

- ***Faecal fat:*** steatorrhoea with >2g/day faecal fat (on a 3 day diet containing 100g total fat) is indicative of malabsorption. Levels <20g/day are more likely to be due to absorptive dysfunction (eg tropical sprue, coeliac disease), whereas severe steatorrhoea (>20g/day faecal fat) is usually due to digestive anomalies (eg pancreatitis) and may warrant abdominal USS, and ERCP. Steatorrhoea may be accompanied by deficiency of fat-soluble vitamins (A, D, E & K). Check the INR.
- ***Carbohydrate absorption:*** plasma glucose is measured after a standard oral dose of glucose (see glucose tolerance test). Malabsorption tends to result in a lower than normal rise, whilst pancreatic disease gives a greater than normal rise. ***Xylose absorption test:*** is a better test; 5g oral dose of xylose is eaten and urinary xylose excretion monitored for 5hrs. Greater than 22% excretion is normal, assuming normal gastric emptying and renal function.
- ***The Schilling test:*** may be used as a measure of ileal function, in the absence of other causes of vitamin B_{12} malabsorption. If a low level is obtained, the test should be repeated, giving intrinsic factor with the vitamin B_{12}. If the result remains low, malabsorption is due to ileal pathology. If it is normal, however, it suggests a diagnosis of pernicious anaemia, or other gastric disease.

Clinical malabsorption

1° hypolactasia (a lactase deficiency of genetic origin) is a common non-infectious cause of watery diarrhoea in the tropics. 2° hypolactasia results from brush border damage during GI infection; it may persist afterwards. Incomplete hydrolysis of lactose results in osmotic diarrhoea, abdominal pain, distension, and flatulence. Colonic bacteria may produce lactic acid by hydrolysing of lactose – this can also cause an irritative diarrhoea.

Diagnosis: rests upon detection of worsening symptoms with increased lactose intake (lactose tolerance test), the hydrogen breath test, or a lactase assay in a jejunal biopsy. ***Management:*** consists of eliminating lactose-containing products from the diet, sometimes attempting their gradual reintroduction after 6 weeks without symptoms.

Causes of chronic diarrhoea:

1. Subclinical malabsorption
2. Hypolactasia (1° and 2°)
3. Tropical sprue
4. Strongyloidiasis
5. HIV enteropathy
6. Enteropathogenic *E.coli*
7. Chronic calcific pancreatitis
8. Intestinal flukes
9. Chronic intestinal schistosomiasis
10. Short bowel disease (eg recovered pigbel disease)
11. Lymphoma – Burkitt's & Mediterranean
12. Ileocaecal TB
13. Acute and chronic liver disease
14. Inflammatory bowel disease and coeliac disease

Causes of malabsorption

- ***Infective***
  acute enteritis, intestinal TB, parasitic infections, traveller's diarrhoea, Whipple's disease.
- ***Anatomical/motility***
  blind loops, diverticulae, strictures, fistulae, small bowel lymphoma, systemic sclerosis, diabetes mellitus, pseudo-obstruction, radiotherapy, amyloidosis, lymphatic obstruction (TB, lymphoma, cardiac disease).
- ***Defective digestion***
  chronic pancreatitis, cystic fibrosis, food sensitivity (lactose, gluten), malnutrition, gastric/intestinal surgery, Zollinger-Ellison syndrome, pancreatectomy, biliary obstruction, terminal ileal disease/resection (short bowel syndrome), parenchymal liver disease, bacterial overgrowth.
- ***Drugs***
  antibiotics, cholestyramine, metformin, methyldopa, alcohol, antacids, purgative misuse, para-aminosalicylic acid.

Post-infective malabsorption (PIM or tropical sprue)

A better name for this syndrome of diarrhoea, malabsorption, and weight loss is post-acute infective malabsorption, since a chronicity of at least 2 months is required for the diagnosis. Malabsorption of nutrients is quantitatively more important than that of water or electrolytes in this condition. It produces an estimated 10% deficit of dietary energy. It is therefore obvious that its impact on individuals (particularly children) living on marginal diets is significant and that it will quickly exacerbate malnutrition. PIM is common in central America, northern S America and Asia; it also occurs around the Mediterranean and in the Middle East.

Aetiology: is thought to involve i) genes – an association with certain HLA antigens has been found; ii) infection – *Klebsiella pneumoniae, Enterobacter cloacae,* and *E. coli* are the organisms most commonly isolated from mucosal biopsy or luminal fluid; they may persist in overgrowth for many months; and iii) jejunal morphology – partial villous atrophy, crypt hyperplasia, elevated jejunal surface pH, and changes in gut hormones and colonic function have been found.

Clinical features: chronic diarrhoea of >2 months duration with large, pale, fatty stools and often flatulence. Other features include weight loss; glossitis; megaloblastic anaemia; fluid retention; depression; lethargy; amenorrhoea, and infertility. Serum folate and vitamin B_{12} may fall to very low levels. Hypoalbuminaemia and oedema are late signs.

Investigations 1hr blood xylose concentration following a 5g or 25g loading dose; 72hr faecal fat estimation; Schilling test; serum B_{12}; RBC folate concentration; serum globin and albumin. Exclude faecal parasites. Barium meal and follow-through will show dilated loops of jejunum with clumping of barium. Jejunal biopsy may show a ridged or convoluted mucosa, depending on the duration of the disease, with T lymphocyte infiltration.

Management

1. Eliminate bacterial overgrowth with tetracycline 250 mg PO qds for at least 2 weeks.
2. Aid mucosal recovery by providing folate supplements.
3. Provide a suitable diet to promote weight gain.
4. Give symptomatic relief in the acute stages:

- codeine phosphate 30 mg PO tds *or*
- loperamide 2mg after each loose stool, to a maximum of 6–8mg daily.

Tropical enteropathy and subclinical malabsorption

Repeated low-grade viral, bacterial, and parasitic infections may also cause damage to the small intestinal mucosa of individuals living in the tropics. Concurrent systemic infections (eg TB, pneumococcal pneumonia), malnutrition, and pellagra have also been implicated in causing subclinical malabsorption. Xylose, glucose and vitamin B_{12} are most commonly malabsorbed.

Distribution of tropical sprue

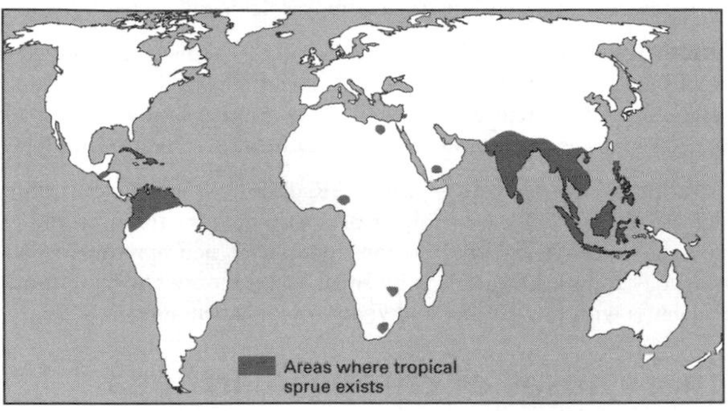

Pathogenesis of tropical sprue

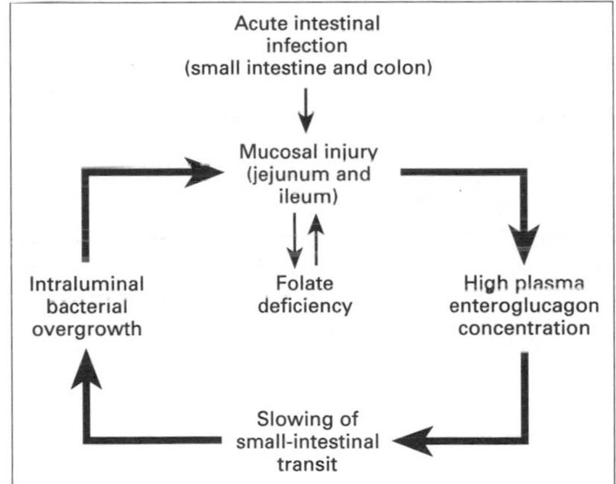

Other causes of malabsorption

Whipples disease – a rare malabsorptive condition characterized by transient migratory polyarthritis, fever, lymphadenopathy, and cardiac and neurological complications. It is caused by *Tropheryma whippei*. Treatment is with penicillin, tetracycline or co-trimoxazole; many patients relapse.

Lymphangiectasia – either 1° or following an abdominal malignancy, it results in lacteal dilatation. Clinically there is peripheral oedema secondary to hypoproteinaemia owing to a protein-losing enteropathy. Diagnosis requires small bowel biopsy. Treatment is with a low fat diet.

Abetalipoproteinaemia – a rare AR disorder, usually presenting in childhood due to defective triglyceride transport from the liver and gut. Eventually neurological dysfunction (peripheral neuropathy, cerebellar ataxia) may follow. Diagnosis is by small bowel biopsy and symptomatic treatment is with low-fat diet and vitamin supplementation.

Other causes of chronic diarrhoea

1. Enteropathogenic *E. coli* (EPEC)

A major cause of infantile diarrhoea that is spread by the faeco-oral route. It is also associated with traveller's diarrhoea. The mucosal brush border is lost by a process of vesiculation resulting in malabsorption and osmotic diarrhoea.

Clinical features: relapsing severe and prolonged diarrhoea, usually with mucus but no blood. Initially there may be vomiting and fever. Fatality in untreated epidemics can reach 50%. Diagnosis rests upon culture of EPEC from the stool or duodenal aspirate.

Management: rehydration. If the diarrhoea is prolonged, enteral or parenteral feeding and antibiotics may be required. Use trimethoprim since ampicillin is unlikely to be effective.

2. Chronic calcific pancreatitis

A syndrome of pancreatic calcification associated with both exocrine and endocrine impairment is commonly encountered in the tropics, especially equatorial Africa, southern India, and Indonesia. Its aetiology is unknown, although childhood kwashiorkor, gastroenteritis, dehydration and ingestion of cassava (*Manhiot esculenta*) have all been implicated.

Clinical features: are of chronic malabsorption with weight loss, often associated with DM (10% of diabetes in E&W Africa) and (sometimes severe) pain. There is an association with pancreatic malignancy.

Management: consists of diabetic control, a low-fat diet, and enzymatic supplementation eg pancreatin BP, 6g orally with food.

Pancreatic dysfunction may also result from schistosomiasis, trichinellosis, cysticercosis, clonorchiasis, opisthorchiasis and hydatid disease. Obstruction is commonly a complication of *A. lumbricoides* infection.

Mechanisms of steatorrhoea

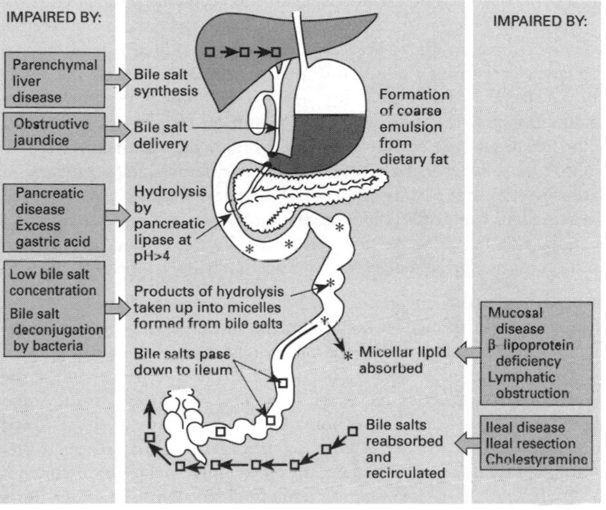

3. Intestinal lymphoma

A wide variety of lymphomas affect the GI tract, originating in either intestinal lymph nodes (eg Hodgkin's lymphoma) or mucosa associated lymphoid tissue (MALT lymphomas). Weight loss is a common feature and nodal disease may be confused with intestinal TB, as X-ray changes appear similar. Diagnosis requires biopsy.

Strongyloidiasis

The nematode *Strongyloides stercoralis* is a common infection of humans worldwide, particularly in parts of S America and SE Asia. It is a serious condition in the immunosuppressed. There are two adult forms of the worm and two larval forms, one of which is infective.

Life cycle: this is complex, since reproduction can take place in either of two cycles; the external cycle involving free-living worms and the internal cycle involving parasitic worms. Contamination of skin or buccal mucosa with larvae-containing soil permits initial penetration of larvae and infection. The larvae travel to the lungs and enter the bronchi, eventually passing onto the small intestine, where they mature into adults. Eggs produced by the female pass out in the faeces and continue the external cycle.

Autoinfection occurs by either bronchial larvae producing progeny or filariform larvae not passing out in the stool, but reinvading bowel or perianal skin. This can produce indefinite (up to 30yrs) multiplication within the host, not requiring further infection. The pre-patent period from infection to the appearance of larvae in the stools is ~1 month.

Clinical features: infection is asymptomatic in most instances, except for autoinfection through perianal skin. The immune response limits the infection to the small bowel and also the number of adult worms.

Larval penetration causes petechial haemorrhages and pruritis at the site of entry, frequently with a linear, red eruption (larva currens) as the larvae migrate under the skin. This is normally transient, but may be followed by congestion and oedema. A creeping urticarial rash may occur in presensitized individuals following reinfection. Symptoms similar to bronchopneumonia with consolidation may result from larval invasion of the lungs which, together with eosinophilia, may resemble TPE. Watery diarrhoea with mucus is a frequent symptom; its intensity is dependent upon the worm burden. It often alternates with constipation. In severe cases, chronic diarrhoea with malabsorption may ensue.

In the immunosuppressed, malnourished or debilitated, massive tissue invasion may occur. Complications include severe diarrhoea, ileus, hepatomegaly, and multisystem disease due to blood/lymphatic spread. Granulomata and/or abscesses occur in the liver, kidneys, and lungs; CNS involvement produces pyogenic meningitis and encephalopathy. Death is usually a result of septicaemia with *E. coli* carried by the larvae.

Diagnosis: detection of adults or rhabditiform larvae in the stool. Also modified Beesmann technique agar plate culture, ELISA and serology.
►Look for *S. stercoralis* infection in the immunosuppressed or those who are about to be immunosuppressed eg put on steroids.

Management – ► treat all infected patients, not just the symptomatic.

1. Albendazole 400mg PO bd for 3 days
   [alternatives: ivermectin 200µg/kg PO as a single dose or thiabendazole 25mg/kg PO bd for 3 days].
2. Massive infection also responds well to albendazole.

Prevention: requires improving hygiene and education on a community level, as well as monitoring and evaluation.

S. stercoralis larva in stool sample. Size 200–300 × 15μm.

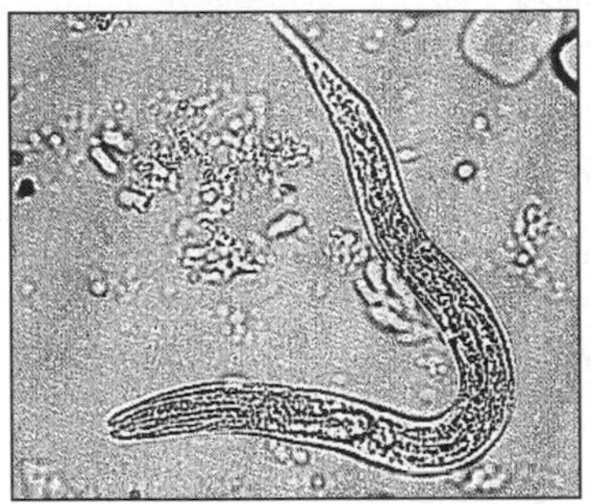

Intestinal flukes

These pathogens are common throughout Asia (particularly SE Asia), where their prevalence may reach 30% in certain populations. Children are more heavily infected and prone to symptoms.

1. Fasciolopsiasis

Caused by *Fasciolopsis buski*, infection is via consumption of metacercaria attached to the seed pods of water plants contaminated by human and pig faeces.

2. Echinostomiasis

At least fifteen *Echinostoma* spp infect humans via the consumption of raw or undercooked freshwater snails, clams, fish, and tadpoles. In NE Thailand, it is commonly associated with *Opisthorchis* infection.

3. Heterophyasis

Numerous species of the small (2.5mm) *Heterophyes* flukes infect humans following consumption of raw aquatic foods and/or insect larvae.

Clinical features: the attachment of parasites to the intestinal mucosa results in inflammation and ulcer formation. Infections are frequently asymptomatic; when symptoms do occur, they are usually mild and non-specific: diarrhoea, flatulence, mild abdominal pains, vomiting, fever and anorexia. Fasciolopsiasis may produce severe disease with ascites, oedema, anaemia, and symptomatic malabsorption. Eggs (and sometimes adult worms) of *Heterophyes* spp may enter the lymphatics after mucosal penetration and be transported to other sites (notably heart, spinal cord, brain, lungs, liver and spleen) where they cause granulomatous reactions. Myocarditis and neurological deficits may result.

Diagnosis: faecal examination for eggs. Differentiation between *Fasciola hepatica*, *F. buski* and echinostomes is often difficult. Similarly, heterophydiae eggs closely resemble those of *Clonorchis* and *Opisthorchis.* Recovery of adult worms from post-treatment faeces allows a definitive diagnosis, although in the case of the heterophyids this is difficult owing to their small size. Extraintestinal cases of heterophyiasis are also difficult to diagnose – they are often only revealed during surgery or autopsy.

Management

1. Praziquantel is the drug of choice, with high efficacy at 10–20mg/kg as a single dose.
2. Mebendazole or albendazole may be used for echinostomiasis although praziquantel is recommended in areas where other trematodes are present, due to its broad efficacy.

Prevention: should concentrate on breaking the faeco-oral cycle (eg stopping the use of human and pig excreta as fertilizer) possibly combined with community-based praziquantel treatment and education regarding the consumption of raw/undercooked foodstuffs.

Eggs of *Fasciolopsis buski* (top, 140 × 85 μm) and *Heterophyes heterophyes* (below, 25 × 15 μm).

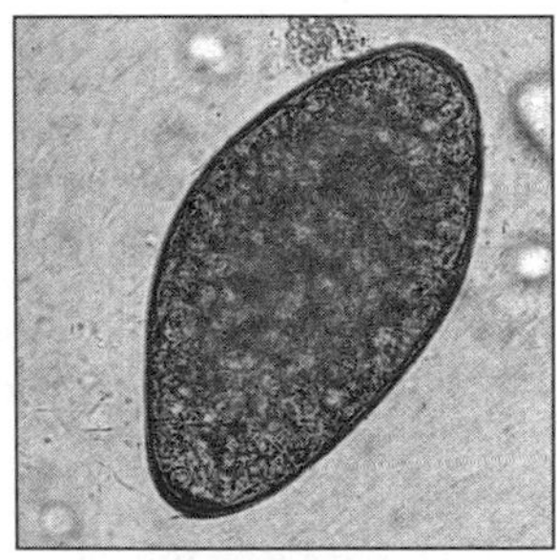

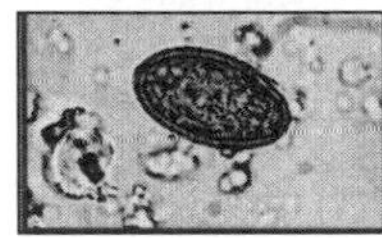

Dehydration[1]

The volume of fluid lost in the stool in 24hrs can vary from 5ml/kg to 200ml/kg, or more. The loss of electrolytes also varies. The total body sodium defect in young children with severe dehydration owing to diarrhoea is usually about 70–110mmol per litre of water lost. The degree of dehydration is graded according to the signs and symptoms which reflect the amount of fluid lost.

- In the early stages of dehydration, there are no signs or symptoms. As dehydration increases, these develop, including thirst, restless or irritable behaviour, decreased skin turgor, dry mucous membranes, sunken eyes, sunken fontanelle (in infants), and absence of tears when crying.
- In severe dehydration, these effects become more pronounced and the patient may develop signs of hypovolaemic shock, including decreased consciousness, anuria, cool moist extremities, rapid and feeble pulse, low blood pressure, and peripheral cyanosis. ► Death may follow swiftly if rehydration is not started at once.

Types of dehydration

1. ***Isotonic dehydration:*** is the most frequently encountered type of dehydration and occurs when the net losses of water and sodium are in the same proportion as is normally found in the extracellular fluid (ECF). The principal features of isotonic dehydration are: a balanced deficit of water and sodium; normal serum sodium concentration (130–150 mmol/l); normal serum osmolality (275–295 mOsmol/l); hypovolaemia as a result of excess ECF losses. Clinical features are those of hypovolaemic shock, ie thirst, reduced skin turgor, dry mucous membranes, sunken eyes, oliguria, and a sunken fontanelle in infants. This progresses to anuria, hypotension, a weak pulse, cool extremities and eventually coma and death.
2. ***Hypertonic (hypernatraemic) dehydration:*** reflects a net loss of water in excess of sodium and tends to occur in infants only. It usually results from attempted treatment of diarrhoea with fluids that are hypertonic (eg sweetened fruit juices/soft drinks, glucose solution) combined with insufficient intake of water and other hypotonic solutes. Hypertonic solutions cause water to flow from the ECF into the intestine, leading to decreased ECF volume and hypernatraemia. The principal features are: a deficit of water; hypernatraemia (>150 mmol/l); serum osmolality >295 mOsmol/l; severe thirst; irritability; and convulsions (especially if serum Na^+ is >165 mmol/l).
3. ***Hypotonic (hyponatraemic) dehydration*** occurs in patients with diarrhoea who drink large amounts of water or other hypotonic fluids containing very low quantities of salt and other solutes. It also occurs in patients who receive IV infusions of 5% glucose in water. It occurs because water is absorbed from the gut while the loss of salt continues, producing a net excess of water and hyponatraemia. The features are: dehydration with hyponatraemia (serum Na^+ <130 mmol/l); low serum osmolality (<275 mOsmol/l); lethargy and, rarely, convulsions.

1. *The Treatment of Diarrhoea. A Manual for Physicians and Other Senior Health Workers*, WHO: Geneva 1990

Assessment of dehydration in patients with diarrhoea

1. Look at:

Condition	well, alert	*restless, irritable	*lethargic [a] or unconscious
Eyes[b]	normal	sunken	very sunken, dry
Tears	present	absent	absent
Mouth[c]	moist	dry	very dry
Thirst	none	*very thirsty	*unable to drink
2. Pinch the skin:[d]			
	goes back quickly	goes back slowly	goes back very slowly
3. Decide:	**no dehydration**	**some dehydration**	**severe dehydration**
		Plans B and C require at least three signs including at least one marked *	
4. Treat:	*PLAN A*	*PLAN B*	*PLAN C*

Notes:

a. A lethargic patient is not simply asleep; the patient's mental state is dull and the patient cannot be fully awakened. The patient may appear to be drifting into unconsciousness.

b. In some infants, the eyes normally appear a little sunken, so ask the mother if the child's eyes appear normal to her.

c. Look at the buccal mucosa and tongue. The mouth may be moist in a dehydrated patient who has recently vomited or drunk fluids.

d. The skin pinch is less useful in malnourished children.

Estimation of fluid defect

Children with dehydration should be weighed without clothing, as an aid to estimating their fluid requirements. If weighing is not possible, the child's age may be used to estimate the weight. Treatment should never be delayed because scales are not readily available.

► A child's fluid defect may be estimated as follows:

Assessment	Fluid defect as % of body weight	Fluid defect in ml/kg body weight
No signs of dehydration	<5%	<50ml/kg
Some dehydration	5–10%	50–100ml/kg
Severe dehydration	>10%	>100ml/kg

Suitable fluids: many countries have designated recommended home fluids which should be used in the *prevention* of dehydration only (ie treatment plan A). Whenever possible, these should include at least one fluid that normally contains salt (oral rehydration solution (ORS); salted drinks eg salted rice water or salted yoghurt; vegetable or chicken soup with salt). Other fluids should be recommended that are frequently given to children in the area, that mothers consider acceptable for children with diarrhoea, and that the mothers would likely give in increased amounts if advised to do so. Such fluids should be safe and easy to prepare. ► If there are signs of dehydration, ORS should be used as in treatment plans B and C.

- Teaching mothers to add salt (about 3g/l) to unsalted drinks or soups during diarrhoea is beneficial, but requires education and (initially) supervision.
- A home made solution containing 3g/l salt and 18g/l of common sugar (sucrose) is effective, but the recipe is often forgotten and/or the ingredients hard to obtain.

Unsuitable fluids: a few fluids are potentially dangerous and should be avoided during episodes of diarrhoea. Especially important are drinks sweetened with sugar which can cause osmotic diarrhoea and hypernatraemia – eg soft drinks, sweetened fruit drinks, sweetened tea.

Oral rehydration solution (ORS)

The formula for ORS recommended by WHO and UNICEF is given in the box opposite. Where bulk preparation is required, multiply the amounts shown by however many litres of solution you wish to make. ORS should be used within 24hrs of preparation.

When given correctly, ORS provides sufficient water and electrolytes to correct the deficits associated with acute diarrhoea.

To make a litre of ORS solution from bulk ingredients

Ingredients:

1.	Sodium chloride	3.5g
	plus	
2.	Glucose (anhydrous)	20g
	or	
	Sucrose (common sugar)	40g
	or	
	Glucose (monohydrate)	22g
	plus	
3.	Trisodium citrate, dihydrate	2.9g
	or	
	Sodium bicarbonate	2.5g
	plus	
4.	Potassium chloride	1.5g

- Completely dissolve the sugar and salts in one litre of clean water – boiled or chlorinated water is best.
- ORS solution should be used within 24hrs, after which time it should be discarded and fresh solution prepared.
- To make 1 litre of rice-based ORS, boil 50g of rice powder in 1.1 litres of water. Mix in sugar and salt in the quantities stated above. Use within 12hrs.

Treatment plan A

► To treat diarrhoea without signs of dehydration at home

Use this plan to teach the mother to:

- continue to treat her child's current episode of diarrhoea at home
- give early treatment for future episodes of diarrhoea.

Explain the 3 rules for treating diarrhoea at home

1. ***Give the child more fluids than usual to prevent dehydration***
Use recommended home fluids (see above) and ORS as described below. NB: if the child is <6 months old and not yet taking solid foods, give ORS solution rather than a food-based fluid. Give as much of these fluids as the child will take. Use the amounts shown below for ORS as a guide. Continue giving these fluids until the diarrhoea stops.

2. ***Give the child plenty of food to prevent malnutrition***
Continue to breastfeed frequently. If the child is not breastfed, give the usual milk.
If the child is 6 months or older, or already taking solid foods, also give cereal or another starchy food mixed, if possible, with pulses, vegetables, meat, or fish. Add 1–2 tablespoons of vegetable oil to each serving. Give fresh fruit juice or mashed banana to provide potassium. Give freshly prepared foods. Cook and mash/grind food well.
Encourage the child to eat; offer food >5 times per day. Give the same foods after diarrhoea stops and give an extra meal each day for 2 weeks.

3. ***Take the child to a health worker if the diarrhoea does not improve within 3 days, or the child develops any of the following:***

- many watery stools
- fever
- repeated vomiting
- eating/drinking poorly
- marked thirst
- blood in the stool

Children should be given ORS at home if:

1. They have been on treatment plans B or C.
2. They cannot return to the health worker, but the diarrhoea gets worse.
3. It is national policy to give ORS to all children who see a health worker for diarrhoea.

How to give ORS

- Give a teaspoon every 1–2 mins for a child <2yrs.
- Give frequent sips from a cup to older children.
- If the child vomits, wait 10mins then give fluid more slowly.
- If diarrhoea persists after all ORS is used, use food based fluids (see above), or return to the health care centre with the child.

Amount of ORS to give according to child's age

Age	*After each loose stool*	*At home*
<2yrs	50–100ml	500ml/day
2–10yrs	100–200ml	1 litre/day
>10yrs	as much as tolerated	2 litres/day

Treatment plan B

►To treat mild dehydration

Approximate amounts of ORS to give in the first 4hrs of treatment

Age	Weight (kg)	ORS (mls)
<4mths	<5	200–400
4–11mths	5–8	400–600
1–2yrs	8–11	600–800
2–4yrs	11–16	800–1200
5–14yrs	16–30	1200–2200
>14yrs	>30	2200–4000

- Use the patient's age only when you do not know the weight. The required amount of ORS in ml can also be calculated approximately by multiplying the patient's weight by 75.
- If the patient wants more ORS than the dose shown, give more.
- Encourage the mother to continue breastfeeding the child.
- For infants <6 months who are not breastfed, give 100–200ml of clean water in addition to these ORS amounts within these 4 hrs.

NB during the initial stages of therapy, whilst still dehydrated, adults can consume up to 750ml per hour if necessary and children up to 20ml per kg body weight per hour.

Observe the patient carefully and help mothers to give ORS

1. Show the mother how much solution to give to her child.
2. Show the mother how to give it – a teaspoon every 1–2 mins for a child under 2 years, frequent sips from a cup for an older child.
3. Check from time to time to see if there are problems.
4. If a patient vomits, wait 10 mins and then continue giving ORS.
5. If the child's eyelids become oedematous, stop ORS and give plain water or breast milk. Give ORS according to plan A once the oedema has subsided.

After 4 hours, reassess the patient using the chart on p 163 and continue plan A, B or C as appropriate.

1. If there are no signs of dehydration, shift to plan A. When dehydration has been corrected, urine will start to be passed and children may become less irritable and fall asleep.
2. If signs indicating some dehydration are still present, repeat plan B, but start to offer food, milk, and juice as in plan A.
3. If signs indicating severe dehydration are present, treat according to plan C.

If the mother must leave the health post or hospital before completing treatment plan B:

- Show her how much ORS to give to finish the 4hr treatment period at home.
- Give her enough ORS packets to complete rehydration and for 3 more days, as in plan A.
- Show her how to prepare ORS.
- Explain to her the 3 rules in plan A for treating her child at home: give ORS until diarrhoea stops; feed the child more to prevent malnutrition; and bring the child back to the health post/hospital if symptoms persist.
- Make sure that all children >6 months are given some food before being sent home. Emphasize to the mother the importance of continuing feeding throughout the diarrhoeal episode.

Monitoring signs of oral rehydration therapy

Check the patient from time to time during rehydration to ensure that ORS is being taken satisfactorily and that signs of dehydration are not worsening. ► If at any time the patient develops severe dehydration, switch to treatment plan C. After 4 hours reassess the patient following the guidelines in the table on p 163. Decide what treatment to give next.

1. If signs of severe dehydration have appeared, IV therapy should be started immediately, following plan C. This is very unusual, however. It tends to occur in children who drink ORS poorly and continue to pass large volumes of watery stool during the rehydration period.
2. If the patient still has signs of mild dehydration, continue oral rehydration therapy following plan B. At the same time start to offer food, milk and other fluids as described in treatment plan A. Reassess the patient frequently.
3. If there are no signs of dehydration, the patient should be considered fully rehydrated. If this is the case: the skin pinch is normal; the thirst has subsided; urine is passed normally and the child is no longer irritable and may fall asleep.

Teach the mother to treat her child at home using ORS following plan A. Give her enough ORS sachets for 3 days and teach her the signs that indicate she must bring her child back to the health post.

Meeting normal fluid needs

While treatment to replace the existing water and electrolyte deficit is in progress the child's normal daily fluid requirements must also be met. This may be done as follows:

1. Breastfed infants: continue to breastfeed as often and as long as the infant wants to, even <u>during</u> oral rehydration therapy.
2. Non-breastfed infants under 6 months of age: during rehydration with ORS, give 100–200ml of plain water by mouth. After completing rehydration, resume full strength milk or formula feeds. Give water and other fluids normally taken by the infant.
3. Older children and adults: throughout rehydration treatment, offer as much plain water, milk, or juice as is accepted, in <u>addition</u> to ORS.

When oral rehydration therapy fails or is inappropriate

In about 5% of patients the signs of dehydration do not improve, or worsen after starting treatment with ORS. The usual causes are:

- continuing rapid stool loss (>15–20 ml/kg/hr), as may occur in cholera
- insufficient intake of ORS due to fatigue, lethargy, or lack of supervision
- frequent severe vomiting.

Such patients should be admitted to hospital and given ORS by NG tube or Ringer's Lactate solution 75ml/kg IV over 4hrs. Look for other signs of cholera infection and take necessary precautions. In most instances it will not be cholera and the patient will improve.

When not to give ORS:

Rarely, ORS should not be given. This is true for children with:

- abdominal distension due to paralytic ileus (often owing to opiate drugs such as codeine or loperamide or to hypokalaemia).
- glucose malabsorption, indicated by a marked increase in stool output as ORS is started. There is no improvement and the stool contains large amounts of glucose.

► In these situations rehydration should be given intravenously until diarrhoea subsides.

Treatment plan C

► For patients with severe dehydration in hospital

Can you give IV fluids immediately? If not, see below.

1. Patients who can drink, however poorly, should be given ORS until the IV drip is running. In addition, *all* children should begin to receive some ORS (5ml/kg/hr) as soon as they can drink without difficulty, which is usually within 3–4 hours. This provides additional base and potassium which may not be adequately supplied by the IV fluid.

2. Start IV infusion of 100ml/kg of Ringer's Lactate[a] (Hartmann's solution) as soon as possible. Divide the dose as follows:

Age	First give 30 ml/kg in:	Then give 70 ml/kg in:
<12 mths	1 hour[b]	5 hours
>12 mths	30 minutes	2.5 hours

3. Reassess the patient every 1–2 hours. If the state of hydration is not improving, give the IV fluid more rapidly.

4. After 6 hours (infants <12 months) or 3 hours (>12 months), evaluate the patient using the assessment chart (p 163). Follow the appropriate treatment plan to continue treatment.

Notes

[a] If Ringer's Lactate solution is not available, isotonic saline is an acceptable substitute – see opposite.

[b] Repeat once if radial pulse is weak or not detectable.

Monitoring IV rehydration therapy

- Patients should be reassessed every 15–20 mins until a strong radial pulse is present.
- Thereafter, they should be assessed hourly to confirm that hydration is improving. If it is not, the IV fluid may be run at a faster rate.
- When the planned amount of IV fluid bas been given (6hrs for infants, 3 hrs for older patients), the patient's state of hydration should be reassessed using the chart on p. 163.
  If there are still signs of severe dehydration, repeat plan C. This is unusual, but may occur in cases of cholera and children who pass frequent, watery stools during the rehydration period.
  If the patient shows signs of mild dehydration, discontinue IV fluid replacement and commence oral rehydration with ORS for 4hrs according to plan B.
  If there are no signs of dehydration, discontinue IV therapy and commence ORS treatment according to plan A.
- Observe the patient for at least 6hrs before discharging.
- For children, ensure that the mother is able to continue giving ORS at home and is aware of the signs that indicate she must bring the child back.

Alternative solutions for IV rehydration

- *Ringer's Lactate solution with 5% dextrose* – provides glucose to help prevent hypoglycaemia. If available, it is preferred to Ringer's Lactate solution without dextrose.
- *Physiological saline* (0.9% NaCl, also called normal saline) – widely available, it is an acceptable alternative to Ringer's Lactate solution, but contains neither a base to correct acidosis nor potassium to correct K^+ losses. Sodium bicarbonate or sodium lactate (20–30mmol /l) and potassium chloride (5–15 mmol/l) may be added.
- *Half strength Darrow's solution* is made by diluting full-strength Darrow's solution with an equal volume of glucose solution (50g/l or 100g/l). Note that it contains less sodium than is required to replace the sodium lost in diarrhoea.

►► Plain glucose (dextrose) solution **should not be used** since it does not contain any sodium, base, or potassium and does not correct hypovolaemia effectively.

When no IV fluid is available

1. Is there the facility for IV infusions within 30mins travelling time? If so transfer the patient, giving ORS as frequently as tolerated.
If not:

2. Is there the facility for nasogastric intubation? If so, insert a NG tube and start rehydration with ORS 20ml/kg/hr for 6hrs (total 120ml/kg). Reassess the patient q2h. If there is repeated vomiting or abdominal distension, give the fluid more slowly. If there is no improvement after 3hrs, send the patient for IV therapy, continuing NG tube rehydration throughout the journey. After 6hrs, reassess the patient and follow the appropriate treatment plan.
If not:

3. Can the patient drink? If yes, start rehydration using ORS, giving 20ml/kg/hr for 6hrs (total 120ml/kg). Reassess the patient every 1–2hrs. If there is repeated vomiting give the fluid more slowly. If the patient has not improved after 3hrs, send her for IV therapy, giving oral ORS throughout the journey. After 6hrs, reassess the patient and follow the appropriate treatment plan.
If not:

4. Refer the patient as urgently as possible for IV/nasogastric rehydration.

Management of persistent diarrhoea

This is diarrhoea, with or without blood, that begins acutely and lasts at least 14 days; it needs to be differentiated from sequential episodes of acute diarrhoea over a prolonged period. It is usually associated with weight loss and, often, with serious non-intestinal infections. Many children with persistent diarrhoea are malnourished *before* the diarrhoea starts. Persistent diarrhoea almost never occurs in infants who are exclusively breastfed. Take a careful history and examine the patient well.

The object of treatment is to restore weight gain and normal intestinal function. In most cases, the patient will need to be admitted to hospital for diagnostic tests, treatment and observation.

Treatment of persistent diarrhoea consists of:

1. Appropriate fluids to prevent/treat dehydration. See above.
2. Appropriate antimicrobial therapy to treat *diagnosed* infections, in particular non-intestinal infections in children eg. pneumonia, otitis media, UTI. If there is persistent, bloody diarrhoea look for evidence of *Shigella, Entamoeba* or *Giardia* infection. See earlier.
3. A nutritious diet that does not cause worsening of the diarrhoea. Children will require a minimum of 110 calories/kg per day, which may have to be given via a NG tube if the child is too weak or refuses to eat. For infants <12 months, encourage *exclusive* breastfeeding. Help mothers who are not breastfeeding to re-establish lactation (see chapter 13).
4. Where possible, replace animal milk with yoghurt or a lactose-free formula. For older infants and young children, use standard diets made from local ingredients. Two diets are given opposite, the first containing reduced lactose, the second being lactose-free for the 30% of children who do not improve with the first.
5. Supplementary vitamins and minerals. All children with persistent diarrhoea should receive supplementary multivitamins and minerals each day for two weeks. Tablets which may be crushed and mixed with food are less costly. One should aim to provide at least two recommended daily allowances (RDAs) of folate, vitamin A, iron, zinc, magnesium and copper. As a guide, the RDAs for a 1-year-old child are:
   - folate 50μg
   - zinc 10mg
   - iron 10mg
   - vitamin A 400μg
   - copper 1mg
   - magnesium 80mg.

Diet 1 (low lactose)	**Diet 2 (lactose-free)**
83 calories/100g 11% of calories as protein 3.7g lactose/kg body weight/day	75 calories/100g 10% of calories as protein
Full fat dried milk 11g (or 85ml whole milk) Rice 15g Vegetable oil 3.5g Cane sugar 3g Water 200ml	Whole egg 64g Rice 3g Vegetable oil 4g Glucose 3g Water 200ml
• 130ml/kg provides 110 calories per kg.	• 145ml/kg provides 110 calories per kg.

Malnutrition and diarrhoea

Diarrhoea is as much a nutritional disease as one of fluid and electrolyte loss. Children who die from diarrhoea, despite good management, are usually malnourished – often severely so.

During diarrhoea, decreased food intake, decreased nutrient absorption, and increased nutrient requirements often combine to cause weight loss and failure to grow. The child's nutritional status declines and any pre-existing malnutrition is made worse. Malnutrition itself makes diarrhoea worse, prolonging it and making it more frequent. This vicious cycle may be broken by continuing to give nutrient-rich foods *during* diarrhoea and giving a nutritious diet, appropriate for the child's age, when the child is well.

► When these steps are followed, malnutrition can be either prevented or corrected and the risk of death from a future episode of diarrhoea is much reduced. See chapter 13 for further information.

Complications of diarrhoea

Electrolyte disturbances: knowing the serum electrolyte concentrations rarely changes the management of patients dehydrated due to diarrhoea. In most cases, hypernatraemia, hyponatraemia, and hypokalaemia are all adequately treated by oral rehydration with ORS or IV rehydration with Ringer's Lactate. In severe dehydration, however, plasma sodium concentrations may reach extremes and hypokalaemia may produce muscular weakness, dangerous cardiac arrhythmias, and paralytic ileus.

Fever: in a patient with diarrhoea may be due to the organism causing the diarrhoea, or, particularly in children, a second infection (eg. pneumonia or otitis media). The presence of fever should prompt a search for other infections, particularly if it persists after the patient is fully hydrated.

In an area where *P. falciparum* malaria is prevalent, children with a fever of 38°C or above should be treated with an appropriate antimalarial. High fevers (>39°C) in children should be brought down with an antipyretic drug such as paracetamol. This may reduce irritability and prevent febrile convulsions.

Convulsions: in a child with diarrhoea and convulsions during the illness, the following diagnoses should be considered:

- *Febrile convulsion:* this usually occurs in children <8yrs old when their temperature exceeds 40°C or rises very rapidly. Treat with paracetamol and tepid water sponging.
- *Meningitis:* needs to be considered in any child or adult following a convulsion. Look for neck rigidity and Kernig's sign. Do a lumbar puncture after checking the retinae for papilloedema (raised ICP) and looking for focal neurological signs.
- *Hypoglycaemia:* this occasionally occurs in children with diarrhoea, due to their small hepatic glycogen reserves and insufficient gluconeogenesis. If suspected, give 1.0ml/kg of 50% glucose solution or 2.5ml/kg of a 20% glucose solution IV over 5 minutes. If hypoglycaemia is the cause, recovery will usually be rapid. In such cases Ringer's Lactate with dextrose should be given to the child for IV rehydration.

Vitamin A deficiency: diarrhoea reduces the absorption of and increases the need for vitamin A. In areas where vitamin A deficiency is already prevalent, young children with diarrhoea have an increased risk of developing eye problems.

Metabolic acidosis: during episodes of diarrhoea, a large amount of bicarbonate may be lost from the stool. If renal function is normal, this will be replaced. However, renal impairment due to hypovolaemia may result in the rapid development of a base deficit and acidosis. Excess lactate production may also occur. Features of metabolic acidosis are: serum bicarbonate (<10 mmol/l); acidaemia (pH <7.3); a compensatory respiratory alkalosis (look for rapid and deep breathing); vomiting.

Antidiarrhoeal drugs

These agents, though commonly used, have no practical benefit and are *never* indicated for the treatment of acute diarrhoea in children. Some of them are dangerous.

Adsorbents: eg kaolin, attapulgite, smectite, activated charcoal, cholestyramine are of no proven value in the treatment of diarrhoea.

Antimotility drugs: (eg. loperamide, diphenoxylate with atropine, tincture of opium, paregoric, codeine). These drugs reduce the frequency of stool passage in adults, but do not do so appreciably in children. Moreover, they may cause severe paralytic ileus and prolong infection by delaying the elimination of the causative organism/toxin. They may be used cautiously in adults in exceptional circumstances (eg required to travel) but should never be used in children or infants.

Other drugs

Antiemetics (eg prochlorperazine, chlorpromazine, metaclopramide). Such drugs should not be given since they often cause sedation and may interfere with ORS treatment. Vomiting will cease as the patient becomes hydrated.

Cardiac stimulants should *never* be used to overcome shock and hypotension which may occur in severe dehydration with hypovolaemia. Cardiac output will be restored as rehydration fluid is infused IV.

Blood or plasma is only indicated if there is proven shock.

Steroids and purgatives are of no benefit and should never be used.

Prevention of diarrhoea

Proper treatment of diarrhoeal diseases is highly effective in preventing death, but has no impact on the incidence of such diseases. It is every medical professional's responsibility to teach family members and motivate them to adopt preventative measures. Do not overload the mother with technical advice, but emphasize the most important points for each particular mother and child.

1. Measures which interrupt the transmission of pathogen

The various infectious agents that cause diarrhoea are virtually all transmitted by the faeco-oral route. Measures taken to interrupt the transmission of the causative agents should focus on the following pathways:

- giving only breastmilk for the first 6 months of life
- avoiding the use of infant feeding bottles
- improving practices relating to the preparation and storage of weaning foods (to minimize microbial contamination)
- using only clean water for drinking
- washing hands after defaecation, disposing of faeces, and before preparing food
- disposing of all faeces in a safe manner.

2. Measures which strengthen host defences

A number of risk factors for frequent or severe diarrhoea reflect impaired host defences. Measures may be taken to improve this:

- continuing to breastfeed for the first 2 years of life
- improving a child's nutritional status by giving more nutritious food, more often
- immunizing against measles.

3. How doctors can help to prevent diarrhoea

- ensure appropriate in-service training of health facility staff
- display promotional material on how to treat and prevent diarrhoea
- be a good role model (breastfeeding, hand-washing, water hygiene, latrine hygiene)
- take part in community-based activities to promote health
- co-ordinate efforts for disease prevention with those of relevant government programmes.

Some difficulties encountered in home therapy for diarrhoea

1. The mother is disappointed because she is not given a prescription for drugs or the child does not receive an injection.

Explain that the diarrhoea will stop by itself after a few days. Also, explain that drugs do not help to stop diarrhoea, but that fluid replacement and continued feeding will help shorten the illness and also maintain her child's strength and growth.

2. The mother believes that food should not be given during diarrhoea.

Ask her to explain her beliefs about how diarrhoea should be treated. Discuss with her the importance of feeding in order to keep her child strong and to support normal growth, even during diarrhoea.

3. The mother does not know what fluids to give her child at home.

Ask her what fluids she can prepare at home and reach an agreement on appropriate fluids for her child.

4. The mother does not have the ingredients to make a recommended fluid.

Ask her if she can obtain the necessary ingredients easily. If she cannot, suggest another home fluid.

5. The child vomits after drinking ORS or other fluids.

Explain that more fluid is usually kept down than is vomited. Tell her to wait 10mins and then start giving fluid again, but more slowly.

6. The child refuses to drink.

A child who has lost fluid will usually be thirsty and want to drink, even when there are no signs of dehydration. If the child is not familiar with the taste of ORS, some persuasion may be needed at first. When a child drinks well to begin with but then looses interest, it usually means that sufficient fluid has been given.

7. The mother is given some packets of ORS for use at home but is afraid they will be used up before the diarrhoea stops.

Explain that after the ORS has been used up she should give a recommended home fluid (eg rice water) or water or she should return to the health facility for more packets of ORS. In any event, she should continue to give extra fluid until the diarrhoea stops.

3E. Acute respiratory infections/ pneumonia

Viral respiratory infections 180
Pneumonia 182
Community-acquired pneumonia (CAP) 184
Atypical pneumonia 184
Pneumococcal pneumonia 186
Nosocomial pneumonia 188
Aspiration pneumonia 188
Recurrent pneumonia 188
Management of pneumonia 190

ARI/pneumonia

Viral respiratory infections

Many cases of bacterial pneumonia appear to be preceded by a relatively harmless viral infection of the upper or lower airways. These infections damage the epithelial cells that line the airway, possibly inhibiting their ability to remove debris with their cilia. The viral infection may also debilitate the person, making them more susceptible to subsequent bacterial superinfection. Whatever the mechanism, the bacterial pneumonia that follows acute respiratory tract infections (ARI) is a major cause of childhood death in the developing world. Their importance is recognized in the WHO's 'Integrated Management of Childhood Illness'.

Aetiology – the viral agents of respiratory infections include:

- measles
- influenza virus
- rhinovirus
- coronavirus
- parainfluenza virus
- adenovirus
- respiratory syncytial virus (RSV).

The viruses are transmitted either in small droplets after sneezing or coughing (eg measles, influenza) or by contact with infected secretions (eg RSV, rhinoviruses).

Upper respiratory tract infections

A group of infections which are normally self-limiting and do not require specific treatment. They include the 'common cold' (coryza), pharyngitis (sore throat), and laryngitis. Signs of coryza include nasal stinging, a watery nasal discharge and a blocked nose – signs which are similar to the prodrome of measles and influenza but without the systemic upset.

Acute bronchitis

A condition that is characterized by mild malaise (the patient does not look ill), retrosternal soreness and a dry, tickly cough which becomes more prominent as the infection progresses and, with 2° bacterial infection, mucopurulent. It may be characterized as a "common cold that has gone into the chest" and is often still accompanied by signs of an upper respiratory tract infection. The severity of the attack is possibly increased by exposure to cigarette smoke and air pollution both inside houses and in the outside environment.

Aetiology: most cases are due to viral infection. Superinfection with *H. influenzae* or *S. pneumoniae* is a common complication. Much more rarely bacteria such as *Bordetella pertussis*, *Mycoplasma pneumoniae*, and *Chlamydia pneumoniae* give rise to a primary bronchitis.

Diagnosis: is one of exclusion – more serious conditions such as pneumonia, and cardiovascular or thromboembolic disease must be ruled out.
► If the cough and wheeze persist, consider the diagnosis of asthma and the use of bronchodilators and steroids.

Management: bacterial superinfection of the trachea or bronchi will often require specific therapy. Antibiotics according to local guidelines are also warranted for 2° bacterial infection affecting the sinuses or middle ear.

Causes of sore throat

- Mild viral infections
- *Streptococcus pyogenes* [→ rheumatic heart disease *and* glomerulonephritis]
- *Corynebacterium diphtheriae*
- Epstein-Barr virus
- *Neisseria gonorrhoea*
- Secondary syphilis
- Herpes simplex virus – especially in AIDS patients
- Lassa virus
- Vincent's angina

Pneumonia

Pneumonia causes between 2 and 5 million deaths per year in young children of the developing world. It remains a major killer in the industrialized world, particularly of the elderly. Even as development reduces the importance of infectious diseases, pneumonia remains important – in the UK, 10× as many people die of pneumonia as all other infectious diseases put together. While viral pneumonia may occur during a severe systemic viral infection, for example with measles or influenza infection, most serious cases are due to bacteria.

Causes: relatively little is known about the causative agents in much of the developing world. Studies from Europe and the USA looking at the aetiological agents of community-acquired pneumonia in hospitalized adult patients have found a mix of agents (see table opposite). *Streptococcus pneumoniae* was the most common microbe identified, but in up to 50% of cases the agent was not identified. *S. pneumoniae* may be the cause of many of these infections – because of its great susceptibility to common antibiotics (especially penicillin), treatment in the community before admission may have removed the bacteria from the blood.

► It will be very important to get similar data for different groups of patients in other areas of the world.

Cases of pneumonia can be classified in a number of ways. The most useful involve determining:

- ***where the pneumonia was acquired*** – community or hospital?
- ***the previous health status of the patient*** – previously healthy (***primary pneumonia***) or chronically ill (***secondary pneumonia***). Important risk factors for pneumonia include: • HIV infection • malnutrition • periods of unconsciousness (alcoholics, surgical patients) • the absence of a functioning spleen (post-splenectomy or due to sickle cell disease) • pregnancy • diabetes.

Both these factors will be important for determining the likely causative agent, disease course and severity, and therefore the patient's management and prognosis. The resulting categories are summarized opposite.

Clinical features

- The patient is systemically ill with malaise, fever, anorexia, body aches and headache. Delerium occurs in severe infections.
- Respiratory symptoms include cough, sputum production, dyspnoea, pleural pain and rarely haemoptysis. Sputum is often initially scanty or absent, becoming purulent later in the infection except in *Legionella* and other atypical pneumonias. Signs include tachypnoea, tachycardia, reduced chest movement on affected side, inspiratory crepitations, pleural rub.
- lower lobe pneumonia may present as an acute abdomen – abdominal pain, ileus, rigidity.

► In the very young, elderly, and debilitated, there may be few signs of systemic illness or respiratory involvement. Look for a raised respiratory rate and perform a careful chest examination. Have a high index of suspicion.

Causes of community-acquired pneumonia (CAP) in adults in Europe and USA[1]

	All CAP % (range) [*n* = 2679]		Severe CAP % [*n* = 233]
No cause found	36	(3–50)	33
S. pneumoniae	25	(9–79)	27
Influenza virus	8	(5–8.5)	2.3
M. pneumoniae	7.2	(2–18)	2.3
Legionella spp	7	(2–8)	17
H. influenzae	5.4	(2–11)	5
Other viruses	5	(1–10)	8
Psittacosis/Q fever	3	(0–6)	1
Gram-neg. enteric bacteria	2.7	(0–8)	2
S. aureus	2	(0–3)	5

Classification of pneumonia[1]

- Community-acquired pneumonia   primary
  secondary
- Nosocomial (or hospital-acquired) pneumonia
- Aspiration and anaerobic pneumonia
- Pneumonia in the immunocompromised host
- AIDS-related pneumonia
- Geographically restricted pneumonias
- Recurrent pneumonia.

The classical division of pneumonia into lobar pneumonia (involvement of whole, sometimes isolated, lung segments) or bronchopneumonia (involvement of many areas in a patchy fashion – commonly due to previous illness) appears to offer little clinical benefit.

1. Both tables are taken from McFarlane JT, *OTM*, pp. 2694–5

Community-acquired pneumonia (CAP)

In a previously healthy person with community-acquired pneumonia, the most likely pathogens are *S. pneumoniae* and, less often, atypical organisms.

► However, since many of the signs of acute pneumonia are similar to those that occur in post-primary *M. tuberculosis* infection, TB should always be considered early in the differential diagnosis.

In the history, consider whether the patient was

- Previously healthy or had chronic lung disease. The latter condition predisposes to colonization of the respiratory tract with pathogenic microbes such as *H. influenzae*.
- Generally debilitated, an alcoholic or an intravenous drug abuser. These patients are commonly infected by microbes that are more typical of nosocomial infection, although they are also at increased risk of pneumococcal infection. The infection may be an aspiration pneumonia.

Common bacterial causes of CAP:

1. ***Streptococcus pneumoniae*** – see page 186.
2. ***Haemophilus influenzae* type B** – occurs particularly in children <5yrs old who often present with lobar pneumonia, pleural involvement, and an effusion. It also occurs in adults both as a 1° infection and in previously damaged lungs. The onset is slower than the other bacteria. Severe dyspnoea may suggest pericarditis. The pneumonia is often accompanied by infection elsewhere, eg meninges, epiglottis. The use of a Hib vaccine in the tropics should markedly reduce its incidence, if the vaccine can be afforded.
3. ***Staphylococcus aureus*** – an important cause of aspiration pneumonia in patients with pre-existing lung disease (eg bronchial CA) or following viral infection, usually influenza or measles. Note that the influenza infection may be subclinical. Alternatively, hematogenous spread from a distant site of infection (eg skin) may produce pneumonia in a previously healthy lung. *S. aureus* can be cultured from the blood in the latter case but not the former. It is always a serious condition with high fever and cyanosis; common complications include pulmonary abscess formation, cavitation, empyema.

Atypical pneumonia

Pneumonias which normally occur in previously healthy children and young adults and which start with a mild sore throat followed by dyspnoea, an often non-productive cough, fever and malaise. Pleuritic chest pain, splinting, and respiratory distress are rare. The CXR picture is often worse than signs would suggest, the WCC normal. The clinical course is normally benign; occasionally they are severe and require ICU admission.

Common causes are *Mycoplasma pneumoniae* and *Chlamydia pneumoniae*. Others include *C. trachomatis* and *C. psittaci*, *Coxiella burnetti*, *Legionella pneumophila*, and viruses such as influenza and adenovirus. Diagnosis is by serology.

A poor prognosis is associated with:

- Presence of bacteraemia. (eg the fatality rate increases from 5% in isolated *S.pneumoniae* pneumonia to 25–35% fatality rate when *S.pneumoniae* can also be cultured from blood.)
- Infections with *S.aureus*, *H.influenzae* and Gram –ve bacteria.
- Previous illness, either chronic (eg COAD, cardiac disease, malnutrition) or acute (influenzae, measles)

Clinical features

- confusion
- respiratory rate >30/min
- diastolic blood pressure <60mmHg
- new atrial fibrillation

Investigations

- blood urea >7mmol/l
- WCC <4 x 10^9/l *or* >30 x 10^9/l
- arterial O_2 <8kPA
- serum albumin <25 g/l
- multilobe involvement on CXR

Legionnaires' disease

The importance of *Legionella pneumophila* in the tropics is unknown. It is transmitted by inhalation of aerosolized water droplets from air conditioning systems, water storage tanks, shower heads and medical equipment such as nebulizers.

Clinical features: vary from subclinical or mild infections to severe pneumonia. In severe infection, after 2–10 days, there is abrupt high fever, rigors, myalgia and headache followed by the onset of a dry cough, dyspnoea and crepitations on auscultation. The patient becomes very ill quickly, appearing toxic, sometimes with delirium or diarrhoea. During the toxic phase, complications include respiratory failure, pericarditis, myocarditis, ARF. CXR shows homogeneous shadowing, often basal initially, subsequently widespread with deterioration. **Diagnosis:** Gram –ve slender rods of variable length in biopsy or sputum samples; bacterial antigen in urine for first 1–3 weeks.

Treatment: erythromycin 0.5–1g/6h IV or PO for up to 2–3 weeks (adding in rifampicin 600mg bd if patient is deteriorating) is recommended. **Prevention:** treatment and maintenance of stored water and tanks to prevent bacteria colonization and spread.

Pneumococcal pneumonia

Although the pneumococcus is an important cause of disease in children and adults across the world, it is the developing world's children who are at greatest risk of dying. It causes 25–50% of ARIs in children admitted to hospital and, each year, at least 1 million children die from pneumococcal pneumonia. The disease is worse in crowded communities with poor living conditions. Adults with debilitating diseases (eg DM, AIDS, alcoholism, asplenia, hypogammaglobinaemia) are also at increased risk of invasive pneumococcal disease.

Historically, *Streptococcus pneumoniae* was extremely sensitive to common antibiotics such as penicillin. However, 1967 saw the identification of pneumococcus isolates with reduced sensitivity to penicillin in Australasia. 10 years later, children in southern Africa were noted to be dying from isolates which were clinically resistant to pencillin. This trend has continued, apparently driven by indiscriminate use of penicillin antibiotics. Now, >50% of pneumococcal isolates in some areas of the world have reduced sensitivity to penicillin. Many of these resistant bacteria have reduced sensitivity to other common antibiotics such as tetracycline. The increase in resistance has worrying implications for the management of invasive pneumococcal disease. Currently, the prevalence of penicillin-resistant pneumococci in many parts of the developing world is unknown.

Transmission: spread is person-person via droplet spread. Many people become long term carriers of the infection in their nasopharynx. Local spread to ear or meninges (particularly after head trauma) can produce *otitis media* or meningitis.

Clinical features: the onset is sudden (sometimes following an URTI) with fever, rigors, malaise, headache, myalgia. [Onset is often less clear at the extremes of age – children show tachypnoea in addition to fever and cough while the elderly may have little fever and present with confusion.] Chest pain (pleuritic, sometimes referred to shoulder if diaphragm is involved) and cough (initially painful and dry, → blood-tinged, → purulent) commonly follow. Lower lobe involvement will result in abdominal pain and guarding. Jaundice may occur due to haemolysis and/or liver damage. The WCC is often raised; leukopenia is a poor prognostic sign.

Complications: pneumococci in the lungs may spread directly to pericardium or pleura producing empyema. Hematogenous spread results in infection of meninges, joints, eyes, or abscess formation in distant organs. Rare complications include: acute septicaemia in patients with underlying conditions, such as asplenia; endocarditis; peritonitis in patients with lowered immunity and ascites (nephrotic syndrome, cirrhosis).

Diagnosis: is most often made on clinical grounds. Bacteria can be cultured from sputum or aspiration of the abscesses in distant organs.

Management: see later. It is essential to follow local guidelines for antibiotic use that are based on knowledge of local antibiotic sensitivities.

Prevention: general improvements in living conditions and reduced air pollution; vaccination.

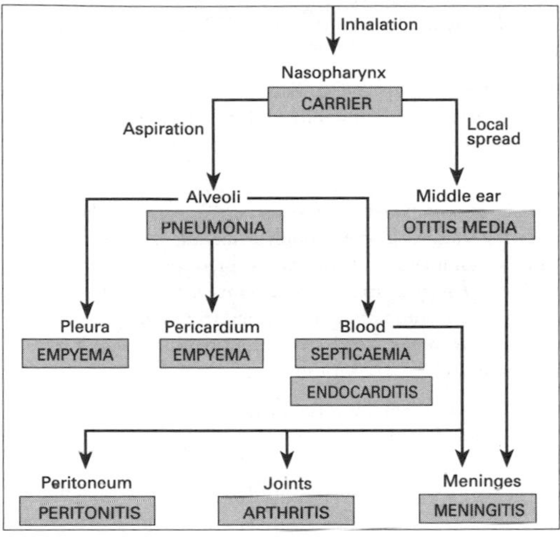

Locally recommended antibiotics for pneumococcal pneumonia:

-
-
-

Rare causes of severe community-acquired pneumonia include:

- meliodosis
- anthrax
- tularaemia
- pneumonic plague
- typhoid
- brucellosis
- paragonimiasis
- fungi – such as histoplasmosis and blastomycosis

Nosocomial pneumonia

Definition: pneumonia that occurs more than 48 hours after admission to hospital.

Signs: development of fever, increased WCC, purulent sputum, lung infiltrate on CXR.

Risk factors: increasing age, obesity, smoking, long preoperative stay, prolonged anaesthesia, intubation, abdominal/thoracic operations plus risk factors for aspiration pneumonia (see below).

Aetiology:

- *Aspiration of nasopharyngeal secretions* – particularly of Gram –ve bacteria that may colonize nasopharynx during hospital stay. Broad spectrum antibiotics and serious illness predispose to such colonization.
- *Inhalation of bacteria from contaminated instruments* – such as ventilators, nebulizers, intubation and nasogastric tubes.
- *Haematogenous spread* – eg from abdominal infection, infected cannulas or catheters left *in situ* for too long.

Prevention: prevent smoking preoperatively, encourage early mobilization. Good hospital staff and respiratory equipment hygiene, and good general infection control measures should decrease the risk. Chest physiotherapy postoperatively may help decrease nosocomial pneumonia.

Aspiration pneumonia

Risk factors: impaired consciousness (eg alcoholics, epileptics), dysphagia, being bed-bound, neuromuscular diseases, decreased ability to clear bronchial secretions or cough after general anaesthesia or abdominal/thoracic surgery.

Aetiology:

- *In the community* – anaerobes from oropharynx and teeth crevices (normally penicillin sensitive).
- *In the hospital* – aerobic bacteria become more important, particularly Gram –ve enterobacteria and *P. aeruginosa.*

It may be possible to diagnose anaerobic infection from a *Hx* of poor dental hygiene, aspiration or impaired consciousness. As the infection proceeds, tissue necrosis results in foul-smelling purulent discharge.

Recurrent pneumonia

Defined as more than two episodes of pneumonia, it may be caused by:

- Localized respiratory disease – bronchiectasis, bronchial obstruction (foreign body, bronchial stenosis, bronchial carcinoma, lymphadenopathy), intrapulmonary sequestration.
- Generalized respiratory disease – COAD +/– bronchiectasis, impaired local defences.
- Non-respiratory problem – recurrent aspiration (see above), immune suppression.

Management of pneumonia

1. Bed rest. The patient should sit up rather than lie flat – except in cases of severe pneumonia where this may exhaust the patient.
2. Give analgesia for pleuritic pain.
3. Give fluids (IV if necessary) to rectify dehydration and maintain an adequate urine output (>1.5 litres/24h). Remember that losses are increased if the patient is febrile. However, free water clearance is impaired, so beware of overhydration.
4. Oxygen.
5. Antimicrobials: see below and opposite.
6. Treat empirically for sepsis if very ill – see chapter 5.
7. Physiotherapy is no longer recommended in the early acute stages of pneumonia.

Antimicrobial use: general points

- if the patient is too ill to wait for blood cultures, or if they are not available, empiric IV antibiotic therapy should be started immediately. Be aware of local guidelines and, if possible, seek advice from a senior colleague. Antibiotic choice in this situation (blind therapy) depends upon the clinical picture/patient history – see opposite.
- empirical therapy may be appropriate in outpatient clinics.
- only give IV therapy if the patient is very ill, cannot swallow, or if the GI tract is not functioning.
- therapy can be given for 3–7 days in mild pneumonia. For those with severe pneumonia, duration needs to be judged according to the clinical response. In the presence of cavitation and abscesses, treatment can be continued for up to 3–4 weeks.

► Change the guidelines given opposite to reflect the most common pathogens, and their antimicrobial sensitivities, in your region.

Chest X-rays in pneumonia:

X-rays are expensive and their interpretation subject to wide variation. Therefore the value of an X-ray for each particular patient should be carefully considered before ordering one. For example

- is the diagnosis already clear from the clinical features?
- will the X-ray change the patient's management?
- Note that CXR changes in pneumonia may take weeks to resolve following successful treatment and clinical improvement by the patient.

►► Gentamicin

This is a very useful but toxic antibiotic. Both the kidneys and ears are damaged by high plasma concentrations. Renal failure reduces excretion of the drug, allowing serum levels to rapidly rise to toxic levels. 5mg/kg is the highest allowable dose – children and the elderly should receive ~3mg/kg daily. Ideally, the drug should be monitored by measuring plasma concentrations one hour after giving a dose (peak level) and just before the next dose (trough level). ► Keep regimens as short as possible in all patients.

Blind treatment of pneumonia[1]

Clinical picture	*Organisms to be covered*	*Antibiotic route PO*	*IV*
I. Primary CAP			
(mild – moderate)	*S. pneumoniae* If 'atypicals' likely	Ay add E	A add E
II. Secondary pneumonia			
• Previous lung disease (eg COAD)	*S. pneumoniae*, *H. influenzae*	Co	Co + E *or* C + E
• If following flu, or associated with URTI	Cover for *S. aureus*	add F	add F
		to above regimen	
• Aspiration	*S. pneumoniae*, *Klebsiella* spp, anaerobes, Gram –ve organisms	x	P + M + G
• Immunosuppression eg leukaemia	*Pseudomonas* spp as well as usual organisms	x	Cz + G
• Nosocomial (especially if 2° disease)	Gram –ve as well as usual organisms	x	Ct + G
• Sepsis elsewhere	Treat as for sepsis	x	F + G + M
III. Severe pneumonia			
	Widest possible range	x	Ct + E + G

For treatment of an HIV[+] patient, see chapter 3B.

Key to antimicrobials

A	Ampicillin 500mg q6h IV
Ay	Amoxycillin 250mg tds PO
C	Cefuroxime 750mg q8h IV
Co	Co-amoxiclav 1 tablet (250mg/125mg) tds PO or 1.2g (1000mg/200mg) q8h IV
Ct	Cefotaxime 1g q8h IV
Cz	Ceftazidime 2g q8h IV
E	Erythromycin 250–500mg qds PO or 500mg q6h **slowly** IV
F	Flucloxacillin 250mg qds PO or 250–1000mg q6h **slowly** IV
G	Gentamicin 2–5mg/kg daily IV (see notes opposite)
M	Metronidazole 500mg q8h IV (for up to 7 days)
P	Benzylpenicillin 600mg q6h IV (dose may be increased)
x	Oral therapy is inappropriate in these situations

1. Hope T. *Oxford Handbook of Clinical Medicine*, 3rd edn, Oxford University Press, 1993.

4. Fevers/systemic signs

Differential diagnosis of fevers 194
Sepsis 198
Sepsis during pregnancy 200
Cancer 202
General rules of management 204
Typhoid and parathyroid fevers 206
Typhus fevers 208
Other rickettsial infections 210
Relapsing fever 212
Leptospirosis 214
Brucellosis 216
Plague 218
Melioidosis 220
Anthrax 220
African trypanosomiasis 222
American trypanosomiasis 226
Visceral leishmaniasis (kala-azar) 228
Influenza 230
Infectious mononucleosis 230
Measles 232
Arboviruses 236
Dengue fever 238
Chikungunya 238
Viral haemorrhagic fever (VHF) 240
Arbovirus haemorrhagic fevers (HF) 242
Dengue haemorrhagic fever 242
Yellow fever 242
Hantavirus haemorrhagic fever 244
Arenavirus haemorrhagic fever 244
Filovirus haemorrhagic fever 244

Fevers/systemic signs

Differential diagnosis of fevers

Fever is an extremely common presentation in much of the tropics. A process is required to work through the differential diagnosis – we have adapted one from the work of Bell.[1]

► It is important to consider locally important causes of fever early in the differential diagnosis.

1. Take a detailed history, including the questions:
- *Where have you been?*
- *What have you been doing?*

2. A careful examination is essential. This must be repeated at regular intervals to look for evolving signs when a diagnosis cannot be made. Particularly examine • skin • eyes • nail beds • lymph nodes • abdomen and • heart.

3. Ideally, the temp should be recorded at least twice each day – 6am and 6pm.

From the history, the fever can be categorized as either acute or chronic (>14 days).

Ask yourself – "Is this presentation unusual or has it become more numerous recently – might an epidemic be occurring?" (p8).

Localizing signs on examination

- dyspnoea, cough, pleuritic pain, discoloured sputum → bacterial pneumonia
- severe sore throat → streptococcal sore throat or diphtheria
- pain & swelling in a joint → septic arthritis
- frequency, dysuria, loin pain → pyelonephritis or UTI
- severe headache & neck stiffness → meningitis
- bone pain (worse at night) → osteomyelitis
- severe lower abdominal pain → see gastroenterology chapter
- bloody diarrhoea → see diarrhoeal diseases chapter
- marked local lymphadenopathy → local sepsis, abscess, plague
- cutaneous inflammation → erysipelas, cellulitis.

All of these conditions are characterized by the presence of an ***acute fever with neutrophil leukocytosis***

Note in particular:

- chronic cough for > 4 weeks or blood in sputum → TB
- woman who has given birth in the last 4 weeks → puerperal sepsis
- a patient who has had any form of recent abdominal or pelvic operation or abdominal/gynaecological disease may have a liver, subphrenic, or pelvic abscess.

1. Bell DR, *Lecture Notes in Tropical Medicine*, 4th ed, Blackwell Scientific Ltd, Oxford 1995

Fever in the absence of localizing signs

In the absence of any localizing signs, the following investigations become essential for diagnosis and treatment:

1. thick and thin blood films for malaria
   (also examine these films for trypanosomes, borrelia, etc)
2. total and differential white cell counts (WCC)
3. if available, blood cultures for anaerobic and aerobic bacteria.

Common causes of fever include:
- infections
- tumours
- connective tissue disease.

In the tropics, infections are the most important since they are the most common and treatable.

Blood films

► Malaria is the most common cause of fever and should be the first diagnosis considered in endemic areas. However, positive blood films are extremely common in these areas and it may be difficult to decide whether malaria is causing the fever. These simple rules may help:

- Low-grade parasitaemia is common, therefore when this is found other causes of fever should be looked for.
- The greater the level of parasitaemia, the more likely it is that the symptoms are caused by malaria.
- Epidemiological studies have attempted to identify a level of parasitaemia above which it is likely that malaria is causing the fever. Has a cut-off point been determined for the local area?
- In clinical practice in non-endemic areas, any level of parasitaemia is clinically relevant and cannot be ignored.

In some areas, malaria is so common that all patients with fever and no localizing signs will receive antimalarial chemotherapy and/or penicillin.
What is the local policy?

Differential white cell counts (WCC)

Differentiation of neutrophil vs lymphocyte leukocytoses is useful in the identification of many causes of fever. The common causes are listed on the next page. ► If there is a neutrophil leukocytosis as well as a positive malarial blood film, it is likely that the fever is caused by something other than malaria.

Differential white cell counts (WCC)

1. Acute fever in the absence of localizing signs

Acute fever, neutrophil leukocytosis →

- bacterial sepsis
- *Leptospira* and *Borrelia* infections:
  - leptospirosis
  - tick-borne relapsing fever
  - louse-borne relapsing fever

Acute fever, lymphocytosis →

- viral fevers
- mononucleosis
- rickettsial fevers
- typhoid fever.

2. Chronic fever (>14 days) in the absence of localizing signs

► First ask yourself – could this patient have either • TB or • HIV infection?

Otherwise:

Chronic fever, neutrophil leukocytosis →

- deep sepsis/abscess*
- amoebic liver abscess
- erythema nodosum leprosum
- cholangitis
- relapsing fever.

* may show spiking fever

Chronic fever, eosinophilia →

- invasive schistosomiasis
- other invasive parasitic infections.

Chronic fever, leukopenia →

- malaria
- disseminated tuberculosis
- visceral leishmaniasis
- brucellosis.

Chronic fever, normal wbc picture →

- localized tuberculosis
- brucellosis
- secondary syphilis
- trypanosomiasis
- toxoplasmosis
- subacute bacterial endocarditis
- systemic lupus erythematosus
- chronic meningococcal septicaemia.

Chronic fever, variable wbc picture →

- tumours
- reticuloses
- drug reactions
- connective tissue disease.

Fever with systemic signs

► For all these signs, it is essential to gain knowledge of the clinically important infections in the local area.

1. Fever accompanied by rash

The history is important since many rashes are transient and have disappeared by the time the patient is seen by a doctor. Some rashes are diagnostic of certain conditions and therefore of great help to the clinician. Palpate the skin; rashes that are not immediately obvious may become apparent by blanching. Be aware that the rash may be the result of drug treatment.

- dengue and other arboviral infections
- typhoid and paratyphoid fevers
- measles
- connective tissue diseases
- rickettsial infections
- secondary syphilis
- HIV seroconversion
- cat scratch disease.

2. Fever with haemorrhagic manifestations

- petechial/purpuric rashes →
  - sepsis, especially meningococcal
  - tick typhus fevers
  - dengue/yellow fever
- frank haemorrhage →
  - viral hemorrhagic fevers
  - malaria with DIC.

3. Fever following tick bites

Find out if there is a history of exposure to tick habitats (will depend on locality – check knowledgeable source) or domesticated animals such as cows or dogs. The patient may not recall having been bitten.

Search the patient's body for **ticks** or **eschar** – ticks may be hidden in hair on the scalp or in axillary/groin regions. Check for lymphadenoapthy.

- tick typhus fevers
- tick-borne relapsing fever
- Lyme disease
- ehrlichiosis
- arboviral infections such as Crimean-Congo haemorrhagic fever, Kyasanur Forest disease, and tick-borne encephalitis.

► Sepsis[1]

Sepsis can be defined as 'clinical evidence of infection plus evidence of a systemic response to the infection'. This systemic response is manifested by >1 of the following:

- temperature >38°C or <36°C
- heart rate >90 beats/min
- respiratory rate >20 breaths/min or $PaCO_2$ <32mmHg (<4.3kPa)
- WCC >12,000 cells/mm^3 or <4,000 cells /mm^3
  or >10% immature band forms.

Sepsis has a high mortality rate, of at least 35% – if the patient progresses into ***septic shock***, then mortality increases to >65%.

Septic shock

This is sepsis plus profound hypotension (systolic BP <90mmHg or a reduction of >40mmHg from baseline) despite adequate fluid resuscitation (>500ml). Evidence of organ hypoperfusion may include lactic acidosis, oligouria, or acute alteration in mental status. Hypotension may not be present due to the use of inotropic or vasopressor drugs.

Causes: septic shock most often results from infection with either

- ***Gram-negative bacteria*** **–** via their release of a toxic cell wall component, lipopolysaccharide (LPS), into the bloodstream, or
- ***Gram-positive bacteria*** **–** via their secretion of toxic proteins called exotoxins (see toxic shock syndrome below).
- Fulminant parasitic infections, miliary TB, and systemic fungal infections may also cause septic shock.

The characteristic features of septic shock include:

- tachypnoea
- acidosis
- fever (or hypothermia)
- profound and prolonged hypotension
- hypoxia (causing mental confusion)
- warm peripheries (since the blood vessels are dilated)– cf cardiogenic shock.

Toxic shock syndrome – is due to protein toxins released into the blood stream by *Staphylococcus aureus* or *Streptococcus pyogenes. S. aureus* can cause shock by releasing toxins from superficial skin or mucosal sites of infection – disseminated infection is not required.

Management

1. Resuscitate the patient.
2. If possible, take blood cultures before starting antibiotics.
3. Start empirical antibiotic regimen.
4. Provide oxygen.
5. Replace fluids with colloid or crystalloid, taking care not to induce pulmonary oedema as the perfusion returns to normal.
6. Treat hypotension – infuse dopamine at 5–20μg/kg/min; adjust according to the response.

1. Young S, 1995, *Mandell's 'Principles and practice of infectious disease'*, p690

Local recommendations

1) For normal immunocompetent patients:

-
-
-

2) For neutropenic patients (<1000 cells/μl):

-
-

Additional Gram-positive cover at 48hrs:

-

Antifungal therapy after a further 48hrs:

-

- ► If the patient is able to take liquids, give antibiotics PO.
- ► If the patient's condition declines rapidly, changes in antibiotic regimen should be considered before waiting 48hrs.
- ► Always consider non-infective causes of rapid deterioration, eg pulmonary embolism.
- ► Due to the toxicity of gentamicin, withdraw this antibiotic at 48hrs if there has been no improvement.
- ► It is imperative in the management of sepsis that treatment options are not narrowed too quickly. In the absence of clear improvement, management should be reconsidered every day and reasons why the patient has not responded explored.

► Sepsis during pregnancy

The risk of a woman dying in the puerperal period varies from 7/100,000 in Scandinavia to 1000/100,000 in some parts of Africa and Middle-East, a horrifying contrast between the industrialized and developing worlds.[1] Most of maternal deaths are due to

- sepsis
- hypertensive disorders of pregnancy
- haemorrhage
- complications of obstructed labour

Causes of sepsis: sepsis is caused by the entry of bacteria into the genital tract through the use of unwashed hands and unsterilized instruments during delivery. Abortion is also a major cause of sepsis – unsafe abortions kill at least 70,000 women each year. Septic abortions are the most common reason for admission to gynaecological wards and may account for 10–30% of maternal deaths in some communities. Such deaths are rare where abortions are both legal and accessible.

Reducing the number of unwanted pregnancies will reduce the number of women dying from illegal abortions. A prerequisite for this will be sexual equality, so that women can avoid coercive sexual relationships and use safe contraceptive methods.

Puerperal sepsis

Puerperal sepsis presents with:

- lower abdominal pain
- fever
- vomiting
- vaginal discharge <4 weeks after childbirth (often within first few days).

Caesarean section and a long delay between membrane rupture and delivery greatly increase the risk. The infections are usually polymicrobial and include streptococci, enterococci, and Gram negative gut bacteria.

► The presence of group A β-haemolytic streptococci (*S. pyogenes*) suggests that health workers are infecting patients – stress rigid adherence to aseptic technique and handwashing, and attempt to identify the infected caregiver.

Septic abortion[2]

The infection is normally polymicrobial. It may include resident bacteria of the vagina and endocervix, sexually-transmitted pathogens, *Clostridium perfringens* and *C. tetani*. Patients present in early to mid-pregnancy with fever and foul-smelling discharge. ► Those with temperature >38°C, pelvic peritonitis, and tachycardia should be admitted to hospital for IV antibiotics and immediate uterine evacuation. Such patients are at high risk of sepsis and ARDS.

Patients presenting with mild illness (low-grade fever; mild lower abdominal pain; moderate vaginal bleeding) require immediate evacuation plus antibiotics such as ciprofloxacin and metronidazole. The patient should be admitted if there is no improvement at 48hrs.

1. *Maternal mortality. A Global Factbook*. Division of Family Health, WHO: Geneva 1991
2. Stubblefield PG 1994, *NEJM*, **331**, 310

Management

Puerperal sepsis

1. Severely ill patients requiring hospital admission should receive IV antibiotics: metronidazole plus ampicillin plus gentamicin (see previous page) until the fever has resolved, the pain has gone, and the WCC has returned to normal.
2. Women with milder infections can receive a 2nd generation cephalosporin (eg cefuroxime).
3. If *Chlamydia* infection is suspected, doxycycline or erythromycin should be given for 10 days even if she has responded to other antibiotics.

Septic abortions

1. These patients require immediate uterine evacuation. ►► Do not wait for her condition to improve since delay may prove fatal.
2. If possible, culture urine, blood, and tissue from uterine aspiration. Gram stain of this aspirate may give some guidance for early management.
3. Give high dose IV antibiotics:
   - benzylpenicillin 5MU IV q6h *plus*
   - clindamycin 900mg IV q8h *plus*
   - gentamicin up to 5mg/kg IV daily (if renal function is normal).

► ***Laparotomy*** is required if there is:

- no response to the above antibiotics
- uterine perforation with suspected bowel damage
- pelvic abscess
- clostridial myometritis.

► ***Total hysterectomy*** is required if there is

- discoloured, woody-appearing uterus
- suspected clostridial sepsis
- pelvic tissue crepitation *or*
- radiographic evidence of air in the uterine wall.

Cancer

Cancer is a common disease worldwide, although there is wide geographical variation in the prevalence of particular cancers. About 6 million people were estimated to have died from cancer during 1990, 3.6 million in the developing world.[1] Lung cancer was the commonest cancer worldwide, followed by stomach, liver, colon and rectum, oesophagus, and breast. Breast cancer was the commonest cause of death from cancer in women. Individual cancers are discussed in the relevant sections.

Cancer requires early intervention for therapy to be effective. Bearing this in mind, some basic rules include:

- cancer should be suspected with any unexplained illness, particularly in the elderly.
- every attempt should be made to get a histological or cytological diagnosis as soon as possible.
- once diagnosed, patients should start a planned regimen of treatment within days, not weeks. Tumours grow exponentially and there is no room for delay.

Signs and symptoms common to many forms of cancer:

- **Pain –** due to direct effect of tumour (eg infiltration of nerves or compression), its treatment, or metastatic spread to the bones. Any patient with unexplained persistent pain should be suspected of having malignant disease.
- **Weight loss –** due to involvement of GI tract (obstruction, metastatic liver involvement) or a poorly understood general cachexia syndrome with anorexia and malaise (? due to factors released by the tumour). May be exacerbated by treatment.
- **Tumour mass –** often ignored by doctors but requiring early Dx by biopsy, preferably by fine needle aspiration.
- **Fever –** while normally caused by superimposed infection, fever may itself be a feature of particular cancers such as lymphomas, renal CA, and tumours metastasizing to the liver. Frequently occur as drenching night sweats without rigors.
- **Anaemia –** normocytic normochromic (sometimes hypochromic) due to bleeding or malabsorption.
- **Hypercalcaemia –** due to widespread metastases to the skeleton or, more commonly, to paraneoplastic syndromes.

Paraneoplastic syndromes – diverse syndromes which, while individually uncommon, are common when taken together. They are due to tumour-derived cytokines or hormones or to a tumour-induced immune response which cross-reacts with normal tissue. The range of syndromes is wide and includes endocrine, neurological, dermatological, musculoskeletal, and haematological syndromes. ► However, unless obviously paraneoplastic in character, symptoms from cancer should initially be considered direct effects of the tumour since this will have important implications for therapy. Most neurological problems are due to metastases, and most endocrine problems due to the endocrine tumours themselves, not paraneoplastic syndromes.

1. Murray CJL, 1997, *Lancet*, **349**, 1498.

World Health Organization performance status – useful for grading the status of cancer patients and determining prognosis.

0 Able to carry out normal activity without restriction

1 Restricted in physically strenuous activity but walking about and able to carry out light work

2 Walking about and capable of selfcare but unable to carry out any work; up and about >50% of waking hours

3 Capable of selfcare; confined to bed or chair more than 50% of waking hours

4 Completely disabled; cannot carry out selfcare; totally confined to bed or chair.

Complications that may occur with various tumours:

- Spinal cord/cauda equina compression.
- Cerebral metastases and raised intracranial pressure.

► Management of either requires immediate administration of dexamethasone 8mg bd IV. Neurological symptoms should settle quickly. Delay in the treatment of spinal cord compression will result in paraplegia.

- Carcinomatous meningitis - leads to headache and increased ICP.
- Pleural and pericardial effusions.

General rules of management

Whenever you see a patient known to have cancer, think of the following points:

1. **Could the patient have neutropenia?** Infection in a neutropenic patient often presents atypically, eg without fever or without chest consolidation. Have a high level of suspicion – anyone who is feeling run-down must have their WCC done immediately and NOT be sent home. Such patients can deteriorate very quickly and be dead in hours.

2. **Could the patient have hypercalcaemia?** Unlike 1° parathyroid disease, the onset is rapid and there are none of the classical 'stones, bones, or groans'. Instead clinical features include: polyuria, thirst, confusion, fatigue, coma. ► Treatment of the hypercalcaemia will produce a marked improvement in the patient's condition.

3. **Is the patient's pain controlled?** Use morphine – it is a good powerful drug. The following regimen is very effective:
   - Give quick-acting morphine 10mg q4h at 07.00, 11.00, etc, until 23.00 at which point give a double dose so that the 0300 dose can be missed out, offering the chance of a good night's sleep.
   - If pain breaks through at any time, always give an extra dose of morphine 10mg (even if the next q4h dose is only 10 minutes away), continuing the q4h dose as normal.
   - As more breakthrough doses are required, increase the q4h dose AND the breakthrough dose – eg to 20mg.
   - (If using long acting morphine eg MST 80mg bd, take total daily dose (160mg) and divide by 6 (q4h doses) to give size of the breakthrough dose – here 160/6 = ~26mg)

4. **Could the patient have early cord compression?**

   Ask: •Can you walk? •When was the last time you walked? •Have you experienced incontinence of urine and/or faeces?

   Do a neurological exam including anal tone and sacral sensation. ► Missing spinal cord compression may result in the patient spending their last few weeks or months in a miserable paraplegic state.

Overview of the managment of acute pain

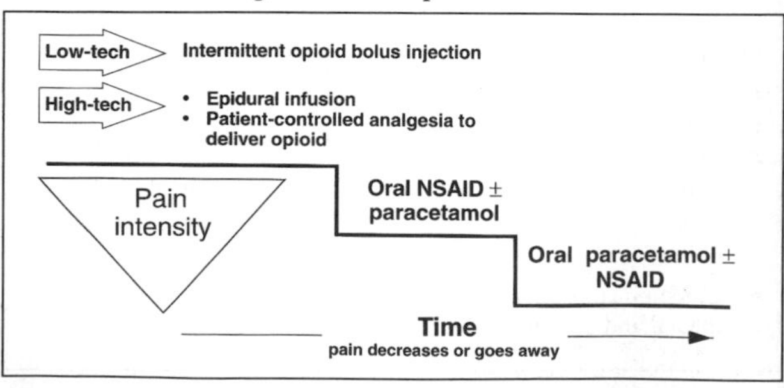

Management of acute pain in hospital[1]

1. Effective relief can be achieved with oral non-opioid and non-steroidal anti-inflammatory drugs (NSAIDs). Studies indicate that ibuprofen 400mg is the most effective of these drugs; paracetamol 1g and the combination of paracetamol with codeine are also highly effective. Ibuprofen is associated with fewer gastrointestinal bleeds than some other NSAIDs.

Initial management of moderate pain, such as in postsurgical patients, should ideally be an oral NSAID such as ibuprofen, supplemented if necessary with paracetamol. In the elderly, paracetamol may be preferred although it is less effective. There is no evidence that giving the drug by routes other than orally is beneficial.

2. Opioids are the first choice treatment for severe acute pain. Additional, often smaller, doses can be given if the patient is still in pain and you are sure that all the previous dose has been delivered and absorbed. More drug can be given 5mins after IV injection, 1hr after IM or SC injection, and 90mins after an oral dose. The route of administration can be changed to achieve faster control if there is no response to the repeated dose.

- ► The key principle for safe and effective use of opioids is to titrate the dose against the degree of pain relief. If the patient is asking for more opioid then it usually signals inadequate pain control resulting from too little drug, too long between doses, too little attention being paid to the patient, or too much reliance on rigid regimens.
- ► It is very important to set up a q4h regimen which prevents the occurence of pain.
- ► It may be safer to use only one opioid in routine practice. Morphine is the most appropriate choice and it is popular amongst pain specialists. It has an action which lasts a reliable four hours and is easier to titrate than opioids with a longer half-life. (See left for an example of a q4h morphine regimen.)

As the pain decreases, the patient can be switched over to ibuprofen and paracetamol (see figure to the left). Supplementation of morphine with an NSAID allows the morphine dose to be reduced.

1. McQuay H, 1997, *BMJ*, **314**, 1531

► Typhoid and paratyphoid fevers

These conditions, also called enteric fever, follow systemic infection with *Salmonella* spp (*S. typhi* – typhoid; *S. paratyphi* types A, B, C – paratyphoid) and, at least initially, show minimal GI involvement. They are endemic and important causes of morbidity throughout the developing world. Typhoid is the most severe, paratyphoid B the mildest, with types A & C falling somewhere inbetween. ► Early antibiotic treatment is essential to decrease mortality – start empirically if clinical suspicion is strong.

Following 1° multiplication in the mesenteric lymph nodes, bacteria infect cells of the reticuloendothelial system where multiplication occurs again. This produces a massive 2° bacteraemia, infection of multiple organs, and clinical illness. If untreated, 20% cases die from overwhelming toxaemia or 2° organ involvement, particularly toxic myocarditis or GI haemorrhage and peritonitis (following infection and ulceration of intestinal Peyer's patches). ► Importantly for infection control, chronic infection of the gallbladder is common – the asymptomatic carrier has highly infectious stools.

Transmission: via the ingestion of food or water contaminated by infected faeces/urine. Gastric acid is protective so any condition that decreases its production increases an individual's susceptibility to infection.

Clinical features: the incubation period is normally between 10–20 days; the illness typically lasts 4 weeks but may be shorter in severe infections (and vice versa). ***1st week*** – non-specific features of malaise, headache, rising remitting fever with mild cough, constipation. ***2nd week*** – patient becomes toxic and apathetic; sustained high temperature with relative bradycardia; rose spots (2–4mm pink papules on central torso, fading on pressure) transiently occur between day 7 & 12 in 50% individuals; distended abdomen; splenomegaly. ***3rd week*** – increasing toxicity with persistent high temp; the patient becomes delirious and weak with feeble pulse, tachypnoea (+/– basal creps); ↑ abdominal distension, ↓ bowel sounds, profuse 'pea soup' diarrhoea; neurological complications may occur at this stage (may rarely be the presenting complaint). Death may occur during week 3 or 4. ***4th week*** –if the patient suvives; GI complications may occur; fever, mental state, and abdominal distension improve over a few days.

Diagnosis: culture of bone marrow (best), blood, stool, or rectal swab.

Management:

1. Give antibiotics – see opposite.

2. Give dexamethasone (3mg/kg IV stat then 1mg/kg 6-hrly for 2 days) ↓ mortality in patients with shock or ↓ mental status.

► Toxic patients must be observed carefully for signs of GI haemorrhage (treat conservatively) or peritonitis (treat with surgery).

Relapse: 10–20% of treated patients relapse after treatment and initial recovery. Relapses are generally milder and shorter than 1° illness; 2nd and 3rd relapses have been reported – therefore follow up if possible. Coinfection with schistosomes may result in chronic/recurrent fever since the bacteria can survive within parasites, being protected from antibiotics.

Control: improved sanitation.

First choice antibiotics vary due to local resistance:

In Asia:

- quinolone eg ciprofloxacin 500mg PO bd for 14 days [alternative: cefotaxime 1g IV q8h for 14 days].

In Africa and the Americas:

- chloramphenicol 500mg PO q4h until afebrile, then q6h for 14 days
  [alternatives: amoxicillin 250mg PO qds or cotrimoxazole 960mg PO bd; both for 14 days].

Dosages for each drug can be doubled initially for severe infections (cotrimoxazole – 1.5×) and given IV.

Typhus fevers

These are fevers caused by members of the *Rickettsia* genus, small obligate intracellular microbes that resemble Gram-negative bacteria. Different *Rickettsia* produce different forms of typhus – these range from the normally subclinical murine typhus to the potentially fulminant louse-borne typhus fever and Rocky Mountain spotted fever. All except mild infections show a macular petechial rash that is caused by endothelial cell destruction. Classical typhus fever is now rare since all the typhus fevers respond rapidly to tetracycline or doxycycline therapy.

Transmission: the various bacteria are transmitted by lice, fleas, ticks or mites. Their natural hosts include herbivores such as deer. The typhus fevers are normally grouped according to their mode of transmission.

1. **Typhus fever** – exists in two forms:
   - ***Epidemic louse-borne typhus*** **–** a potentially severe disease of overcrowded populations in mountainous areas of Asia, Africa and the Americas. Brill-Zinnser disease is late reactivation of dormant infection.
   - ***Endemic murine typhus*** **–** a much milder disease which occurs in people in close contact with rodents. Neither form shows an eschar at the site of infection.

2. **Spotted fever or tick typhus** – occurs in two main forms:
   - ***American tick typhus*** (Rocky Mountain spotted fever [RMSF] and S. American tick typhus).
   - ***Old World tick typhus*** (Fièvre Boutonneuse, African tick typhus, tick typhus fevers of Asia).

   The rickettsia are transmitted by the bite of Ioxdid ticks. The different fevers follow a similar clinical course except that RMSF is much more severe and lacks an eschar. Long-term complications are rare. Immunity to all the tick-borne fevers is short-lived, resulting in relapses and reinfections.

   Rickettsialpox is a mite-borne typhus fever that is similar to the tick typhus fevers. It is important because its rash is similar to varicella.

3. **Scrub or mite typhus** – is a severe infection, indigenous to south and east Asia and northern Australasia, that kills up to 30% of untreated patients. Complications include meningoencephalitis and myocarditis. An eschar develops at the site of infection.

Diagnosis: of any of the rickettsial infections is by serology (including Weil-Felix reaction and rickettsial agglutination tests) or isolation of rickettsia from the blood or tissues early in infection. ► Rickettsia cannot be grown on normal bacterial plates; they must be inoculated into animals or eggs. If culture is an option, warn the laboratory in advance.

Prevention: reduction of vector populations and improvements in hygiene (including delousing); avoidance of contact with vectors by using tick repellants and protective clothing. (If a tick is found attached to the skin, remove it by grasping its anterior parts and pulling steadily until it comes away.) Although vaccines against particular rickettsia do not offer complete protection, they may decrease the severity of disease.

Management:

1. Give antibiotics: • doxycycline 200mg PO in a single dose.
   Alternatives:
   - chloramphenicol 500mg PO q6h *or*
   - tetracycline 500mg PO q6h,
     both for 7 days.

   Drugs can be given IV in severe cases.
   Continue treatment for 2–3 days after the patient is afebrile to prevent recrudescence.
2. Severe cases require prednisolone 40mg PO loading dose, then 20mg daily tailing off over several days.
3. Louse-borne typhus infected patients (& clothes) must be washed and disinfected (or autoclaved/burnt), and then deloused weekly with 1% malathion or 10% DDT. Regular treatment of medical/nursing staff is recommended.
4. Nursing involves cold sponging for temp >40°C; replacement of fluids; mouth toilet; and prevention of bed sores.

Other rickettsial infections

1. **Trench fever** – a usually mild systemic illness caused by *Bartonella quintana* infection transmitted by the human body louse. The fever may be self-limiting, recurrent every 5th day, or prolonged. Full recovery is usual but bacteraemia and endocarditis have been noted.
2. **Q fever** – a worldwide infection caused by very small, rickettsia-like bacteria – *Coxiella burnetti*. Transmission is from domestic cattle and goats via milk, placental products, or dried faeces in dust; very occasionally via ticks. Most infections produce a mild fever without rash. Some patients have a chronic course with involvement of lungs (atypical pneumonia), liver, pericardium & heart. Cardiac involvement occurs in 10% of cases; destructive valve lesions (often aortic) occur many months after the acute illness.
3. **Human ehrlichiosis** – a disease caused by infection with coccobacilli *Ehrlichia* spp via tick bites. It occurs in two forms – monocytic and granulocytic. Patients present with flu-like symptoms; complications include pneumonitis, encephalopathy, renal failure, and sepsis. Thrombocytopenia and leukopenia are common.

4. **Cat scratch disease** – is caused by *Bartonella henselae* infection and normally presents as a self-limiting regional lymphadenopathy with fever following contact with cats, particularly kittens. A small papule may be found at the inoculation site. Complications occur in <5%, in the liver, CNS and peripheral nerves, lungs, eyes, bones and skin (erythematous, maculopapular or papulovesicular rashes; petechiae). Blood film may show thrombocytopenia; ultrasound may show multiple lesions in an enlarged liver or spleen.
5. **Bartonellosis** – occurs in two forms following infection with *Bartonella bacilliformis*:
   - an acute febrile haemolytic illness (Oroya fever)
   - cutaneous hemangioma-like growths (verruga peruvana) which develop several weeks after recovery from the 1° illness (they may develop without any apparent 1° illness if this was subclinical).

   Without treatment, Oroya fever is commonly fatal due to massive haemolysis and necrosis of the reticuloendothelial system. Complications include *S.typhimurium* superinfection, pleurisy, parotitis, thromboses, and meningoencephalitis. The fever may last 3–4 months in survivors.

   It is restricted to the western slopes of the Andes where it is transmitted by the bite of *Lutzomyia* spp sandflies. Prevention is by controlling the sandfly vectors and preventing human exposure.

Diagnosis

- Serology and/or culture for trench fever, Q fever, ehrlichiosis, CSD.
- Examination of peripheral blood films for morulae within neutrophils/monocytes (ehrlichiosis) or bacilli within erythrocytes (Oroya fever).
- For cat scratch disease, large rods can be seen in tissue sections stained with Warthin-Starry silver stain (not Gram or ZN stains).

Management:

Give antibiotics:
- Doxycycline 200mg PO as a single dose, then 100mg daily for 7–14 days. The dose can be doubled in severe infections.
- [Alternatives as for typhus fever]

- Bacteraemia with *B. quintana* requires 4 weeks therapy, longer in HIV^+ patients
- Endocarditis with *C. burnetti* requires long-term combination therapy. The best regimens have not yet been identified; try rifampicin plus either tetracycline or doxycycline.
- Cat scratch disease can be managed symptomatically in most cases; however, severe infection probably warrants gentamicin or a quinolone (the best treatment regimens have still to be identified).
- Chloramphenicol (500mg PO qds for 7 days) is probably best for bartonellosis since it also covers *Salmonella* infection in this region.

Relapsing fever

Louse-borne RF is caused by *Borrelia recurrentis;* it has caused massive epidemics in deprived populations. Untreated mortality is ~70%. Tick-borne RF is a less severe disease that is due to infection with one of 7 *Borrelia* spp, particularly *B. duttoni*. The bacteria invade the skin without causing an eschar and multiply in the blood. The fever falls as the immune system removes bacteria but recurs as antigenic variation allows bacterial numbers to recover. Platelets are sequestered in the bone marrow producing thrombocytopenia → petechial rashes & widespread haemorrhage.

1. Louse-borne relapsing fever

Transmission: is human-human via the body and head lice (*Pediculus humanus* var. *corporis* and *capitis*). Humans are the only host. Lice become infected by feeding on human blood during a febrile period and infect other humans by being crushed onto the skin, not via a bite.

Clinical features: chills, high fever and N&V develop rapidly 4–8 days after infection. Temp can be >40.5°C; the patient is delirious, with a severe headache and generalized pains. Dyspnoea is characteristic – hissing, loud, and audible from a distance – as are: cough with *B. recurrentis*$^+$ sputum, hepatosplenomegaly, jaundice. An erythematous upper-body rash may occur during 1st attack. Bleeding occurs into the skin (petechial rash), mucous membranes (epistaxis), or conjunctivae.

The fever lasts 5–7 days at which point it falls to 36°C → state of collapse (termed a 'crisis') and relief from symptoms. The second attack is less severe; >1 relapse occurs in 25% patients; never >4.

Death is due to DIC, myocarditis, or hepatic encephalopathy during the first febrile period or hyperpyrexia with shock, heart failure, and cerebral oedema during the first crisis. Death may also occur after antibiotic treatment due to a Jarisch-Herxheimer reaction.

2. Tick-borne relapsing fever

Transmission: is via the bite of *Ornithodoros* soft ticks. Humans are the only source for tick infection, although rodents and other animals may become infected.

Clinical features: after an incubation period of up to 14 days (possibly as few as 2), there is severe fever and headache (rarely this continues to coma & death). Splenomegaly and splenic infarction are common (hepatomegaly less so, jaundice rare); as are diarrhoea; bronchitis; pneumonia; haematuria. Neurological complications without long-term sequelae are common: cranial & spinal nerve involvement, meningitis +/– sub-arachnoid haemorrhage, encephalitis, hemiplegia. Other rare complications include bronchitis, liver failure, arthritis.

Fever may recur up to 11×, separated by a gap of a few days to 3wks.

Diagnosis: spirochaetes in a Giemsa-stained thick blood film, or culture, during febrile periods; serology (?unreliable due to cross-reactivity).

Prevention: control of ticks and rodent vectors (TBRF); use of insecticides and improved hygiene (LBRF).

Management:

1. Give tetracycline 500mg PO as a single dose.
   Alternatives:
   - tetracycline 500mg PO q6h plus procaine penicillin 300mg IM q12–24h for seven days
   - tetracycline 250mg IV q6h
   - erythromycin 500mg PO as a single dose.
2. Louse infected patients must be washed and disinfected, and then deloused weekly with 1% malathion or 10% DDT. Regular treatment of medical/nursing staff is recommended. The patient's clothes should be autoclaved or burnt.

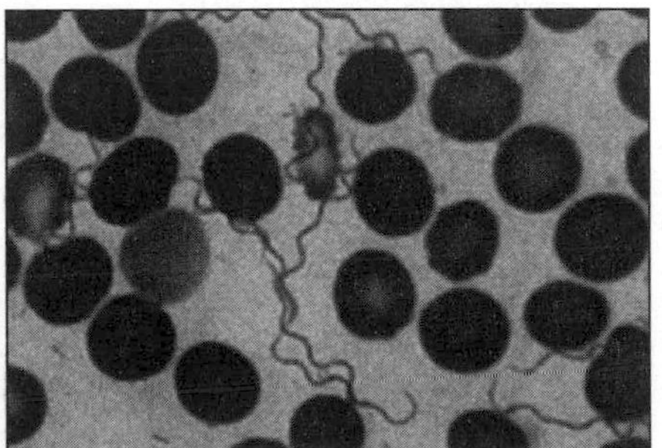

Borrelia **in a blood film**

Leptospirosis

This condition is caused by spirochaetes of the *Leptospira interrogans* complex. Following infection, the spirochaetes spread to multiple organs and cause direct damage to parenchymal and endothelial cells. Further damage in the form of immune complex glomerulonephritis and vasculitis then results from the host's immune response.

Many infections are subclinical. Clinical disease varies from mild, low-grade chronic febrile illness, with or without meningitis, to the classical **Weils disease** with hepatitis and nephritis. Recent epidemics in C America have presented with pulmonary haemorrhage. Death in leptospirosis is due to hepatorenal failure or to haemorrhage secondary to endothelial damage (rather than to consumption of clotting factors).

Transmission: follows contact of broken skin (or ? mucous membranes) with rat urine in contaminated water (particularly pools, canals, rivers) or through close contact or bites during agricultural work. Although rats are responsible for most human infection, many animals can be infected with *Leptospira* and dogs and foxes may be rare sources of human infection.

Clinical features: 1–3 weeks post-infection, there is sudden onset of fever, headache, myalgia, anorexia, N&V, eye discharge, subconjunctival haemorrhage, and sore throat. In severe infections, the patient becomes prostrate with high fever and marked myalgia; cough, haemoptysis, dyspnoea; persistent vomiting, abdominal pain, constipation, mild hepatomegaly and jaundice. Other signs which may be present include meningism, a transient non-specific rash, and purpura (indicative of underlying endothelial damage and 2° thrombocytopenia).

In mild cases, a 2-day remission occurs after 4–7 days but this may usher in a second immunopathologic phase. If this is severe, the patient's condition worsens with the development of persistent high fever, myocarditis, widespread haemorrhage (into lungs, GI, skin), renal failure, and shock.

Diagnosis: during days 1 to 4, it is possible to culture *Leptospira* from the blood and visualize it on blood films under dark field microscopy. They can also be seen after day 10 in fresh alkaline urine. Look for motile, viable fine spiral bacteria with hooked ends. Serology.

Management:

1. Give antibiotics: • benzylpenicillin 1.2g IV/IM q6h
[alternatives: doxycycline 200mg PO stat then 100mg PO bd, *or*
erythromycin 500mg bd PO]

2. Severe disease may warrant transferring the patient to an intensive care ward. Haemodialysis is often required.

3. ► Beware a Jarisch-Herxheimer reaction after antibiotic treatment early in the disease.

Prevention: education of at risk groups to ↓ exposure; control of rodent population and vaccination of domestic animals; chemoprophylaxis in very high risk groups (eg sewerage workers).

Fevers/systemic signs

Brucellosis

A worldwide disease of people in close contact with domesticated animals caused by Gram-negative bacilli of the *Brucella* genus, particularly *B. melitensis*. The bacteria are zoonoses in cows, camels, sheep, and pigs, causing lifelong infections and abortions during 1° infection. Latent infections reactivate during pregnancy, resulting in the production of infected milk.

Following an initial bacteraemia, macrophages become chronically infected in multiple organs. Granulomas form in many of these tissues, with variable progression to i) microabscesses and ii) clinically apparent abscesses. The infection is normally controlled by T cells but it is probable that some organisms persist and reactivate from time to time, producing frequent relapses. ► It is difficult to eradicate the bacteria once a chronic infection has been established – it is essential to treat early during the acute infection.

Transmission: occurs via the consumption of infected unpasteurized milk or soft cheese. Aerosols of milk/amniotic fluid and bacteria surviving in dry dusts may also be infectious via inhalation – the bacteria survive 40 days in dry soil, longer in damp soil. Other routes include sexual; transfusion; skin abrasions; congenital; breast milk. ► Live attenuated animal vaccines are not attenuated in humans.

Clinical features: after a 2–4 week incubation period, a non-specific illness occurs with fever, lethargy, anorexia, night sweats; (hepatosplenomegaly and lymphadenopathy occur in ~30%). The fever subsides but will recur with a periodicity of 2–4 weeks ('undulant fever') if the patient remains untreated. Bones and joints are frequently involved in 2° disease: reactive and septic arthritis (commonly of large weight bearing joints, but any possible); sacroiliitis; vertebral and disc infection with paravertebral abscesses (similar to TB). Other organs involved include the heart (endocarditis), testes; kidneys; (less commonly: lungs, CNS and PNS). **Ix**: show a normochromic normocytic anaemia; the WCC is often normal.

Diagnosis: culture of blood or, better, bone marrow aspirate taken during the acute illness, or pus taken during 2° disease. Serology: agglutinating titre >1/160 (if titre falls after serum treatment with β2-mercaptoethanol [due to destruction of IgM], then infection is 1° and treatment will probably prevent chronic infection).

Prevention: pasteurization (boiling) of milk prevents infection in endemic areas. Brucella-free certified cattle and the use of animal vaccines are other useful elements of disease control. There is no human vaccine.

Management of brucellosis

1. Give antibiotics:
- streptomycin 1g (0.5–0.75g in patients >45yrs) IM daily *plus*
- doxycycline 200mg PO daily, for 1 month,

followed by:
- doxycycline 200mg PO *and*
- rifampicin 600–900mg PO, daily for 6–12 weeks.

2. Longer courses are required when the heart or other organs are involved. Gentamicin can be used for hospitalized patients.

3. Children <8 yrs should receive rifampicin and cotrimoxazole for 8wks; doxycycline and gentamicin can be used for serious complications.

4. Pregnant women should receive rifampicin and cotrimoxazole daily for 8wks.

Plague[ND]

An acute disease caused by the Gram negative coccobacillus, *Yersinia pestis*, which can be rapidly fatal. ►► It thus requires empirical antibiotic therapy, as soon as cultures have been taken, when clinical suspicion is high.

Although some infections are asymptomatic, most fall into two groups:

- ***bubonic plague*** following a fleabite, and
- ***pneumonic plague*** following inhalation of a bacteria-filled respiratory droplet coughed out by an infected human.

Pneumonic plague has a very short incubation period and can kill in 1 day.

Transmission: of bubonic plague is via the bite of infected rodent fleas. Plague is a zoonosis, being maintained in wild rodents. Most human infection comes from urban rats (spectacular die offs of these rodents are the precursors of plague outbreaks), occasionally from domestic cats or dogs.

Clinical features of bubonic plague: the first specific sign is often local lymphadenitis in the nodes draining the site of the flea bite. After 2–7 (always <15) days, a bubo forms in these nodes. There is typically a short prodrome of fever, malaise, headache and, in some cases, a dull ache in the nodes for up to 24 hrs before the bubo is apparent. The enlarged nodes are extremely painful and swollen, the overlying skin warm, red, oedematous and adherent. The mass is non-fluctuant and immobile.

Onset of high fever is rapid with prostration, hepatomegaly (but no splenomegaly), and sometimes D&V. Skin lesions (pustules in bubo-draining area which may become an eschar/carbuncle; patchy purpuric dermal necrosis) are uncommon. Complications include bacteraemia, sepsis; meningitis; pneumonia; and pharyngeal or tonsillar abscess.

Clinical features of pneumonic plague: initially intense headache, malaise, fever, vomiting, prostration, ↓ consciousness. Later: cough, dyspnoea, bloodstained sputum with few chest signs. Patient soon dies from respiratory failure. CXR shows multilobar consolidation or bronchopneumonia – paucity of chest signs compared with the CXR is characteristic. This picture needs to be distinguished from ARDS which may occur in bubonic and septicaemic forms of plague.

Diagnosis: fever plus localized lymphadenopathy in endemic area; aspiration of a bubo → culture and Giemsa/Gram-stained smear (bipolar coccobacillus); blood, sputum, CSF for culture; serology (after a week?).

Prevention: via control of flea and rodent populations with public health measures and public education; vaccination; surveillance including the use of sentinel animals; active case finding.

► Suspected cases should be reported to both local health authorities and the WHO.

► Pneumonic plague patients are highly contagious and must be isolated until after >3 days of antibiotics <u>and</u> clinical improvement. Prophylaxis with tetracycline may be considered for contacts and medical staff.

Management: antibiotics must be given for the pneumonic form within 24 hrs if it is not to prove fatal:

- gentamicin 5mg/kg IV daily (ensure good renal function), *or*
- streptomycin 15mg/kg IM bd.

- For milder cases: tetracycline 250–500mg PO qds or doxycycline 100mg PO bd.
- For meningitis: chloramphenicol 25mg/kg IV stat as a loading dose then 25mg/kg IV qds (PO when clinical condition permits).

All regimens are for 10 days.

Melioidosis

A disease caused by the bacterium *Burkholderia pseudomallei* which is endemic to specific localities – S and SE Asia, and N Australasia. It is a major cause of septicaemia in certain parts of its range eg NE Thailand. The bacterium is stable in mud and surface water (rice paddy); people in regular contact with either are probably infected by inoculation or inhalation.

Infection is often subclinical; clinical illness commonly presents as septicaemia or infection localized to lung (cavitating pneumonia with profound wt loss), bone (particularly spine), or (in children) parotid glands. Septicaemia causes rapid deterioration with production of abscesses in lung, liver and spleen. The infection does not respond to common empiric regimens for sepsis – this diagnosis must be borne in mind in endemic regions. Diagnosis is by culturing blood, pus, sputum, etc.

Glanders is a similar disease caused by *Burkholderia mallei* which normally occurs in horses but may be transmitted to humans.

Anthrax

Anthrax is a disease of herbivores caused by the bacterium *Bacillus anthracis*. Humans acquire it via contact with diseased animals – eg eating or skinning livestock (such as cattle or sheep). It is currently uncommon in most of the world. The bacterium produces spores which can survive almost any environmental condition (except 5–10% formalin for 4hrs, or boiling for >10 mins). The spores may be transported around the world in hides and wool, infecting people and initiating disease in non-endemic areas. Animals which have died from the disease are highly infectious.

Clinical features: cutaneous infection produces a rapidly growing papule that ulcerates and becomes a dry black scab – the anthrax sore. It is of variable size and surrounded by purple vesicles, sometimes massive local oedema, and lymphadenopathy. Pus indicates secondary infection or a different aetiology. There is usually little pain. ► The lesion should not be incised; most sores resolve with or without treatment in 2–6 weeks – oedema and lyphadenopathy may take longer. ► Neck sores with extensive oedema may lead to laryngeal obstruction – consider early tracheotomy.

Serious infections may become generalized, leading to shock and GI haemorrhage. Pulmonary and GI infection may result in sudden onset of severe illness followed by haemorrhage, shock and death in 2–3 days if left untreated.

Diagnosis: visualization of capsulated, dark, square-ended bacilli in short chains using the M'Fadyean stain in smears made from vesicular fluid, fluid from under the eschar (lift edge and extract fluid with capillary tube), blood, lymph node biopsy, or CSF.

Prevention: veterinary public health measures – disposal of infected carcases, disinfection of contaminated areas, and vaccination of herds after single cases. Mass vaccination of animals should also be effective.

Antibiotics for melioidosis:

Treat sepsis with:

- ceftazidime 40mg/kg IV q8h until clinical improvement
  alternatives: • co-amoxiclav 1.2g IV q6–8h
  • imipenem 20mg/kg q8h.

Then give oral therapy to prevent relapse:

- doxycycline 100mg PO bd for 20wks ***plus***
- TMP/SMX 960mg (child 480mg) PO bd for 20wks ***plus***
- chloramphenicol 500mg PO qds for the first 8wks.

Resistance to these drugs has been recognized. Adapt according to local circumstances.
The oral regimen can be used IV for sepsis in β-lactam allergic patients but it is not as effective as ceftazidime.

Management of anthrax

1. Early use of antibiotics may save lives in generalized, pulmonary, and GI disease.
   - give benzylpenicillin 600 mg q6h IV for 3-5 days

The sore becomes sterile in less than 2 days. In late cases, bacterial toxins may cause severe shock and death even with use of antibiotics.

African trypanosomiasis

African trypanosomiasis, or **human sleeping sickness**, is a protozoal disease caused by *Trypanosoma brucei* spp. It exists in two forms: **Gambian** and **Rhodesian**, which are caused by *T. b. gambiense* and *T. b. rhodesiense*, respectively. The former is decreasing in incidence in the west of its range (possibly as a result of decreased vector-human contact), while the incidence of both diseases is increasing in central and east Africa due to breakdown in treatment and vector control measures.

Initial infection is followed by bouts of fever with intervening afebrile periods due to immune-mediated parasite clearance. Variation in the trypanosome antigens allows a few parasites to escape the immune response and cyclically repopulate the blood. Multiple organs become infected, inducing a strong inflammatory reaction and tissue damage.

- The disease course is rapid in *T. b. rhodensiense* infection – patients die during the 1° toxic phase of the illness or in the subsequent few months due to damage to the heart or other viscera.
- Gambian sleeping sickness is a chronic disease which may remain asymptomatic for long periods (although patients remain infective to the tsetse fly). Death occurs after many months or years due to meningoencephalitis.

Transmission: is by the bite of a tsetse fly, genus *Glossina*. *T. b. gambiense* is an endemic infection of humans and riverine tsetse flies. In contrast, *T. b. rhodesiense* is a natural infection of game animals and cattle and is less well adapted to humans. Human infections are sporadic on the E African plains but human epidemics can occur. *T. brucei* is a major killer of cattle and therefore of great economic importance.

Clinical features

1. Rhodesian sleeping sickness: a large tender boil, the primary chancre, may develop at the bite site, in association with localized lymphadenopathy. It subsides to leave a hyperpigmented scar or eschar.

After a 1–3 week incubation period, entry of the trypansomes into the peripheral blood causes severe fever, accompanied by malaise, severe headaches, weight loss, deep hyperaesthesia (Kerandel's sign), myalgia, and arthralgia. An erythematous rash is sometimes apparent; as the infection continues, the skin may become itchy. Subcutaneous oedema produces a puffy face swelling and transitory swelling elsewhere.

The infection proceeds rapidly causing carditis, hepatitis with tender hepatomegaly, and nephritis. Death may occur within weeks or months due to visceral involvement, particularly of the heart (pancarditis, pericarditis, pericardial effusion, heart failure), and often before involvement of the CNS. Infection during pregnancy causes abortions and stillbirths.

2. Gambian sleeping sickness: *T. b. gambiense* infection is not associated with the development of a chancre.

The early stages of the infection are similar to Rhodesian sleeping sickness but less severe; patients tend not to die from acute toxicity. Low-grade fevers recur irregularly before drying out, leaving few signs except lymphadenopathy, often in the posterior cervical triangle, and splenomegaly.

Distribution of African trypanosomiasis

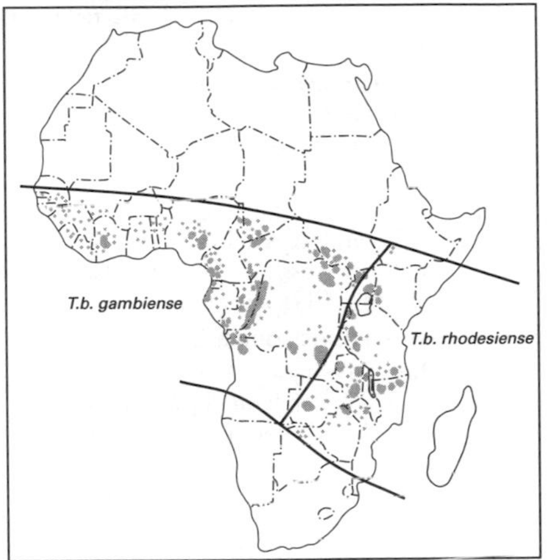

Gambian disease is characterized by severe CNS involvement – the terminal stage is due to encephalomyelitis with headache, ↓ mental function, and ultimately coma. Changes in personality precede changes in sleep pattern. Extrapyramidal signs develop, notably fixed face and tremor or choreic movements of hands, limbs, or tongue. The patient becomes withdrawn, sleeps increasingly during the day, does not eat, and becomes cachetic. The patient dies from starvation, 2° infections, hyperpyrexia, or convulsions.

Diagnosis: microscopic analysis of lymph node aspirate (in Gambian trypanosomiasis), blood (Giemsa-stained thick film) or CSF. Examination of buffy coat preparations is particularly sensitive. Serology is useful: serum and CSF IgM levels are raised.

Management: requires specialist knowledge. All patients should be treated in a specialized centre. Pentamidine and suramin are effective during early disease, but do not cross the blood-brain barrier. Melarsoprol is a very toxic arsenical used for CNS infection.

1. Acute Gambian trypanosomiasis

- Pentamidine **isethionate** 4 mg/kg IM every other day for 7–10 injections (► note isethionate form of pentamidine), *or*
- Suramin 5 mg/kg by slow IV injection on day 1 followed by 10 mg/kg on the 3rd day and 20 mg/kg on days 5, 11, 17, 23 and 30. Improve the patient's condition as much as possible before suramin treatment and administer under close medical supervision.

► A patient exhibiting an anaphylactic reaction after the first dose must never receive suramin again.

2. Acute Rhodesian trypanosomiasis

- Use suramin, as above.

3. Trypanosomiasis with CNS involvement

- Give melarsoprol by slow IV injection with a fine needle, taking care not to allow extravasation. Several treatment regimens are currently used, each comprising 3 or 4 series of daily injections with intervening rest periods of 7–10 days. See opposite for an example.
- 5–10% of patients treated with melarsoprol die due to a drug-induced arsenical encephalopathy. At the onset of encephalopathy, patients should be removed to a quiet area and given a bolus of mannitol over 10mins via an isotonic glucose infusion. This can be repeated every 6hrs. Give prednisolone 50mg IV or an ACTH substitute 25IU IV (beware anaphylaxis with the latter). Beware onset of haemorrhage and seizures.

► Jarisch-Herxheimer reactions resulting from massive destruction of parasites may occur during melarsoprol therapy. Preliminary injections of pentamidine or suramin should be given to clear the majority of parasites from the bloodstream.

Control: reduce exposure to tsetse flies with screens, fly traps, and insecticides; and by detecting and treating human cases. In endemic regions, all suspected cases should be referred to specialized treatment centres for confirmation of the diagnosis and management.

T. brucei as seen on a blood film

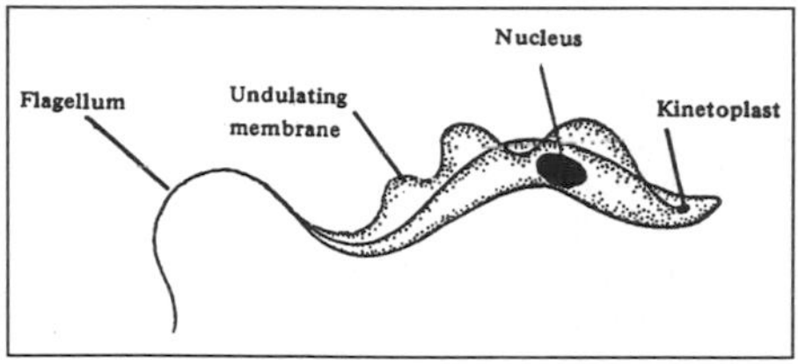

Day	*Drug*	*Dose (mg/kg)*
01	suramin	5.00
02	suramin	20.00
04	melarsoprol	0.36
05	melarsoprol	0.72
06	melarsoprol	1.10
13	melarsoprol	1.40
14	melarsoprol	1.80
15	melarsoprol	1.80
22	melarsoprol	2.20
23	melarsoprol	2.90
24	melarsoprol	3.60
31	melarsoprol	3.60
32	melarsoprol	3.60
33	melarsoprol	3.60

American trypanosomiasis

A parasitic disease of south and central America, also called **Chagas disease**, which is caused by the protozoa *Trypanosoma cruzi*. It may result in fatal cardiomyopathy and GI tract dilatation. The acute infection is often subclinical in adults, although severe and potentially fatal in children. Persistent infection in adults will cause chronic disease in only ~30% of cases. The parasites invade mesenchymal tissues such as heart muscle and intestinal smooth muscle, where the immune response and parasite toxins destroy the autonomic ganglia. This produces chronic dilatation of hollow viscera and, in the case of the heart, arrhythmias. Once in the tissues, the parasites persist there in their amastigote form, without necessarily re-entering the blood, thus making detection and chemotherapy difficult.

Transmission: through contamination of mucous membranes, conjunctivae, and skin by the faeces of nocturnal house-dwelling reduviid bugs. Both domestic and wild animals are reservoirs for the infection, although repeated infection of humans and vector in the absence of natural hosts can occur. Transmission may also be congenital or via blood transfusion.

Clinical features:

- ***Acute disease*** – parasites invading the bite site cause a local swelling, the chagoma, and lymphadenopathy. If the bite is close to the eye, unilateral eyelid oedema may occur, a characteristic feature of Chagas disease (Romaña's sign). 14–28 days postinfection, parasite entry into the blood coincides with the onset of fever. Other features include: a non-pruritic rash of sharply-defined, small macules on the trunk which fades after 7–10 days; swelling, particularly of the face; hepatosplenomegaly; cardiac arrhythmia or insufficiency; meningoencephalitis (often mild, but fatal in ~10% children).
- ***Chronic disease*** – sequelae of autonomic ganglia destruction include • cardiomyopathy → cardiomegaly, tricuspid incompetence, arrhythmias, conductance disorders (often RBBB & L ant hemiblock), heart block (→ sudden death); • megaoesophagus → late dysphagia, oesophagitis and regurgitation of food • parotid hypersalivation, • recurrent aspiration pneumonia, • megacolon → chronic constipation, abdominal pain and, rarely, acute obstruction.

Diagnosis: detection of parasites in wet mount or Giemsa-stained blood films or CSF precipitates; serology. *T. rangeli*, which is not a cause of clinical human disease, may be mistaken for *T. cruzi*.

Management: current treatment is effective during the acute stage – benznidazole 2.5–3.5 mg/kg (children 5mg/kg) PO bd for 60 days or nifurtimox 2.6–3.6 mg/kg PO tds (children 3–5mg/kg PO qds) for 90 days. Benznidazole is also effective in early chronic disease as occurs in children in endemic areas.[1] Symptomatic treatment is often necessary for later complications: CCF, arrhythmias (see chapter 5, but ▶ β blockers are contraindicated), AV block, and sick-sinus syndrome. Megaoesophagus and megacolon may require surgery.

Control: improve the construction of and chemically disinfect houses, so that the vector cannot live in close contact with humans. Screen blood. Promote the use of mosquito nets.

Distribution of American trypanosomiasis

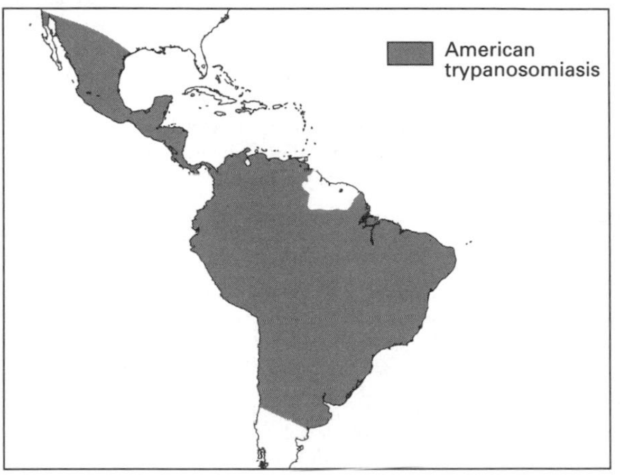

T. cruzi as seen in a blood film

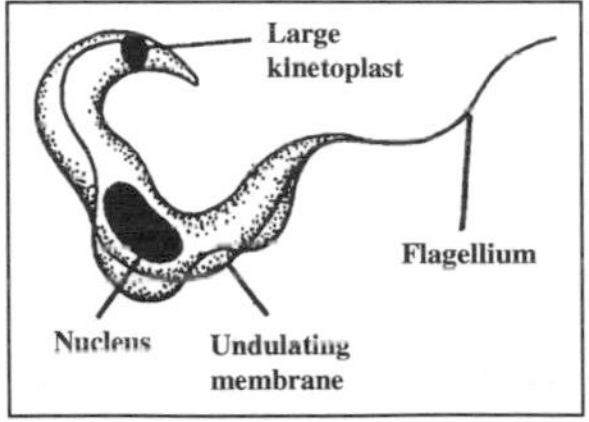

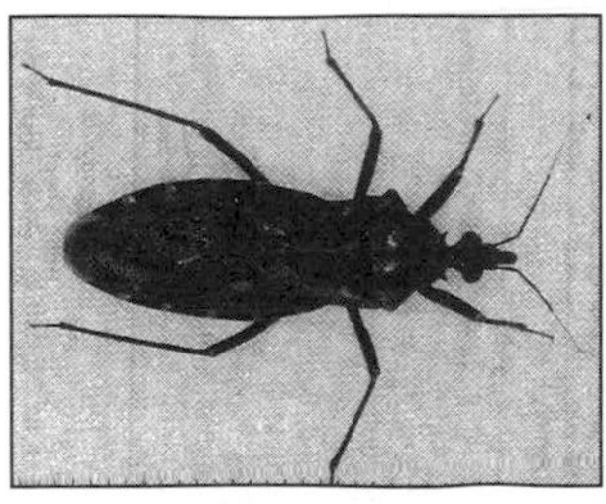

Reduviid bug *Panstrongylus megistus* (cone-nose or kissing bug) responsible for transmission of *T. cruzi.* (25mm long).

1. Sgambatti de Andrade A, 1996, *Lancet*, **348**, 1407

Visceral leishmaniasis (kala-azar)

A endemic parasitic disease caused by infection with *Leishmania donovani* or *L. infantum* (called *L. chagasi* in S. America) which is increasing in incidence and causing major epidemics with high mortality. At infection, the promastigote form invades macrophages which spread the infection to multiple organs, particularly spleen and liver. Many infections are subclinical, being controlled by an efficient cell-mediated immune response. Latent infections may be reactivated during immunosuppression, eg AIDS. In clinically overt disease, this cellular response is ineffective and the parasite continues to multiply, resulting ultimately in pancytopenia and immunosuppression. The patient dies from malnutrition or intercurrent infection. Treatment is normally effective.

Transmission: is by the evening or nocturnal bite of female *Phlebotomus* and *Lutzomyia* sandflies. Dogs are the major reservoirs of *L. infantum* infection. Humans appear to be the major reservoir of Indian and E. African *L. donovani* parasites, particularly during epidemics, when peripheral parasites in infected individuals are taken up by biting sandflies. Patients with post kalar dermal leishmania (PKDL) act as long-term reservoirs of infection.

Clinical features: a small papule (1° leishmanioma) may mark the site of infection in a few cases. Incubation is 2–6 months.

- ***In visitors or during epidemics***, the onset is sudden with high intermittent fever that persists. Initially, the patient appears well, is ambulant, and has a good appetite. Dry cough and epistaxis are common. The spleen enlarges rapidly and can reach the RIF. Rapidly developing anaemia causes fatigue.
- ***In endemic areas***, the acute phase is less common, patients presenting late with low grade fever and abdominal distension or pain due to the splenomegaly. Other features include diarrhoea, moderate hepatomegaly, lymphadenopathy (in Africa), pedal oedema, brittle hair; darkened skin. Hypersplenism produces pancytopenia – petechial and mucosal haemorrhages are late manifestations. Bacterial diarrhoea, pneumonia, and TB infections may develop due to immunosuppression. There is hypoalbuminaemia and hypergammaglobulinaemia due to polyclonal B cell activation. Renal and liver biochemistry is otherwise normal.

Diagnosis: detection of parasites in Giemsa stained smears of spleen aspirates (best) or bone marrow biopsy. Aspirates should also be cultured for *Leishmania* on special media and for other differential diagnoses: eg typhoid, brucellosis, TB. In HIV-infected patients, parasites are very numerous and may be found accidentally in biopsies of skin, gut, or liver or on bronchioalveolar lavage. Serology is useful.

Prevention: via reduction of sandfly vectors and canine/rodent reservoirs. In areas of human-to-human spread, case identification and treatment is essential.

Distribution of visceral leishmaniasis

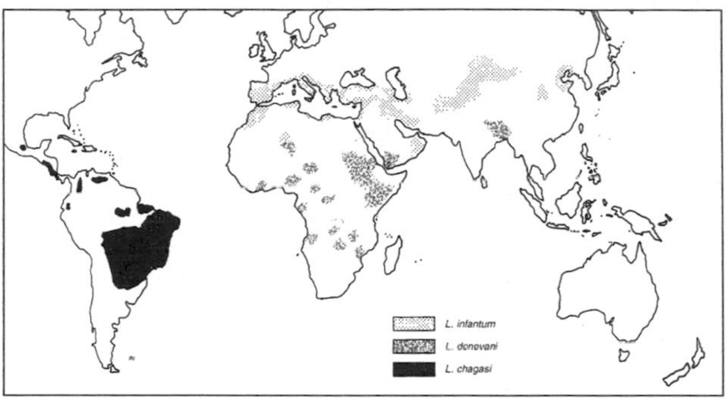

Management:

1. The parasite is usually responsive to IM or IV pentavalent antimony (Sb^v) – 20mg/kg IM daily for >20 days as either meglumine antimoniate (85mg Sb^v/ml) or sodium stibogluconate (100mg Sb^v/ml) – generic stibogluconate have been shown to be as effective as Brand-name preparations (*TMIH* 5; 312). Duration of therapy may need to be prolonged if there is local Sb^v resistance. Primary resistance is a problem in India; secondary resistance occurs in relapsed patients.
2. Patients who relapse following the 1st course can be immediately retreated with the same daily dosage of Sb^v. An alternative is to give amphotericin B 0.3–0.5mg/kg/day (or 1mg/kg on alternate days) for 21 days or liposomal amphotericin B 2–3mg/kg/day to a total of 21mg/kg over 7–10 days. (WARNING – a test dose of amphotericin B and close supervision throughout therapy are required.)
3. Second choice drugs include pentamidine isethionate: 4mg/kg IM (or IV) 3×/week for 5–25 weeks or aminosidine/paromomycin 15mg/kg/day IV for 21 days. The WHO/TDR are working with researchers in an attempt to bring further anti-leishmanial drugs, such as miltefosine, into clinical practice.
4. Clinical response should be evident in 7–10 days. Response can be monitored by fever, haemoglobin, and spleen size. A parasitological response can be verified by a negative splenic aspirate (bone marrow if spleen is now small) at the end of treatment. Clinical follow-up is important after 3 and 6 months to detect relapse; by 12 months the person can be considered cured. Relapse rates should be <5% except in HIV^+ patients almost all of whom will relapse.

► Influenza

A viral cause of respiratory tract infections that produces local epidemics every year and worldwide pandemics at regular intervals – see opposite.

Transmission is probably in large droplets spread via sneezes and coughs. People secrete influenza (particularly type A) for up to 6 days before becoming symptomatic and for 1–2 weeks after the onset of illness.

Clinical features: sudden fever, chills, headache, dry cough, myalgia +/– sore throat, nasal stuffiness lasting from 3 days up to a week. Children may have abdominal pain and vomiting. Influenza B is associated with eye involvement (conjunctivitis, eye pain, photophobia). Influenza may cause 1° pneumonia in patients with weakened immune systems or pre-existing heart disease. A 2° bacterial pneumonia may also occur, normally due to pneumococci or *S. aureus*, the latter of which can be rapidly fatal. Other complications include myocarditis, pericarditis, myositis (? if myalgia severe) and rarely Reye's or Guillain-Barré syndromes.

Diagnosis: serology if a firm diagnosis is required. Epidemics occur at regular intervals and can basically be predicted – during these epidemics care must be taken to not misdiagnose other conditions as influenza.

Treatment: is basically symptomatic although amantidine, rimantidine and ribavirin (all expensive antivirals) are effective in treatment of the infections. Patients should be nursed carefuly and observed for signs of pneumonia and bacterial superinfection. Early treatment of pneumonia with antibiotics and intensive care may save lives.

Prevention: vaccination of those at risk (elderly, immunocompromised, children with heart disease).

Infectious mononucleosis

An acute syndrome of fever, sore throat, malaise, headache and lymphadenopathy that is most commonly caused by the herpesvirus Epstein-Barr virus (EBV). The condition is named after the characteristic mononuclear lymphocytosis that accompanies the infection. A number of lymphocytes are atypical and represent activated virus-specific lympocytes. A few patients (~5%) show a variable rash during the infection; however, treatment with ampicillin produces a maculopapular rash in >90%. Complications include mild hepatitis and thrombocytopenia, and less commonly: autoimmune haemolytic anaemia, splenic rupture (prevent trauma to patients with mononucleosis), and self-resolving encephalitis.

Mononucleosis is normally a self-limited illness lasting 2–3 weeks, although there may be a long post-infection convalescence; very rarely it is a devastating infection with major complications.

Other causes:

- CMV
- hepatitis viruses
- *Toxoplasma gondi*
- *Ehrlichia sennetsu*
- HIV,
- rubella.

Streptococcal sore throat may be confused clinically with the sore throat of mononucleosis.

The influenza virus's genetic elements are packaged as RNA into 8 separate segments. They encode 8 proteins including neuraminidase (NA) and haemaglutanin (HA) – NA is particularly important since antibodies against this protein protect humans from reinfection. RNA viruses mutate their genome rapidly – with influenza this results in small changes in the NA protein every year that allows the virus to avoid the immune response elicited by infection the previous year. This is termed genetic drift and accounts for the yearly influenza epidemics. Every 30 years or so, RNA segments containing the NA gene from avian influenza viruses recombine with human viruses when pigs are simultaneously infected by both sorts of influenza. Humans are then infected by an influenza virus that has a NA protein which has never been 'seen' by humans before and a worldwide 'pandemic' occurs – this is termed 'genetic shift'. The single pandemic that occured in war-torn Europe in 1918–20 killed over 20 million people.

► Measles

This paramyxovirus is a major cause of childhood illness and death in the developing world. In addition to sporadic disease with a fatality rate of ~5%, it also occurs in devastating epidemics that can kill up to 40% of infected children in unvaccinated populations. In contrast, it tends to be a self-limiting infection in industrial societies. Although the reasons for the severity of infection in the developing world are still debated, two possible reasons stand out:

1. *Overcrowding* – measles is a very contagious virus: up to 90% of non-immune people who come into contact with a case will be infected. Transmission rates are therefore high in areas of overcrowding. Secondary cases resulting from household contact are also more severe – in one epidemic, case fatality rates were 23% for 2° cases vs 1% for the first case in a household; 85% of deaths were due to 2° household infections.[1] This may be because of more intense exposure in crowded multifamily dwellings.

2. *Malnutrition* – cellular immunity is important for the host's response to the measles virus. Since this is impaired in the severely malnourished child, poverty and malnutrition may predispose to severe and persistent infections.

The virus infects and lyses epithelial cells of the respiratory and GI tracts, leading to 2° bacterial pneumonia and enteropathy that produces further malnutrition. It also attacks and depresses the immune system itself, encouraging both the 2° infections and reactivation of dormant pathogens such as TB. Death mostly occurs from respiratory and CNS complications. Infection of pregnant women is associated with a subsequent marked increase in infant and child death.

Immunity: an infant receives passive immunity from an immune mother. Once this immunity wanes between 6–9 months, a live vaccine can be given – it is highly effective in protecting infants and children.

Non-immune infants <16 months old have a high mortality rate (over 50% in some epidemics). Vaccination limits both the extent of epidemics and the mortality by increasing herd immunity and decreasing the number of children susceptible to 2° infection. The standard measles vaccine also produces a far greater decrease in child mortality than is expected from simply reducing measles infection[2] – the mechanism for this is unclear.

Transmission: is directly from humans via inhalation of virus in respiratory droplets following face-to-face exposure. Exposure to airborne virus may also be important in areas of high density. Medical clinics are recognized sources of infections. There is no animal reservoir or vector.

Clinical features: after 10–14 days, fever and coryza develop over 24hrs followed by severe conjunctivitis and cough. During this prodromal phase, infants often lose a lot of weight. By day 3, Kopliks spots (bright red blobs with bluish/white centre) become visible on the buccal mucosa. 24–48hrs later, a rash appears on the forehead and neck, spreading to the trunk over 2–4 days. On dark skin, the maculopapular rash is deep-red or purple and ultimately desquamates; on pale skin, it is initially reddish, becoming brown. The patient is most ill during the first day or two of the rash; if the infection is uncomplicated, the fever abates several days after the rash's appearance.

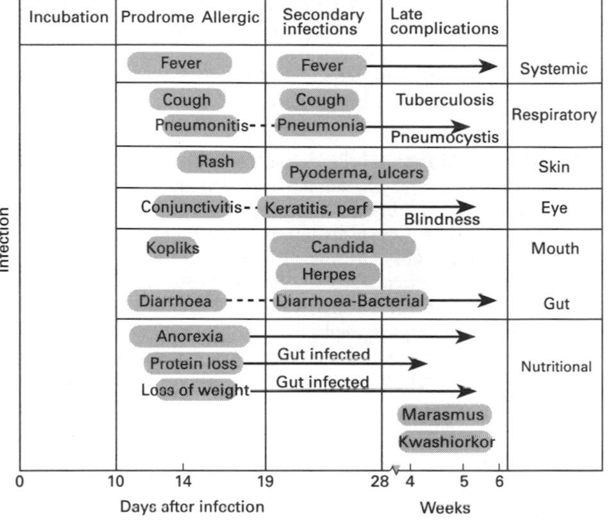

Timecourse of measles infection

1. Aaby P, 1988, *Rev Infect Dis*, **10**, 474 2. Aaby P, 1995, *BMJ*, **311**, 481

Complications include

- Laryngitis (both 2° bacterial and viral) → upper airway obstruction
- 2° bronchopneumonia (normally ? bacterial) – may be difficult to recognize since patients already have fever, cough, ↑ RR: ? prophylactic antibiotics? – see management.
- Sore mouth (decreases feeding by infant); otitis media.
- Corneal ulceration and keratomalacia (+ 2° HSV infection) → blindness (exacerbated by Vit A deficiency).
- Diarrhoea (+/– tenesmus, blood) → ***dehydration & malnutrition***
- Haemorrhagic measles with purpuric rash and mucosal haemorrhage (very rare but has a high mortality rate).

CNS complications: febrile convulsions are the most common. Encephalitis is a rarer manifestation, occuring in three forms:

- Acute postinfectious measles encephalitis – occurs in older children (>2yrs) 4–7 days after the rash's appearance; it has a 10–20% fatality rate and many survivors have neurological sequelae.
- Acute progressive encephalitis – occurs in immunosuppressed patients; manifests with lethargy, seizures, motor and sensory defects.
- Subacute sclerosing panencephalitis (SSPE) – very rare late complication of 5–15 yr olds, M > F , slow progressive disease developing over months with subtle changes in personality and intellect due to continuing infection; later: myoclonic jerks → chorioathetosis; ataxia; coma; focal retinitis → blindness. There is no specific treatment.

Diagnosis: the clinical features of cough, conjunctivitis, coryza and morbilliform rash are often diagnostic. Otherwise: serology, (rarely multinucleate giant cells in Giemsa-stained smears of urine/sputum by light microscope). The virus is present in blood, urine, respiratory secretions, and on conjunctivae from onset of symptoms until ~4th day of the rash.

Management:

1. ► Give vitamin A 200,000IU PO immediately. It may well save the child's eyesight and also decrease the severity of the disease in general.
2. Give topical antibiotics to patients with conjunctivitis or corneal dryness to prevent 2° bacterial infection.
   - chloramphenicol eyedrops, preferably q2h, but at least q6h.

   These eye problems are normally due to the child being unable to close her eyelids adequately.
3. Give symptomatic care, with particular regard to hydration & nutrition.
4. Give antibiotics for 2° infections.

   Studies from Senegal have also suggested that prophylactic antibiotics markedly decrease mortality during an epidemic.

Control: active immunization. Passive immunization with human γ-globulin (0.25mg/kg) is effective up to 5 days postexposure.

Hospital admission

During an epidemic, decide which clinical signs should determine whether a patient is ill enough to warrant admitting to hospital. The following criteria were used by Lamb in a Gambian epidemic to grade severity of illness.[1]

	Degree of severity of infection			
	Severe	***Mod/Sev***	***Moderate***	***Mild***
Oral lesions				
Buccal mucosa	+	+	+	+
Gingiva	+	+	+/–	–
Tongue/palate	+	+	–	–
Haemorrhagic	+	–	–	–
Rash				
Haemorrhagic	+	–	–	–
Confluent	+	+	–	–
Desquamating	+	+/–	–	–
Widespread	–	–	+	–
Scattered	–	–	–	+
Systemic upset				
Bronchopneumonia	+	+	–	–
Cough	+	+	+	–
Coryza	+	+	+	+
Diarrhoea	+	+	+	–
Bloody diarrhoea	+	–	–	–

Other signs that may warrant admission include:

- severe mouth or skin ulceration
- convulsions/LOC
- marked dehydration.
- corneal ulceration
- laryngeal obstruction

► If the child is malnourished or underweight, these signs should be considered with greater seriousness.

1. Lamb WH, 1996, *Rev Infect Dis*, **10**, 457

Arboviruses

Arboviruses, (RNA viruses from the Togaviridae, Flaviviridae, and Bunyaviridae families), are a common cause of non-specific viral fever throughout the tropics. Although there are hundreds of these viruses, relatively few are known to cause clinical disease in humans. Some are geographically restricted; others are important in many parts of the world. A number of arboviruses infect humans but do not cause clinical disease – the resulting immunity may be important in protecting populations from similar cross-reactive viruses that do cause disease.

The illnesses that these viruses cause can be roughly divided into 4 syndromes: • fever +/– rash, • fever with arthralgia, • haemorrhagic fever and • encephalitis. While the first two syndromes are generally self-limiting, haemorrhagic fever and encephalitis can cause immense morbidity and mortality, particularly in children and the elderly.

Epidemics occur when a virus meets a non-immune population (except DHF), for example when climatic changes alter a vector's range, eg after the flooding of normally dry areas. A vector may also be introduced into new areas by human activity, as has happened with the inadvertent introduction of the dengue vector, *Aedes albopictus* (Asian tiger mosquito), into

the Americas in a shipment of tyres from Asia.

Transmission: almost all ***arbo***virus are ***ar***thropod-***bo***rne, ie transmitted by the bites of blood-sucking insects – mostly mosquitos, sandflies and ticks. Transmission can also occur when people, such as butchers or vets, come into direct contact with infected animal tissues, or when people drink milk from infected animals.

Most arboviruses naturally infect a specific animal host (commonly birds, rodents or primates – termed 'maintenance hosts') in which they cause little disease. Infection of humans is normally incidental and non-productive. Some viruses have 'amplifier' hosts – animals such as pigs in which the virus is amplified before possible exposure to humans. The presence of such animals in close proximity to human habitation will increase the risk of human infection.

Diagnosis: is difficult with sporadic cases since the clinical features may be non-specific – it is often, therefore, a diagnosis of exclusion. During epidemics, diagnosis becomes easier. Virus is present in the blood early in the illness with some infections. If there are no facilities for viral culture or immunohistochemistry (for visualization of virus in peripheral cells – used for dengue fever[1]), then acute and convalescent sera are required for retrospective serological analysis.

Prevention: involves breaking vector-human contact by controlling vectors and maintenance or amplifier hosts. Knowledge of the arboviruses that cause disease in any particular region, and their life cycle, is desirable for setting up control measures – this is a good reason for determining the aetiology of 'viral fever' in each area.

Vaccines have been developed for a few infections, notably yellow fever, Rift valley fever, Omsk HF.

1. Myint KS, 1991, *Am J Trop Med Hyg*, 45, 173

Local arboviruses

Each region will have its own set of arboviruses. This box can be used to list the arboviruses that are known to occur in the local area along with their distinctive clinical signs.

- **fever +/– rash**

- **fever with arthralgia**

- **haemorrhagic fever**

- **encephalitis**

Dengue fever

Dengue fever is the classic arboviral systemic febrile illness. A similar syndrome is caused by a variety of other arboviruses.

Dengue fever is caused by the dengue virus, which is endemic throughout the tropics where its principal mosquito vector *Aedes aegypti* occurs. This self-resolving illness needs to be distinguished from malaria. The four serotypes each produce an identical syndrome. Although immunity to one serotype is absolute, protection across serotypes is partial and transient, leading to recurrent episodes of dengue. It has caused vast epidemics affecting whole communities in SE Asia, India, Central and S America. In endemic areas, children are almost exclusively affected and seroprevalence approaches 100% by young adulthood.

Transmission: by the daytime bite of *A. aegypti* (and *A. albopictus*) mosquitos; the cycle is continued when mosquitos bite viraemic humans. There does not appear to be an intermediate animal host.

Clinical features: classical dengue fever occurs in adults and older children (in young children, upper respiratory symptoms may occur and dengue not be suspected). Incubation period is 2–8 days, followed by sudden onset of fever (up to 41°C, with relatively slow pulse), severe headache, malaise, chills, retro-orbital, lumbrosacral, and generalized severe muscular pains. A *transient* macular rash may occur during the first 2 days of illness. A further, maculopapular rash of the trunk, limbs and face occurs after 3–6 days, as the fever settles. This resolves after a few days, often with desquamation. Anorexia, generalized lymphadenopathy, altered taste sensation and upper respiratory tract symptoms are common. Some patients show signs of altered haemostasis – see dengue haemorrhagic fever on page 242. Blood films show leukopenia (neutropenia with relative lymphocytosis) and mild (occasionally severe) thrombocytopenia. The acute illness resolves after ~10 days.

Management: of dengue is symptomatic except for dengue shock syndrome/haemorrhagic fever – see following pages. Salicylates should be avoided since they can exacerbate problems of haemostasis and because dengue has been associated with Reye's syndrome.

Chikungunya

An arbovirus that causes an acute self-limiting febrile illness in Africa, south-east Asia, Middle East and south Asia. It is also the prototypic arbovirus causing arthralgia and fever. The patient's temperature suddenly climbs to 40°C with chills; it may fall after a few days only to climb back up again. Presentation typically involves severe polyarticular arthralgia – symmetrically affecting small joints and sites of previous injury, with joint swelling. The patient will try not to move at all. This presentation is more common in adults; children may present with signs of CNS involvement. A macular rash appears on the face and neck and works down towards the soles of the feet, becoming pruritic as it does so. The other clinical features are similar to dengue fever. Convalescence is complicated by the intermittent presence of a crippling arthralgia.

Distribution of dengue fever

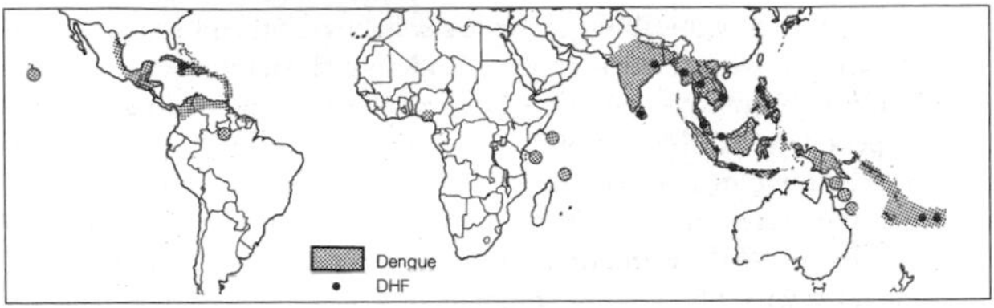

Viral haemorrhagic fever (VHF)

A potentially fatal complication of infection with a variety of viruses. Although most of these viruses cause mild disease, all can produce severe disease with haemorrhagic manifestations and fatality rates of >50% during epidemics. The viruses infect and disrupt vascular endothelial cells causing increased permeability, complement activation and immune complex deposition with further damage. Widespread haemorrhage and fluid loss results in haemoconcentration, hypovolaemia, tissue hypoxia, acidosis, and hyperkalaemia which may result in irreversible shock. Some viruses damage the bone marrow and liver.

Since the early clinical features are often non-specific, experience of locally relevant VHFs is important for early diagnosis. More specific signs include fever with pharyngitis, conjunctivitis, D&V, abdominal pain and haemorrhage.

► It is important to consider treatable causes of fever, shock, and haemorrhage such as malaria, sepsis, leptospirosis, rickettsial infections and meningococcaemia before diagnosing VHF.

General precautions

1. Patients should, if at all possible, be isolated in separate rooms. Otherwise, only essential medical personnel should approach within 1 metre (3.5 feet) – draw a red line around the bed to mark out this distance.
2. Body fluids are highly infectious in the early stages of most VHFs (not dengue HF). All nursing and medical staff need to take great care not to expose themselves to infectious fluids, particularly during blood sampling, surgery, and post-mortem procedures. Some of the viruses can be transmitted in aerosols – avoid generating them.
3. Minimize the use of invasive procedures to avoid the potential for injury and accidental exposure. Use oral rather than injectable drugs whenever possible
4. Scrupulous adherence to universal precautions should decrease exposure but may not prevent it.
5. Unless there is an epidemic going on, many patients with VHFs are not diagnosed until they have been in hospital for a few days. Any hospital which does not practice universal precautions at all times is putting its health workers and patients at great risk.

Management Patient management is predominantly supportive. It requires careful nursing and, most of all, careful monitoring and management of fluid balance and electrolytes. For specific therapy, see box opposite.

6. Careful fluid replacement by mouth should be started before the onset of shock.
7. Loss of vascular fluid to the extracellular space will produce hypovolaemia – watch for an increase in packed cell volume and replace fluids to maintain the circulating blood volume.
8. Beware acidosis and hyponatraemia.
9. Transfuse blood if there are signs of severe haemorrhage and give FFP (5 units for an adult) to manage thrombocytopenia.

Curative therapy:
- Convalescent serum has been used to treat the infection.
- Ribavarin (2.0g loading dose IV, then 1.0g IV q6h for 4 days, then 0.5g IV q8h for 6 days) also appears to be of value in many of the hemorrhagic fevers, particularly if it is used early. It is very expensive but it may be lifesaving.

The following surveillance case definition was produced by the CDC and WHO for the Kikwit Ebola outbreak during 1995. With some adaptation, it may be relevant for other viral haemorrhagic fevers.

Surveillance case definition for patients with suspected Ebola virus haemorrhagic fever

1. An illness characterized by fever (>38.5°C) for more than 3 days, diarrhoea, and at least 1 of the following 5 clinical signs: myalgia, arthralgia, back pain, headache, intense weakness after rehydration.
2. The patient has no response to treatment with antibiotics and anti-malarials for a minimum of three days
3. The patient's illness can be classified into one of the following categories:
   a) presence of at least three additional clinical signs (sore throat or dysphagia, red eyes, hiccups, burning sensation of the skin, or rapid respiration).
   b) bleeding signs (nose, mouth, urine, black or bloody stools, black or bloody vomit).
   c) reported history of recent care for another person, likely a family member or hospitalized patient, who died of a disease with features similar to those listed above.

Patients fulfilling the surveillance case definition for Ebola VHF can be tested for infection by immunohistochemistry on formalin-fixed tissue biopsy samples (preferably liver, although for Ebola VHF any tissue will do). Full information from the patient's notes is required for this test to be done by the CDC.

Arbovirus haemorrhagic fevers (HF)

1. Dengue haemorrhagic fever (DHF)

A serious complication of dengue infection that mostly affects indigenous children in endemic dengue areas. Visitors to these areas are rarely affected since prior exposure to dengue virus is thought to be necessary in the great majority of cases. Low-affinity antibodies against one serotype of virus interfere with the immune response raised against a second serotype during a later infection. This results in immunopathology and, in some cases, circulatory failure and disseminated intravascular coagulation – the **dengue shock syndrome**. Capillary leak is the major difference between DHF and dengue shock syndrome. Mild DHF can be similar to dengue fever and is only recognised by checking the haematocrit. DHF is now common throughout SE Asia and has spread to tropical America.

Clinical features: initially identical to dengue fever, after 2–5 days the patient's condition worsens rapidly with signs of hypotension, circulatory shock, and haemorrhage (petechiae, echymoses, needlesite bleeds, gross GI bleeds; significant bleeding is uncommon in children). The patient is prostrate, restless and dehydrated if shocked; some show facial flushing, and have abdominal pain. Examination commonly shows tender hepatomegaly (jaundice is rare), shallow pulse, tachypnoea. Rarely, there may be neurological signs, particularly those of encephalopathy. Blood samples show thrombocytopenia ($<100 \times 10^9$/l), and haemoconcentration (haematocrit ↑ by >20%) due to diffuse capillary leakage of plasma.

2. Yellow fever

A disease restricted to S America and Africa that is caused by a flavivirus transmitted by the bite of *Haemagogus* and *Aedes* mosquitos. Mosquitos transmit the virus between monkeys or rodents in the forest; human outbreaks occur when urban mosquitos become infected and intiate an urban human-mosquito-human cycle.

Most endemic infections are mild or subclinical; a minority of endemic infections plus many epidemic infections are serious and may kill due to liver or renal failure, or haemorrhage. Although jaundice occurs, it is rarely as deep as that of hepatitis or relapsing fever.

Clinical features: after 3–6 day incubation, there is a sudden onset of fever and headache (severe cases + myalgia, N&V, abdominal pain) which lasts up to 48hrs. The fever may decrease for a few hours at this point before recurring with widespread haemorrhage. This includes: haematemesis (coffee ground or fresh), melaena, diarrhoea; jaundice; heavy proteinuria cardiac changes, rarely CNS signs of meningoencephalitis. Death occurs around the 7–10th day; recovery may be after 3–4 days or protracted over weeks. Post-recovery death is rare but may occur due to cardiac complications.

WHO criteria for diagnosis of DHF

Useful for diagnosis before critical shock stage:

1. high continuous fever for 2–7 days
2. haemorrhagic manifestations
3. hepatomegaly
4. thrombocytopenia ($\leq 100 \times 10^9$/l)
5. haemoconcentration (↑ by 20% or more).

Distribution of yellow fever

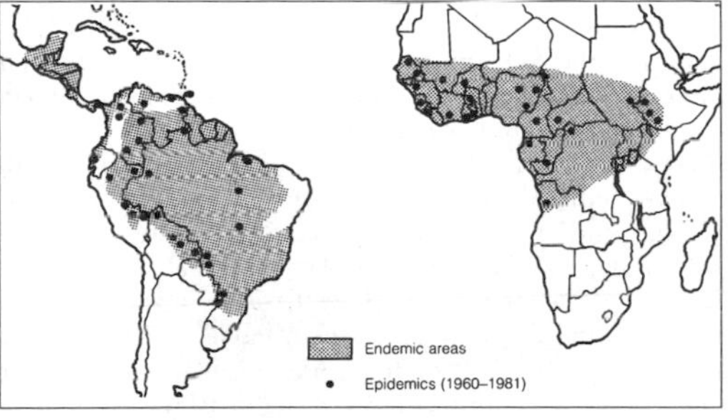

Hantavirus haemorrhagic fever

Caused by four hantaviruses (incl. Hantaan and Puumala) that may cause severe haemorrhagic, renal, or pulmonary disease via immunopathology. Most infections are mild or inapparent; occasionally, outbreaks occur with a high mortality, particularly in the Far East. The viruses are transmitted from chronically infected rodents via aerosol or in food or water which has become contaminated with rodent urine.

Clinical features: after a 2–3 week incubation period, there is a sudden onset of fever, retro-orbital headache and eye pain, photophobia, mild myalgia, abdominal pain, and N&V. An erythematous rash develops which may → petechial on face, neck, shoulders, and upper thorax. After 5 days, proteinuria and shock occur, followed at around day 9 by oliguria and signs of haemorrhage (this is only rarely serious). The patient recovers with diuresis but convalescence may be protracted.

Arenavirus haemorrhagic fever

An expanding family of RNA viruses that cause severe haemorrhagic disease. Three viruses are well characterized: **Lassa** – cause of Lassa fever in west Africa, **Junin** – cause of Argentinian HF, and **Machupo** – cause of Bolivian HF. The former is often subclinical, while AHF and BHF appear to always be overt. They produce similar diseases but the severity differs: Junin ≥ Machupo > Lassa. Humans are infected by direct contact with the rodent vector, by food or water contaminated by rodent urine, or by aerosol contact with urine. The Lassa and BHF rodent vectors are peridomestic; in contrast, the AHF rodent vector lives in maize fields and AHF is therefore an infection of agricutural workers. Human-human infection can occur via blood or body secretions.

Clinical features: onset is insidious after a 7–14 day incubation, with fever, chills, N&V, retro-orbital pain, periorbital and facial oedema, proteinuria, myalgia and/or severe body pains. Other features include pharyngitis with tonsillar patches (Lassa), axillary petechial rash, generalized lymphadenopathy & conjunctivitis (A/BHF). After a week, there is sudden deterioration with collapse, hypovolaemia, and in severe cases signs of haemorrhage and oligouria. In Lassa fever, AST >150U/ml is a marker of poor prognosis. Neurologic disturbances occur in AHF and BHF – clonic seizures and coma indicate a very poor prognosis. Infection of pregnant women with any of the viruses commonly leads to abortion and maternal death. Uterine evacuation may improve maternal prognosis.

Filovirus haemorrhagic fever

Two African viruses – **Ebola** and **Marburg** – that can cause severe haemorrhagic disease. Ebola infection may be subclinical. Ebola epidemics have occurred in hospitals through re-use of needles – nosocomial transmission appears to have a higher fatality rate than community-acquired disease. The only identified mode of community transmission is from contact with body fluids of an acutely ill patient. No vectors have been identified.

Clinical features: include an acute fever after a 7–14 day incubation period, headache, myalgia, sore throat with ulceration of mouth & pharynx, diarrhoea (marker of severity); followed after the 5th day by GI bleeding, morbilliform rash, CNS signs, and commonly death.

VHFs caused by high hazard agents

►► These viruses all require isolation precautions (see above and chapter 1) to reduce the risk of nosocomial transmission.

- Hantaviruses – see opposite
- Arenaviruses – see opposite
- Filoviruses – see opposite
- Phlebovirus – rift valley fever (RVF) virus causes a simple febrile illness in most patients; 10% develop macular retinitis that may progress to blindness. Fulminant disease develops after 4–6 days in up to 1% of infections, the patient has hepatitis, jaundice, and haemorrhage; 50% die. Fatal encephalitis may also occur.
- Nairovirus – Crimean–Congo haemorrhagic fever (CCHF) virus causes a severe haemorrhagic fever with icteric hepatitis, DIC and haemorrhage. The mortality rate is 30–50%.

Distribution of arenaviruses

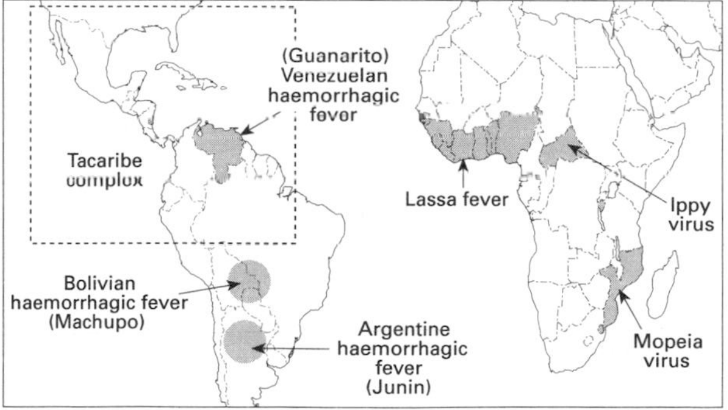

5. Cardiology

Cardiology in the tropics 248
Chest pain 248
Summary of praecordial signs in common heart conditions 250
ECG abnormalities 252
Angina 254
Myocardial infarct (MI) 256
Immediate management of an MI 258
Post-infarct management 258
Complications of MI 260
Advanced life support (ALS) protocols 262
Peri-arrest ALS protcols 264
Arrhythmias and conduction disturbances 266
Atrial fibrillation (AF) 266
Bradycardia 266
Peripartum cardiac failure 267
Heart failure 268
Management of heart failure 270
Shock 272
Hypertension 274
Rheumatic fever 276
Infective endocarditis 278
Cardiomyopathies 280
Pericardial disease 282

Cardiology

Cardiology in the tropics

As certain populations in developing countries relinquish traditional ways of life in favour of more 'Western' practices, they are it seems also adopting the accompanying heightened risks of cardiovascular disease. Prevention, detection and treatment of such diseases is likely to consume already scarce resources in countries where life expectancy is increasing due to better control of communicable diseases and malnutrition and where in most instances the birth rate is increasing. To say that a new epidemic is beginning may well be no exaggeration and it remains to be seen whether the developing world will be able to cope with it.

Chest pain

Central chest pain

Nature:

- a constricting pain suggests angina, oesophagitis, or anxiety
- a sharp pain may be from the pleura or pericardium (both may be exacerbated by deep inspiration – ie pleuritic)
- a prolonged, intense pain suggests myocardial infarction (MI).

Pains which are unlikely to be cardiac in origin include:

- short, sharp stabbing pains
- pains lasting <30s, however intense
- well localized left submammary pain ("In my heart, doctor")
- pains of continually varying location.

Ask about:

- Radiation (to shoulders, neck, jaw, or arms suggests MI).
- Precipitating and exacerbating factors (exercise, emotion, or palpitations suggest MI, whereas food, lying flat, hot drinks, or alcohol suggest oesophagitis).
- Alleviating factors (NB glyceryl trinitrate relieves both cardiac pain and oesophageal pain, but acts much more rapidly in the former) Pericardial pain classically improves on leaning forward.
- Associations (eg dyspnoea and/or palpitations, pallor, nausea and vomiting).

Non-central chest pain: may still be cardiac in origin, but other conditions enter the differential diagnosis (see opposite). The more common conditions include:

- pleuritic pain
- musculoskeletal pain
- varicella zoster infection (shingles)
- ankylosing spondylitis
- gall bladder disease
- pancreatic disease.

Causes of chest pain

Cardiovascular
Myocardial ischaemia
Myocardial infarct
Aortic dissection
Aortic aneurysm

Airway
Intubation
Central bronchial carcinoma
Inhaled foreign body
Tracheitis

Mediastinal
Oesophageal spasm
Oesophagitis
Mediastinitis
Sarcoid lymphadenopathy
Lymphoma

Pleuropericardial
Pericarditis
Infective pleurisy
Pneumothorax
Pneumonia
Autoimmune disease
Mesothelioma
Metastatic tumour

Chest wall
Rib fracture
Muscular strain
Thoracic nerve compression
Rib tumour
Thoracic herpes zoster
Coxsackie B infection

Summary of praecordial signs in common heart conditions

Mitral stenosis

Pulse: can be in AF
JVP: only raised in heart failure
RV: can be hypertrophied if accompanied by pulmonary hypertension
LV: normal, but tapping apex
HS: loud I (+ opening snap), loud PII if pulmonary hypertension present
Murmurs: mid-diastolic at apex only (duration is directly proportional to severity). There may be a presystolic accentuation murmur (atrial contraction), absent in AF.

Mitral incompetence

Pulse: can be in AF
JVP: only raised in heart failure
RV: may be dilated
LV: dilated, apex beat is diffuse and displaced
HS: soft S_1, loud PII if pulmonary hypertension is present
Murmurs: pan-systolic radiating to the axilla.

Ventricular septal defect

RV and LV: both hypertrophied
Murmurs: pan-systolic murmur at left sternal edge (loud if defect is small).

Patent ductus arteriosus

Murmur: systolic & diastolic machinery murmur loudest below L clavicle.

Third heart sound S_3

This occurs shortly after S_2 and is normal in young, fit people. It also occurs in heart failure, mitral incompetence, and constrictive pericarditis.

Fourth heart sound S_4

This occurs just before S_1 and is due to atrial contraction against a stiff ventricle (aortic stenosis, hypertension).

Aortic stenosis

Pulse: plateau or anacrotic, narrow pulse pressure
JVP: only raised in heart failure
LV: hypertrophied, apex beat may be sustained
HS: soft AII (+/– ejection click), with paradoxical split (widening of S_2 on expiration)
Murmurs: harsh midsystolic murmur radiating to the carotids

Aortic incompetence

Pulse: water-hammer with wide pulse pressure; may be collapsing at wrist
JVP: only raised in heart failure
LV: dilated, apex may be displaced and diffuse
Murmurs: early diastolic murmur radiating to lower sternum (there may also be an ejection systolic murmur from increased flow).

Atrial septal defect

JVP: only raised in heart failure or tricuspid incompetence
RV: hypertrophied
HS: fixed split S_2
Murmurs: pulmonary ejection murmur (+/– tricuspid diastolic flow murmur).

Acute pericarditis

Murmurs: scratchy, superficial noise heard throughout cardiac cycle, which may be brought out by stethoscope pressure and may vary with respiration.

Chronic constrictive pericarditis

Pulse: may be pulsus paradoxus (>10mmHg ↓ BP upon inspiration)
JVP: ↑, may be Kussmaul's sign (JVP ↑ on inspiration)
LV: apex may be unpalpable
HS: reduced heart sounds, may have S_3 and pericardial knock (due to rapid ventricular filling being abruptly halted).

Abnormalities of the JVP

- ↑ JVP with a normal waveform: RHF, fluid overload, bradycardia.
- ↑ JVP with absent pulsation: SVC obstruction.
- Abnormal *a* wave: tricuspid stenosis, pulmonary hypertension, pulmonary stenosis, complete heart block, atrial flutter.
- Absent *a* wave: atrial fibrillation.
- JVP ↑ on inspiration: constrictive pericarditis/pericardial tamponade (high JVP plateau, with deep *x* and *y* descents).

ECG chest leads

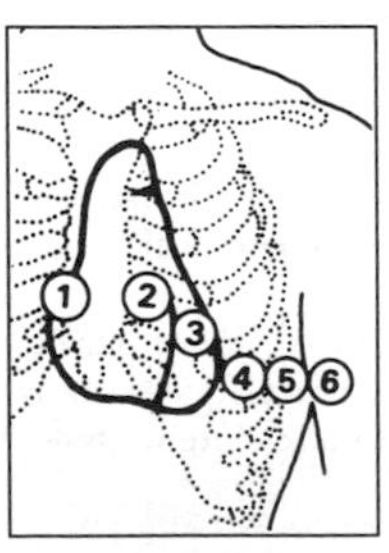

Cardiac axis from ECG

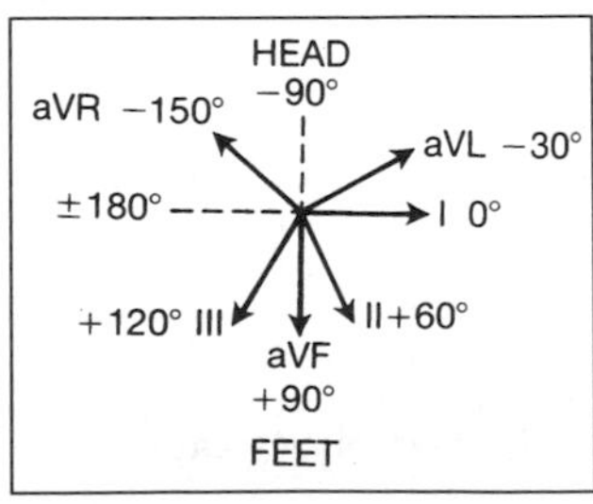

ECG abnormalities

Rate defects: *Bradycardia* = <60/min. *Tachycardia* = >100/min.

Normal durations: PR interval = <200ms (5 small squares); QRS duration = <120ms (3 small squares); QT interval = <400ms (2 large squares).

Axis: *Right axis deviation* (pulmonary stenosis, pulmonary hypertension, congenital L→R shunts) the QRS in lead I is negative (ie downwards). *Left axis deviation*, (hypertension, aortic stenosis) the QRS in leads III and II are negative, leaving only lead I as positive.

Conduction defects:

- *First degree block:* one P per QRS, but PQ > 200ms (5 small squares).
- *Second degree block: Wenckebach* = a cycle of progressive PR lengthening, then one non-conducted P wave. *Mobitz type II* = a pattern of non-conducted P waves eg 2:1 block (2 P waves to each QRS, with a normal P wave rate). Can be 3:1.
- *Right bundle branch block (RBBB):* QRS >120ms, an RSR pattern in V1. Dominant R in V1, inverted T in V1–3/4, deep and wide S wave in V6. '**M**a**RR**o**W**' is a way to remember the changes; an **M**-shaped QRS in V1 and a **W**-shaped QRS in V6 = **R**ight bundle branch block.
- *Left bundle branch block (LBBB):* QRS >120ms, an RSR pattern in V6. Inverted T waves in I, VL, V5–6. Similarly to above, think of '**W**i**LL**ia**M**' as a way of remembering the changes.

Supraventricular arrhythmias

These all have a narrow QRS and normal T waves (unless there is bundle branch block or the Wolff-Parkinson-White syndrome).

- *Extrasystoles:* single, early beats suppressing the sinus beat.
- *Sinus arrhythmia:* RR interval varies with respiration (↑ on inspiration).
- *Atrial tachycardia:* QRS rate >150/min, abnormal P with short PR. May be 2:1 block.
- *Atrial flutter:* P wave rate 300/min with a 'saw-tooth' pattern and 2:1, 3:1 or 4:1 block. The block is ↑ by carotid sinus pressure or adenosine.
- *Atrial fibrillation (AF):* QRS rate usually > 160/min, no P waves and a varying, completely irregular baseline.
- *Escape rhythms:* bradycardias with the above characteristics (except that AF does not occur as an escape rhythm).

Ventricular arrhythmias

These all have a wide QRS (>120ms, or 3 small squares) and abnormal T waves.

- *Ventricular extrasystole:* early, wide QRS with abnormal T wave. Next QRS is 'on time'.
- *Ventricular tachycardia (VT):* no P waves. Rate >160/min (accelerated idioventricular rhythm = VT at a rate <120/min). ►► **Pulseless VT needs emergency treatment.**
- *Ventricular fibrillation (VF):* rule out any muscular movement eg patient is brushing teeth. The trace is totally irregular, as there is no organized ventricular contraction and no cardiac output. ►► **VF needs emergency treatment.**

Pulmonary embolus: the most common ECG feature is a sinus tachycardia (+/– right axis deviation, RBBB, a dominant R in V1, inverted Ts in V1–3/4, a deep S in V6). The 'classical' changes of a deep S in I with Q wave and inverted T in III ('S1Q3T3') are rare.

Digoxin effect: ST depression and inverted T in V5–6. Changes are more extensive in digoxin *toxicity* (any arrhythmia, but ventricular ectopics and nodal bradycardia are most common).

Hyperkalaemia: tall, tented T waves with wide QRS and absent Ps.

Hypokalaemia: small T waves with prominent U waves (a flattened T wave with a hump on the end). There may be ventricular bigemini (a premature extrasystole coupled to each sinus beat).

Hypercalcaemia: shortened QT interval (<400ms).

Hypocalcaemia: prolonged QT interval (>400ms).

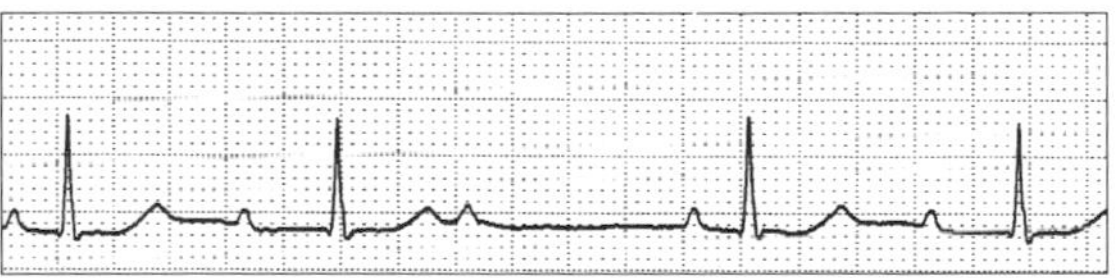

Mobitz type I (Wenkebach) second degree AV block

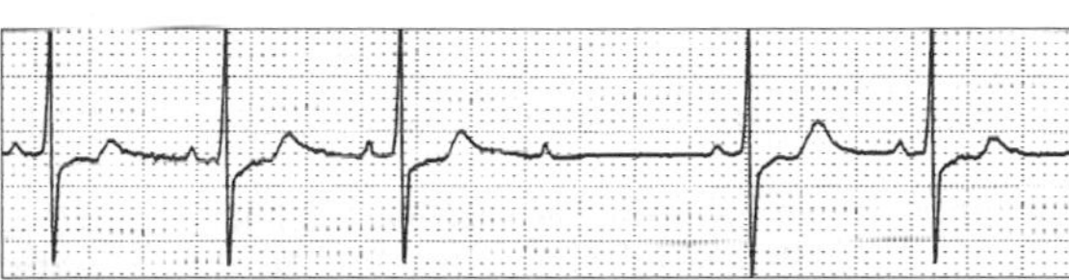

Mobitz type II second degree AV block

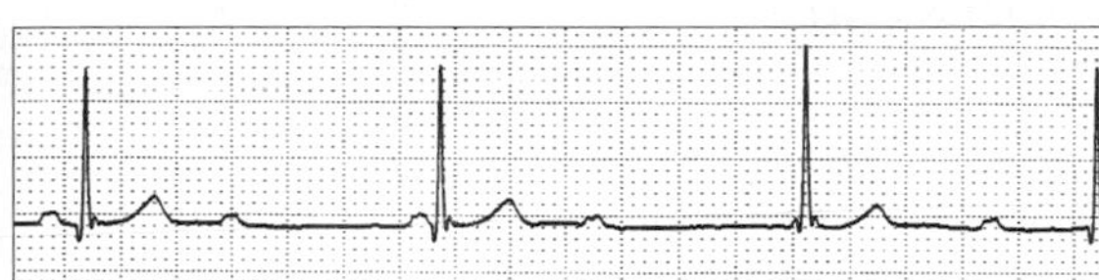

Third degree AV block (complete AV dissociation)

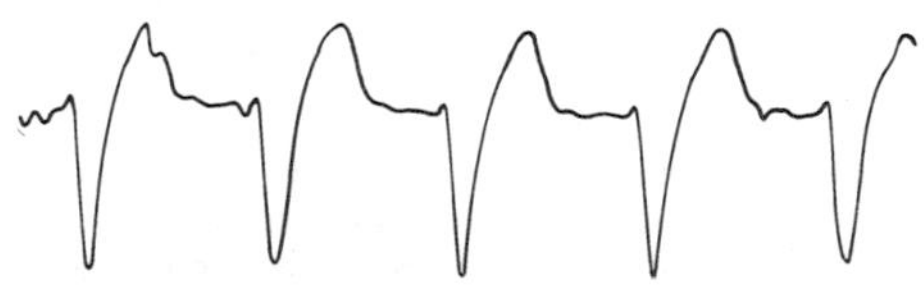

Hyperkalaemia

Angina

This, classically, is central, crushing chest pain which may radiate to the jaw, neck or one or both arms. It may only be felt in the jaw or arm, or be felt as a tightness across the chest. It represents myocardial ischaemia and may be precipitated by exertion, anxiety, cold or a heavy meal and be associated with dyspnoea, pallor and faintness. It is relieved by rest and nitrates. In most cases it is caused by coronary artery disease, but may be due to aortic stenosis, hypertrophic obstructive cardiomyopathy, hypoperfusion from arrhythmias, arteritis, or anaemia. Indigestion is the most common differential diagnosis.

The incidence of ischaemic heart disease shows significant variation amongst ethnic groups, being particularly common in people of south Asian origin (who also have $\uparrow$ incidence of NIDDM). The incidence is also higher in black than in white Americans.

Investigations: on the ECG look for ST depression, flattened (or inverted) T waves and evidence of old infarcts (Q waves). If available, do an exercise ECG 48hrs after the angina settles. Take bloods for FBC and ESR to exclude non-atheromatous causes (as above), U+Es and CK to exclude infarct.

Management

1. Encourage the patient to give up smoking, improve her diet to reduce lipids and weight, and exercise more.
2. Improve diabetic control.
3. Start with glyceryl trinitrate (GTN) either sublingually, or as a spray at 0.5mg per dose, up to every hour. When this is no longer adequate, work up to a functioning dose of quadruple therapy:
   - Aspirin 75mg daily as an anti-platelet agent.
   - β-blockers: eg atenolol 50–100mg PO daily. *CI:* asthma, LVF, bradycardia.
   - Slow release calcium antagonists: eg nifedipine modified release 20mg PO daily. *CI:* fertile women. Short acting Ca^{2+} blockers $\uparrow$ cardiac events.
   - Isosorbide dinitrate modified release 30–120mg PO once or twice daily.
4. When drugs fail to control angina, surgical options are available. Coronary artery bypass grafts (CABG) improve the overall prognosis, but pain returns to 50% of patients in 5yrs. It carries a 2% mortality risk. Angioplasty gives symptomatic relief, but with no overall improvement in prognosis. 30% go on to require CABG in the UK.

Unstable angina is new onset angina or angina which is rapidly worsening and present on minimal exertion, or at rest.

Management: is as for angina, with diltiazem added where available. In the acute state, isosorbide dinitrate should be infused intravenously. To the above, also add aspirin 75mg PO daily and consider using heparin (IV or SC). 15% of patients will die if untreated and even those treated have a 0.5–4% per year risk of death (from MI or LVF).

Preventing ischaemic heart disease (IHD)

Hypercholesterolaemia, smoking and hypertension are the main risk factors for IHD. Others include male sex, family history, diabetes, alcohol, obesity and use of the OCP. Geographic, environmental, and social factors are also clearly involved.

Dietary manipulation can lower lipids; aim for a body mass index (see nutrition chapter) of 20–25, on a diet which has <10% of calories derived from saturated fats and which is high in fibre. Encourage exercise (↑ HDL). If the plasma cholesterol is raised, look for a cause: alcohol abuse, DM, hypothyroidism, cholestasis, renal failure, nephrosis, oestrogen use.

Drug treatment should begin if the cholesterol remains >6.5mmol/l (or triglycerides >2.3mmol/l) after 3 months of diet and exercise. Fibrates (eg *bezafibrate*), nicotinic acid or resins (eg *colestipol*) may be used. The diet should continue and lipid-raising drugs (eg diuretics, unselective β-blockers, norgestrel) should be stopped, or an alternative sought. Statins are expensive but highly effective drugs for treating hyperlipidaemia. Beware turning healthy people into patients chronically anxious about hyperlipidaemia.

Myocardial infarct (MI)

This is the irreversible necrosis of part of the heart muscle, almost always due to coronary artery atherosclerosis. Although not as common in the tropics as it is in the West (5/1000/year in England), the mortality in the tropics is probably higher.

Clinical features: the pain is usually of greater severity and duration (>30mins) than angina, though similar in nature and usually associated with nausea and vomiting, sweating, pallor and extreme distress. In the elderly, small MIs may be painless. There may be tachycardia, tachypnoea, cyanosis, mild pyrexia (<38.5°C). The BP may be ↑ or ↓. There may also be features of the complications, eg dyspnoea, basal lung crepitations, pericardial rub, or the pan-systolic murmur of mirtal incompetence (after rupture of the chordae tendinae).

Investigations: an *ECG* is essential. The absence of Q-waves in a proven infarct is associated with a higher risk of subsequent infarcts and a poorer long-term prognosis. On *CXR* look for signs of heart failure, changes in cardiac size (ventricular aneurysm) and aortic dissection. Monitor FBC, U&E, glucose and ESR (may be up to 80mm/hr and take some weeks to return to normal). Lipids may also be raised for several weeks. *Cardiac enzymes*, where available, are a useful aid in the diagnosis of MI. Creatinine kinase is the first to rise (within 12–24hrs), followed by aspartate transaminase (24–36hrs) and finally, lactate dehydrogenase (48hrs–10 days). See graph opposite. Try to make the diagnosis on the basis of 2 out of 3 of history, ECG changes, and cardiac enzymes.

ECG changes in myocardial infarction

An initially normal ECG progresses to tall T waves and ST elevation. Within 24hrs, the T wave inverts as ST elevation begins to resolve. Pathological Q waves (>1 small square in width and >2mm in length) form within a few days. These may persist, or completely resolve in 10%. T wave inversion may or may not persist. ST elevation rarely persists, unless there is a ventricular aneurysm.

Site of infarct:

- *Anterior:* changes occur in V2–5.
- *Septal:* usually in V3 & 4 (depends on axis).
- *Inferior:* changes occur in III and VF.
- *Lateral:* changes in I, VL and V6.
- *Posterior:* look for the reciprocal (ie inverted) changes in the anterior leads V1–5; dominant R wave (= inverted Q wave) and ST depression (= inverted ST elevation) with the clinical features of an infarct. Always ask for posterior leads (V7–9) if you suspect a posterior infarct.

Non-Q wave infarcts: (formerly called subendocardial infarcts) do not involve the whole thickness of the myocardium and thus have the ST changes, without Q waves.

Differential diagnosis: angina, oesophagitis, peptic ulcer, pericarditis, pulmonary embolus, pleurisy, aortic dissection, pancreatitis, cholecystitis, chest wall pathology.

ECG changes following MI

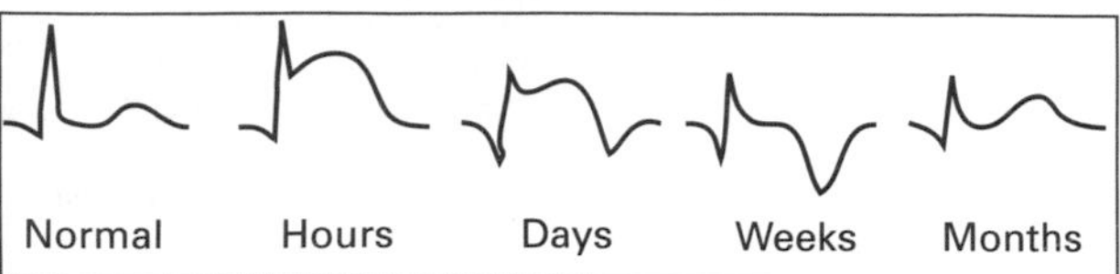

Cardiac enzyme changes following MI

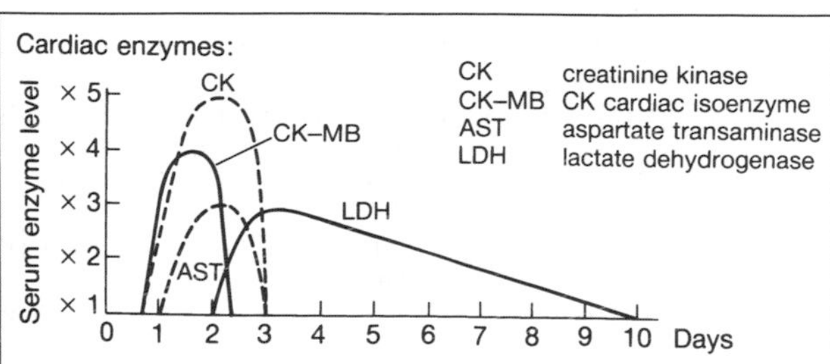

Immediate management of MI

The greatest risk of death is in the first hour – prompt action can save lives.

1. Try to calm and reassure the patient.
2. Give 100% oxygen via face mask (if you suspect chronic obstructive airways disease, give less concentrated O_2 and check ABGs).
3. Insert an IV line and give pain relief (morphine 10mg IV).
4. Give glyceryl trinitrate 0.5mg sublingual for coronary artery vasodilation.
5. Give aspirin 300mg PO stat and continue on 75mg daily thereafter.
6. If possible, refer to a centre where the patient may be given streptokinase within 16hrs.
7. Give a β-blocker eg atenolol 10mg IV then 50mg PO daily unless the patient has heart failure or asthma. It will ↓ cardiac O_2 demand and may ↓ infarct size.
8. Give heparin 5000 units SC then 5000 units BD until mobilized (as prophylaxis against DVT).
9. Start the patient on an oral ACE inhibitor eg captopril 24hrs after the infarct. Do **not** give a calcium channel blocker.
10. Discontinue any pre-infarction cardiac drugs.
11. Prohibit smoking.
12. Give at least 24hrs bedrest with continuous ECG monitoring and q4h temp, pulse, RR, BP. Perform frequent checks for complications.
13. Daily ECG, cardiac enzymes, U&Es (and CXR if there is deteriorating lung function) for the subsequent 2–3 days.

Post-infarct management

If the post-MI period is uncomplicated, the patient may be mobilized by day 2–3 and the SC heparin may be stopped on day 5. All being well, the patient may return home after 5–7 days and gradually increase the amount of exercise done over 1 month. The patient should not drive during this period. Strongly discourage smoking and advise about diet.

Prognosis depends upon: the degree of LV dysfunction, presence of significant arrhythmias, heart size on CXR, presence of post-MI angina, and the presence of pulmonary oedema. In the UK, mortality rates for the first year after discharge are 6–8% with over half these deaths occurring in the first 3 months.

Long term treatment Patients with no complications and good prognostic indices should be discharged without long term medication. All patients should be advised to modify their risk factors and have a follow up appointment at 6–8 weeks for CXR, ECG and an exercise treadmill test if there post-infarct angina.

All patients with one or more poor prognostic signs should take

- β-blocker for at least 18mths (eg atenolol 50mg od) to ↓ incidence of further cardiac events (use caution in those with unstable diabetes; β-blockers are contra-indicated in patients with asthma or heart failure)
- low dose aspirin (eg 75mg PO od) for life
- an ACE inhibitor should be prescribed if there is ↓ LV function.

Streptokinase contraindications

Streptokinase should not be given if the patient:

- has had a stroke or active bleeding (eg peptic ulcer) within the last 2 months;
- has systolic BP>200mmHg
- has had surgery or trauma in the past 10 days
- has a bleeding disorder or uses anticoagulants
- is pregnant
- is menstruating
- has had previous streptokinase treatment – between 4 days and 1 year previously.

Complications of MI

1. **Infarct extension:** occurs in ~10% (↑ in non-Q wave infarcts) in the first 10–14 days, with varying severity. Treat as a new infarct (ie as above).
2. **Post-infarct angina:** is associated with ↑ mortality and occurs in ~30% (↑ if there was pre-infarct angina or non-Q wave infarct). Treat vigorously with nitrates, β-blockers, Ca channel blockers, and aspirin.
3. **Arrhythmias** (see ECG section, above and ALS protocols, below):

- ***Sinus bradycardia*** – may be due to infarct or to medication (β-blocker). It may require atropine and, rarely, temporary pacing.
- ***Supraventricular tachycardia*** – a sinus tachycardia is common post-MI. Atrial fibrillation (***AF***) occurs in ~10% and should be rapidly controlled to avoid the onset of ventricular tachycardia (VT) and infarct spread. Use digoxin after excluding hypokalaemia (0.5mg initially, then 0.25mg every 90–120mins up to 1–1.25mg as a loading dose; followed by 0.25mg daily – assuming normal renal function). AF is usually transient, but if necessary conversion back to sinus rhythm can be achieved by DC cardioversion (presence of heart failure, hypotension, or refractory to other treatments), IV sotalol or IV amiodarone.
- ***Ventricular arrhythmias*** are most common in the first few hours post-MI and may be heralded by ventricular premature beats. ***VT*** >120 bpm may progress to ventricular fibrillation (VF). Treat early with lignocaine IV, or synchronized cardioversion. ***VF*** may occur in the first few hours or days and needs emergency treatment. It carries a poor prognosis in the presence of cardiogenic shock or failure. ***Accelerated idioventricular rhythm*** can occur after any MI and is usually benign, not affecting the cardiac output.
- ***Nodal rhythms:*** have a narrow QRS complex but have no associated P wave (or it may come after the QRS). They are usually intermittent and self-limiting, but in a large MI may ↓ both cardiac output and BP. Treat with atropine or a temporary pacemaker.

4. **Conduction disturbances:** all degrees of AV block may occur and are most common in inferior MIs (20%). First degree block needs no treatment. Second degree block is usually Wenckebach and only requires treatment if there is symptomatic bradycardia. Third degree block often follows second degree block and is usually temporary. Again, treat with atropine or isoprenoline if symptomatic. In anterior MIs, extensive damage to the His-Purkinje system will cause complete and progressive AV block which will require pacing, possibly permanent.
5. **Myocardial dysfunction:**

- ***Left ventricular failure*** (see below).
- ***Cardiogenic shock:*** severe failure causing hypotension, tachycardia, oliguria, distress, and peripheral shut-down. It may be due to: acute MR, severe LV dysfunction, cardiac rupture, VSD, arrhythmias, RV infarct. Treatment is with 100% O_2, IV diuretics (if LVF), fluids (if RVF), GTN, inotropes.

6. **Right ventricular infarct:** occurs in 1/3 of inferior infarcts but is clinically significant in less. There is ↓ BP and ↑ JVP with clear lungs. Lead V4 on the ECG may show ST elevation. Treatment is with fluids to ↑ LV filling. Inotropes may be useful.
7. **Mechanical defects** (MR and VSD): papillary or septal rupture occurs in <1% of all MIs and may occur 1–7 days after an anterior or inferior MI (MR most commonly after infero-lateral MIs, VSD after septal MIs). Listen for new murmurs and basal crepitations, and watch for clinical deterioration.
8. **Left ventricular aneurysm:** occurs in 10–20% of anterior MIs. The apex beat is diffuse and there may be atypical/stabbing chest pain, accompanied by ST elevation lasting 4–8 weeks. They rarely rupture but are associated with emboli, arrhythmias, and CCF. Patients may require life-long anticoagulation.
9. **Cardiac rupture:** usually results in rapid death 2–7 days post-MI. It occurs in <1% of MIs. A small or incomplete rupture may be sealed by the pericardium, forming a pseudoaneurysm (this needs prompt surgical repair).

10. **Pericarditis:** 20% of patients have a pericardial rub after 24hrs. There is chest pain, relieved by sitting up and varying with respiration. It is usually self-limiting but may require analgesia.

- ***Dressler's syndrome:*** is an autoimmune pericarditis occurring 1–10 weeks post-MI in 5% of patients. There is fever, leucocytosis and occasionally pericardial or pleural effusion. Treatment is with NSAIDs +/– corticosteroids. Watch for signs of constrictive pericarditis.

11. **Mural thrombus:** is common in large MIs and may cause arterial emboli, leading to strokes, gut infarcts, or renal infarcts. The patient should be heparinized and long-term warfarin considered in all anterior MIs.

Advanced life support (ALS) protocols

The majority of sudden deaths result from arrhythmias associated with acute MI or chronic ischaemic heart disease. Successful resuscitation following a cardiopulmonary arrest is most likely if:

- the arrest is witnessed,
- basic life support is started promptly, *and*
- defibrillation (if appropriate) is carried out as early as possible.

Basic life support (BLS): the purpose of BLS is to maintain adequate ventilation and circulation until a means can be obtained to reverse the underlying cause of the cardiac arrest.

Remember **A**, **B** & **C** – Airways, Breathing and Circulation.

► Ensure that it is safe to approach the patient – eg risk of being hit by traffic or being electrocuted.

A. Remove foreign bodies from the airways (including false teeth); use suction if necessary. Tilt the head back (unless a neck injury is suspected) or do jaw thrust.

B. Is the patient breathing? If not, assist via a mask (with 100% O_2) and bag ventilation if available, or mouth-to-mouth resuscitation until intubation is possible. If there is upper airway obstruction a cricothyrotomy may be needed. If there is a tension pneumothorax, relieve it before proceeding further.

C. Is there a pulse in the carotid arteries? If not, begin external cardiac massage until defibrillation under the guidelines below is possible.

► If you are alone and the patient is unconscious, assess whether going/calling for help would be of more benefit than attempting resuscitation alone. It is hard to leave an injured/unconscious person, but their only realistic hope of survival may be if you go straight for help.

ALS treatment algorithms for cardiopulmonary arrest

The algorithm opposite is merely a summary of the methods used in the advanced life support training scheme. The methods involve skilled procedures which should only be attempted by qualified staff, since improper use of defibrillators could result in more harm being done to the arrested patient, as well as harm to those carrying out the resuscitation. It is strongly recommended that all medical staff read the ALS (or equivalent) course book and practise arrest protocols in 'mock' arrest scenarios.

► Notes: If at any stage a pulse is felt, defibrillation should stop and the patient be ventilated. Watch for peri-arrest arrhythmias (see below). Intubation and IV access should take no longer than 30 seconds. If difficult, they should be delayed until the next loop of the cycle. If defibrillation remains unsuccessful, consider changing the paddle positions or the defibrillator.

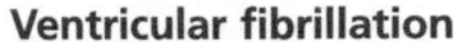

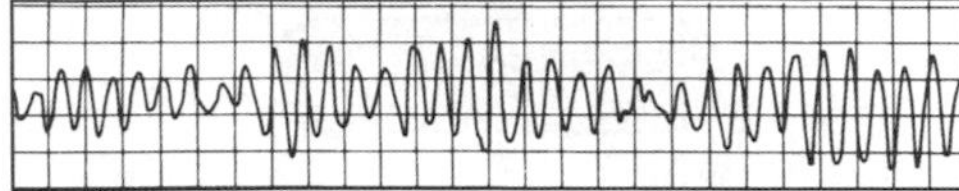

Ventricular tachycardia at 235 beats/min

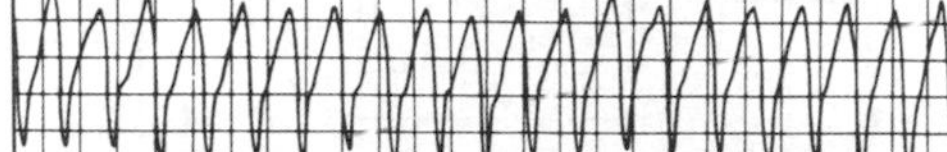

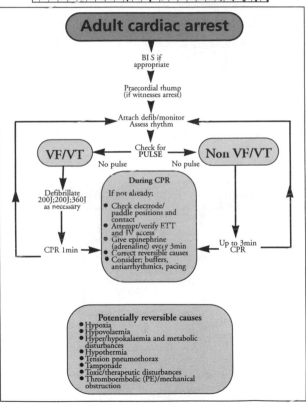

Adult cardiac arrest

↓

BLS if appropriate

↓

Praecordial thump (if witnesses arrest)

↓

Attach defib/monitor
Assess rhythm

↓

Check for PULSE

- No pulse → **VF/VT**
  - ↓ Defibrillate 200J;200J;360J as necessary
  - ↓ CPR 1min → During CPR
  - → back to Attach defib/monitor, Assess rhythm
- No pulse → **Non VF/VT**
  - ↓ Up to 3min CPR → During CPR
  - → back to Attach defib/monitor, Assess rhythm

During CPR

If not already;

- Check electrode/paddle positions and contact
- Attempt/verify ETT and IV access
- Give epinephrine (adrenaline) every 3min
- Correct reversible causes
- Consider; buffers, antiarrhythmics, pacing

Potentially reversible causes

- Hypoxia
- Hypovolaemia
- Hyper/hypokalaemia and metabolic disturbances
- Hypothermia
- Tension pneumothorax
- Tamponade
- Toxic/therapeutic disturbances
- Thromboembolic (PE)/mechanical obstruction

NB: Each successive step is based on the assumption that the one before has been unsuccessful.

Peri-arrest ALS algorithms

Arrhythmias that occur during the peri-arrest period may be divided into bradycardias, and broad or narrow complex tachycardias:

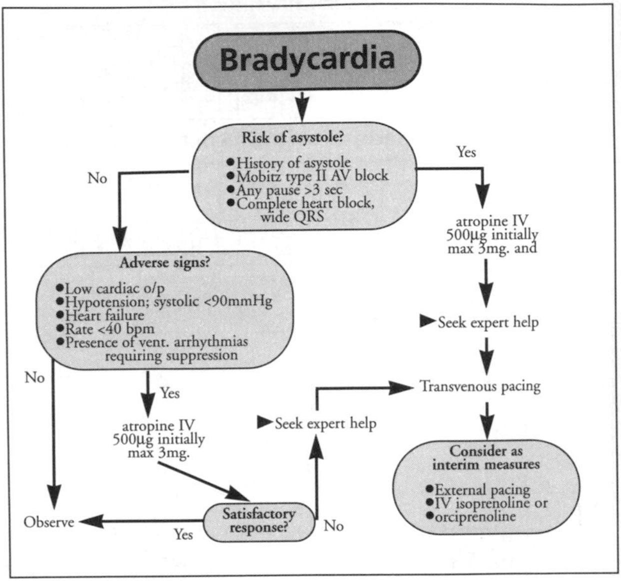

Bradycardia

Risk of asystole?

- History of asystole
- Mobitz type II AV block
- Any pause >3 sec
- Complete heart block, wide QRS

Yes

atropine IV 500μg initially max 3mg. and

▶Seek expert help

Transvenous pacing

Consider as interim measures

- External pacing
- IV isoprenoline or
- orciprenoline

No

Adverse signs?

- Low cardiac o/p
- Hypotension; systolic <90mmHg
- Heart failure
- Rate <40 bpm
- Presence of vent. arrhythmias requiring suppression

No

Yes

atropine IV 500μg initially max 3mg.

Satisfactory response?

Yes

Observe

No

▶Seek expert help

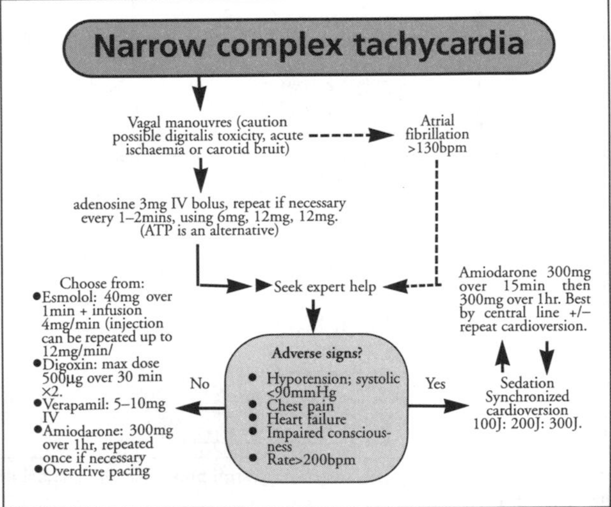

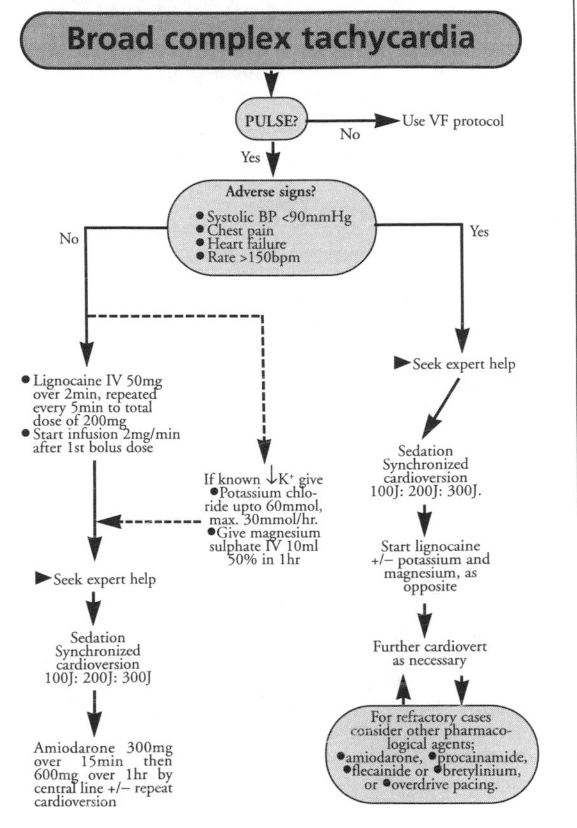
Broad complex tachycardia
PULSE?
No
Use VF protocol
Yes
Adverse signs?
• Systolic BP <90mmHg
• Chest pain
• Heart failure
• Rate >150bpm
No
Yes
• Lignocaine IV 50mg over 2min, repeated every 5min to total dose of 200mg
• Start infusion 2mg/min after 1st bolus dose
If known ↓K+ give
• Potassium chloride upto 60mmol, max. 30mmol/hr.
• Give magnesium sulphate IV 10ml 50% in 1hr
Seek expert help
Sedation
Synchronized cardioversion
100J: 200J: 300J
Amiodarone 300mg over 15min then 600mg over 1hr by central line +/− repeat cardioversion
Seek expert help
Sedation
Synchronized cardioversion
100J: 200J: 300J.
Start lignocaine +/− potassium and magnesium, as opposite
Further cardiovert as necessary
For refractory cases consider other pharmacological agents;
• amiodarone, • procainamide,
• flecainide or • bretylinium,
or • overdrive pacing.

Arrhythmias and conduction disturbances

See also preceding algorithms

These most commonly occur in the setting of an acute MI, but may also occur during chronic ischaemia.

Clinical features: are usually of 'funny turns', collapse, palpitations. Distinguish from epilepsy – a witness may help in this.

Investigations: FBC, U&E, Ca^{2+}, glucose, TFTs, CXR, ECG. Arrange echocardiography if cardiomyopathy or valvular disease is suspected.

Atrial fibrillation (AF)

AF is an ineffective, irregular atrial tachycardia, which results in totally irregular ventricular contraction. The commonest causes are MI, ischaemia, MV disease, hyperthyroidism, hypertension. Also: cardiomyopathy, pericarditis, sick sinus syndrome, Ca bronchus, endocarditis, atrial myxoma, and haemochromatosis. It is a significant risk factor for stroke.

Clinical features: an irregularly irregular pulse with a first heart sound of varying intensity and the apex rate greater than the radial rate. The patient may be breathless. ECG shows a chaotic baseline with no P waves and irregularly irregular QRS complexes of normal shape.

Management

- ***Acute AF:*** anticoagulate with warfarin for 1 month, then attempt DC cardioversion.
- ***Chronic AF:*** The aim is to control the ventricular rate, not the atrial rhythm. Give 3 doses of digoxin 0.5mg PO over 2 days as a loading dose, then continue on maintenance of 0.25mg PO daily for life (if renal function is normal). Use half these doses in the elderly. If still tachycardic, assess compliance, check serum level, and cautiously ↑ digoxin dose. If this fails, add in a low-dose β-blocker (eg propanolol 10–20mg tds po). Give warfarin anticoagulation (INR 2–3) to minimise the risk of embolic stroke.
- ***Paroxysmal AF:*** refer for specialist treatment; requires oral quinidine or amiodarone.

Bradycardia

If the bradycardia is acute and symptomatic (usually post-MI):

- treat or remove the underlying cause (eg β-blockers);
- give atropine 0.3–0.6mg slowly IV, repeating to a max. of 3mg in 24hrs;
- alternatively, try isoprenaline 0.5–10µg/min IV;
- temporary pacing may be needed for unresponsive bradycardia. Chronic bradycardia necessitates permanent pacing.

Other causes of arrhythmias and conduction disturbances

Drugs (mostly those used to *treat* arrhythmias), cardiomyopathy, myocarditis, cardiac dilatation, thyroid disease, electrolyte disturbances.

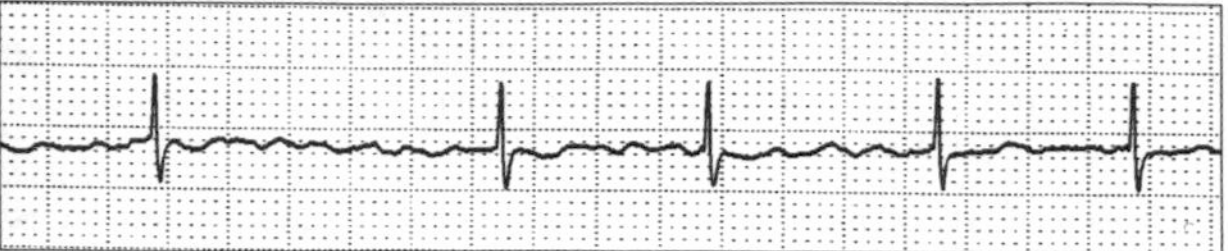

Atrial fibrillation

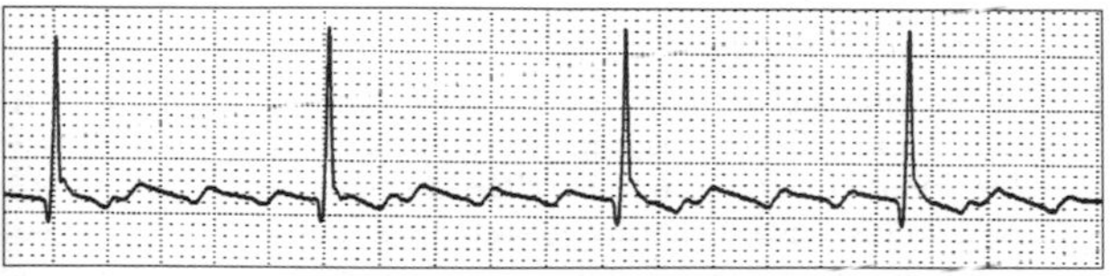

Atrial flutter

Heart failure

Heart failure occurs when the heart fails to maintain sufficient circulation to provide adequate tissue oxygenation in the presence of a normal filling pressure. It may be classified as high output, low output, or fluid overload heart failure, or as right or left ventricular failure. Heart failure is a syndrome and not a diagnosis – ie the patient may have features consistent with heart failure, but what is the *cause*?

1. **High output failure:** occurs when the heart fails to maintain a normal or increased output in the face of grossly increased requirements. It can occur with a normal heart, but will occur earlier if there is cardiac disease eg anaemia, hyperthyroidism, Paget's disease, A–V malformation, or pregnancy. Features are usually of RVF before LVF.
2. **Low output failure:** is when the heart fails to generate adequate output or can only do so with increased filling pressures. Causes:
   - ***Intrinsic heart muscle disease:*** ischaemia, infarction, myocarditis, cardiomyopathy, Chagas disease, beri-beri, amyloid.
   - ***Chronic excessive after-load:*** aortic stenosis, hypertension.
   - ***Negatively inotropic drugs:*** eg any anti-arrhythmic drug.
   - ***Chronic excess pre-load:*** eg mitral regurgitation.
   - ***Restricted filling:*** constrictive pericarditis, tamponade, restrictive cardiomyopathy.
   - ***Inadequate heart rate:*** β-blockers, heart block, post-MI.
3. **Fluid overload** involves pushing the myocardium too far over the Starling length-tension relationship (initially, stretching results in ↑ contractile force, but beyond the apex of the curve, further stretch results in ↓ force), resulting in a lower cardiac output. The features are of LVF and do not normally occur unless there is renal impairment leading to fluid retention, or gross over-hydration.
4. **Left ventricular failure (LVF):** is dominated by pulmonary oedema, resulting in exertional dyspnoea, orthopnea, paradoxical nocturnal dyspnoea, wheeze, cough, haemoptysis, and fatigue.
   The signs are tachypnoea, tachycardia, basal lung crackles, a third heart sound, pulsus alternans, cardiomegaly, peripheral cyanosis, pleural effusion, reduced peak expiratory flow.
   CXR signs are shown opposite.
   ECG will show changes according to the particular cause.
   Echocardiography, where practicable, may differentiate between valvular and pericardial lesions.
5. **Right ventricular failure (RVF):** causes dependent oedema (ie in the legs if standing, in the sacrum if supine), abdominal discomfort, nausea, fatigue and wasting.
   Signs: ↑ JVP, hepatomegaly (may be pulsantile), pitting oedema, peripheral cyanosis.

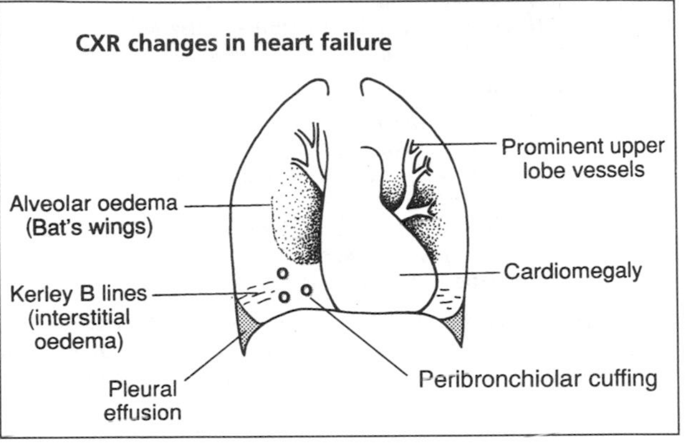

Peripartum cardiac failure

Cardiac failure beginning in pregnancy or up to 6 months postpartum, of up to 6 months duration, with no other history of heart failure and with no discernible cause for the failure other than anaemia or hypertension, presumed to be acute.

Aetiology: commonest in multiparous, hypertensive black women. Myocarditis was found in 50% of cases in some series, but the mechanism was unclear. Cultural practices such as eating Na^+ and K^+-rich foods in hot climates during pregnancy may have a role. One theory is that the combination of ↑ circulatory demands during pregnancy (+/– anaemia), heat (peripheral vasodilatation) and ↑ salt load (volume retention and ↑ renal artery flow required) lead to a high output dilated cardiac failure, with accompanying systemic and pulmonary symptoms.

Investigation and management: are as for other forms of heart failure. In a few cases there is permanent cardiac damage. Do not use an ACE inhibitor, so that the mother may continue breast feeding. A poor prognosis is heralded by any arrhythmia, a persistently dilated heart, and systemic or pulmonary emboli. In those with myocarditis, if there is no improvement after 1 week of a diuretic, a course of immunosuppression may be beneficial.

Management of heart failure

1. Treat the cause if possible.
2. Treat reversible exacerbating factors, eg anaemia, hypoxia.
3. Restrict salt and alcohol intake.
4. Avoid NSAIDs as they cause fluid retention. They may also interact with diuretics and ACE inhibitors to cause renal failure.

5. Drug treatment:

- Start with a diuretic (usually frusemide) – monitor U&Es.
- Once stabilized, begin an **ACE inhibitor** (see opposite).
- If this is inadequate, add a **vasodilator** such as isosorbide dinitrate 10–20mg od (not in RVF).
- Consider low dose spironolactone (25mg od) if available and the patient is not hyperkalaemic *and/or*
- Adding an **inotrope** such as digoxin.

Treatment resistant heart failure: search for other causes and check patient compliance with drug regimes. Admit to hospital for bed-rest, anti-thromboembolic stockings, heparin 5000units SC tds and frusemide IV up to 4mg/min. Increase the ACE inhibitor or venodilator dose to the maximum tolerated; consider metolazone where available. In extreme circumstances, consider using IV inotropes for a short time (eg dopamine 2–10μg/kg/min), though these should not be used in the long term.

Sometimes the patient must accept mildly swollen ankles and exercise limitation in order to avoid unacceptable symptoms of low output.

One treatment protocol:

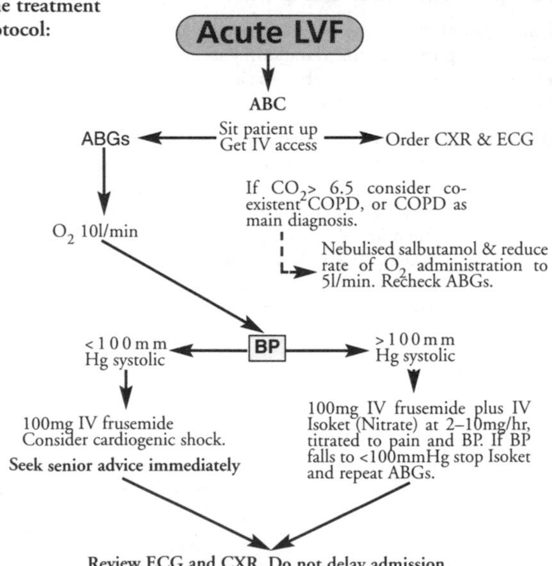

Starting an ACE inhibitor

- Watch for hypotension after the 1st or 2nd doses:
- Check the BP (if <100mmHg systolic, give the first doses in hospital).
- Ensure that the patient is not salt or volume depleted (eg due to D&V).
- Check for aortic and renal artery stenosis.
- Stop or reduce all diuretics and hypotensives a few days before. If there is symptomatic hypotension, give a 0.9% sodium chloride infusion (*plus* atropine if the patient is bradycardic).
- Start with captopril 6.5mg PO bd (short $t_{1/2}$) building up to 25mg bd or tds.
- Change to other ACE inhibitors once stabilized, if side effects (cough, D&V) are troublesome, or if a once daily dose is needed.

Contraindications ↓BP, angio-oedema, renal artery/aortic stenosis, pregnancy, breastfeeding, collagen disease, porphyria.

Other precautions:

- Check U&Es and creatinine routinely and stop the ACE inhibitor if there is worsening renal function (↑ urea thought to be due to a diuretic is not an indication to stop, however).
- Weigh the patient regularly to monitor the response.
- Monitor WCC and urine protein if there is co-existent connective tissue disease.
- Beware of other interactions; Li^+ (levels ↑), digoxin (levels may ↑), NSAIDs (urea↑ K^+↑), anaesthetics (BP ↓).
- Watch for K^+ derangement (usually ↓) through diuretic action. Mild hypokalaemia is well tolerated without the need for K^+-sparing diuretics as long as: the K^+ is >3.5mmol/l, there is no predisposition to arrhythmias, and there are no other K^+-losing conditions (eg cirrhosis, chronic diarrhoea).

However, do not be put off trying a patient on ACE inhibitors by these cautions. Most patients tolerate ACE inhibitors very well and gain a significant benefit from them.

Shock

Shock is the inadequate perfusion of vital organs due to hypotension.

Clinical features: are of tachycardia (unless on β-blockers, or in spinal shock), hypotension (although in fit adults there may be ~10% blood loss before any BP change, which is often an initial *rise* in diastolic pressure ie a narrowing of the pulse pressure), pallor, faintness, sweating, and cold peripheries with poor capillary refill.

Causes of shock

1. Cardiogenic shock

Failure of the heart to pump sufficient blood around the circulation. It may occur rapidly or after progressive heart failure. It carries a high mortality and may be due to arrhythmias, tamponade, pneumothorax, MI, myocarditis, endocarditis, PE, aortic dissection, drugs, hypoxia, sepsis, and acidosis.

Management: treat the cause if known. Give morphine 2–10mg IV and O_2 mask. Monitor ECG, urine output, ABGs, U&Es, CVP. Consider inotropic agents eg dobutamine 2.5–10μg/kg/min IV adjusted to keep the systolic BP >80mmHg. Promote renal vasodilatation with dopamine 2–5μg/kg/min IV. Refer to a specialist if possible.

2. Anaphylactic shock – see opposite.

3. Endocrine failure – see Addison's disease and hypothyroidism.

4. Septic shock – see chapter 4.

5. Hypovolaemic shock

Due for example to trauma, ruptured aneurysm, or ectopic pregnancy.
Management: prevent further blood loss and aim to restore circulatory volume as quickly as possible until the pulse rate falls and the BP starts to rise. Give whole blood where possible (crossmatched if there is time, otherwise use O Rh–ve blood). Whilst waiting for blood to arrive, give warmed crystalloids such as Hartmann's solution.

► For the last two causes of shock, the immediate need is for rapid IV fluid replacement.

Points on fluid resuscitation:

- Use the largest vein and largest cannula possible.
- Add pressure to the fluid bag to speed the infusion.
- If access is difficult it may be necessary to cut down to a vein, eg 2cm above and anterior to the medial malleolus.
- If this fails intraosseous infusion is possible using specific cannulae below and medial to the tibial tuberosity.
- Give extra fluid if there are fractures: ribs ~150ml, tibia ~650ml, femur ~1500ml, pelvis ~ 2000ml.
- Double these estimates if there are open fractures.
- Remember to splint fractures and apply traction to reduce blood loss.

Anaphylaxis[1]

Anaphylactic shock requires prompt energetic treatment of laryngeal oedema, bronchospasm, and hypotension. It may be caused by exposure to insect venom (eg bee stings), food (eg eggs, peanuts), drugs (antibiotics, aspirin; especially if given IV) and other medicinal products (eg vaccines, antivenom).

Management

1. Stop infusion if this has caused the anaphylaxis.
2. Secure the airway, give oxygen.
3. ►►Give epinephrine 0.5–1.0mg (0.5–1ml of 1:1000 solution) IM
   Repeat every 10 minutes until BP & pulse both increase.
   [Patients on non-cardioselective β-blockers may not respond to epinephrine; they require salbutamol 250μg IV over 10 mins]
4. Give an antihistamine eg chlorpheniramine 10–20mg by slow IV injection. Continue this PO for 48hrs.
5. Continuing deterioration requires additional treatment with IV fluids, IV aminophylline, and nebulized salbutamol. Assisted ventilation and emergency tracheostomy (for laryngeal oedema) may be required.
6. Give hydrocortisone 100–300mg IV to prevent further deterioration.

- If there is doubt about the adequacy of the patient's circulation, it may be necessary to give the epinephrine IV as a dilute solution.
- Anaphylactic reactions require prior exposure to the antigen. Anaphylactoid reactions appear clinically similar but occur when large quantities of allergen are infused IV eg antivenoms rich in Fc antibody portions. Prior skin testing does not exclude the possibility of a subsequent anaphylactoid reaction since the reaction is dependent on the quantity of antigen injected. Always have epinephrine already drawn up when injecting antivenoms.

1. *British National Formulary*, 1998, 3.4.3

Hypertension

Hypertension (HT) is an increasing problem in the tropics, particularly in urban areas, where lifestyles are becoming similar to those in the West. In S Africa, there is evidence suggesting a greater prevalence of HT amongst black as against white people (up to 20% in some African urban studies). Environmental factors are chiefly involved in this process, since in these same countries the disease is virtually unheard of in rural populations, living traditional lifestyles. It is a major risk factor in the development of MI, stroke, renal failure, heart failure and peripheral vascular disease.

Clinical features: people are usually asymptomatic until irreversible damage has been done. Symptoms include dizziness, fatigue, headache, palpitations. Signs: ↑ BP (though if there is heart failure, the BP may be normal); if 2° HT, there may be signs of the cause; end-organ damage eg LV hypertrophy, heart failure, retinopathy, proteinuria, uraemia.

Who to treat?[1]

1. Where the BP is systolic ≥200mmHg or diastolic ≥110mmHg, treat if these values are confirmed on 3 separate occasions over 1–2 weeks (► if severe or in the presence of associated conditions, eg heart failure, treat immediately – see opposite).
2. Where the initial BP is systolic 160–199mmHg or diastolic 90–109mm Hg (or when higher initial values fall into this range) take one of the following courses of action:
   - If vascular complications or end-organ damage or diabetes are present, treat if systolic ≥160mmHg or diastolic ≥90mmHg is confirmed on at least 3 separate occasions.
   - If there are no vascular complications, no end-organ damage, and no diabetes, repeat BP measurements at monthly intervals for 3–6mths and treat if the average value during this period is systolic ≥160mmHg or diastolic ≥100mmHg.
   - If the average value is systolic <160mmHg and diastolic 90–99mm Hg, treatment may be withheld but continue to monitor; however, consider treatment if this BP is sustained in patients >60yrs and those at particularly high risk of cardiovascular complications.
3. Isolated systolic hypertension (systolic >160mmHg, diastolic <90mm Hg) in persons >60yrs should be monitored over 3mths and then treated, preferably with a low dose thiazide diuretic +/– low dose β-blocker.
4. Hypertension during pregnancy can be treated with methyldopa; β-blockers can be used during the third trimester.

Investigations: recheck the BP on at least 3 separate occasions. Search for a cause (particularly in the young). U&E, Cr, glucose, plasma lipids, MSU (twice), renal USS, urinary VMA, ECG, CXR, fundoscopy.

Accelerated HT

This is heralded by sudden onset heart failure, renal failure, encephalopathy (convulsions/coma), or a diastolic BP >140mmHg. Untreated, its mortality is ~90%; treated, it carries a 5yr survival of only 60%. See opposite.

Management of hypertension[1]

Aim to reduce the incidence of stroke, heart and renal failure, and MI.

1. Non-drug therapy

- stop smoking (not itself a risk factor for HT; only for MI/stroke)
- ↓ (Na^+ salt) intake
- ↓ alcohol intake
- ↑ physical exercise
- ↑ K^+ intake (fresh vegetables & fruit)
- ↓ weight in the obese
- encourage relaxation therapy.

2. Drug therapy: explain that the patient may need to be on tablets for life, even though she has had no symptoms and may, indeed, feel worse on the medication. Encourage her to return to a doctor if there are unacceptable side effects and not simply to stop taking the medication.

► Aim to reduce systolic BP to <160mmHg and diastolic BP to <90.

Suggested approach:

- Start with a thiazide diuretic (eg bendrofluazide 2.5mg/24hrs PO). Use lowest possible dose; check plasma K^+ 4wks after starting therapy (however K^+ supplements or K^+-sparing diuretics are rarely required).
- If not controlled, add a β-blocker eg atenolol 50mg PO daily (contra-indicated in patients with asthma or heart failure).
- If still uncontrolled, start either an ACE inhibitor (see page on heart failure) eg captopril initial dose 6.25mg PO daily or a Ca^{2+} channel blocker eg modified-release nifedipine 20mg PO bd.
- If the HT is still not resolved (<10% will not respond to one or a combination of these drugs) seek expert help before starting centrally acting α-agonists, peripheral α-antagonists, or hydralazine.

► Always try to stop ineffective drugs – this helps patient compliance.

Management of accelerated hypertension[1]

This requires urgent treatment in hospital but not normally IV therapy. IV therapy risks causing a very rapid fall in blood pressure, resulting in: cerebral hypoperfusion, occipital infarction and blindness; renal hypoperfusion exacerbating any renal failure present; or myocardial ischaemia.

- Give either a β-blocker eg atenolol 50mg PO or a Ca^{2+} channel blocker eg modified release nifedipine 20mg PO bd.

1. *British National Formulary* 2.5

Rheumatic fever[1]

Rheumatic fever is an important cause of cardiovascular mortality throughout the developing world. Group A streptococcal (*Streptococcus pyogenes*) pharyngitis leads in about 0.3–3% of cases to rheumatic fever, due to an immune cross-reactivity between the bacteria and connective tissue.

It is a disease of the poor, the overcrowded, and the poorly housed, with children being chiefly affected. Although the disease is often more severe in the developing world than in the West, with a higher incidence of severe carditis and earlier development of chronic valvular heart disease, it is not a different disease. Instead, this severity reflects a failure of developing world health services to prevent recurrences of acute rheumatic fever. ► If these recurrences can be prevented, 70% of patients who have carditis in their 1st attack will eventually lose their murmurs and have normal hearts.

Clinical features

- Arthritis – occurs in 80% of cases. It is typically asymmetrical and migratory, affecting large joints; the pain is severe while swelling is often modest. Onset is acute and subsides over a week; as one joint improves, a second gets worse. This process may continue for 3–6 weeks. There is a dramatic response to aspirin.
- Carditis – occurring in 40–50%, this is the most serious manifestation of acute RF, causing death acutely in <1% of cases. It may affect only the endocardium (valvulitis, often MR +/– AR, 'mild carditis') or the myocardium and pericardium may also be involved ('severe carditis').
- Chorea – occurs in ~10% after a longer incubation period. Sydenham's chorea is emotional lability and involuntary movements (face, limbs).
- Erythema marginatum – <5% cases.
- Subcutaneous nodules – now rare.

Diagnosis: is based upon the revised Jones criteria (see opposite) and requires i) evidence of recent streptococcal infection *plus* ii) either two major criteria *or* one major and two minor criteria.

Management:

1. Bedrest for at least 2 weeks, *and* until the child feels better.
2. Anti-inflammatory drugs to suppress the inflammatory process:
   - Aspirin 20–25mg/kg PO qds. Continue for 3–6 weeks if heart is not involved; 3 months in mild carditis; 4–6 months in severe carditis.
   - In severe carditis, give prednisolone 0.5mg/kg qds for 2 weeks.
3. In heart failure, give frusemide.
4. Sodium valproate 7.5–10mg/kg PO bd for 3 months for chorea [alternative haloperidol 0.05mg/kg daily].

►► Secondary prophylaxis is essential for all patients

Give benzathine penicillin G 1.2MU IM every 3–4 weeks for:

- >10yrs after last episode and at least until age 40 (sometimes for life) for patients with carditis and residual heart (valvular) disease.
- 10yrs or well into adulthood, whichever is the longer for patients with carditis but no residual heart disease.
- 5yrs or until age 21yrs, whichever is the longer for patients who did not have carditis.

[Alternative for penicillin-allergic patients is erythromycin 250mg bd PO]

Revised Jones criteria

A. *Evidence of recent group A streptococcal infection*

- positive throat culture or rapid streptococcal antigen test
- elevated or rising streptococcal antibody titre.

B. *Major manifestations*

- carditis
- polyarthritis
- chorea
- erythema marginatum
- subcutaneous nodules.

C. *Minor manifestations*

Clinical findings

- arthralgia
- fever.

Laboratory findings

- elevated acute-phase reactants (ESR or C-reactive protein)
- prolonged PR interval.

Any effort which will make the IM injection less painful, and therefore less frightening for the child, will make secondary prophylaxis more successful. Painful monthly IM injections for a young child can be a very frightening prospect which could make the child unwilling to take this life-saving treatment.

Prevention of rheumatic fever: requires improvements in housing conditions, as well as better methods of primary prevention. These can include early detection of streptococcal sore throats and their selective treatment or treatment of all children with pharyngitis with a single IM dose of benzathine penicillin.

1. Majeed HA, 1997, *Medicine*, 25, 12

Infective endocarditis

► *Fever + changing murmur = endocarditis until proven otherwise.*

50% of endocarditis in the UK is on normal valves. It follows a more acute course when accompanied by heart failure. The course is more sub-acute on rheumatic or otherwise damaged valves. It may also occur on prosthetic valves (~2%), in which case the involved valves usually need replacing.

Pathogenesis: any bacteraemia, especially following dental procedures, GU manipulation, or surgery may expose the valves to colonization. In the UK, the commonest organisms are *Streptococcus viridans, Enterococcus faecalis,* and *Staphylococcus aureus*. Rarely fungi, *Coxiella,* or *Chlamydia* species may infect heart valves. Non-infective causes include Libman-Sachs endocarditis of SLE and malignancy. Right sided disease is more common in IV drug abusers and may lead to pulmonary abscesses.

Clinical features include evidence of:

- ***Infection:*** fever, malaise, night sweats, finger clubbing, splenomegaly, anaemia.
- ***Heart murmurs*** and ***heart failure***.
- ***Embolic events:*** (since vegetations on the valves may embolize and cause stroke).
- ***Vasculitis:*** microscopic haematuria, splinter haemorrhages, Osler's nodes (painful lesions on finger pulps), Janeway lesions (palmar macules), Roth's spots (retinal vasculitis), and renal failure.

Classically fever, haematuria, splenomegaly, and murmurs = endocarditis.

Diagnosis: take 3 blood cultures from different sites at different times (at least one of these will be positive in 99% of endocarditis cases) ESR, FBC, U&E, Cr. Echocardiography (where available) may show the vegetations on valves. Perform urinalysis for haematuria.

Management:

1. For streptococcal infection, give benzylpenicillin 1.2g IV q4h (or vancomycin) *plus* gentamicin 60–80mg IV bd (see warning p190), for 2 weeks, then amoxycillin 1g PO tds for 2 weeks.
2. For *Staphylococcus aureus* infections, give flucloxacillin 2g IV q6h and gentamicin as above, then just flucloxacillin for 2 weeks.
3. For *Staphylococcus epidermidis* infections, use vancomycin and rifampicin for at least 4 weeks
4. If 'blind' empirical therapy is required, give benzylpenicillin and gentamicin and add in flucloxacillin if the endocarditis is acute in onset. Wait for blood culture results. This recommendation is based on streptococcal infections being the most common cause of endocarditis. Alter these recommendations according to the local circumstances.

Prognosis: There is 30% mortality in the UK from staphylococcal endocarditis, 14% with anaerobic infection, and 6% with endocarditis due to sensitive streptococci.

Prophylaxis before dental procedures

Patients with cardiac defects (congenital, rheumatic, etc), or who have had a prosthetic replacement of a damaged valve, are at risk from infective endocarditis following dental procedures. Those who have had one or more episodes of infective endocarditis in the past are particularly susceptible. There is no evidence that patients with prosthetic valves are any more susceptible to endocarditis after dental operations than those with damaged natural valves, but if endocarditis develops therapy may be more difficult.

Antibiotic cover should be given just before high risk dental procedures (see below for regimens). These include tooth extractions, scaling, and surgery involving gingival tissues. Particular care must be taken not to delay the procedure after giving antibiotics.

- All patients who have had previous infective endocarditis should be referred to hospital for high risk dental procedures.
- * Special risk patients are those who have received antibiotics in the previous month, who have a prosthetic valve, or who are allergic to penicillin.
- The teicoplanin dose is 400mg IV.
- An alternative regimen for penicillin-allergic patients in hospital is clindamycin 300mg IV over >10mins at induction (or 15mins before the procedure), then clindamycin 150mg PO/IV 6hrs later. Children <5yrs require a quarter of the adult dose; children 5–10yrs require half the adult dose.
- Similar prophylaxis will be needed for other invasive procedures eg endoscopy.

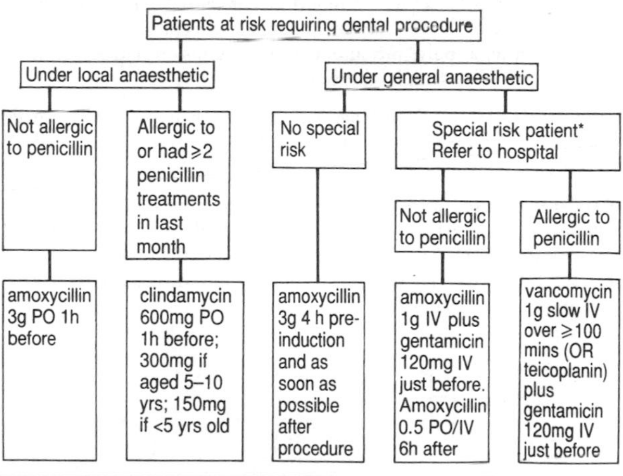

Cardiomyopathies

Diseases of the heart muscle are classified as follows:

1. Congestive (dilated) cardiomyopathy

This is common throughout the tropics. Often there is no identifiable cause, though aetiological factors may include heart failure (anaemia, hypertension), toxins (? wheat fungi), alcohol, beriberi, myocarditis.

Clinical features: are usually of heart failure although there is a poor response to treatment. The apex beat is diffuse and displaced and there is often valvular incompetence giving rise to murmurs. There may be AF and associated embolic events. Typically the patient is a man of 40–50yrs.

Investigations and management: echocardiography shows a dilated, hypokinetic heart. The cause may be difficult to ascertain if there is accompanying ↑ BP (hypertensive failure), mitral incompetence (rheumatic heart failure), or endomyocardial fibrosis. The distinction is, however, academic, since treatment is for the underlying heart failure (see above). The mortality is high – ~40% by 2yrs.

2. Restrictive cardiomyopathy

This is due to endomyocardial stiffening and clinically resembles constrictive pericarditis. It is almost always due to endomyocardial fibrosis. It is thought that hypereosinophilia (possibly triggered by a helminthic infection, especially filariasis) leads to cellular damage in the myocardium. This in turn causes mural thrombus formation, producing a fibrotic mass. It may rarely be caused by amyloid or carcinoid.

Clinical features: may begin with a febrile illness, facial oedema, and dyspnoea (which may be progressive and fatal in a few months). LV disease consists of MR (never stenosis, or aortic incompetence – cf rheumatic fever) with an S_3, and progressive pulmonary HT. RV disease (usually tricuspid incompetence) results in gross ascites and ↑↑ JVP, but often no peripheral oedema. There may be exophthalmos, central cyanosis, delayed puberty, ↓ arterial pulse pressure, pericardial effusion and AF. Murmurs may be heard (cf pericardial disease).

Investigations: CXR findings vary from a massive cardiac shadow (aneurysmal R atrium or pericardial effusion), to an almost normal film. Echocardiography may be helpful.

Treatment: in the acute stage, treatment is purely supportive. If there is eosinophilia, look for and treat the cause. In established disease resist the temptation to drain the ascites, since it may cause the patient to lose a lot of protein. Digoxin may be used to control the ventricular rate if there is AF. Surgery may be curative.

3. Hypertrophic (obstructive) cardiomyopathy

There is asymmetrical hypertrophy of ventricular muscle (50% are inherited as autosomal dominant – screen other family members).

Clinical features: are of dyspnoea, angina, syncope, palpitations. There may be a double impulse at the apex, jerky pulse, S_3/S_4, late systolic murmur. The ECG may show LBBB or RBBB; echocardiography is usually diagnostic.

Management Give β-blockers for angina and treat any arrhythmias. Uncontrolled AF should prompt life-long anticoagulation.

4. Acute myocarditis

Inflammation of the myocardium which may present similarly to MI. Causes are: viral (coxsackie virus), diphtheria, rheumatic fever, drugs, and other infections. There is angina, dyspnoea, arrhythmia, tachycardia, and heart failure. Exclude MI and pericardial effusion.
Management: is supportive, or for heart failure if it ensues.

5. Left atrial myxoma

A rare, benign, primary tumour, presenting with left atrial obstruction (as in mitral stenosis), systemic emboli, AF, fever, weight loss, and ↑ ESR. Rarely, one may hear a tumour 'plop' on auscultation. Atrial myxoma is twice as common in females than in males. Differentiate from mitral stenosis by the occurrence of emboli in the absence of AF, or on echocardiography.
Management: is by surgical excision.

Pericardial disease

1. Pericarditis

In the tropics, this is commonly due to TB or pyogenic infection.

- **Tuberculous pericarditis** is especially important in areas of high HIV prevalence. Spread is probably from the adjacent lymph nodes and pleura.
- **Acute pyogenic pericarditis** results from generalized bacteraemia derived from, or associated with, a primary focus elsewhere.
- **Other causes:** any infection (especially coxsackie virus), malignancy, uraemia, MI, Dressler's syndrome, trauma, radiotherapy, connective tissue diseases, and hypothyroidism.

Clinical features: there is often an associated pericardial effusion (see below). There is sharp, constant sternal pain, relieved by sitting forward, which may radiate to the left shoulder, down the left arm, or to the abdomen. It may be made worse by lying on the left, coughing, inspiration, and swallowing. Auscultation may reveal a scratchy, superficial pericardial rub, loudest at the left sternal edge.

Diagnosis: is by ECG which classically shows upwardly concave (saddle-shaped) ST segments in all leads except AVR, with no reciprocal changes. Unless there is an effusion or TB changes, the CXR will be normal.

Management: find and treat the cause. Give analgesia and consider systemic steroids for unresolving cases (2mg/kg daily for 11 weeks). For TB pericarditis, commence anti-TB treatment and consider an HIV test.

2. Pericardial effusion

This is an accumulation of fluid in the pericardial space, caused by any of the causes of pericarditis.

Clinical features: depend upon the speed at which the effusion has formed. If formed quickly, the pericardium cannot stretch and so pressure ↑ and the heart is compressed to produce ► **tamponade**. There is a fall in cardiac output (↓ BP), the JVP is ↑↑, Kussmaul's sign (JVP ↑ with inspiration), tachycardia, inpalpable apex, pulsus paradoxus, peripheral shut down, and quiet heart sounds. In more chronic effusions, signs of heart failure predominate, with severe ascites and hepatosplenomegaly.

Diagnosis: CXR shows a large, globular heart (may show pericardial fluid). ECG has ↓ voltages and changing QRS complexes. Echocardiography is diagnostic. Differentiate from an MI and PE.

Treatment: Find and treat the cause eg antibiotics for bacterial infections, antituberculous drugs for TB.

►Tamponade requires urgent drainage. Aspirate with a 50ml syringe, fitted with a long needle and two-way tap, inserting upwards and to the left of the xiphisternum, with the patient sitting up. Watch an ECG monitor to note when the myocardium is touched. If pus is drained, instillation of antibiotics into the pericardial space may prevent recurrence.

ECG changes in pericarditis

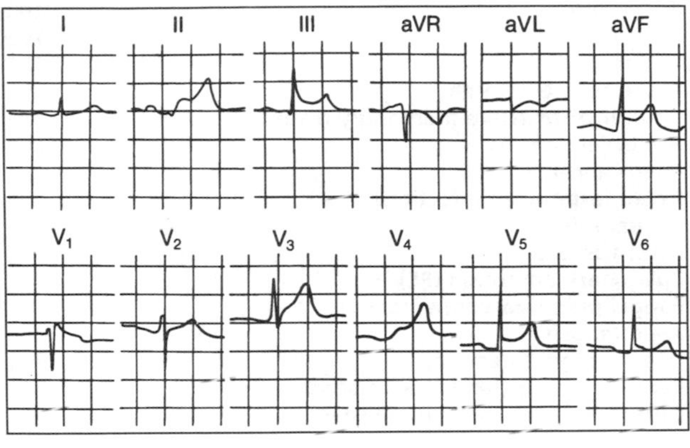

3. Constrictive pericarditis

This is encasement of the heart in a non-expansile pericardium, usually following TB infection. Features are as for chronic effusion, however the heart is small on CXR and may show calcification. The condition requires surgical excision of the pericardium.

6. Chest medicine

Cough 286
Haemoptysis 286
Dyspnoea/breathlessness 288
Wheezing/stridor 288
Pneumothorax 290
Pleural effusion 292
Asthma 294
Acute severe asthma 296
Chronic obstructive pulmonary disease (COPD) 298
Bronchiectasis 300
Lung cancer 302
Acute respiratory infections *see chapter 3E*
Pneumonia *see chapter 3E*
Lung abscess 304
Pulmonary embolism (PE) 304
Fungal pulmonary infections 306
Aspergillosis 306
Other fungal infections 308
Paragonimiasis (lung fluke disease) 310
Diffuse parenchymal lung disease 312

Chest medicine

Cough

A cough in isolation is common. It is often due to mild viral infection and needs only symptomatic relief or more often no therapy. In contrast, a productive cough or one associated with dyspnoea may be more ominous and requires further investigation. A careful search for cardiac or pulmonary causes should be started.

- ► A cough without associated signs or symptoms may be due to diphtheria or TB pleurisy. Both will require specific management.
- A cough by itself does not warrant a CXR.
- TB, pertussis, smoking, lung cancer, and a foreign body can each cause a chronic cough.
- A change in cough habit is significant, particularly in a smoker.

Pulmonary causes of cough:

- smoking
- bacterial pneumonia
- asthma
- reflux
- bronchitis.
- lung cancer
- drugs eg ACE inhibitors
- TB
- COPD

Other infective causes include: typhoid, *P. falciparum* malaria (due to pulmonary oedema), measles, bronchiectasis (post-measles or pertussis), amoebic liver abscess, pulmonary hydatid disease, AIDS, rickettsial infections, paragonimiasis, tropical pulmonary eosinophilia, Loffler's syndrome, plague.

Nocturnal coughing is characteristic of asthma.

Haemoptysis

- ► Consider TB in anyone with a chronic cough and haemoptysis.
- ► Be careful to distinguish haemoptysis from haematemesis, or blood from the gums/throat.

Causes

Acute – pneumonia, bronchitis, pulmonary embolism.
Chronic – TB, lung cancer, bronchiectasis.

Other causes include:

Lung infection: parasitic disease (eg paragonimiasis), bronchitis, lung abscess, fungal disease (eg aspergillosis, paracoccidioidomycosis).
Trauma: contusion, foreign body, post-intubation.
Vascular disease: vasculitis.
Parenchymal disease: diffuse parenchymal diseases, haemosiderosis, CF.
Cardiovascular disease: pulmonary oedema, mitral stenosis, aortic aneurysm.
Bleeding diatheses: sepsis, DIC, viper bites, haemorrhagic fevers.

Chest medicine

Dyspnoea/breathlessness

A subjective sensation of difficulty with breathing.

Causes:

1. **Cardiac:** left heart failure (eg due to ischaemic heart disease, anaemia, myocardial infarction, cardiomyopathy, myocarditis, pericarditis). Normally occurs on exertion, associated with orthopnoea and paroxysmal nocturnal dyspnoea. A dry cough may be present.
2. **Pulmonary diseases** eg asthma, COPD, effusions, pneumothorax, pulmonary embolism (PE), foreign body, parenchymal disease, pulmonary hypertension.
3. **Diseases** of the chest wall and muscles, spine, diaphragm, or pleura.
4. **Miscellaneous:** thyrotoxicosis, ketoacidosis, gross ascites.

Of value in finding a cause for the breathlessness is determining the rate of onset. Dyspnoea has an acute onset in PE, pneumothorax, pulmonary oedema, pneumonia, asthma, and LVF. Dyspnoea with a more chronic or insidious onset may be due to pleural effusions, lung cancer or metastases, and subacute pulmonary infiltrations. COPD, diffuse fibrosing diseases and anaemia may come on over months. Try to determine any initiating and resolving factors.

Both asthma and LVF tend to cause intermittent dyspnoea.

Sudden onset or exacerbation of dyspnoea

► Immediately sit the patient up and give O_2.
In COPD give O_2, but monitor ABGs for signs of CO_2 retention.

Causes:

- pulmonary oedema
- pneumonia
- pneumothorax
- asthma
- acute toxin inhalation
- allergic airways disease
- pulmonary embolism
- cardiac tamponade
- ARDS
- exacerbation of COPD
- pulmonary haemorrhage
- pulmonary effusion.

Take a *Hx* (looking for pre-existing disease; exposure; travel; operations; chest pain) and investigate to exclude particular conditions.

► Treat pulmonary oedema, asthma, and tension pneumothorax before continuing to do CXR or blood gas analysis if these are indicated.

Wheezing/stridor

Stridor is the harsh inspiratory sound that arises from obstruction in the larynx or major airways. Wheezes are sounds which may occur during inspiration and/or expiration. They can be heard externally and are of polyphonic nature in patients with asthma, obstructive bronchitis (and cardiovascular dyspnoea). Forced expiration may reveal wheezes when tidal breathing is silent.

A foreign body or tumour mass in a major airway produces a wheeze with a single pitch (monophonic). This wheeze cannot be altered by coughing to shift mucus.

Chest medicine

Pneumothorax

Rupture of an alveolar bullus or traumatic chest injury may produce a pneumothorax – air entering the pleural space. Part of the lung subsequently collapses, reducing the vital lung capacity and ventilation of the affected lung. Where there is pre-existing pulmonary disease, this additional insult may be sufficient to cause respiratory failure. In many cases, however, there is little functional impairment.

- ***Primary pneumothorax*** – occurs spontaneously in previously healthy individuals, often tall young men. It is commonly small with little functional deficit. There is ~20% risk of recurrence.
- ***Secondary pneumothorax*** – is a consequence of pre-existing lung disease, often COPD, necrotizing infections such as *S. aureus*, TB, or anaerobic bacteria; less often asthma or malignancy.
- ***Traumatic pneumothorax*** – common cause following road traffic injuries and assault.
- ***Iatrogenic pneumothorax*** – common complication of percutaneous lung biopsy. Also occurs during mechanical ventilation and after transbronchial lung biopsy.

Clinical features: a small pneumothorax may be asymptomatic. Otherwise, common features include pleuritic chest pain of sudden onset; dyspnoea (partly due to ventilatory deficit but also due to the pain of breathing → small breaths; in 2° disease, it may be an acute exacerbation on top of pre-existing respiratory distress); reduced breath sounds; percussive resonance; reduced chest movements. ►► A tension pneumothorax will also present with deviated trachea and marked respiratory distress.

Management

1. A 1° pneumothorax, if small, does not require aspiration; watch and wait. A large pneumothorax should be aspirated through the 2nd intercostal space in the midclavicular line with a catheter and 50ml syringe. If >2 litres of air is aspirated, it is likely that there is a continuing air leak. Where there are significant symptoms or simple aspiration fails, a chest drain can be inserted
2. For a pneumothorax complicating pre-existent lung disease, attempt simple aspiration even for a small pneumothorax. Symptomatic pneumothoraces require insertion of chest drain.
3. A pleurodesis may be required once the lung is fully inflated again – see opposite. Surgery may be indicated for patients with air leakage that continues for >1 or 2 weeks.

►► Tension pneumothorax

Loose tissue at the site of a penetrating chest injury may act as a flap, allowing air to enter during inspiration but preventing it leaving during expiration. As air accumulates in the pleural space, mediastinal shift across into the opposite hemithorax results in lung compression and respiratory compromise. Unless relieved quickly, cardiorespiratory arrest will occur. If suspected, insert a wide bore needle into the affected side (2nd intercostal space, midclavicular line; opposite side to direction of tracheal deviation) before doing anything else. There should be rapid relief of the respiratory distress. Get a CXR both before and after going on to insert a chest drain.

Pleurodesis

Give the patient 10mg morphine IM. This will take effect as you instil 20ml of 1% lignocaine into the chest drain and clamp it off. Ask the patient to roll from side to side. After 20mins, instil 500mg of tetracycline dissolved in 30–50ml of normal saline and leave clamped off for 2–3hrs, again with the patient rolling intermittently, to spread the solution around the pleura. This can be very painful, so don't hesitate to provide good analgesia quickly. After 3hrs max, unclamp and allow fluid to drain through the underwater seal. Once no longer bubbling, remove the drain after 12hrs and recheck CXR to see whether the lung has remained inflated.

Pleural effusion

The accumulation of fluid in the pleural space. The fluid may be transudate, exudate, blood, pus, or lymphatic fluid (chyle).

- **Transudates** are serous fluids, low in protein, that form when the capillary hydrostatic pressure forcing fluid out of the capillaries is not balanced by the colloid osmotic force drawing the fluid back in (Starling's equation). Transudates may also occur if fluid passes across the diaphragm in patients with ascites.
- **Exudates** are serous fluids which flow into the pleural space because of leaking capillaries – they have the normal plasma level of protein (> that of transudates).
- **Chylothorax** results from leakage of lymphatic fluid from the thoracic duct.

Clinical features: pleuritic chest pain (worse if 'dry pleurisy', decreases as fluid accumulates); dyspnoea (often only apparent if patient has low reserve or as the fluid accumulates); decreased chest movement on affected side; stony dull percussion decreased breath sounds on auscultation (although there may be signs of consolidation at the top of the effusion).

Diagnosis: is confirmed by CXR and/or ultrasound. Aspiration of 50–100mls of pleural fluid across the thoracic wall (thoracentesis) may indicate the underlying cause – see opposite. ***Best site:*** 10cm lateral of the spine and one intercostal space below the top level of the effusion as determined by percussion. If this fails to draw fluid the effusion may be loculated or the aspiration too high-ultrasound may help. Note macroscopic appearance of the fluid and stain for organisms and cells; culture. If neoplasm or TB is suspected a pleural biopsy is often useful.

Management: if relevant, treatment of the underlying condition (eg heart failure, RA) will often resolve the effusion. Aspiration of 1–2 litres provides at least temporary relief from dyspnoea. With recurrent effusion, an intercostal drain may be useful. In malignant disease, the effusions will continue to recur unless prevented with pleurodesis – see above and opposite. NB more than 2l should not be drained in 24hrs, as this increases the risk of reactive pulmonary oedema.

Empyema

An infected pleural effusion that is normally 2° to bacterial pneumonia, pulmonary TB, or lung abscess. Empyema should be suspected if a patient with pneumonia has persisting fever after adequate antibiotic therapy. Ultrasound may guide aspiration with a wide-bore needle for both drainage and culture/microscopy of pus. Treat with antibiotics – high-dose ampicillin plus metronidazole 500mg IV q6h until antibiotic sensitivities are known. If antibiotic treatment is unsuccessful, fibrin deposition leading to fibrosis of the interpleural space may require thoracotomy and surgical removal of pus.

TB effusions present as pulmonary TB plus pleuritic pain and dyspnoea.

Causes of pleural effusion

Transudate:	• cardiac failure • hepatic cirrhosis • nephrotic syndrome	• peritoneal dialysis • myxoedema • hepatic/renal failure.
Exudate:	• infections eg pneumonia, TB • subphrenic abscess, infection • metastatic CA • PE	• lymphomas • collagen vascular diseases (RA, SLE) • pancreatitis • drug reactions • mesothelioma.
Chylothorax:	• trauma • lymphatic filiarisis	• metastatic CA • lymphomas.
Haemothorax:	• trauma.	

Diagnostic effusion features

- neutrophils → pyogenic infection
- lymphocytes → TB, lymphoma, malignancy
- malignant cells → malignancy
- >30g/l protein → exudate
- <4mmol glucose → RA, infection, malignancy
- high amylase → pancreatitis

Asthma[1]

Now recognized to be a chronic inflammatory disorder of the airways, asthma is a syndrome of reversible airflow obstruction.

Asthma is caused by a combination of genetic susceptibility and a triggering factor:

- allergens (eg food, dust, in an atopic individual)
- infections (particularly viral in children eg RSV, or aspergillus)
- environmental or occupational pollutants, particularly cigarette smoke.

Each of these stimuli will also trigger acute excerbations of asthma. ► Severe asthmatic attacks can be provoked by β-blockers (including eye-drops) and NSAIDS.

Pathology: a triggering factor elicits chronic mucosal inflammation. This has two consequences which result in asthmatic attacks:

- it makes the bronchi more prone to constrict in response to irritants such as cold dry air, pollen, fumes, paints – termed bronchial hyper-responsiveness, *and*
- the inflammation produces mucosal oedema and intraluminal mucus which block the airway during this bronchoconstriction.

Current treatment for asthma therefore aims primarily to control the inflammation.

Clinical features: polyphonic wheeze on both inspiration and expiration (often only present during exertion or forced expiration); chest tightness; cough (often producing mucoid sputum); dyspnoea; difficulty breathing in.

Asthma has diurnal variation – it is worse in the early hours of the morning. If the asthma is severe, the patient may wake up between 3 and 5am. If less severe, she will sleep through this period but find her symptoms worse on waking up – morning cough. The patient gradually gets better through the day. Into this daily rhythm are interspersed episodic attacks, the stimulus for which may not be recognized. These attacks can be acute and over in minutes to hours or drawn out, initiating a deterioration in symptoms that lasts days.

Diagnosis: from characteristic clinical features and >20% change in peak expiratory flow (PEF) either on exercise or stimulus challenge or, if PEF normally <80% of predicted value, after therapy with β_2-agonists or steroids. Serial PEF measurements are also extremely valuable in following the course of the condition and its response to therapy. Every ward requires a meter such as the mini-Wright PEF meter.

Management: involves identification of and subsequent avoidance of allergens and triggers, prophylaxis, and relief of symptoms during an acute attack. Most attacks will respond to adequate doses of β_2-agonists, steroids, and O_2.

Aims of treatment: • freedom from symptoms, particularly nocturnal awakening • lung function within the normal range, varying by <20% during 24hrs • normal quality of life.

1. Adapted from Lane D, *OTM*, p2738, 1996

Notes

1. Patients should start treatment at the step most appropriate to the initial severity. A rescue course of prednisolone may be needed at any time and at any step. The aim is to achieve early control of the condition and then to reduce treatment.
2. Until growth is complete, any child requiring beclomethasone or budesonide >800µg daily or fluticasone >500µg daily should be referred to a paediatrician with an interest in asthma.

Step 1

Occasional use of relief bronchodilators
Inhaled short acting β agonists "as required" for symptom relief are acceptable. If they are needed more than once daily, move to step 2.
Before altering a treatment step ensure that the patient is having the treatment and has a good inhaler technique.
Address any fears.

Step 2

Regular inhaled anti-inflammatory agents
Inhaled short acting β agonists as required
plus
beclomethasone or budesonide 100–400 µg twice daily or fluticasone 50–200 µg twice daily.
Alternatively use cromoglycate or nedocromil sodium, but if control is not achieved start inhaled steroids.

Step 3

High dose inhaled steroids or low dose inhaled steroids plus long acting inhaled β agonist bronchodilator
Inhaled short acting β agonists as required
plus either
beclomethasone or budesonide increased to 800–2000 µg daily or fluticasone 400–1000 µg daily via a large volume spacer
or
beclomethasone or budesonide 100–400 µg twice daily or fluticasone 50–200 µg twice daily plus salmeterol 50 µg twice daily.
In a very small number of patients who experience side effects with high dose inhaled steroids, either the long acting inhaled β agonist option is used or a sustained release theophylline may be added to step 2 medication. Cromoglycate or nedocromil may also be tried.

Step 4

High dose inhaled steroids and regular bronchodilators
Inhaled short acting β agonists as required with inhaled beclomethasone or budesonide 800–2000 µg daily or fluticasone 400–1000 µg daily via a large volume spacer
plus
a sequential therapeutic trial of one or more of

- inhaled long acting β agonists
- sustained release theophylline
- inhaled ipratropium or oxitropium
- long acting β agonist tablets
- high dose inhaled bronchodilators
- cromoglycate or nedocromil.

Step 5

Addition of regular steroid tablets
Inhaled short acting β agonists as required with inhaled beclomethasone or budesonide 800–2000 µg daily or
fluticasone 400–1000 µg daily via a large volume spacer
and one or more of the long acting bronchodilators
plus
regular prednisolone tablets in a single daily dose.

Review treatment every three to six months. If control is achieved, a stepwise reduction in treatment may be possible. In patients whose treatment was recently started at step 4 or 5 or included steroid tablets for gaining control of asthma, this reduction may take place after a short interval. In other patients with chronic asthma, a three to six month period of stability should be shown before slow stepwise reduction is undertaken.

British Thoracic Society, BMJ Group

►►Acute severe asthma[1]

Find out what the normal PEFR is, what the current medication is, when the last severe attack was.

Features of severe asthma

- unable to finish sentences in one breath
- pulse >110 beats/min
- PEFR <50% normal
- RR>25 breaths/min.

►► Life-threatening features

- silent chest or cyanosis
- PEFR <33% normal
- exhaustion, confusion, or decreased consciousness,
- bradycardia or hypotension
- arterial blood gases: PaO_2 <8kPa, $PaCO_2$ normal or increased, low pH.

Rule out respiratory obstruction from; inhaled foreign body, epiglottitis, mediastinal/neck lumps.

Immediate management

1. Sit the patient up and give 100% O_2.
2. Give salbutamol 5mg by O_2-driven nebulizer.
3. Give hydrocortisone 200mg IV.
4. Do ABGs, CXR, PEFR (may be too breathless), pulse oximetry.

If there is no improvement or there are severe signs

1. Contact an anaesthetist concerning possible emergency intubation.
2. Add ipratropium 0.5mg to the nebulized salbutamol.
3. Give aminophylline 250mg by IV infusion over 20min or salbutamol 250μg IV over 10min.
► Do not give aminophylline to patients already taking theophyllines.
4. Give prednisolone 30–60mg PO.

Subsequent management

If patient is improving continue:

1. 100% O_2.
2. Prednisolone 30–60mg PO daily or hydrocortisone 200mg IV q6h.
3. Salbutamol 5mg by O_2-driven nebulizer q4h.

If patient is not improving:

1. Continue 100% O_2 and steroids.
2. Give nebulized salbutamol more frequently, up to every 15–30mins.
3. Repeat ipratropium q6h.
4. If still no improvement, give aminophylline 750–1500mg IV over 24hrs (monitor blood concentrations if continued over 24hrs). Salbutamol infusion can be given as an alternative.

Monitoring treatment

- PEFR 15–30min after starting treatment, then at least q6h.
- Maintain SaO_2 >92% by oximetry.
- Repeat ABG within 2hrs of starting treatment if initially abnormal.

1. British Thoracic Society guidelines 1997, *Thorax*, 52 (suppl 1), S12

On discharge from hospital, a patient should have:

1. Been on discharge medication for 24hrs and have had inhaler technique checked and recorded.
2. PEFR >75% of predicted or best and PEFR diurnal variability <25%, unless discharge is agreed with a respiratory physician.
3. Treatment with oral and inhaled steroids in addition to bronchodilators.
4. Their own PEFR meter and written self-management plan.
5. Follow-up arranged within 1 week.

Chronic obstructive pulmonary disease (COPD)

A chronic, predominantly irreversible, condition that variably affects both the intrathoracic airways and terminal alveoli of much of the lungs. It is considered obstructive since it is this aspect of the disease that produces its clinical features. It is mostly a disease of smokers, ex-smokers, and people who live or work in smoke-filled, poorly ventilated buildings.

Pathology: inhaled smoke elicits an inflammatory response with recruitment of neutrophils. An imbalance between neutrophil-derived proteinases and lung-derived proteinase inhibitors (which control and dampen the inflammatory response) is believed to predispose towards chronic inflammation and lung damage. The disease process also impairs lung defences, leading to recurrent infection and colonization of the normally sterile central airways.

- **Airways disease** – inflammation and mucosal gland hyperplasia results in mucous hypersecretion into the central conducting airways, producing a chronic productive cough (previously termed *chronic bronchitis*) and narrowing of the peripheral airways (due to fibrosis, stenosis, gland hyperplasia, and intraluminal mucus). Both chronic cough and airways obstruction can exist without the other.
- **Alveolar disease** – the alveolar walls become destroyed, probably due to chronic inflammation – a process termed *emphysema*. Macroscopic emphysema (ie visible by imaging) is associated with a loss of lung function since perfusion and ventilation of these areas is decreased. In microscopic disease, the attachments between terminal bronchioles and alveoli are lost. The bronchioles are then no longer held open as the lung expands, producing further airways obstruction.

Clinical features: occur after a period of gradual decline in lung function. The first feature is decreased FEV_1 but this is often asymptomatic – dyspnoea on exertion may not develop until FEV_1 is <50% of normal.

Patients often present with recurrent bronchial infections, chronic productive cough, and/or dyspnoea on exercise. Lung function deteriorates during acute infections and takes some weeks to recover. Increased dyspnoea at this time may bring the patient to medical attention. The lung fields are normal on CXR. With progression, the chest shows signs of hyperinflation (barrel-shaped; laryngeal prominence lower than normal; loss of cardiac/hepatic dullness to percussion; typical CXR). There may also be tachypnoea; use of accessory muscles; wheeze; and later: cyanosis, pursed lip breathing, ankle oedema, left- or right-sided heart failure, and respiratory failure.

Management: ► **Stop smoking**. Give a trial of • bronchodilators and • steroids – prednisolone 30–40mg PO daily for 2–3 weeks. Continue at lowest maintenance dose if effective. Physiotherapy to increase respiratory muscle strength can benefit some patients.

Prevention: Stop patients smoking and ► actively dissuade people from starting. Decrease smoke in the workplace and house.

Oxygen therapy

If the patient has a PaO_2 <8kPa on air, give a trial of oxygen at 2l/min via a mask. Recheck ABG after 1hr. If there is no rise in $PaCO_2$, increase the oxygen to 4l/min and recheck ABGs after another hour. If there is still no rise, the patient is not CO_2 retaining, and may have oxygen therapy without risk. If CO_2 does rise, reduce oxygen delivery to the level before which CO_2 was retained.

Bronchiectasis

A condition that is characterized by chronic dilatation of bronchioles and inflammation of airways +/– parenchyma. The normally sterile airways may become persistently infected with bacteria such as *H. influenzae, Strep. pneumoniae, M. cattarhalis,* or *P. aeruginosa.* Lung pathology is normally widespread but may be localized – eg distal to bronchial obstruction, or in a lung apex following TB.

Aetiology: appears to be due to defects in the lungs' defense systems → chronic self-perpetuating inflammation after an initial trigger. Primary inherited causes include Kartagener's syndrome. Immunosuppression in AIDS or hypogammaglobulinaemia also predispose to bronchiectasis. Secondary disease can follow TB, pneumonia, whooping cough, a foreign body, aspergillosis.

Clinical features: patients may be asymptomatic except during exacerbations – purulent cough; fever; chest pain; dyspnoea; haemoptysis. Hx may suggest a trigger for these episodes – eg infection or other lung injury. Between exacerbations, she may produce mucoid sputum; in more severe disease, the sputum is continuously purulent and there may be clubbing. Other features include: recurrent or chronic sinusitis; otitis media; post-nasal drip. Complications include: cor pulmonale, respiratory failure; brain abscesses; 2° amyloidosis; arthropathy.

Diagnosis: CXR shows a variety of changes including cysts and atelectasis. Because of persistent airway infection, sputum culture is rarely valuable but Gram stain of the sputum may indicate a likely causative agent. Also check immune status, neutrophil function.

Management:

1. Treat any underlying condition which can be identified. Surgery is only warranted for focal obstruction or severe persistent haemoptysis.
2. Regular physiotherapy, particularly during exacerbations, can offer symptomatic relief.
3. Check for airflow obstruction – treat if reversible.
4. Give antibiotics – amoxycillin 500mg PO tds either for a minimum of ten days for an acute exacerbation or continually as prophylaxis for recurrent disease (>6 episodes/year).
5. Persistent purulent sputum or unresponsive exacerbations may require higher doses – amoxycillin up to 3g PO bd. If unresponsive, attempt to culture *Pseudomonas* spp from sputum. If positive, this may respond to oral fluoroquinolones or IV antipseudomonal antibiotics.

Prevention: reduce smoking, reduce infections (education, better housing, antibiotics).

Chest medicine

Lung cancer

Bronchial carcinoma is almost completely related to tobacco smoking. While once an uncommon disease in much of the developing world, the recent boom in cigarette smoking in these areas will soon make it an all too common diagnosis. Importantly,

- it is preventable by reducing exposure to tobacco smoke, *and*
- it is often a condition which presents late with a very poor prognosis (7/8ths of a lung tumour's life may have passed before it is diagnosed; the vast majority will be disseminated at time of diagnosis).

Different tumour types

- ***Squamous cell carcinoma*** – slow-growing tumours that often present with obstruction. Metastatic spread is relatively uncommon.
- ***Small-cell (oat-cell) carcinoma*** – fast-growing tumours that often present with disseminated disease. They may secrete hormones.
- ***Adenocarcinoma*** – the most common peripheral tumour, it may produce mucin and will surround associated bronchi, stenosing the lumen. Not smoking related.
- ***Large-cell carcinoma*** – large, necrotic, pleomorphic, mucin-producing tumours. They are frequently peripheral and locally invasive; while metastatic spread is common, survival rates post-surgery are good.
- ***Carcinoid tumours*** – a group of tumours which are unrelated to smoking and occur in a younger age-group. They may be malignant and metastasize to distal organs. Most occur in proximal airways.
- ***Metastases*** – often from primaries in the breast; colon; kidney, lung. Less often choriocarcinoma; testicular cancer; sarcomas; melanoma.

Clinical features: can be grouped as follows:

1. ***Pulmonary features*** **–** cough; sputum (often grey and viscous if there is no infection; contains malignant cells in ~60% of cases); dyspnoea; haemoptysis; chest pain/discomfort; wheeze; stridor; pleural effusion; pneumonia due to proximal airway obstruction.

► Cough and haemoptysis are early signs of lung cancer. If the cancer is recognized at this stage, there may be some hope of a cure.

2. **Due to local invasion** – Horner's syndrome; vocal cord paralysis; unilateral diaphragmatic paralysis; pain due to branchial root involvement; superior vena caval obstruction; dysphagia; cardiac dysfunction; bone pain (ribs/spine).
3. **Due to metastatic spread** – signs relate to the organs which are involved: lymph node enlargement (particularly scalene and supraclavicular); bones (especially ribs, vertebrae, femora, humeri); brain; liver; adrenal gland; skin (blue umbilicated lesions).
4. **Systemic effects** – tiredness; lack of energy; weight loss; fever and night sweats (normally due to 2° infection).
5. **Endocrine and metabolic abnormalities** – caused by secretion of a variety of hormone-mimicking peptides by the tumour. They include SIADH; ectopic ACTH secretion; hypercalcaemia (mostly due to bone metastases; sometimes secretion of a parathyroid-like hormone); gynaecomastia, testicular atrophy. Other endocrine effects are uncommon.
6. **Other complications** include neuromyopathy; finger clubbing; hypertrophic pulmonary osteoarthropathy, dermatomyositis.

Diagnosis: lesions or 2° consolidation/collapse may be seen on CXR. Lateral CXRs are often useful. Normal CXRs do not exclude the diagnosis since the tumour may be central. Microscopy of sputum (particularly if induced with warm saline aerosol) often reveals malignant cells – take at least 3 early morning samples to increase diagnostic yield. Bronchoscopy, BAL and CT if available are valuable for diagnosis and staging.

Management

This depends on the performance status of the patient (see chapter 4) and the tumour type.

1. Patients with performance status 3 or 4 require palliative treatment.
2. Other patients should be referred for specialist treatment.

- Non-small-cell tumours, if localized (~20%), respond well to surgery. Many other patients gain symptomatic relief from palliative radiotherapy for haemoptysis, cough, dyspnoea, dysphagia, superior vena caval obstruction, and less often bone pain. The benefit of chemotherapy is currently unclear.
- Small-cell tumours – careful staging almost always rules out surgery since most are disseminated. Chemotherapy is worthwhile for most patients, markedly increasing median survival from ~6wks to 9–12 months in extensive disease. Radiotherapy has a useful palliative role and may also have an additive effect in a few patients.

Prevention: decrease active and passive smoking; decrease exposure to smoke and chemicals in workplace and home environments.

Lung abscess

A suppurative infection with necrosis of lung parenchyma. The box opposite lists the main causes of lung abscesses.

Clinical features: acute onset of fever, shivers, cough, and pleuritic pain often followed >1 week later by production of large quantities of blood-stained sputum as the abscess discharges into a bronchus. Finger clubbing occurs rapidly, the patient remaining febrile and ill. Empyema develops in 20–30% of cases.

If the abscess is formed as a consequence of septicaemia, the clinical features of this condition will predominate. The onset may also be chronic over months. Short courses of antibiotics will result in only temporary improvement if the diagnosis is not suspected.

Diagnosis: A cavitating opacity with fluid level on CXR. The location of the abscess may suggest its aetiology (see box). Take blood cultures. Examine sputum for anaerobes, mycobacteria, fungi.

Management: give antibiotics – benzylpenicillin 1.2–1.8g IV qds changing to the PO route as the patient's condition improves. Continue for 4–6 weeks. Metronidazole can be added if anaerobes are considered unlikely to respond to penicillin alone. Abscesses 2° to bacteraemia require broad spectrum antibiotics. The possibility of a lung CA should be explored where this is considered a possible cause.

Pulmonary embolism (PE)

Most pulmonary emboli consist of thrombi which have formed in the deep veins of the legs and pelvis, or from mural thrombi post-MI. Rarely, they may be due to material from tumours, amniotic tissue, fat, and parasites. Conditions which predispose to the formation of deep vein thrombi (DVT) therefore also predispose to the occurrence of PEs.

The clinical effects of PEs vary greatly.

- In many cases, the PEs occur without clinical manifestations as small thrombi pass deep into the pulmonary vasculature. Over time, however, repeated damage from these silent PEs results in pulmonary hypertension and cor pulmonale.
- Acute minor embolism will cause dyspnoea, pleuritic pain if the damaged tissue lies close to the pleura, and in ~30% of cases haemoptysis. Heparin therapy is required for 4–5 days; warfarin should be started at least 2 days before ending the heparin. Aim for INR 2.5–3.5 and continue for 3 months (6 months or more if there is no obvious cause/recurrent PE).
- Acute massive embolism is rare. It follows obstruction of >50% of the pulmonary vascular tree in a previously well person. The person collapses and becomes severely breathless, +/– central chest pain. In contrast to LVF, dyspnoea is not relieved by sitting the patient up and there are no crackles on auscultation. The patient requires heparin; if the circulatory state worsens, thrombolysis, or surgery should be urgently considered. Long-term warfarinization will often be needed.

Causes of lung abscesses

- **Pulmonary aspiration** – Most occur in the right lung; aspiration while supine results in abscesses in apical segment of the lower lobe or posterior segment of the upper lobe. Often caused by anaerobes, *Actinomyces* spp.
- **Bronchial obstruction** – due to lung CA or inhaled foreign body. Caused by mixed anaerobes.
- **Bacteraemia/septicaemia** – often multiple abscesses from sites such as right-sided endocarditis, infected IV cannulas, IV drug abuse. Common causes are *S.aureus*, *Streptococcus milleri*.
- **Primary infection with cavitation** – TB, or as a complication of severe pneumonia with *S.aureus*, *Klebsiella pneumoniae*, *Nocardia asteroides*.
- **Spread from subphrenic or hepatic abscess** – produces 2° abscess, often in the right lower lobe. Due to *Entamoeba histolytica*, coliforms, *Streptococcus faecalis*.
- **Immunosuppression** – such as malignancy, AIDS. Predisposes to unusual infections.

Cavitating lesions seen on CXR may be caused by:
lung abscess; TB; paragonimiasis; fungal infection; cavitating squamous cell CA; pulmonary infarct; pulmonary vasculitis.

Fungal pulmonary infections

A number of fungi infect the lung after inhalation of their spores. The infections manifest in a variety of ways, depending on the immune status of the individual and also the level of exposure. While many cases are asymptomatic, others may present as:

- **Self-resolving pneumonitis (acute pulmonary form)** – cough, chest pain, fever, joint pains, malaise, occasionally erythema nodosum or multiforme. Specific therapy may be required in addition to bed rest.
- **Localized cavitation** – this may be asymptomatic and found on CXR for other reasons. No treatment is required. However, since they can be similar to lung tumours, they may be diagnosed only at surgery.
- **Persisting or spreading cavitation** – the cavitation results in chest pain, cough, and sometimes haemoptysis (which can be heavy). Surgery and antifungal therapy may be required. These manifestations look similar to, and can be mistaken for, pulmonary TB.
- **Acute or chronic systemic dissemination** – to organs characteristic of each infection. Patients present with fever, often marked weight loss, skin lesions. If acute, there may be signs of lung disease and purpura due to thrombocytopenia. Disseminated disease is fatal in the absence of systemic antifungal therapy.

►Moderate immunosuppression associated with DM predisposes to spreading cavitation in some infections. Immunosuppression or neoplasia predispose to acute disseminated disease. The elderly, pregnant women, and children are also at increased risk of disseminated disease.

Aspergillosis

Most infections are caused by *Aspergillus fumigatus*, *A. flavus*, or *A. niger* in predisposed hosts. The fungus is ubiquitous; infection and disease occur sporadically throughout the world.

Transmission: is via inhalation of fungal spores. The spores occur in the environment in the soil and, in the case of histoplasmosis, bat faeces. Human–human transmission does not appear to be a problem. Accidental transmission may occur through the skin.

Clinical forms and management:

- ***Allergic bronchopulmonary aspergillosis (APBA)*** – persistent endobronchial infection elicits a chronic hypersensitivity response in atopic individuals. This produces asthma and with time a chronic cough (producing mucoid plugs) and dyspnoea. CXR may show shadowing in the peripheral fields. Manage with steroids.
- ***Aspergilloma*** – a fungal ball that develops in a pre-existing cavity (commonly due to TB). Intermittent cough is often the only sign but haemoptysis may develop. If this is severe, the aspergilloma should be surgically excised.
- ***Invasive disease*** – occurs in brain, kidney, liver, and skin of the severely immunocompromised. Attempt to reduce immunosuppression, if possible. Immediately give amphotericin B 1–1.5mg/kg IV daily, to a total dose of 2–2.5g. ► This is a toxic drug, check local formulary.

Diagnosis of aspergillosis

This is often difficult. Microscopic analysis of skin lesion scrapings, sputum, or pus for evidence of fungal infection. Serology, culture. In disseminated disease, yeasts may be seen in Giemsa-stained bone marrow. In acute primary lung infection, the radiographic appearances may give a clue, being typically more severe than expected from clinical examination. Isolated chronic lung lesions (mycetomas) may only be distinguished from lung tumours at surgery.

Other fungal infections

1. Histoplasmosis – a disease which occurs in two forms: i) small form histoplasmosis (caused by *Histoplasma capsulatum* var.*capsulatum*) which occurs in the Americas plus Africa and Asia and ii) large form or African histoplasmosis (*H.capsulatum* var.*duboisii*.) which occurs in central Africa.

- Acute disseminated ***small form histoplasmosis*** particularly affects bone marrow, spleen, liver, lymph nodes, and skin (papules, ulcers). A chronic form in immuncompetent patients presents with persistent painful oral ulceration and/or hypoadrenalism. Complications include laryngeal ulceration, endocarditis, and meningitis.
- ***African histoplasmosis*** is either a focal disease affecting bone, skin, and lymph nodes or a progressive disseminated disease affecting mucosal surfaces, particularly the GI tract and lungs.

2. Blastomycosis – a systemic infection caused by *Blastomyces dermatitidis* that occurs in northern America, Africa, India, and Middle East. It causes chronic pulmonary or disseminated disease (involving both lung and skin of face and forearm). Skin lesions are commonly an initial single nodule, then crusted plaques, ulcers, and abscesses. Complications include lytic bone lesions (particularly axial skeleton) and GU tract disease (particularly epididymitis).

3. Coccidioidomycosis – a disease of semi-arid regions of the Americas, caused by the fungus *Coccidioides immitis*. It is inhaled into the distal air-spaces, where it rounds up and divides to form a large spherule with thick outer wall. The clinical features are typically varied with dissemination occurring particularly to meninges, joints, and skin.

4. Paracoccidioidomycosis – a granulomatous disease caused by the fungus *Paracoccidioides brasiliensis*. It occurs sporadically in south and central America where it is the commonest systemic mycosis. An acute form of the disease occurs in children and adults <30yrs while a chronic form is more common in 30–50 year olds, particularly agricultural workers living in endemic areas. The M:F ratio is ~10.

- The ***acute form*** presents with generalized lymphadenopathy, moderate hepatosplenomegaly, fever, and weight loss over several months. The nodes are hard but may become fluctuant. Involvement of mesenteric and hepatic perihilar nodes may produce an appendicitis-like picture or obstructive jaundice. Complications include lytic bone lesions, small bowel disease, multiple mucocutaneous lesions (lymphatic/haematogenous spread). Pulmonary involvement is uncommon. Immunosuppression can lead to severe superinfection (eg TB, cryptococcus, pneumonia).
- ***Chronic disease*** normally presents with lung disease: dyspnoea, cough, (rarely haemoptysis and fever), with extensive involvement on CXR. Mucocutaneous lesions are common on skin (face, limbs); painful lesions in the mouth, pharynx, or oesophagus inhibit eating, producing marked weight loss. Other features: ulcerated tongue, hypoadrenalism. Chronic inflammation and fibrosis may result in tracheal/laryngeal fibrosis, pulmonary fibrosis, and bowel obstruction due to enlarged lymph nodes. Tumours may arise in the skin or lung lesions.

Management

►Follow local guidelines

1. Amphotericin B 0.6mg/kg IV daily for 7 days, then 0.8mg/kg every second day, up to a total of 15mg/kg.
   [alternative: fluconazole 200–400mg PO daily for 6–18 months depending on specific fungus]
2. Meningitis due to coccidioidomycosis requires fluconazole 400–600mg PO daily for 9–12 months
3. Surgery may be required for management of chronic sequelae in paracoccidioidomycosis

Paragonimiasis (lung fluke disease)

A persistent lung disease, occurring widely around the globe, which is caused by >15 different species of *Paragonimus* trematodes. Humans are infected by eating undercooked crustaceans infected with the metacercariae.

The flukes pass out of the intestine into the peritoneum, where they mature and then tunnel their way into the lungs. Here they cause inflammation, haemorrhage, and necrosis of the lung parenchyma. Turbid fluid accumulates in the pleural cavity, and abscesses, which later become encapsulated, form in the lungs. Ova are released from cysts that lie close to bronchi and are expelled out of the body either in expectorated sputum or in the faeces after being swallowed.

Flukes which miss the lungs produce extrapulmonary symptoms (due to cysts, granulomas, and abscesses) in muscles, abdominal viscera, brain, genitalia.

Clinical features: a few days to weeks after eating infected food, migration of the flukes within the peritoneal and pleural cavities causes signs of inflammatory and allergic responses – fever, rashes, urticaria, abdominal and chest pain or discomfort.

The classic feature of chronic pulmonary disease is a persistent cough with production of a thick brownish-red sputum (due to the presence of ova and flukes). While diverse lesions can be found on CXR (including infiltration; consolidation; effusion; cysts +/– calcification), physical examination of the chest often reveals little and the patients appear quite well.

Aberrant migration of the flukes may produce signs of a cerebral space occupying lesion (epilepsy; raised ICP; psychiatric syndromes; meningeal irritation) or spinal space occupying lesion, necrosis of abdominal viscera, or transitory subcutaneous swellings. Extrapulmonary disease may occur in the absence of pulmonary signs but this is uncommon.

Diagnosis: presence of ova or adult flukes in the sputum, faeces, or effusion; serology.

Management: is contentious.

1. Follow local guidelines.
2. Praziquantel 25mg/kg PO tds for 2–3 days often produces rapid symptomatic improvement, although radiological changes may take some months to improve.
3. However, treatment of cerebral infection may result in neurological deterioration, in some cases producing seizures and coma. Beware ↑ ICP due to dying parasites. Treat cautiously and consider using dexamethasone 4mg IV q6h as cover.

Prevention: improve health education to decrease consumption of under-cooked crustaceans; mass treatment of persons in endemic areas.

Figure – the WHO figure presented opposite shows an egg of *Paragonimus westermani* for comparison with other helminth species (from *Bench Aids for the Diagnosis of Intestinal Helminths*, WHO: Geneva 1994)

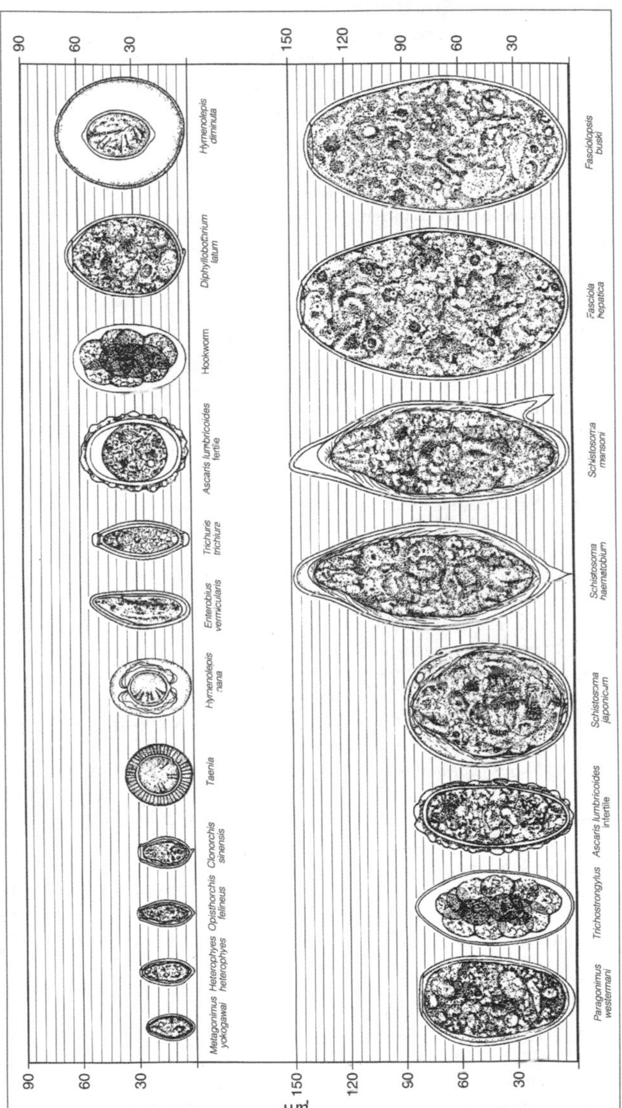
Hymenolepis diminuta
Diphyllobothrium latum
Hookworm
Ascaris lumbricoides fertile
Trichuris trichiura
Enterobius vermicularis
Hymenolepis nana
Taenia
Clonorchis sinensis
Opisthorchis felineus
Heterophyes heterophyes
Metagonimus yokogawai
Fasciolopsis buski
Fasciola hepatica
Schistosoma mansoni
Schistosoma haematobium
Schistosoma japonicum
Ascaris lumbricoides infertile
Trichostrongylus
Paragonimus westermani
90
60
30
150
120
90
60
30
μm

Diffuse parenchymal lung disease

A vast array of different diseases which can often only be distinguished by a specialist examining a lung biopsy. Also called interstitial lung disease, this condition covers over 180 different causes of inflammatory or infiltrative damage to the pulmonary interstitium, alveoli, and capillaries.

It is essential to identify a triggering factor, so take a detailed history, particularly of occupational and domestic exposure.

Presentation is often with a chronic dry cough or progressive dyspnoea. Haemoptysis, pleural disease, clubbing, and other extrapulmonary signs are common features of some diseases. Typically, there are few signs on chest examination (sometimes fine end-inspiratory crackles) but the CXR shows diffuse alveolar shadowing. Lung function studies reveal a restrictive defect in most conditions.

Specific conditions include (following the ordering of the OTM):

- *Cryptogenic fibrosing alveolitis.*
- *Bronchiolitis obliterans* – follows pneumonia (also called BOOP – bronchiolitis obliterans organising pneumonia), presenting with fever +/– malaise, or an immune response directed against the lung.
- *Systemic collagen-vascular diseases* – many have pulmonary involvement eg RA; SLE; systemic sclerosis; polymyositis and dermatomyositis; Sjogren's syndrome; ankylosing spondylitis, Behcet's disease.
- *Granulomatous vasculitides* – includes Churg-Strauss syndrome (triad of asthma, eosinophilia, systemic vasculitis) and Wegener's granulomatosis (triad of URT and LRT granulomas and necrotising glomerulonephritis).
- *Hypersensitivity vasculitides* – includes Henoch-Schonlein purpura and essential mixed cryoglobulinaemia.
- *Pulmonary haemorrhagic disorders* – show triad of haemoptysis, diffuse alveolar opacities on CXR, and anaemia. Result from chronic pulmonary venous congestion; idiopathic pulmonary haemosiderosis; pulmonary vasculitis; Goodpasture's disease.
- *Pulmonary eosinophilia* – diffuse alveolar shadowing with peripheral eosinophilia. Includes tropical eosinophilia.
- *Lymphocytic pulmonary infiltrations* – lymphomas often infiltrate into the lung at some stage (low grade non-Hodgkin's lymphoma has a bad prognosis). Lymphoid granulomatosis is a benign T-cell lymphoma; other forms are even more benign.
- *Extrinsic allergic alveolitis.*
- *Sarcoidosis* – a condition that is very rarely diagnosed in the tropics. It is a chronic granulomatous disease of unknown aetiology which affects multiple organs (particularly lungs, eyes, skin) and may result in premature death.
- *Lipoid pneumonia* – chronic low grade pneumonia due to buildup of ingested vegetable or mineral oil → to 2° fibrosis.
- *Pneumoconioses* - due to inhalation of harmful material such as coal dust, silica or asbestos, particularly by miners. Local forms will depend on local industrial activity, in particular mining.
- *Drug, toxic gas, or radiation-induced parenchymal disease.*

Management: ► stop or do not start smoking (since this will often exacerbate the condition). If causative factor has been identified, reduce exposure (preferably completely). More specific management will require a clear diagnosis – this is often difficult in even the best centres.

7. Renal disease

Urine	316
Haematuria	318
Chyluria	318
Urinary schistosomiasis	320
Micturition dysfunction	322
Genitourinary pain	322
Prostatic carcinoma	323
Kidney lumps	324
Kidney tumours	324
Glomerular disease	326
Acute nephritic syndrome	326
Interstitial nephritis	326
Nephrotic syndrome	328
Urinary tract infection (UTI)	330
Acute renal failure (ARF)	332
Clinical syndromes causing ARF	334
Chronic renal failure (CRF)	336
Renal calculi and renal colic	338
Renal manifestations of systemic diseases	340

Creatinine clearance

The kidney controls the elimination of many substances. It also produces erythropoietin, renin and 1,25-dihydroxycholecalciferol. Sodium in the urine is exchanged with potassium and hydrogen ions by a pump in the distal tubule. Glucose spills over into urine when plasma concentration is above threshold (~10mmol/l).

Renal function is measured by calculating the creatinine clearance. Because creatinine is only slightly reabsorbed in the kidney, its clearance is a measure of glomerular filtration rate (GFR) which is the volume of fluid filtered by the glomeruli per minute. It can be expressed as follows:

$$[\text{creatinine}]_{\text{plasma}} \times \text{creatinine clearance} = [\text{creatinine}]_{\text{urine}} \times \text{urine flow rate}$$

To measure creatinine clearance (usually ~100ml/min) collect 24hr urine (empty bladder before start). Take blood sample for plasma creatinine once during the 24hrs. Use the formula above. Major sources of error are incorrect units and failure to collect all urine. If urine collection is unreliable, use the formula:

$$\frac{(\text{age in years}) \times (\text{weight in kg})}{72 \times \text{serum creatinine in mg/dl}}$$

(for women multiply result by 0.85).

This formula is unreliable if there is unstable renal function, or the patient is obese or oedematous.

Urine

In any patient with suspected renal, gastroenterological, diabetic or other major system disease, a fresh midstream urine sample should be collected for microscopy, culture and analysis (with 'dipstick' tests, where available).

1. **Colour** • *Pale/colourless:* overhydration, excessive beer consumption, diabetes insipidus, post-obstructive diuresis. • *Yellow/orange:* dehydration, bilirubin, tetracycline, anthracene, sulphasalazine, riboflavine. • *Brown:* bilirubin, nitrofurantoin, phenothiazines. • *Red:* haematuria, haemoglobinuria, myoglobinuria, porphyrins, rifampicin, beetroot consumption. • *Black:* severe haemoglobinaemia, methyldopa, melanoma, ochronosis.
2. **Transparency** cloudiness is usually due to bacteria, but may be due to blood, pus or chyle, whilst crystals of phosphate (white) and urate (yellow) can also produce cloudy urine.
3. **Smell** an unpleasant smell is characteristic of a UTI. Antibiotics may also cause a smell.
4. **Specific gravity (SG)** is normally 1.002–1.025. A consistently low SG suggests chronic renal failure or diabetes insipidus. A high SG suggests dehydration or DM (large amounts of dissolved glucose).
5. **Chemical analysis**

   • ***pH:*** the urine is normally acidic. UTIs can cause an alkaline urine, which favours calcium stone formation. Suspect distal renal tubular acidosis if the early morning urine cannot be acidified.

   • ***Protein:*** Up to 150mg of protein is normally lost in the urine daily. Gross proteinuria may make the urine appear frothy. NB: Bence-Jones proteins (immunoglobulin light chains produced in myeloma) are not detected by chemical dipsticks.

   Causes of persistent proteinuria: **1.** Renal disease, especially glomerular diseases producing the nephrotic syndrome. **2.** Non-renal causes: exercise, UTI, vaginal mucus, severe hypertension, DM, pregnancy, CCF, burns, blood transfusions, operations, haemolytic-uraemic syndrome, SLE, myeloma, amyloid. **3.** Postural (orthostatic) proteinuria occurs in 2–5% of adolescents; there is mild proteinuria (<1g/24hrs) when upright, reverting to normal when reclining.

   • ***Glucose:*** glycosuria usually indicates DM, but may be caused by metabolites of salicylates, ascorbic acid, galactose or fructose, as well as tetracycline and levadopa ingestion. Renal glycosuria is an impaired ability of the kidney tubules to reabsorb glucose (eg Fanconi syndrome).

   • ***Ketones:*** are found in diabetic patients (where there may be hyperglycaemia, but without insulin glucose is unable to enter cells) and in starving patients (due to a lack of glucose). They are metabolites of fatty acids which are produced by the liver in an attempt to produce an alternative source of energy for the brain to utilize.

   • ***Nitrites:*** their presence suggests a UTI, but may be falsely positive after a protein-rich meal or vitamin C ingestion.

Radiology of the urinary tract

Plain abdominal film: look for **1.** the renal outlines (10–12cm long and situated at T12–L2) and **2.** abnormal calcification – renal stones; tumour; TB; nephrocalcinosis.

Ultrasound: is good for demonstrating urinary tract obstruction and renal size and for guiding renal biopsy. Doppler ultrasound may be used to look for renal vein thrombosis.

Intravenous urography (IVU): the nephrogram is the image of contrast diffusing through the kidney – it is usually immediate and brief. It is *intense* in obstruction and glomerulonephritis (GN); *prolonged* in obstruction, acute tubular necrosis (ATN), chronic GN, and renal vein thrombosis; *absent* in a non-functioning kidney (infarct, severe GN); and *delayed* in renal artery stenosis.

Micturating cysturethrogram the bladder is catheterized and filled with contrast. It is used to show ureteric reflux during micturition.

Haematuria

Blood in the urine is always abnormal. It can be seen with the naked eye if >0.5ml of blood is present per litre of urine. While almost half of patients presenting with haematuria in the West have neoplastic lesions, this is not the case in the developing world where a large number of other diseases can present with bleeding from the urinary tract. See opposite.

Haemoglobinuria: is caused by intravascular haemorrhage due to, for example, microangiopathic haemolytic anaemia, haemorrhagic toxins/venoms (certain snake venoms), march haemoglobinuria, paroxysmal nocturnal haemoglobinuria, chronic cold agglutinin disease.

Myoglobinuria: is caused by rhabdomyolysis (muscle destruction) following, for example, muscle infarction (trauma), excessive contraction (convulsions, hyperthermia, very heavy exercise), viral myositis (influenza, Legionnaire's disease), and drugs/toxins (alcohol, haemorrhagic snake venoms). Myoglobinuria may also be idiopathic.

Investigations: microscopy, culture, and cytology of a midstream urine sample; IVU; renal USS; cystoscopy (where available).

Chyluria

Chyluria is the presence of chyle in the urine, which is described as milky or as rice-water. It is relatively common in the tropics, especially where filariasis is prevalent. It must be differentiated from pyuria, phosphaturia, and lipuria. A rose or pink coloration to the urine may mean that there is concurrent haematuria.

- It is commonly caused by parasites blocking the lymphatics. Causative parasites include: *W. bancrofti, Eustrongylus gigas, T. echinococcus, Taenia nana, Ascaris lumbricoides, S. haematobium* and *Plasmodium* spp.
- Non-parasitic chyluria is rare and usually involves stenosis or obstruction of the thoracic duct for other reasons, eg tuberculosis, abscess, neoplastic infiltration, trauma, and pregnancy.

Clinical features: usually relapse and remit over a long period. There may be loin pain, ureteric colic, passage of clots (may cause retention), and fever.

Investigations: urine microscopy reveals chylomicrons. Look for a cause. Measure 24hr urinary creatinine and LFTs (to assess albumin loss). Perform an IVU with or without cystoscopy (2hrs after a fatty meal) or lymphography.

Treatment: >50% resolve spontaneously, therefore initial treatment should be conservative. Advise a low fat diet and a high fluid intake to minimize the risk of urinary stasis and clot formation. If the chyluria is severe and/or accompanied by episodes of dysuria, colic, retention and/or weight loss, surgical treatment should be considered.

Investigating haematuria:

Ask the following questions:

1. Is it **true** haematuria? Look for and ask about other causes of red urine (see p316).
2. What is the **timing** of the red coloration in relation to micturition? Early haematuria suggests a low (urethral/genital) bleeding site, while late haematuria (ie at the end of voiding) suggests a bladder site; red coloration throughout micturition implies a ureteric or renal lesion.
3. Is the haematuria **painful**? Carcinoma and schistosomiasis tend to be painless, whilst cystitis, obstruction (eg stones), and infection are commonly painful.

Causes of haematuria

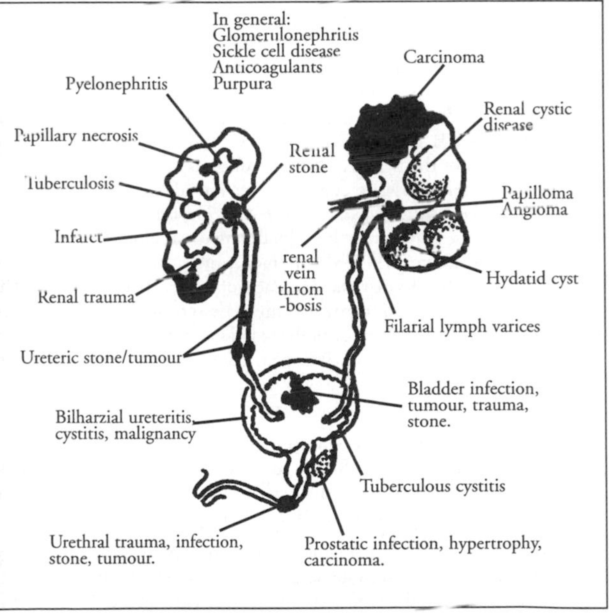

Urinary schistosomiasis

Schistosomiasis (bilharzia) affects ~200–300 million people in 76 countries and is the second most common parasitic cause of death, after malaria. It is mainly a disease of rural populations. *Schistosoma haematobium* causes urinary schistosomiasis and is found in Africa and SE Asia. *S.intercalatum* sometimes produces urinary symptoms and the known natural hybrid species between *S. haematobium* and *S. intercalatum* can produce atypical clinical pictures, with ectopic localization of worms. For distribution and life cycle, see p386.

Transmission: depends on • human (definitive host) availability and water-contacting activities, • snail (intermediate host) prevalence and species, • the *S. haematobium* strain, • the host-parasite relationship and • the host's immune response.

Prevalence increases with age up to a peak at 15yrs, after which there is a plateau until ~30yrs, at which point it begins to decline. Reasons for the decline are age-related changes in water-contact, increased immunity, the death of adult worms, and a reduced output of eggs in the urine due to extensive bladder wall fibrosis and scarring.

Pathology: eggs of the worm stimulate a T-cell-mediated immune response, resulting in eosinophil granulomata in the bladder, uterus, and genitals. They may also involve the GI tract, lungs, liver, skin, and CNS.

Clinical features of urinary schistosomiasis

Egg deposition – begins ~3 months after infection; it is often accompanied by painless haematuria which may persist for months. It may be accompanied by dysuria, pain, lassitude, and mild fever.

Established infection – haematuria often decreases in the chronic stage, unless there is 2° infection, ulceration, and/or malignancy. Fibrosis and calcification of the bladder tend to reduce its volume, producing frequency and dribbling. Other complications include perineal fistulae and 2° bacterial infection (*Salmonella* spp, *E. coli, Klebsiella* spp, *Pseudomonas* spp). In severe cases, there may be urinary retention, stasis, and eventually renal failure or stone formation. In men, involvement of the seminal vesicles correlates well with the presence of obstructive uropathy. The prostate, epididymis, and penis are much less commonly affected. In women, ulcerating, polypoid, or nodular lesions may be seen in the vulva, vagina, and cervix. The ovaries, Fallopian tubes, and uterus are much less commonly affected. There are, however, suggestions that *S. haematobium* infection is associated with ectopic pregnancies and infertility.

Diagnosis: is by direct visualization of parasite eggs in the urine. Schistosome antigens may also be detected immunologically. Radiologically, one should look for bladder calcification on AXR. IVU may also be useful. Exclude other causes of haematuria.

Treatment: see p389. Praziquantel is the only drug which is effective against all species of schistosomes and is the drug of choice. It is also effective against other snail-borne trematode infections and certain cestode infections. Whichever drug is used, the patient should be followed up at 2 and 6 months for urinalysis and clinical assessment of improvement.

S. haematobium and bladder cancer

The close association between bladder cancer and *S. haematobium* infection has been known for many years. While once thought to be caused directly by the parasites, this now seems unlikely, particularly since there is no associated increase in bowel cancer in GI schistosomiasis. Instead it is believed that environmental or locally-produced chemicals excreted in the urine cause neoplastic change in the mucosa. Tumour growth is then accelerated by the schistosome egg-induced inflammation and irritation. There is a lag period of at least 20yrs between infection and the development of cancer. 75% of patients in Egypt are <50yrs old; in contrast most patients are >65yrs in non-schistosome areas. It is commoner in men (although this may reflect exposure to schistosomes during work); smokers and those working with aromatic amines (eg in the rubber industry).

Clinical features: haematuria, cystitis and obstruction. Spread is local to pelvic structures, via the lymphatics to the iliac and para-aortic nodes, and via the blood to liver and lungs.

Investigation: urinalysis, FBC. AXR may show a calcified bladder wall. IVU, cystoscopy and biopsy. Staging is as follows:

- T1 – tumour in mucosa or submucosa. Not felt at EUA.
- T2 – superficial muscle involved. Rubbery thickening at EUA.
- T3 – deep muscle involved. Mobile mass at EUA.
- T4 – invasion beyond bladder. Fixed mass at EUA.

Management: T1 & T2: cystoscopic diathermy. Consider intra-vesicular chemotherapy or BCG administration. T3: Radical surgery and radiotherapy. T4: Palliation (long-term catheterization).

Micturition dysfunction

• ***Frequency:*** implies a decreased bladder capacity (chronic cystic TB, schistosomiasis, prolonged catheterization) or polyuria (DM, diabetes insipidus, polydipsia, hypercalcaemia, chronic renal failure, congestive cardiac failure). When present with dysuria it suggests lower tract disease.
• ***Urgency:*** suggests irritation of the bladder neck.
• ***Urge incontinence:*** is seen in severe inflammatory states, with a stone impinging at the bladder neck, or a neurogenic bladder. • ***True incontinence,*** for example due to epispadias, vesicovaginal fistula, neurogenic bladder or sphincter damage, must be differentiated from ***stress incontinence*** which only occurs upon coughing, straining or lying down and is due to sphincteric weakness. • ***Overflow incontinence*** is leakage of urine from a full, flaccid, chronically obstructed bladder.
• ***Nocturnal enuresis*** is normal below 2 years of age, but may continue for many years due to functional or psychosomatic causes. When persisting beyond 7 years of age, investigate to exclude organic disease.
• ***Hesitancy, poor flow and terminal dribbling*** are features of prostatic disease and may progress to retention. In a young patient, it may signify a urethral/meatal stricture, or urethral valves in an infant. A normal flow which is periodically interrupted suggests a stone in the bladder. ***Oliguria*** (urine <400ml/24 hrs) or ***anuria*** should prompt urgent investigation for bilateral obstruction, acute renal failure or severe dehydration.
• ***Pneumaturia*** is pathognomic of a urinary-intestinal fistula, usually in the bladder or urethra. Certain gas-forming bacteria can also, rarely, cause mild and transient pneumaturia.

Genitourinary pain

• *Renal pain* is felt maximally in the renal angle (except for ectopic kidneys). It is constant and dull, radiating anteriorly to the hypochondrium. • *Ureteric pain* is usually acute, very intense and colicky in nature. Upper ureteric pain often radiates around the loin and down to the testicles/ vulva; it is sometimes only felt in the genitalia. Mid-ureteric pain may localize to the iliac fossa, and on the right, mimic appendicitis. Lower ureteric obstruction may cause bladder dysfunction due to trigone irritation. • *Bladder pain* is usually only evident in acute distension states (retention, obstruction) and specific infections such as schistosomal and TB cystitis. Chronic bladder distension may, however, be pain-free even when there is overflow incontinence. • *Dysuria* is the commonest symptom with inflammatory and other conditions involving the bladder, prostate, or urethra. Often described as a burning sensation, the pain is localized to the distal urethra and worse during the act of voiding. • *Stranguary* is spasms of pain, continuing after voiding has finished and is due to severe inflammation. • *Prostatic pain* and pain from the posterior urethra may manifest as an ache in the perineum, or a fullness in the rectum, almost always accompanied by dysuria. • *Testicular pain* and pain from the epididymis are usually localized, but if severe may radiate up the line of the spermatic cord to the abdomen.

Acute retention

Complete failure of micturition is nearly always due to obstruction due to enlarged prostate, stones, blood clot, or urethral stricture. Rare causes include anticholinergic drugs, holding on, constipation, alcohol, pregnancy, pelvic tumour/fracture, perineal trauma, and infection. Palpate for a stricture or stone and do a PR examination to assess the size of the prostate and exclude constipation.

Treatment and investigations: give analgesia and catheterize (should give instant relief). Test the urine for blood/pus, take blood for FBC, Hb, U&E and Cr, and do an AXR to look for renal calcui. Assess perineal sensation (to exclude cauda equina compression).

Chronic retention

This is more insidious. The bladder capacity may be stretched to 1.5l or more. Presentation is with overflow incontinence, acute on chronic retention, a low abdominal mass, UTI, or renal failure. Prostatic enlargement is the common cause. Others include pelvic malignancy and CNS disease. Only catheterize the patient if there is pain, UTI, or renal impairment (eg urea >12mmol/l). Treat the cause.

Suprapubic catheterization: is sometimes necessary in retention when long-term indwelling catheters are needed. Define the distended bladder, then cleanse the skin. Infiltrate local anaesthetic above the symphysis pubis and make a small superficial incision in the skin. Insert the trocar down vertically until urine is draining, then advance the catheter down over the trocar and secure it. Suprapubic catheterization is contraindicated if there is haematuria, a midline abdominal scar, or a bladder malignancy.

Prostatic carcinoma

Evidence suggests that the incidence of prostatic CA is increasing in developing countries, as they westernize and industrialize.

Clinical features: hesitancy, frequency, dribbling. Bone pain may signify metastasis. Spread is to bone (sclerotic or lytic lesions), bladder, and rectum.

Investigation and management: FBC, ESR, U&E, Cr, Ca^{2+}. Acid phosphatase is a marker of disease activity. Bladder USS, IVU, bone X-rays. Provide analgesia. If there is obstruction, the treatment of choice is a transurethral resection of the prostate (TURP). The prognosis is very variable; 10% die within 6 months, 10% live >10 years.

Kidney lumps

Enlarged kidneys tend to bulge forwards, whilst perinephric abscesses or collections tend to bulge posteriorly. A tender loin mass may suggest an obstructed kidney, but, if there is evidence of psoas muscle spasm, a perinephric abscess is more likely. With acute obstruction, or development of a pyonephrosis, guarding is common and the mass difficult to define. With chronic obstructed states and tumours, the mass is usually better defined and less tender. Bilateral, irregular kidneys suggest polycystic renal disease. A horseshoe kidney may present as a central abdominal mass, whilst ectopic kidneys may be felt lower in the loins, in the iliac fossae, or even suprapubically.

Polycystic kidney disease

In adults, this is an autosomal dominant condition (on chromosome 16). Cysts develop in the kidney, causing a gradual decline in renal function.

Clinical features: haematuria, UTI, abdominal mass (~30% have cysts in the liver or pancreas), lumbar and abdominal pain, hypertension. Aneurysms of intracerebral arteries and subarachnoid haemorrhages are associated.
Diagnosis: uraemia and polycythaemia. IVU or USS show large cystic kidneys with spidery calyces.
Management: is supportive. Treat infection and ↓ the BP. CRF is the usual cause of death unless there is access to dialysis or transplantation. Check family members.

Kidney tumours

There are three main types of 1° renal tumours:

- ***Nephroblastoma (Wilm's tumour):*** is an undifferentiated mesodermal tumour of children which may be sporadic or familial (in the latter case it may be associated with aniridia, GU malformations and mental retardation). 95% are unilateral.
- ***Renal carcinoma (hypernephroma):*** rare in the tropics, these tumours are either clear cell or adenocarcinomas. Spread is direct to nearby tissues and via the blood to bone, liver, and lung.
- ***Urothelial tumours:*** may arise in the renal pelvis, ureters, urethra or bladder and may be of different histological types. In the West, transitional cell carcinoma account for 90% of urothelial malignancies, whilst in Africa squamous carcinoma predominates due to the high incidence of urinary schistosomiasis (see above), chronic urethral strictures, obstruction, and recurrent infection.

Clinical features: include fever, flank pain, abdominal mass, haematuria. IVU shows renal pelvis distortion and hydronephrosis. There may be polycythaemia due to increased erythropoietin secretion.

Investigation and management: avoid renal biopsy. Perform urinalysis, CXR, renal USS, IVU, angiogram. Nephrectomy and immunotherapy are the only treatments.

Renal masses:

Unilaterally palpable	*Bilaterally palpable*
Renal cell carcinoma	Nephrotic syndrome
Hydro/pyonephrosis	Polycystic kidneys
Acute pyelonephritis	Bilateral renal cell carcinoma
Acute renal vein thrombosis	Early diabetic nephropathy
Polycystic kidneys (asymmetrical enlargement)	Bilateral hydro/pyonephrosis
Hydatid disease	Amyloid, lymphoma, acromegaly

Genitourinary hydatid disease

After passage through the portal system, right heart, and pulmonary circulation, eggs of the tapeworms *Echinoccocus granulosus* and *E. multilocularis* may come to rest in the genitourinary system. Cysts may form in the kidney, bladder, prostate, seminal vesicles and epididymis, in descending frequency. For details, see p392.

Glomerular disease

Glomerulonephritis (GN) is common in the tropics, with the incidence of the nephrotic syndrome being up to 100 times higher in some countries than it is in the West. In many cases, infection is the underlying cause and the GN resolves after treating the infection. However, the damage associated with chronic parasitic infections such as malaria may be permanent.

Infection associated glomerulonephritis

- ***Membranous nephropathy***
  hepatitis B, *Schistosoma mansoni*, leprosy, *Loa loa*, syphilis.
- ***Mesangiocapillary GN***
  S. mansoni, leprosy, TB, *Loa loa*, onchocerciasis, candidiasis.
- ***Focal segmental GN***
  HIV, *S. mansoni*.
- ***Proliferative GN***
  Streptococcus spp, *Staphylococcus* spp, leprosy, filariasis, onchocerciasis, syphilis, amyloid, leprosy, *S. mansoni*.

Presentation of glomerulonephritis: persistent microscopic haematuria and proteinuria, nephrotic or acute nephritic syndromes, ARF.

Acute nephritic syndrome

Presentation: classically follows 1–3 weeks after a throat, ear or skin infection with Lancefield group A β-haemolytic streptococcus. There is haematuria (+/– red cell casts) and an acute fall in GFR leading to fluid retention, oliguria, hypertension and variable uraemia. Proteinuria is usually present. Complications include hypertensive encephalopathy, pulmonary oedema, and acute renal failure.

Management: strict bed rest if there is severe hypertension or pulmonary oedema. Restrict dietary salt and fluid intake if oliguric. Give diuretics (eg frusemide) IV or PO, appropriate antihypertensive treatment (β blockers may precipitate pulmonary oedema) and a course of penicillin to eradicate any residual infection. Acute renal failure may require specialist treatment. The prognosis is usually good, though some proteinuria and urinary sediments may persist. Rapidly progressive glomerulonephritis and CRF are rare complications.

Interstitial nephritis

This is an important cause of acute and chronic renal failure. It consists of inflammatory cells infiltrating the renal interstitium and tubules due to drug hypersensitivity, analgesic nephropathy, reflux nephropathy, DM, sickle cell disease, or Alport's syndrome. However, the cause is unknown in many cases. Acute disease is often due to drugs (eg antibiotics, diuretics, NSAIDs) or infection, usually with staphylococci, streptococci, brucella, or leptospira (in which ARF develops in up to 50% of cases). Presentation is with renal failure, fever, arthralgia, and/or eosinophils in urine or blood. The diagnosis requires renal histology from a biopsy. Treat as for ARF, plus corticosteroids. The prognosis is usually good.

Patterns of glomerular disease

1. **Minimal change GN:** may account for up to 70% of nephrotic syndrome in India. It is more common in children in any country and is also associated with Hodgkin's disease.
2. **Membranoproliferative GN** (mesangiocapillary GN): 50% present with nephrotic syndrome, usually post-infection. Most have low C3.
3. **Membranous GN:** is common in children in Zimbabwe and adults in Sudan and Pakistan. It accounts for 50% of nephrotic syndrome in adults and is frequently a complication of hepatitis B infection. 50% progress to CRF in 10 years.
4. **Proliferative GN:** is particularly common in Thailand and SE Asia, usually following 10–14 days after streptococcal infection. ↓C3 is common. The prognosis is good.
5. **Focal segmental GN:** is a non-specific response to a variety of insults. It is often associated with HIV and/or schistosomal infection; other associations include SLE, PAN, SBE, Wegener's.
6. **IgA nephropathy (Berger's disease):** is common in SE Asia; 75% of patients in Singapore with >1g proteinuria/24hrs have IgA nephropathy. 10% progress to CRF.
7. **Crescentic GN** (rapidly progressive GN): presents with haematuria, hypertension, and oliguria. It rapidly progresses to renal failure and is associated with anti-basement membrane antibodies, Wegener's granulomatosis, microscopic polyarteritis, Henoch-Schonlein purpura, and rarely streptococcal infection.
8. **Focal segmental glomerulosclerosis:** is particularly common in Ghana and Senegal, usually presenting with proteinuria and nephrotic syndrome. >50% progress to CRF.
9. **SLE nephritis:** lupus nephritis is common in Malaysia, Singapore, and other parts of SE Asia, usually affecting people of Chinese origin. It also affects American Blacks and Jamaicans.

Nephrotic syndrome

The nephrotic syndrome occurs when there is glomerular basement membrane damage sufficient to allow proteins to pass into the kidney tubules. The resulting proteinuria (>3.6g/24hrs) causes hypoalbuminaemia and oedema, often with hypercholesterolaemia.

Clinical features: facial and peripheral oedema, ascites. The urine may be frothy. ***Complications*** include:

- Venous thrombosis and pulmonary embolism (due to urinary loss of anti-thrombin III, fluid, clotting factors).
- Infection (especially pneumococcal peritonitis – consider vaccination if the nephrotic state persists).
- Hypercholesterolaemia – consider treating this in prolonged cases.
- Hypovolaemia and renal failure.
- Loss of specific binding proteins, presenting as iron-resistant hypochromic anaemia.

Causes: certain types of glomerulonephritis (see above), DM, amyloid, neoplasia (especially lymphoma and carcinoma), SBE, PAN, SLE, sickle-cell, malaria, drugs (eg. penicillamine, gold).

Investigations for nephrotic syndrome and GN

Urine microscopy:	RBC casts and dysmorphic RBCs.
Urine:	24hr protein and creatinine clearance.
Serum:	U&E, FBC, ESR, CRP, albumin, autoantibody screen, complement (C3 & C4), ASO titre, HBsAg.
Culture:	blood, throat, ears (if otitis media), skin (if cellulitis).
Radiology:	CXR, renal USS, IVU.
Renal biopsy:	this is not indicated in a child unless the illness is complicated by high BP or haematuria, or treatment failure.

Treatment

1. Bed rest.
2. High protein diet (though of no proven benefit).
3. Restrict salt and fluid intake.
4. Diuresis – give frusemide 40–80mg PO with amiloride as K^+-sparing agent (or spironolactone 100mg/24hr); diuretics relieve oedema but do not treat the underlying disorder. Beware IV diuretics as patients are often intravascularly depleted and they may precipitate pre-renal failure. In general, only give IV diuretics with IV plasma protein, at least until diuresis is established.
5. Monitor U&Es and weight daily (aim to lose 1kg/day).
6. Consider anticoagulation.

Renal vein thrombosis: occurs in 15–20% of those with nephrosis, 30% of patients with membranous GN, and in children with severe, acute dehydration. There may be no symptoms, or mild abdominal or back pain. Others develop severe pain and loin tenderness. Suspect it if there is sudden loss of renal function with haematuria.
Management: anticoagulate; consider streptokinase if the onset is acute. Beware development of pulmonary emboli.

Algorithm for investigating proteinuria

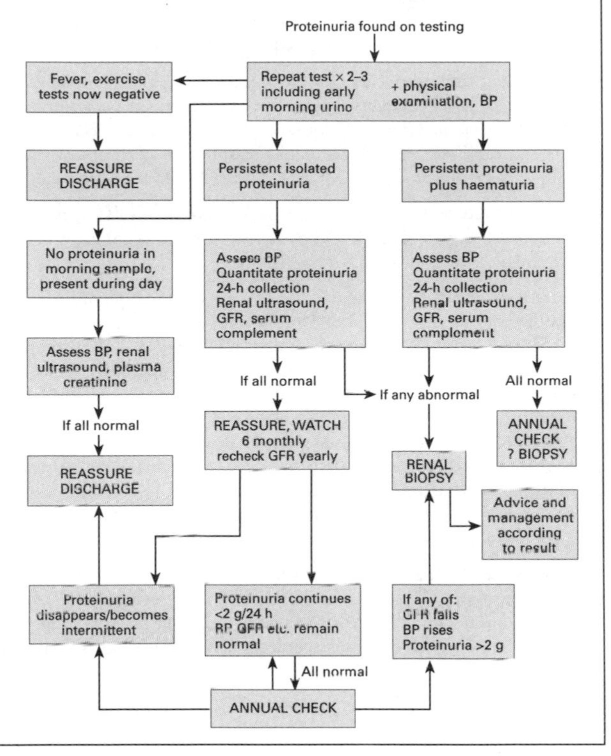

Urinary tract infection (UTI)

The incidence of uncomplicated UTI varies little around the world, though in the tropics disease may progress more rapidly and complications are more common, especially in the malnourished. Urine is a good bacterial culture medium and infection is commonly due to gut bacteria.

Clinical features: frequency, dysuria, haematuria, incontinence, retention, urgency, RIF/loin/suprapubic pain, fever, D&V (in children). Ask about previous infections. Examine for: large prostate, renal mass, meatal ulcers, vaginal discharge, loin tenderness, hypertension, signs of CRF.

Diagnosis: if the urine *looks* clear, it probably *is* clear. Two clean-catch, mid-stream urine specimens will give ~95% sensitivity for bacteriuria. The sterile bag and clean-catch techniques are variably accurate, but useful in infants and children. Suprapubic bladder aspiration is the most reliable technique. Send specimens for MCS. Consider U&E, Cr, blood cultures.

Management: only treat if the patient is symptomatic. Treatment may be: **1.** curative **2.** prophylactic and **3.** suppressive. Look for signs of renal failure and alter drug doses accordingly.

1. **Curative treatment:** advise the patient to drink plenty of water, double-void (going again after 5 mins) and urinate after intercourse.
   - ***Single-dose treatment:*** amoxycillin 3g PO (NB widespread resistance), or trimethoprim 300mg PO, or co-trimoxazole 1.92g PO.
   - ***Three-day treatment:*** trimethoprim 200mg PO bd for 3 days, or nitrofurantoin 50–100mg PO qds for 3 days, or nalidixic acid 1g PO tds for 3 days. Quinolones and cephalosporins are alternatives.
   - ***For complicated cases:*** treat for 5 days (IV if necessary). Monitor fluid balance and provide analgesia. Take blood cultures before starting antibiotics. If there is evidence of pyelonephritis, treatment should continue for 2 weeks. Any of the above drugs are of use.

2. **Prophylactic treatment:** may be beneficial to women suffering from recurrent UTIs. Advise as above and give nitrofurantoin 50mg, or trimethoprim 100mg, or co-trimoxazole 0.24g at night. (Some trials suggest equally good effects giving doses on alternate nights, 3 nights a week, or even weekly.)

3. **Suppressive treatment:** some patients have abnormalities which make it impossible to sterilize the urinary tract (eg calculi, neurogenic bladder, ileal conduit) and have incessant UTIs. Such patients are candidates for long-term suppressive treatment with individually-tailored regimes. Once-weekly nitrofurantoin is a good starting point.

Reasons for referral for IVU or cystoscopy: recurrent UTI (or first UTI in men), overt haematuria, pyelonephritis, persistent haematuria, unusual organism, persisting fever, child <2yrs old, pyuria.

Follow-up: see all patients 10–14 days after treatment has stopped, possibly repeating the MSU. In practice, most recurrences are actually re-infections with different bacterial species.

Special treatment problems

- **Bacterial prostatitis:** presents with symptoms of general infection, often with pain in the perineum. The prostate is very tender, boggy and swollen. The condition usually responds well to standard regimes, but may need 4–12 weeks of treatment to eradicate bacteria from the prostatic tissue. Give erythromycin 500mg qds or trimethoprim 200mg bd or tetracycline 250–500mg qds.
- **Asymptomatic bacteriuria in pregnancy:** treat first infection with a standard single or 3-day regime, as above. Any recurrence will need eradication, followed by a prophylaxis with nitrofurantoin until delivery.
- **Elderly women:** atrophic vaginitis is a risk factor, as ↓ acid in vaginal secretions promotes bacterial overgrowth. Symptoms may be atypical. Treat symptomatic infections as above, adding oestrogen creams to promote lactic acid production by *Lactobacillus* spp.
- **The urethral syndrome:** occurs in women only. Urgency, frequency and dysuria occur in the absence of demonstrable bacteriuria – often called abacterial cystitis. It is induced by cold, intercourse, stress, or nylon underwear, but its cause is unknown.
- **Urinary catheters:** where possible, avoid long term catheterization. Bacteria reside in the catheter tubing and this is not penetrated by antimicrobials. Avoid frequent changing, unless the catheter becomes blocked.
- **Sterile pyuria:** causes: inadequately treated UTI, TB or other atypical organisms, calculi, bladder tumour, prostatitis, papillary necrosis (the elderly, NSAID over-use), polycystic kidneys, appendicitis.

Acute renal failure (ARF)

Acute renal failure may complicate a wide variety of diseases in the tropics. It often presents as uraemia, with ↑ serum Cr and K^+, fluid and electrolyte imbalances, oliguria (<15ml urine/hr) or anuria, vomiting, confusion, bruising, and GI bleeding. It carries a high mortality.

Causes: are pre-renal, renal, and post-renal; see opposite.

Management: The three main problems are

- fluid balance
- electrolytes
- pH

► Refractory pulmonary oedema, pericarditis, and cardiac tamponade need urgent treatment and may require dialysis.

► Always check whether any drugs used are safe for use in ARF.

1. **Optimize fluid balance:** try to avoid precipitating/worsening acute tubular necrosis by maintaining renal perfusion. Monitor the JVP, urine output (via catheter) and, where possible, central venous pressure. If fluid depleted, 24hr fluid maintenance = [estimated deficit + 24hr urine output + diarrhoeal/vomiting losses + 500ml for insensible losses (more if febrile)]. If oligouric, give frusemide 250mg slowly over 1 hour +/– renal dose dopamine; 2–5μg/kg/min. If in pulmonary oedema, think of removing one unit of blood as a temporary measure before dialysis.

2. **Electrolyte imbalance:** serum K^+ can rise rapidly in patients who are hypercatabolic and/or acidotic. Look for typical ECG changes. Treat hyperkalaemia with 10ml of 10% calcium gluconate IV slowly, for cardioprotection, then 15 units of soluble insulin with 50ml glucose 50% in dextrose by IV infusion thereafter according to blood glucose measurements. Cation exchange resins (polystyrene sulphate) 15g/6hr PO, or as enema, increase faecal K^+ excretion.

► If K^+ level is >6.0mmol/l dialysis is urgently required.

3. **Acidosis:** most patients with ARF have a metabolic acidosis and this can be severe if there is hypercatabolism. Give bicarbonate according to level of acidaemia – start with 100ml of a 4.2% solution IV at pH 7.0.

4. **Further management**

- Treat sepsis with antibiotics after cultures have been collected. There is no need to treat prophylactically, but watch IV access sites and temperature chart for signs of infection.
- Exclude an obstructive cause – see below.
- Give a high protein diet (2000–4000kJ/day). Consider NGT or parenteral feeding if the patient is too ill to eat.
- If there is GI bleeding, give a H_2 blocker such as ranitidine 150mg bd PO.

ARF in pregnancy: obstetric problems account for 10–25% of all cases of ARF in the Tropics. Common causes are post-abortion septicaemia, pre-eclampsia and eclampsia, puerperal sepsis, haemorrhage, and *abruptio placentae.*

Causes of renal failure

Pre-renal

Renal hypoperfusion	Hypovolaemia (any cause)
Septicaemia	Obstetric accidents
Massive intravascular necrosis	Rhabdomyolosis
Renal artery emboli	Renal artery stenosis (ACE inhibitors)
Hepato-renal syndrome	

Renal

Acute tubular necrosis (ATN)	Acute interstitial nephritis
Acute cortical necrosis	Diffuse glomerulonephritis
Acute pyelonephritis	Nephrotoxins & drugs
Haemolytic-uraemic syndrome	Vasculitis
Renal vein thrombosis	Myeloma kidney

Post-renal

Obstructive uropathy	Renal tubule blockage
Myeloma	Uric acid
Bilateral urinary tract blockage	Calculi
Schistosoma haematobium	Urethral stricture
Prostatic hypertrophy	Pelvic malignancy
Posterior urethral valves	

Dialysis

Dialysis may be the only remedy for serious cases of ARF. Various alternatives exist.

- ***Intermittent peritoneal dialysis*** is effective in patients with milder ARF who are not hypercatabolic. It involves periodically introducing dialysate into the peritoneal cavity via a catheter for 10–30 mins, then withdrawing it.
- ***Continuous ambulatory peritoneal dialysis*** requires the permanent insertion of a catheter into the peritoneal cavity. Up to 5 litres of dialysate is introduced and exchanged, up to 5 times a day.

In both methods, there is an increased risk of peritonitis, catheter blockage, pleural effusion and leakage.

Clinical syndromes causing ARF

Acute tubular necrosis (ATN): due to tubular cell damage, results from any cause of renal ischaemia. ATN has also been reported with some nephrotoxic drugs (eg aminoglycosides) and certain herbal remedies. It is usually recoverable, but may need up to 6 weeks dialysis. If prolonged, it can lead to permanent cortical necrosis. There is typically oliguria with urinary sodium >40mmol/l, urine: plasma urea >8, and urine: plasma creatinine >40. It is vital to monitor and correct any fluid imbalance.

Renal parenchymal disease: acute glomerulonephritis and interstitial nephritis can precipitate ARF. It may follow leptospirosis, prolonged use of NSAIDs, reflux nephropathy, DM, sickle cell disease and Alport's syndrome.

Rhabdomyolosis (massive myoglobinuria): may occur following: crush injuries, heat stroke, alcohol, heroin, hypokalaemia, convulsions, electric shock, eclampsia, status asthmaticus, burns, snake bite, insect stings, and a variety of infections. Muscular pain and swelling may not be prominent, but the diagnosis should be suspected if there is dark brown urine, positive for blood, but without red cells on microscopy. Large-volume alkaline diuresis is said to promote myoglobin excretion, but poses problems for fluid and electrolyte control.

Hepato-renal syndrome: is the association of severe, progressive liver disease with ARF and no other cause. The disease mechanism is poorly understood, but is thought to involve renal hypoperfusion.

Nephrotoxins and drugs: exogenous agents which cause an adverse alteration in renal structure or function *not* mediated by hypoperfusion or obstruction may result in any of the clinical syndromes of renal disease. They include: animal toxins (certain snake venoms, insect, spider and scorpion stings, bile from the grass carp – a traditional remedy for visual acuity in Taiwan), plant toxins (eg hemlock), metal poisoning, paraquat, copper sulphate, hydrocarbons, organic solvents and other chemical poisoning (including radiographic contrast media). Drug-induced renal disease is not uncommon in countries where drug sales are unrestricted by prescription. Always check drug information when prescribing for patients with renal disease.

Haemolytic-uraemic syndrome (HUS): is a syndrome of thrombocytopaenia, microangiopathic haemolytic anaemia, and ARF. In children it is frequently associated with verotoxin-producing strains of *E. coli* and *Shigella*, which cause dysentery. Clinical features are usually a diarrhoeal illness followed by worsening renal function and GI bleeding, +/– hypertension, convulsions, and confusion. Treatment is as for ARF, plus plasma or prostacyclin infusion. Treat any gastroenterological cause.

Pre-eclampsia is the association of hypertension, proteinuria and oedema in pregnancy. With severe disease there is headache, epigastric pain, visual disturbances and hyperreflexia. Investigation may reveal the *HELLP* syndrome: *h*aemolysis, *e*levated *l*iver enzymes and *l*ow *p*latelet counts. ***Treat*** with bed rest, antihypertensives, and induction of labour if severe.

Effects of uraemia on the body

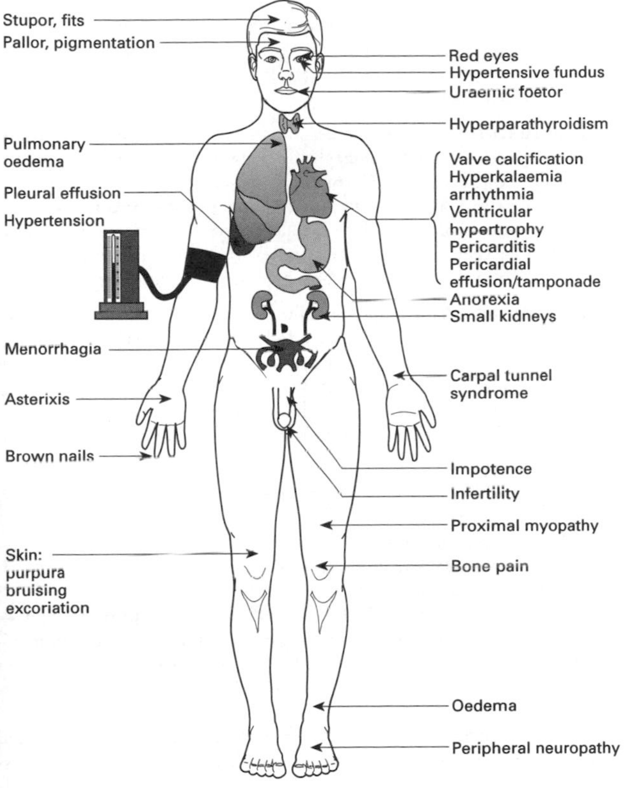

Chronic renal failure (CRF)

Chronic renal failure results from the progressive and irreversible loss of renal function and is characterized by an inability to concentrate urine. It is commonly a result of malarial, schistosomal or lepromatous nephropathy in the tropics where it tends to affect young adults.

► Ask yourself why the patient has presented *now*; is there any factor which may be reversed (infection, dehydration, fasting, drugs)?

Causes: hypertensive renal disease, glomerulonephritis (malaria), pyelonephritis, diabetic nephropathy, obstructive uropathy, renal calculi, tuberculosis, polycystic kidneys. Others include amyloid, myeloma, SLE, PAN, gout, hypercalcaemia.

Clinical features: a small number of patients progress into CRF from an acute episode of glomerulonephritis. However, the majority present insidiously with a variety of symptoms: weakness, refractory anaemia, anorexia, vomiting, hiccups, skin pigmentation, pruritis, nocturia, impotence, dyspnoea, confusion. Signs include pallor, a lemon tinge to skin, (with uraemia there is uraemic frost on skin), pulmonary or peripheral oedema, pericarditis, pleural effusions, hypertension, and retinopathy.

Investigations: ***Urine:*** dipstick, 24hr collection if there is proteinuria. Assess electrolytes, protein, osmolality and Cr clearance. MCS.
Blood: serum Cr and urea do not rise above normal until the GFR falls below 50ml/min (~50% of renal function), U&E, glucose, $\downarrow Ca^{2+}$, $\uparrow PO_4^{3}$, ↑urate, protein, FBC, ESR, protein electrophoresis.
Radiology: AXR or USS (renal size). Consider IVU, renal biopsy.

Management

1. Conservative management is effective in patients with a GFR of 10ml/min or greater.
2. Treat any reversible cause or contributing factors – eg relieve obstruction, avoid nephrotoxic drugs, treat infections.
3. Treat hypercalcaemia and hyperuricaemia.
4. Give advice about diet – high fluid and electrolyte intake (though ↓ Na^+ if hypertensive), whilst restricting protein (the chief source of toxic metabolites) to a degree determined by the severity of renal failure.
5. Monitor and treat hypertension and hyperlipidaemia.
6. Give a trial of iron supplements for anaemia.
7. Fluid and electrolyte balance should be monitored carefully – weigh the patient often and check plasma electrolyte levels. In the terminal stages of CRF, water excretion diminishes, and oedema and dilutional hyponatraemia may develop – fluid restriction will be necessary.

Dialysis and transplantation

Once the GFR falls to 10ml/min or less, life can only be maintained with renal replacement therapy – either dialysis or transplantation. Relatively few tropical countries have established centres for long-term dialysis due to the high costs involved, as well as technical and cultural difficulties. Transplantation is expensive and likely not to be an option for the vast majority of patients.

Bone disease in CRF (renal osteodystrophy)

The commonest features of renal osteodystrophy are 2° hyperparathyroidism, osteomalacia, and osteoporosis, leading to ↓ bone strength and mechanical dysfunction.

Hyperparathyroidism: as serum phosphate ↑ (and thus calcium ↓) in CRF, PTH release is stimulated, which promotes bone resorption and Ca^{2+} release.

Renal osteomalacia: in CRF, vitamin D is not converted to 1,25-dihydroxycholecalciferol. This further promotes release of Ca^{2+} from the bones. The bone disease is therefore vitamin D resistant.

Other factors which exacerbate bone disease include acidosis, PTH metabolism, and concentrations of various trace elements.

Clinical features: bone pain and tenderness (↑ with exercise), fractures, retardation of growth, joint disease, soft tissue calcification, and proximal muscle weakness.

Diagnosis: *radiology:* may show subperiosteal erosion (look at the proximal end of the middle phalanges of the hand), indolent fractures (particularly ribs, pelvis, spine and femoral neck), soft tissue calcification (eg the eye – band keratopathy – skin, aorta), generalized radiolucency, Looser's zones, osteosclerosis, periosteal new bone and formation. *Blood:* Ca^{2+} is initially low but rises as CRF progresses, there is increased PO_4^{3-}, alkaline phosphatase, and PTH.

Management: treat the CRF. Give dietary supplements of vitamins and minerals, particularly vitamins D, B_6 and C, but *not* vitamin A (since this increases bone resorption and may augment PTH action).

Renal calculi and renal colic

► Beware infection above the stone.

► Obstruction may be due to tumour, chronic infection (TB, schistosomiasis), acute gonococcal infection, or fungal infection.

Renal stones are common in the Middle East, Gulf states, Egypt and Israel. Bladder stones are common in Rwanda, Sudan, Niger, Chad, the Middle East, India and SE Asia.

Aetiological factors include: high temperature and decreased fluid intake (increases urinary Ca^{2+} concentration due to ↓ urinary volume and sunlight increasing vitamin D production by the skin); a high dietary animal protein intake (↑ Ca^{2+}, oxalate, and urate in the urine); consumption of beer (high in Ca^{2+}, oxalate, and guanosine); congenital renal abnormalities; GU schistosomiasis; and GU TB.

Stone formation correlates with social class and occupation, but this may reflect dietary differences. Disorders known to promote urolithiasis include gout, nephrocalcinosis, hyperparathyroidism, Cushing's syndrome, sarcoidosis, Wilson's disease, and renal tubular acidosis.

Clinical features: stones in the kidney cause loin pain, whilst stones in the ureter cause renal colic which often radiates from loin to groin (however this may only be felt at the tip of the penis). Bladder stones cause stranguary – the distressing desire to pass something which will not pass. Attacks of pain may occur upon sudden movement or exercise. Urethral stones may cause an interruption of the urine flow and in severe cases lead to anuria.

Classically, renal colic is relieved by curling up, but patients cannot lie still. There is abdominal or loin tenderness with microscopic or macroscopic haematuria. Symptoms do not always correlate with stone size.

Diagnosis: has the patient got a UTI? Test urine for blood; do culture and microscopy for infection, and pH (urate stones cause the urine pH to be <5.5). Do a plain AXR, looking along the line of the ureters. Consider performing an IVU, cystogram or USS. Blood tests: U&E, uric acid, Ca^{2+}, bicarbonate.

Management:

1. Increase fluid intake. Treat any UTI.
2. Provide adequate pain relief – NSAIDs (beware in patients with poor renal function) or opiate analgesia for severe pain.
3. Modify the diet to avoid oxalate-rich foods (parappu keerai, chenopodium, spinach, orach, cocoa, almonds, cashew nuts, beetroot, green peppers, grapefruit juice, orange juice, black tea).
4. Most stones will pass spontaneously. If, however, there are signs of obstruction or infection, or both tracts are involved, seek urgent urological advice. The longer a stone remains impacted at one site, the greater the chance of either infection or obstruction.
5. Drug therapy includes allopurinol for calcium oxalate stones, thiazide diuretics and/or phosphate preparations for calcium stones, penicillamine for cystine stones, and urine alkalization for uric acid stones. Other treatments include litholapaxy, lithotrypsy (ultrasonic dissolution), or surgery.

Composition of stones: 80–90% of stones in the West consist of ammonium acid urate and calcium oxalate; all these are radioopaque. These types account for 50–70% of stones in the tropics. Cystine stones are semi-opaque and account for 1–3% of all stones in the tropics, while uric acid/urate stones account for 10–20%, typically occurring in older men. These stones are radiolucent. Xanthine, silica and 2,8-dihydroxyadenine stones occur, but they are very rare.

Renal manifestations of systemic diseases

Diabetic nephropathy

Results from microangiopathy and occurs in ~30% of type I and type II diabetics, particularly those diagnosed before age 25yrs. Diabetics are prone to atherosclerosis, UTIs, and papillary necrosis, but glomerular lesions cause most of the problems, with a gradual decline in renal function.

Treatment

1. ***Metabolic control:*** good glycaemic control is vital.
2. ***Blood pressure control:*** lower the BP to within the normal range. ACE inhibitors (eg enalapril 20mg/day PO) have been shown to prevent nephropathy and renal failure even in normotensive diabetics.
3. ***Low protein diet:*** restriction of dietary protein to 0.6–0.8g/kg body weight/day reduces the rate of loss of GFR. However, be careful to prevent malnutrition, particularly if there is intercurrent illness.

Diabetics in renal failure need careful monitoring, as above, especially for glycaemic control, since the requirements for insulin and oral hypoglycaemics tends to fall in CRF, due partly to ↓ excretion by the kidney (also true for most of the sulphonylureas) and partly to ↑ insulin resistance. Such patients are also at risk of hypertension, as salt and volume loads are less well handled. There may be a need for massive diuretic therapy, unless dialysis is possible. Advanced nephropathy in the diabetic patient is also strongly correlated to the risk of coronary disease and cardiovascular death. Watch for the abrupt onset of pulmonary oedema or congestive heart failure, which may be the first signs of severe ischaemic heart disease.

Nephritis associated with current infection

Many forms of nephritis complicate active infectious diseases. The most important causes include infective endocarditis, infection of hydrocephalic ventriculoatrial shunt, visceral abscesses, staphylococcal septicaemia, typhoid fever, legionnaire's disease, tuberculosis, hepatitis B, hepatitis C, HIV, schistosomiasis (*S. mansoni*), leprosy, filariasis, malaria and syphilis. A number of infections are associated with renal artery vasculitis including hepatitis B and streptococcal upper respiratory tract infections.

Amyloid

Renal involvement is found in ~50% of patients with AL disease and nearly all those with AA disease. Proteins are deposited in the glomeruli, vessels and, later, in the tubules and interstitium. Proteinuria may lead to nephrotic syndrome (+/– renal vein thrombosis) and renal failure. Postural hypotension (due to amyloid autonomic neuropathy) may be marked. **Diagnosis** is by staining biopsy material (rectal mucosa, abdominal fat, kidney) with Congo red.

Systemic diseases with renal manifestations

- diabetes mellitus
- malignant and chronic hypertension
- connective tissue diseases
- sickle cell disease
- amyloidosis
- multiple myeloma and other malignancies.

Multiple myeloma

ARF or CRF occurs in >20% of patients with myeloma due to the light chains they produce being toxic to renal tubular cells. Treatment is as for renal failure, with measures to avoid precipitating factors (dehydration, hypercalcaemia, acid urine, UTI, or long-term NSAID use) and chemotherapy for the underlying malignancy. Other protein-depositing diseases which may involve the kidneys include; light-chain deposition disease, fibrillary glomerulonephritis, and cryoglobulinaemia.

Renal manifestations of malignant disease

These may occur in patients with benign or malignant tumours or lymphoproliferative or myeloproliferative disorders. They are due to both direct and indirect effects, sometimes as a result of treatment.

- ***Direct:*** metastases (usually multiple and bilateral), infiltration (leukaemia/lymphoma), reduced renal blood flow (hilar tumours), ureteric or bladder obstruction (colonic/cervical carcinoma).
- ***Indirect:*** electrolyte disorders (hypercalcaemia, hypokalaemia, hyponatraemia), ARF, nephropathy, DIC, renal vein thrombosis, hyperviscosity syndrome, Fanconi syndrome, amyloidosis.
- ***Treatment:*** drug nephrotoxicity (NSAIDs, antibiotics, cytotoxics), uric acid nephropathy (tumour lysis syndrome), radiation nephritis.

Miscellaneous

- **Sarcoidosis:** renal involvement is usually a consequence of deranged calcium metabolism, but may be due to acute or chronic interstitial nephritis, glomerulopathy, or obstructive uropathy.

- **SLE:** commonly affects the kidneys (histologically 100% are involved), usually in the form of proteinuria and nephrotic syndrome +/– microscopic haematuria. At renal presentation, 40% of patients have hypertension and 50% have ↓GFR.
- **Systemic sclerosis** (scleroderma): renal involvement occurs in ~33% of patients, leading to proteinuria, haematuria, hypertension, and CRF. There may be accelerated hypertension and ARF – known as the 'scleroderma crisis'. Treatment is with ACE-inhibitors.
- **Rheumatoid arthritis:** occurs through amyloidosis (thought to be present in up to 15% of RA patients) or drug-induced nephropathy (penicillamine, certain gold compounds, NSAIDs). Rheumatoid arthritis may cause proteinuria, nephrotic syndrome and CRF. There have been rare reports of rheumatoid glomerulonephritis.
- **Sickle-cell disease:** renal involvement is worse in homozygous individuals. There may be enuresis (children), haematuria, increased incidence of UTIs, post-streptococcal glomerulonephritis, nephrotic syndrome and CRF – the latter 3 occurring in homozygous carriers only.

Renal disease

8. Gastroenterology

Mouth and pharynx 346
Dysphagia 348
Reflux oesophagitis 348
Oesophageal carcinoma 348
Upper GI bleeding 350
Oesophageal varices 351
Peptic ulcer and gastritis 352
Dyspepsia 352
Gastric cancer 353
Acute abdomen 354
Appendicitis 356
Peritonitis 358
Acute pancreatitis 360
Chronic pancreatitis 361
Ascariasis 362
Right upper quadrant pain 364
Liver disease, jaundice, and hepatomegaly 366
Pre-hepatic causes of jaundice 366
Viral hepatitis 368
Hepatitis A 368
Hepatitis E 368
Hepatitis C 369
Hepatitis B 370
Hepatitis D 371
Chronic hepatitis 372
Primary biliary cirrhosis 372
Haemochromatosis 373
Wilson's disease 373
Cirrhosis and alcoholic liver disease 374
Indian childhood cirrhosis 374
Liver failure 376
Hepatic neoplasia 378
Hepatocellular carcinoma (HC) 378
Post-hepatic causes of jaundice 380
Fascioliasis 380
Opisthorchiasis and clonorchiasis 382
Amoebic liver abscess 382
Hepatomegaly without jaundice 384
Portal hypertension 384
Schistosomiasis (bilharzia) 386
Toxocariasis 390
Hydatid disease 392
Lower GI bleeding 394
Around the anus 396
Enterobiasis (threadworm, pinworm) 396
Visible 'worms' in stool 398

Gastroenterology

Mouth and pharynx

Viral, bacterial and mycotic infections may all give rise to oropharyngeal pathology. It is often more pronounced in malnourished children.

Gingivostomatitis and aphthous ulcers

HSV, EBV and many of the enteroviruses can cause gingivostomatitis. Oral ulceration is also found in Behcet's syndrome (common in the Middle East and Japan), Crohn's disease, coeliac disease and Stevens-Johnson syndrome. Malignancy should be excluded (eg by biopsy) in any ulcer which does not heal after 3 weeks since typical features of a rolled edge and induration may be absent.

Treatment: often not needed. Hydrocortisone 2.5mg lozenges or tetracycline mouth wash (125mg/5ml) held in the mouth for 3mins, three times a day for 3 days, may help.

Oral candidiasis

Appears as small, white mucosal flecks surrounded by a ring of erythema, often in AIDS patients. Treat with nystatin or amphotericin lozenges sucked q6h. Severe infection may need systemic treatment. **Hairy leukoplakia** is associated with a rapid progression of HIV infection/AIDS. It appears as a poorly demarcated, slightly raised and corrugated white patch on the side of the tongue or on the buccal mucosa. Unlike candida, it cannot be scraped off. High dose acyclovir may sometimes cause the lesions to regress, although the condition may be premalignant.

Other diseases with buccal manifestations

Any acute bacterial infection, TB, leprosy, syphilis, yaws, histoplasmosis, blastomycosis, and coccidioidomycosis may all produce buccal lesions. Cancrum oris is a gangrenous condition involving the gums and cheeks following infection by *Borrelia vincenti* or *Fusiformis fusiformis*, most commonly in malnourished W. African children. Angular stomatitis is a feature of iron-deficiency anaemia and ariboflavinosis.

Tongue

Glossitis is a feature of the post-infective malabsorption syndrome (tropical sprue), vitamin B deficiency (a raw, red and fissured tongue), amyloidosis, and iron deficiency. The tongue may be furred and dry in dehydration and Sjogren's syndrome. Overgrowth of papillae and *Aspergillus niger* result in a black, hairy tongue. Carcinoma of the tongue typically appears as a raised ulcer with firm edges and surrounding induration. Check the draining lymph nodes for spread.

Gingivitis and gingivorrhoea

Gingivitis may occur with certain drug treatment (phenytoin, cyclosporin or nifedipine), AML, Vincent's angina, and pregnancy. In the latter stages of vitamin C deficiency (scurvy), it may be accompanied by haemorrhage. Massive gingivorrhoea may follow envenoming by certain snake species. Periodontal disease and caries are a major problem in developing countries; oral hygiene should be encouraged at all times.

Acute necrotizing ulcerative gingivitis

This is characterized by swelling and gingivorrhoea, severe pain and an ulcerated, foul-smelling mouth. It is commonly found in malnourished children in poor housing and should be managed with warm saline mouth washes, metronidazole 7.5 mg/kg tds, and penicillin V 125–150mg qds for 5–7 days. Any underlying malnutrition should be treated.

Buccal mass

Buccal carcinoma and Burkitt's lymphoma are numerically the most important, especially in India and SE Asia (possibly due in part to betel nut consumption). Nasopharyngeal carcinoma is common in the Far East and S China. Malignant change may be preceded by fibroelastosis of the submucous tissues and epithelial atrophy. Salivary gland hypertrophy is common in malnourished children but may also be associated with *Ascaris lumbricoides* infection and chronic calcific pancreatitis. A **rannula** is a bluish salivary retention cyst to one side of the frenulum.

Pigmented buccal lesions

Blue/brown patches in the mouth suggests Addison's disease; a dark line below the gingival lining suggests heavy metal poisoning. Brown spots on the lips suggest Peutz-Jeghers' syndrome. Malignant melanoma should also be borne in mind – particularly with raised, painless, pigmented lesions. Lead, bismuth and iron poisoning may all cause pigmented lesions on the palate.

Pharyngitis

Typically due to viral infection or overgrowth of normal commensual bacterial fauna – the classical 'sore throat'. *Fasciola hepatica* (ingested in raw sheep or goat liver) causes acute pharyngitis. Lasssa fever, diphtheria and rabies can all have pharyngeal involvement.

Dysphagia

A difficulty in swallowing food or liquid. Unless associated with a sore throat it is a serious symptom and merits further investigation, including ESR, FBC, barium swallow, endoscopy with biopsy. In severe cases it may lead to malnutrition. Dysphagia for fluids implies severe narrowing of the oesophageal lumen and may indicate imminent complete obstruction. The 5 questions presented opposite will supply many diagnoses.

Reflux oesophagitis

Heartburn and regurgitation are the hallmarks of gastro-oesophageal reflux. It is due to lower oesophageal sphincter malfunction (smoking, fatty meals, pregnancy, gastric surgery, hiatus hernia); ↑ intra-abdominal pressure (obesity, big meals); drugs (eg tricyclics, anticholinergics); irradiation and ingestion of corrosive agents (including tablets taken without water). It is regarded as a precursor to Barrett's oesophagus and hence important in the aetiology of oesophageal carcinoma. It may also cause anaemia. Symptoms may closely resemble those of ischaemic heart disease.
Diagnosis: history (worse with hot drinks and stooping, relieved by eating). Endoscopy, Ba studies, CXR (fluid level in hiatus hernia).
Management: minimize precipitating factors, raise the bed head at night. Antacids (eg magnesium trisilicate mixture 10ml q6h PO) or alginates (Gaviscon 10ml q8h PO) may be used. Severe cases may require H_2 receptor antagonists, metaclopramide, or omeprazole.

Oesophageal carcinoma

Oesophageal CA is common in C and E Africa, NE Iran, SE Asia and N China, affecting adults in their 4th & 5th decades. In most areas, the M:F ratio is 3:1, although the incidence amongst females in S Africa is rising.

Aetiology: alcohol and smoking, (? eating commercial maize or drinking maize-brewed beers), malnutrition, vitamin A, C or riboflavin deficiency, consumption of Chinese pickled vegetables. Pre-malignant associations include Barret's oesophagus (columnar replacement of squamous oesophageal epithelium), achalasia, and Plummer-Vinson syndrome.

Clinical features: dysphagia, weight loss, retrosternal pain, hoarseness or lymphadenopathy. Disease progression is usually rapid. Extensive oesophageal carcinoma can result in Horner's syndrome, recurrent laryngeal nerve palsy (hoarse voice), and coughing. Episodes of coughing when swallowing may also be due to oesophago-tracheal fistulae, 2° to carcinoma or traumatic perforation.

Management and prognosis: long term survival is poor (4% 5yr survival in UK) since many patients present late. Treatment is mainly palliative, consisting of nutritional and respiratory support, pain relief, and occasionally intubation. Surgical resection may increase survival to 8–22% at 5yrs. Adjuvant trials with chemotherapy are underway. Radiotherapy may cause strictures and fistulae.

5 key questions for dysphagia:

1. Can fluid be drunk normally, except if food is stuck?
   Yes: suspect a stricture (benign or malignant).
   No: possible motility disorder (achalasia, neurological).
2. Is it difficult to make the swallowing movement?
   Yes: suspect bulbar palsy, especially if there is coughing upon swallowing.
3. Is the dysphagia constant and painful?
   Yes: suspect a malignant stricture.
4. Does the neck bulge or gurgle upon swallowing?
   Yes: suspect a pharyngeal pouch.
5. Are there signs of systemic infection or illness?
   Yes: oesophageal symptoms may be a local manifestation of a systemic disease.

Causes of dysphagia

Neoplastic

- oesophageal CA
- gastric CA
- pharyngeal CA
- extrinsic pressure (eg lung CA, goitre)

Neurological

- bulbar palsy
- lat. medullary syndrome
- myasthenia gravis
- syringomyelia
- globus hystericus

Others

- benign strictures
- Chagas disease
- systemic sclerosis
- Fe-deficiency anaemia
- pharyngeal pouch
- TB
- trauma
- achalasia
- mucormycosis
- oesophageal varices
- candidiasis (HIV)

Upper GI bleeding

Upper GI bleeding manifests as either haematemesis or melaena. A methodical approach to management can result in the successful treatment of most patients.

Resuscitate if signs of shock are present:

1. Give IV fluids, high flow O_2, keep nbm.
2. Take bloods for Hb, group & save (or Xmatch), LFTs, U&Es.
3. Monitor vital signs and watch for signs of fluid overload.
4. Insert a urinary catheter and ensure output is >30ml/hr.
5. When the systolic BP is >100mmHg, aspirate gastric contents using a wide-bore NG tube and follow by washing out with ice-cold saline and antacids every 2hrs. If bleeding persists, instil a solution of noradrenaline (8mg in 100ml saline) via the NG tube every 30min for 4 hrs.
   ►Do not insert a NG tube if you suspect oesophageal varices to be the cause of the bleed.
6. Tell the patient what is happening and when haemodynamically stable, proceed towards determining a diagnosis.

Diagnosis

- If there is splenomegaly, suspect oesophageal varices caused by portal hypertension.
- If the spleen is not enlarged, check Hb levels; if <10g/100ml the patient is likely to be bleeding from a peptic ulcer.
- If >10g/100ml there is probably erosive mucosal disease.
- Other (less likely) causes include: Mallory-Weiss tear (oesophageal tear owing to repeated vomiting); drugs (NSAIDs, steroids, thrombolytics, anticoagulants); epistaxis (swallowed blood); upper GI malignancy; haemobilia (triad of haematemesis, jaundice and biliary colic); oesophagitis; angiodysplasia; haemangioma; Ehlers-Danlos syndrome; Peutz-Jeghers syndrome; bleeding disorder; aorto-enteric fistula.
- Where possible, endoscopy is the Ix of choice.

Control of bleeding

Low-risk group – these patients make up ~70% of patients and will normally stop bleeding spontaneously. They have the following characteristics: non-variceal bleeding, <40yrs old, melaena, no haematemesis, not shocked on admission. They may be treated at home with bed rest, ice-cold antacid sips every 2hrs, and followed up with a barium meal/endoscopy 1 week later.

High-risk group – contains all patients who are not considered low risk. They should be managed as an inpatient according to the diagnosis made.

Bleeders/rebleeders – patients who continue to bleed, or who rebleed, should be admitted and treated as for the high risk group.

Indications for surgery in peptic ulcer: i) Continuous bleeding after 4 or more units of blood given. ii) Rebleeding in hospital. iii) Shocked on admission. iv) If blood of that group is in short supply.

Oesophageal varices

In the presence of portal hypertension oesophageal veins may dilate and consequently bleed, with frequently fatal results. Hepatic fibrosis from schistosomiasis is the major cause. ► **Bleeding varices constitute an emergency.**

Aetiology: portal hypertension due to

- Pre-sinusoidal disease: portal vein thrombosis; pancreatic tumours or pseudocysts; myelofibrosis; Hodgkin's lymphoma; schistosomiasis; sarcoidosis.
- Post-sinusoidal disease: cirrhosis; Budd-Chiari syndrome (hepatic vein thrombosis, eg during pregnancy or with OCP use).

Assessment: if the patient is bleeding, check for signs of shock. Look for indications of chronic liver disease and schistosomiasis. Endoscopic visualization is better than barium radiography.

Treatment: the treatment of choice is endoscopic ligation or sclerotherapy using absolute or 50% alcohol. Oesophageal compression is possible with a Sengstaken tube. Shock should be treated appropriately. Oral β-blockade (propanolol) may reduce bleeding and mortality. ► The cause of the underlying liver disease should be sought and treated. Where available, Ocreotide (50μg/hr IV) should be given for 2–5 days.

Prognosis: In the UK, 40–70% of those bleeding from varices for the first time will die. Signs of a poor prognosis include jaundice, ascites, hypoalbuminaemia, and encephalopathy.

Peptic ulcer and gastritis

Both are common in populations where there is heavy smoking, high alcohol intake, and very spicy foods. Infective causes are TB, *S. typhi*, *Shigella spp*, hookworm and roundworms. *Helicobacter pylori* is a cause of ulcers and also possibly gastric carcinoma. However, almost 100% of individuals in developing countries are seropositive for *H. pylori* by early childhood. Ulceration normally occurs in the oesophagus, stomach and duodenum, but may develop in the jejunum (Zollinger-Ellison syndrome) or ileum (Meckels diverticulum with gastric mucosa).

Clinical features: epigastric pain (often worse in the day, cf duodenal ulcers which are worse at night, radiate to the back, and are relieved by eating); waterbrash (the mouth fills with saliva); haematemesis; melaena.

Diagnosis: endoscopic biopsy is the best method, although barium radiography will show most ulcers. *H. pylori* may be demonstrated. All ulcers visualized on endoscopy must be biopsied to exclude cancer.

Management: is based on 3 levels.

1. Reduce exacerbating factors, use antacids. If relapse occurs, exclude malignancy (repeat biopsy).
2. Give 'triple therapy' for *H. pylori* infection: 1 week of ranitidine 400mg bd (lansoprazole or omeprazole are alternatives) plus amoxycillin 1g bd and metronidazole 400mg bd.
3. Surgery is now rarely necessary. Other drug treatments include omeprazole, sucralfate, H_2-antagonists (eg cimetidine) and misoprostol.

Hiatus hernia – a herniation of the stomach through the oesophageal hiatus of the diaphragm; it is rare in the tropics. There are two sorts: sliding and rolling (para-oesophageal). Presentation may be with acute chest pain and/or epigastric pain. A fluid level behind the heart on upright CXR, or on Ba meal, is diagnostic. Management is as for reflux oesophagitis, with surgery reserved for serious complications.

Dyspepsia

Dyspepsia is upper GI pain associated with eating. It can be of 4 types:

- ulcer – epigastric pain, night waking and relief by eating food, drinking milk or taking antacids.
- Gastro-oesophageal reflux – retrosternal discomfort, heartburn and regurgitation/acid. It is worse on lying flat or after large meals.
- Dysmotility – early satiety, bloating and nausea.
- Idiopathic – upper GI pain related to meals but without specific features on history or examination.

Diagnosis: stool microscopy, diagnostic trial of antacids, barium meal or gastroscopy, depending upon the patient's age and symptom severity.

Parasitic infections are a common cause of dyspepsia in the tropics. They include: hookworm, *Taenia* spp, *Ascaris lumbricoides*, *Giardia intestinalis* and *Entamoeba histolytica* – see chapter 3D. ► Detection of parasites does not necessarily exclude other causes of GI pain.

Gastric cancer

The incidence of gastric cancer varies throughout the tropics. It is common in certain regions such as Costa Rica and NE Brazil. Aetiological factors include: chronic gastritis, bile reflux from previous gastric surgery, corrosive ingestion, infection with *H. pylori,* pernicious anaemia, and dietary factors such as high salt intake, lack of fresh fruit, and ingestion of toxic nitrosamines from fish.

Clinical features: patients present with dyspepsia, abdominal mass, left supra-clavicular lymph nodes (Virchows node) or metastatic spread (to umbilicus = Sister Mary Joseph's nodule; to ovary = Kruckenberg tumour). There may be melaena, deranged liver function (from metastatic involvement), anaemia, acanthosis nigricans, and peritonism. Occasionally the presenting picture is one of a protein-losing enteropathy.

Diagnosis and management: definitive diagnosis requires biopsy material for histology and staging. Gastric cancers remain extremely difficult to treat and surgical resection offers the only hope of cure. Palliation should be aimed at relieving pain and obstruction, and controlling haemorrhage.

Acute abdomen

The patient has one or more of: pain, tenderness, vomiting, distension, fever, and constipation. Such symptoms are also features of diseases outside the GI tract so thorough history-taking and examination are essential. Abdominal pain may be misinterpreted as body aches and treatment given for malaria, only for generalized peritonitis to be found several days later.

Two clinical syndromes may require immediate laparotomy:

1. **Organ rupture** (eg spleen, aorta, ectopic pregnancy). Shock and abdominal swelling may be seen. Note any history of trauma (especially if there has been pre-existing splenomegaly, however be aware that splenic rupture can occur several weeks after trauma). Peritonism may be surprisingly mild.
2. **Peritonitis** eg due to perforated peptic ulcer, diverticulum, appendix, bowel, or gall bladder. The patient lies still and has signs of shock, abdominal tenderness, guarding, rebound tenderness, board-like abdominal rigidity, and absent bowel sounds. ► Acute pancreatitis also produces this clinical picture but *does not* require laparotomy, so do not omit doing a serum amylase.

Immediate management consists of

- resuscitation with saline, colloid, or blood as appropriate
- taking bloods for analysis and/or culture
- inserting an NG tube
- giving broad spectrum antibiotics if infection is suspected, until specific sensitivities are known.

►Blood is lost a lot faster from a ruptured ectopic pregnancy or aortic aneurysm blood than it can be replaced. Such patients should be rushed to theatre as soon as possible.

Medical causes of acute abdominal symptoms:

Gastroenteritis	UTI	Pneumonia
Typhoid fever	Sickle-cell crisis	TB
Malaria	Herpes zoster	*Yersinia enterocolitica*
Others:	PAN	Epidemic myalgia
Cholera	MI	Pneumococcal peritonitis
Porphyria	Thyroid storm	Diabetes mellitus
Heroin addiction	Lead colic	Henoch-Schonlein purpura

Causes of painless abdominal distension: large cysts (ovarian, dermoid, pancreatic pseudocyst, or renal), megacolon (Hirschsprung's, anorectal atresia with fistula, idiopathic, Chagas disease), solid tumours (ovarian, fibroids, teratoma), organomegaly (spleen, liver), fluid (ascites, hydronephrosis).

Causes of painful abdominal distension: peritonitis, intra-abdominal abscess, obstruction, paralytic ileus, haematoperitoneum (ruptured ectopic, bleeding hepatoma, ruptured aneurysm, abdominal trauma).

Causes of acute abdominal pain

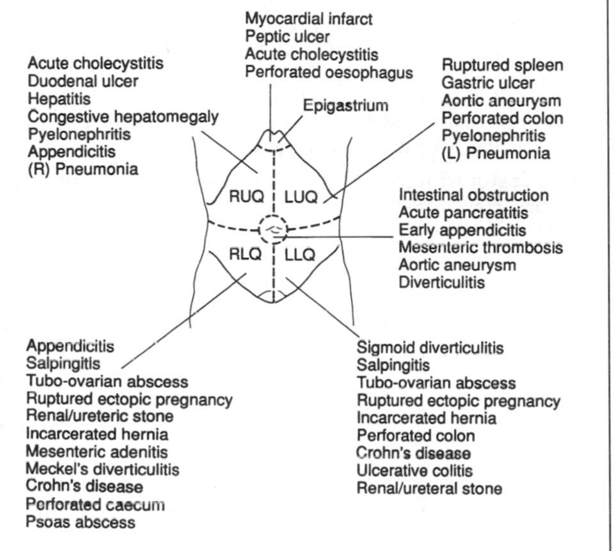
Myocardial infarct
Peptic ulcer
Acute cholecystitis
Perforated oesophagus
Epigastrium
Acute cholecystitis
Duodenal ulcer
Hepatitis
Congestive hepatomegaly
Pyelonephritis
Appendicitis
(R) Pneumonia
Ruptured spleen
Gastric ulcer
Aortic aneurysm
Perforated colon
Pyelonephritis
(L) Pneumonia
RUQ
LUQ
RLQ
LLQ
Intestinal obstruction
Acute pancreatitis
Early appendicitis
Mesenteric thrombosis
Aortic aneurysm
Diverticulitis
Appendicitis
Salpingitis
Tubo-ovarian abscess
Ruptured ectopic pregnancy
Renal/ureteric stone
Incarcerated hernia
Mesenteric adenitis
Meckel's diverticulitis
Crohn's disease
Perforated caecum
Psoas abscess
Sigmoid diverticulitis
Salpingitis
Tubo-ovarian abscess
Ruptured ectopic pregnancy
Incarcerated hernia
Perforated colon
Crohn's disease
Ulcerative colitis
Renal/ureteral stone

Appendicitis

The commonest emergency abdominal operation. It may progress to gangrene and perforation with peritonitis in up to 20% of cases. Mortality is highest at the extremes of age, but also ► in young adults in malaria-endemic areas, where non-specific symptoms may be misinterpreted.

Aetiology: appendicitis follows obstruction of the appendiceal lumen normally due to either lymphoid hyperplasia (hence common in adolescents) or faecolith impaction. Inflammation occurs together with superimposed infection; this is bacterial in the vast majority of cases (although amoebae and helminths such as *S. mansoni, S. stercoralis, T. trichuria, A. lumbricoides* and *Taenia spp*. have also been implicated). Very rarely, appendiceal tumours may present as appendicitis.

Clinical features: as the inflammatory process begins, there is colicky, central abdominal pain. Once the peritoneum becomes involved (via transmural inflammation) the pain shifts to the RIF (classically localized at McBurneys point; 2/3 of the way from the anterior superior iliac spine to the umbilicus). Anorexia is common, but vomiting rarely prominent. The patient lies still, is flushed, and takes shallow breaths (coughing hurts). Common signs include tachycardia, mild fever, furring of the tongue, RIF tenderness, guarding, rebound tenderness and Rosving's sign (LIF palpation causes pain in RIF). An appendix mass may be palpable, due to encasement of the appendix in peritoneum, omentum, small bowel or mesentery. An appendix abscess may form when escaping pus is enclosed by these tissues.

Diagnosis: is made on the clinical picture. Examine the patient often, since the severity may change rapidly. Do ESR, FBC, U&E, urine culture and microscopy, pregnancy test, and thick film if in doubt. AXR and USS are useful only to exclude other pathology and may take up vital time. Do a PR (painful on right side) and a PV in women to exclude pelvic disease.

***Differential diagnosis*:** see opposite. USS may differentiate between an appendix mass and an abscess.

Management:

1. Prompt appendicectomy to avoid perforation unless there is a mass or surgery is otherwise contraindicated. ► Surgery is well tolerated during pregnancy, but perforation carries a 30% foetal mortality, so prompt assessment is vital.
2. Give metronidazole 500mg IV or 1g PR *plus* cefuroxime 1.5g IV prior to surgery.
3. If an appendix mass is present try conservative management alone to begin with. Give metronidazole 1g PR tds *plus* either gentamicin 3–5mg/kg IV daily *or* chloramphenicol 500mg IVq8h.
4. Any abscess should be drained.
5. Surgery is indicated if the patient's condition deteriorates, so monitor vital signs and size of the mass regularly. Elective appendicectomy is carried out once inflammatory adhesions have subsided, usually at ~3mths.

Mesenteric adenitis

A viral inflammation of the mesenteric lymph nodes affecting children. Suspect it if there is high fever, vomiting, a history of URTI and cervical lymphadenopathy. Abdominal signs are usually less severe than in appendicitis and usually subside within 48hrs. Exclude meningitis.

Differential diagnosis of RIF pain

Inflammation	*Clinical features*
Mesenteric adenitis (children)	High fever, vomiting, cervical nodes; improvement with observation.
Meckel's diverticulitis	Usually discovered at appendicectomy; rarely bleeds or causes obstruction.
Caecal diverticulum	May be inflamed, perforate, or bleed; blood PR cannot be attributed to other causes.
Inflammatory masses	?Abdominal mass, weight loss.
Tuberculosis	Other systemic signs of TB.
Crohn's disease/UC	Caucasian patient with systemic, eye, joint, and/or anorectal manifestations.
Infestation	Worms or ova in stool. Chronic history +/– weight loss; pruritis ani.
Amoebic colitis	Diarrhoea with blood and mucus; cysts in stool; patient may be critically ill.
Malignancy	
Lymphoma	Weight loss; lymphoma elsewhere.
Caecal carcinoma	Anaemia, weight loss, intermittent pain.
Large bowel tumour	Diarrhoea; blood PR; eventually obstruction with caecal distension.
Genital tract pathology	
Salpingitis	Vaginal discharge; pelvic pain.
Ectopic pregnancy	2° amenorrhoea, vaginal bleeding, abdominal distension; may be shocked.
Pelvic abscess	Previous salpingitis; ?history of an illegal abortion.
Torsion/bleeding ovarian cyst/fibroid	Severe pain, minimal signs; requires USS.
Testicular torsion	Testis is swollen and very tender +/– referred pain.
Intra-abdominal testis	Torsion/malignancy (teratoma/seminoma).

Peritonitis

Peritonitis in the tropics is most commonly due to appendicitis, perforated duodenal ulcer, tubo-ovarian infection, typhoid perforation, or amoebic colitis.

Clinical features: the patient is immobile, anxious, febrile, and in obvious pain. There may be sweating, tachycardia, and tachypnoea with use of accessory breathing muscles. Septicaemia results in hyperdynamic peripheral circulation initially, but shock may develop as fluid is extravasated into the peritoneal cavity. The abdomen may be rigid and distended, move poorly or not at all with respiration, have signs of tenderness, rebound tenderness, guarding; bowel sounds are absent. In chemical peritonitis (bile, gastric acid, or pancreatic enzymes) the pain is intense; the abdomen may be so rigid that distension is minimized. The reaction to blood is more variable and often produces more subtle signs. Signs of peritonism may also be vague in the very young or critically ill (eg post-op) and present as unexplained renal or respiratory failure, or hypotension. Abdominal signs are also absent in 1/3 of cirrhotic patients with infected ascites.

Diagnosis: is usually evident from history and examination. CXR may show gas or fluid under the diaphragm; sub-phrenic abscesses often have atelectasis or small pleural effusions at the adjacent lung base. Supine AXR may show fluid between thickened loops of bowel if peritonitis is long-standing; an erect AXR with distended bowel and fluid levels at the same level is characteristic of paralytic ileus. USS may show intra-peritoneal fluid or abscesses. Paracentesis with a fine (21-gauge) needle, aspirating in all four quadrants, should be reserved for doubtful cases with abdominal distension and suspected free fluid. Do FBC, ESR, U&E, serum amylase, blood cultures. Cross-match blood if the patient is likely to go to theatre.

Treatment: resuscitate the patient. Start broad spectrum IV antibiotics immediately eg cefuroxime 750mg q8h and metronidazole 500mg q8h. Monitor vital signs and urine output. Give fluid as necessary. Where facilities allow, intra-abdominal/sub-phrenic abscesses should be drained under ultrasound or CT guidance. If the patient's condition deteriorates or the pus is too thick to aspirate, drainage by laparotomy will be required.

Female genital tract sepsis

In tubo-ovarian sepsis where peritonitis is localized to the pelvis, a trial of 48hrs of antibiotic therapy may be indicated in stable patients. Again, if the patient's condition deteriorates, the mass continues to expand, or it is suspected that the uterus is perforated, urgent laparotomy (+/– hysterectomy) should be carried out as soon as the patient is resuscitated. Rupture of tubo-ovarian abscesses carries a high mortality.

Amoebic colitis

Failure to respond within 48hrs to metronidazole (800mg tds PO, or 500mg/8hrs IV) indicates that transmural disease, with likely ischaemic necrosis is present and urgent surgery is required. See chapter 3D.

Causes of gas under the diaphragm

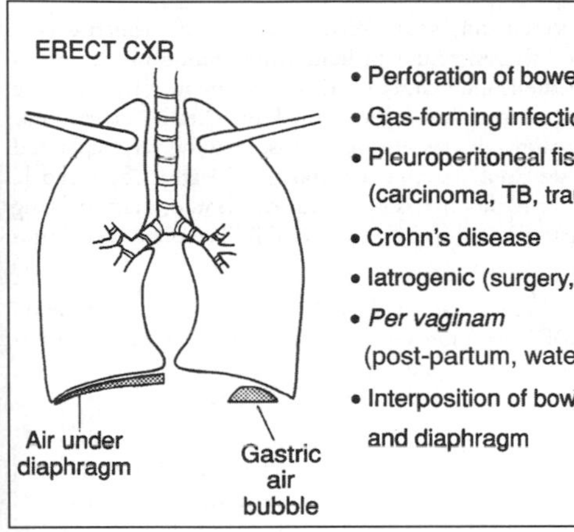

- Perforation of bowel
- Gas-forming infection
- Pleuroperitoneal fistula (carcinoma, TB, trauma)
- Crohn's disease
- Iatrogenic (surgery, laparoscopy)
- *Per vaginam* (post-partum, waterskiing)
- Interposition of bowel between liver and diaphragm

Acute pancreatitis

Acute pancreatitis is rare in most tropical countries and tends to follow trends in alcohol consumption, gallstone incidence, and more infrequently roundworm-induced obstruction. It is common in SE Asia and amongst Australian Aborigines.

Pathology: self-perpetuating acute inflammation of the pancreas (+/– other retroperitoneal tissues) results in fluid sequestration (up to several litres) in the gut, peritoneum, and retroperitoneum. Acute attacks may be isolated incidents, recurrent, or superimposed on chronic pancreatitis. Progression to haemorrhagic, necrotizing disease may be very rapid and mortality is high (see Ronson's criteria, opposite). Death is from shock, renal failure, sepsis or respiratory failure, with contributory factors being protease-induced activation of complement, kinin, fibrinolytic and coagulation cascades.

Causes: alcohol, gallstones, trauma, duct obstruction (eg *Ascaris*, tumour, hydatid cysts in CBD), scorpion venom, autoimmune (eg PAN), hypercalcaemia, hyperlipidaemia, hypothermia, viruses (mumps, coxsackie, EBV, HAV, HBV), drugs (eg thiazides, steroids, tetracycline).

Clinical features: acute epigastric pain (often radiating to the back, especially on the left); sitting forward may give relief; vomiting. Peritonism may develop, but since the pancreas is retroperitoneal, tenderness and rigidity are often not marked. 30% of patients have jaundice due to oedema around the common bile duct. In severe disease there may be discoloration around the umbilicus (Grey Turner's sign) or flank (Cullen's sign).

Diagnosis: serum amylase raised 3–4 fold in the first 48hrs (though may be normal even in severe disease[1]). AXR may show absent psoas shadow due to retroperitoneal fluid. Exclude other causes of an acute abdomen and also a myocardial infarction.

Treatment: is as for the acute abdomen plus strong analgesia eg pethidine 100mg/4hr + prochlorperazine 12.5mg q8h IM; take blood for Ca^{2+}, Cr, amylase, glucose, and arterial blood gasses. Consider USS to look for gallstones and/or pseudocyst.

Antibiotics and peritoneal lavage are of unproven value.

Complications

Early: acute respiratory distress syndrome, acute renal failure, DIC, hypocalcaemia (may require albumin replacement or 10ml of 10% calcium gluconate IV slowly), transient hyperglycaemia (5% require insulin).
Late (>1 week): pseudocyst (fluid in lesser sac, presenting as a palpable mass, persistently raised amylase or LFTs, and/or fever). It may resolve or require drainage into bowel. If it becomes infected, it requires drainage. A small number of patients have persisting diabetes mellitus.

1 Bouchier I, 1985, *BMJ*, **ii**, 1669

Ronson's criteria of severity of acute pancreatitis

At presentation	*During the first 48hrs*
Age >55yrs	Haemocrit fall >10%
WCC >16×10^9/l	Urea rise >4mmol/l
Glucose >11mmol/l	Serum Ca^{2+} <2mmol/l
LDH >450IU/l	Base defect >4
AST >60IU/l	PaO_2 <8kPa
	Plasma albumin <32g/l
	Estimated fluid sequestration >6l

Prognosis

0–2 criteria = 2% mortality (in UK), 3–4 = 15%
5–6 = 40%, 7–8 = 100%

Chronic pancreatitis

Destruction of the pancreas with atrophy results in permanent loss of both exocrine and endocrine function, either partially or totally. It is characterized by pain, diabetes, and malabsorption with steatorrheic diarrhoea. There are 3 main types: chronic obstructive, minimal change (often post acute), and chronic calcific.

Ascariasis

Ascaris lumbricoides is a soil-transmitted roundworm, thought to infect ~25% of the world's population. Prevalences reach 95% in parts of Africa; infection is also very common in C and SE Asia, and S America. Infection is acquired via the faeco-oral route. Eggs are killed by direct sunlight and temperatures >45°C but are resistant to cold and normal detergents.

Clinical features: most infections are asymptomatic. However, heavy infection, especially of children, may produce symptoms roughly proportional in severity to the worm burden.

- ***Larval ascariasis*** – 1–7 days after infection, larvae cause pulmonary symptoms (Loffler's syndrome or pneumonia). Circulating larvae reaching the CNS cause convulsions, meningism, epilepsy, and insomnia; those reaching the eye cause ocular granulomas similar to those of *T. canis*. Larvae may wander anywhere in the body causing acute symptoms.
- ***Adult worms*** – in the small intestine may cause intestinal colic, vomiting, intussusception, volvulus, obstruction, perforation; plus anaemia and malabsorption. Death of adult worms in the liver causes abscess formation, recurrent cholangitis, or acute biliary obstruction, with fever, RUQ pain and jaundice. Worm, larva or egg presence may initiate stone formation; eggs released into the peritoneum may cause granulomas resembling TB peritonitis. High fever and exposure to tetrachloroethylene or anaesthetics can cause adult worms to migrate (eg to Eustachian tubes) hence it is important to deworm patients in such circumstances.
- ***Nutritional effects*** – a child may lose 10% of dietary protein to parasites. Look for kwashiorkor and vitamin A or C deficiency.
- ***Immunopathology*** – hypersensitivity conjunctivitis, urticaria and asthma may occur in pre-sensitized individuals upon re-exposure. It may occur upon passing worms, producing intense anal pruritis.

Diagnosis: is made by identifying worms or eggs in faeces (see opposite). WCC will show a marked eosinophilia during larval disease; persistent eosinophilia implies concurrent *Toxocara* or *Strongyloides* infection. Worms may be seen on CXR or contrast AXR (look for string-like shadows, where the worms take up contrast medium). The differential diagnosis of larval ascariasis includes toxocariasis, hookworm, strongyloidiasis, schistosomiasis, and tropical pulmonary eosinophilia.

Management is only effective against adult worms.

1. Albendazole 400mg PO as a single dose (half dose in children 2–5yrs) [alternative: mebendazole 100mg PO bd for 3 days]
2. Pneumonitis is treated with prednisolone, followed by an antihelminthic 2–3 weeks later.
3. Biliary and intestinal obstruction are best managed conservatively (analgesia, NG tube, antispasmodics, IV fluids, liquid paraffin) followed by antihelminthic treatment once the acute phase is over.
4. If symptoms of intestinal obstruction worsen or persist >48hrs, surgical intervention will be necessary.

Prevention: requires improved hygiene, proper faecal disposal, education and chemotherapy (since man acquires only partial immunity to reinfection).

Life cycle of *A. lumbricoides*

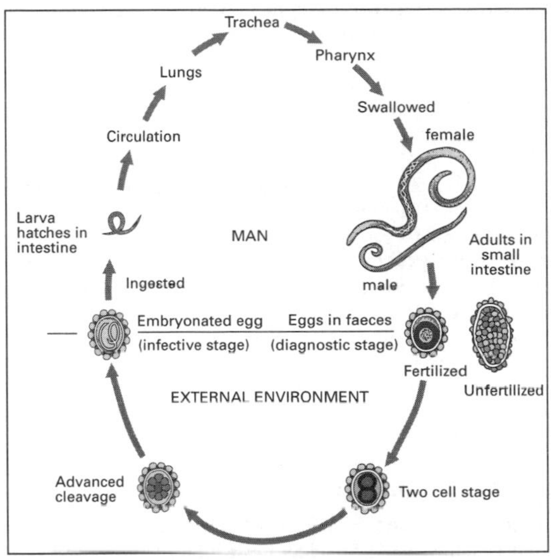

Faecal microscopy of *A. lumbricoedes* eggs

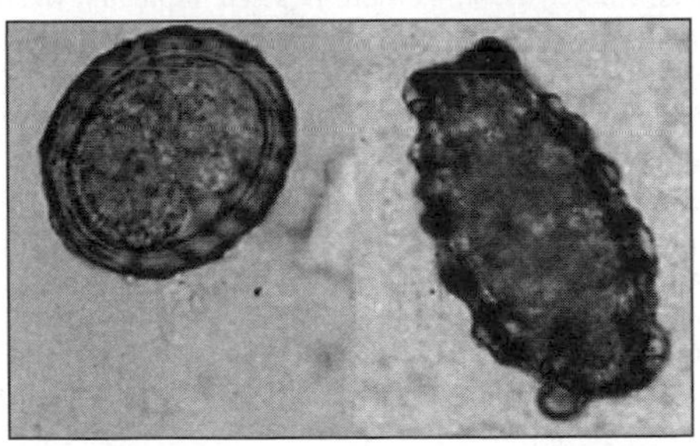

Fertile egg (~60×40μm)   Infertile egg (~90×50μm)

Right upper quadrant pain

RUQ pain is normally due to pathology in the liver or gallbladder; occasionally the heart in congestive cardiac failure or the right lung in R lower lobe pneumonia may be the source.

Biliary 'colic': occurs when a stone impacts in the gallbladder outlet. It is severe, constant pain lasting several hours, with associated nausea and vomiting, that may radiate to the interscapular region of the back. Treatment consists of strong pain relief +/– antispasmodics (eg buscopan 40mg IM) until the stone frees itself, which may be only during surgery.

Cholecystitis

In nearly all cases, this involves gallstones although acalculous cholangitis can be a feature of any severe disease, especially in the malnourished, in typhoid fever, and gas gangrene. Cholecystitis can be acute or chronic.

Acute cholecystitis: follows impaction of a stone in the cystic duct. Features include RUQ pain, vomiting, fever, local peritonism, gall bladder mass and/or jaundice. The gallbladder may rupture resulting in peritonitis or form an abscess. Superimposed infection of the bile ducts produces cholangitis; this classically presents with RUQ pain, fever, and jaundice (Charcot's triad). It is common throughout Asia.

Chronic cholecystitis: intermittent colic and chronic inflammation, with abdominal discomfort, distension, flatulence, nausea, and fat intolerance. Differential diagnosis includes reflux, ulcers, irritable bowel syndrome, pancreatitis, and abdominal masses.

Other complications: mucocele (when impaction occurs in an empty gallbladder), empyema (gallbladder fills with pus), gallbladder carcinoma, gallstone obstruction (gallstone ileus; stone ulcerates through gallbladder into the duodenum, blocking the ileocaecal junction).

Diagnosis: *Murphy's sign*: pain during deep inspiration when the RUQ is palpated, without pain following the same procedure at the LUQ. Tests include: USS, WCC, AXR, ERCP. Differential diagnosis: appendicitis, perforated duodenal ulcer, pancreatitis, R basal pneumonia, hiatus hernia.

Management:

1. Most will settle on bed rest, fluid, and pain relief, *plus*:
2. Broad-spectrum antibiotics covering Gram-ve bacteria (eg cefuroxime 750mg IV q8h).
3. For cholangitis add metronidazole 500mg PR/IV q8h.
4. Cholecystectomy is carried out within 48hrs if the patient's condition allows, otherwise in 6–10 weeks. Without surgery, recurrence occurs in ~18%. Chronic cholecystitis requires elective cholecystectomy.
5. Asymptomatic (silent) gallstones do not require treatment unless the gallbladder wall is calcified, in which case there is a significantly increased risk of gallbladder carcinoma.

Sclerosing cholangitis

A rare condition, frequently associated with ulcerative colitis. It predisposes to cholangiocarcinoma; transplantation is the only cure.

Gallstones are uncommon in the tropics. They are most often encountered when there is a parasitic nidus for their formation (especially *Ascaris* infection) or there is biliary stasis due to pregnancy. Pigment stones occasionally complicate sickle-cell disease. ***Courvoisier's law*** states that a palpable gallbladder in the presence of jaundice is not likely to be due to gallstones.

Type of stone:

pigment	***cholesterol***	***mixed***
small, friable,	large, freq. solitary	faceted
irregular, radiolucent	10% radiolucent	radio-opaque
Fem., >60, obesity	haemolysis, black	clofibrate,
infection, brown	pregnancy	OCP use

Other causes of RUQ pain: include acute hepatitis, liver abscesses, hydatid cyst, hepatoma, *Trichuriasis* (whipworm), duodenal ulcer, congestive hepatomegaly, pyelonephritis, appendicitis and right lower lobe pneumonia.

Liver disease, jaundice, and hepatomegaly

Liver disease is common in the tropics due not only to the widespread consumption of alcohol but also, since the organ is in effect a filter of blood coming from the portal circulation, it is far more frequently exposed to bacteria, viruses, parasites, ova, and toxins.

Although the patient will often complain of other symptoms, jaundice and/or hepatomegaly are almost always encountered clinically in hepatic disease. More subtle dysfunction can be demonstrated by liver enzyme abnormalities; such tests are often useful in differentiating between possible diagnoses. Determine the liver size (normally <12cm) and feel whether it is soft, smooth, non-tender, regular, and non-pulsantile (all normal).

Jaundice (icterus) refers to the yellow pigmentation of the skin, sclerae, and mucosae due to a raised plasma bilirubin (>35µmol/l). Examine the sclerae in good light since these are the most sensitive indicators. Jaundice also causes itching, which may be severe (look for scratch marks); the stools may be pale, offensive or float on the water (steatorrhoea).

Other signs of liver disease

Hands: leuconychia, clubbing, palmar erythema, bruising, asterixis.
Face: scratch marks, spider naevi, hepatic fetor.
Chest: gynaecomastia, loss of body hair, spider naevi, bruising, pectoral muscle wasting.
Abdomen: splenomegaly, ascites, signs of portal hypertension, testicular atrophy.
Legs: oedema, muscle wasting.

Pre-hepatic causes of jaundice

Pre-hepatic causes of jaundice

- falciparum malaria
- sepsis
- pneumococcal pneumonia
- ineffective erythropoiesis
- drugs
- haemolytic diseases (G6PD, favism).
- haemolytic-uraemic syndrome
- filoviruses
- Q fever
- Gilberts syndrome
- Crigler-Nagar

For haematological and infective causes see the relevant chapters.

Acute systemic bacterial infections: are important tropical causes of jaundice, particularly pneumococcal pneumonia and pyomyositis.

Gilberts syndrome: is an inherited metabolic disorder of bilirubin uptake and conjugation, leading to an unconjugated hyperbilirubinaemia. The prognosis is excellent.

Crigler-Nagar syndrome: has two forms. In type I disease, the defect lies in the conjugating enzymes and leads to early death; type II disease is a partial lack of the enzyme. It is treated in infants with phototherapy; adults are given phenobarbital to reduce plasma bilirubin.

An understanding of the (simplified!) biochemistry involved in bile metabolism enables the clinician to determine whether the jaundice has a pre-hepatic, hepatocellular, or post-hepatic origin. As is often the case, however, laboratory test results seldom fit the classical pattern for a given disease and one should view such results in the context of the patient's symptomatology.

Haemoglobin
(from RBC breakdown)
↓
Unconjugated bilirubin in plasma
(water-insoluble, bound to albumin)
↓
Glucoronyl transferase in hepatocytes
↓
Conjugated bilirubin
(water-soluble, passed in bile into gut)
[if bile is blocked, it builds up in plasma and is excreted in urine]
↓
Bacteria in gut
↓
Urobilinogen
(partly reabsorbed into plasma; excreted by the kidneys)
(partly metabolized in the gut to stercobolin)
↓
Stercobilin
(passes out with the faeces)

Investigation of jaundice

Substance	***Pre-hepatic***	***Hepatocellular***	***Post-hepatic***
Urine			
Bilirubin			
(conjugated)	normal	normal/raised	raised
(unconjugated)	raised	raised	normal
Urobilinogen	raised	normal/raised	absent/reduced
Faeces			
Stercobilinogen	raised	absent/reduced	normal

Viral hepatitis

A major public health problem, viral hepatitis is estimated to affect several hundred million people worldwide, causing extensive morbidity and mortality through either acute infection or its chronic sequelae.

Hepatitis A

The hepatitis A virus (HAV) is spread via the faeco-oral route. It is endemic throughout the world and hyperendemic in areas of poor sanitation. Spread frequently occurs in institutions and travellers. It is an unenveloped, symmetrical RNA virus, now classified as a hepatovirus.

Clinical features: replication occurs in the liver after an incubation period of 2–6 weeks, during which time large amounts of virus are excreted in the faeces. Jaundice is usually preceded by a prodrome of anorexia, arthralgia, nausea and fever. Tender hepatomegaly, splenomegaly and lymphadenopathy may follow. However, the majority of infections pass unnoticed in childhood – symptoms tending to be more severe in older, non-immune individuals. Chronic liver disease does not occur.

Diagnosis: specific IgM is detectable at the onset of symptoms; IgG rises 1–2 weeks later and remains elevated for life. AST/ALT rise after ~1mth.

Treatment: is supportive since the infection is normally self-limiting. Avoid alcohol until LFTs return to normal. There is no carrier state.

Prevention: is difficult, since the faecal shedding of the virus is at its highest during the asymptomatic incubation stage. Isolation of patients is therefore unnecessary. Improvement of sanitary conditions and the safe disposal of excreta will reduce transmission.

After infection, immunity is probably lifelong. Normal human immunoglobulin (0.02ml/kg IM) gives ~3 months passive protection and may be given to those at risk (travellers, close contacts, outbreak control) and even during the prodromal stage of the illness in an attempt to prevent/reduce symptoms. Vaccines are available although rarely indicated in the tropics since most children in endemic areas will have acquired immunity. It is most useful for staff in institutions, particularly food handlers.

Hepatitis E

Hepatitis E virus is a non-enveloped, single-stranded RNA virus, similar to caliciviruses. The disease is similar to HAV in transmission and clinical features, although the incubation period is slightly longer, ~6 weeks. Many cases occur in epidemics – these have occurred in India, the former USSR, SE Asia, N Africa and Mexico. The highest attack rates are found in young adults; although many cases are self-limiting, mortality is high (~20%) in women in the 3rd trimester of pregnancy. Diagnosis relies on detection of HEV RNA or specific IgG/IgM antibodies. Treatment is as for HAV but there is no protection from gammaglobulin and no vaccine yet available.

Hepatitis F and G viruses – are not believed to be clinically important.

Hepatocellular causes of jaundice

- Viral hepatidies A-E, EBV, CMV, Lassa fever, yellow fever
- Other infections eg malaria, leptospirosis, syphilis, typhoid fever, bartonellosis, hydatidosis
- Cirrhosis and alcoholic liver disease
- Hepatocellular carcinoma
- Primary biliary cirrhosis
- Autoimmune chronic hepatitis
- Drugs (eg paracetamol, dapsone, methyldopa, barbiturates, halothane)
- Rare syndromes (Rotor, Dubin-Johnstone, Wilson's)

Hepatitis C

The virus is an enveloped, single-stranded RNA flavivirus. Spread is similar to HBV (although there is little evidence for sexual transmission). Up to 50% of cases progress to chronic hepatitis, with increased risk of hepatocellular carcinoma, and abnormal liver histology even in asymptomatic carriers. Disease is worse in patients with concurrent HIV infection and/or alcoholic cirrhosis.

Diagnosis: antibodies become detectable at 3–6 months; they do not indicate whether the patient is either infective or currently infected.

Management: is the same as for acute HBV hepatitis. Gammaglobulin provides some (temporary) passive immunity. There is no vaccine available. Only 20% of patients show complete viral clearance post-infection.

Hepatitis B

This is the most common form of parenterally transmitted viral hepatitis and an important cause of both acute and chronic hepatitis. Spread is via blood products, secretions, and sexual intercourse. Risk groups are therefore: health workers, haemophiliacs, homosexuals, IV drug abusers, patients on haemodialysis, and those in institutions. HBV is also heavily implicated as a causative agent in hepatocellular carcinoma. About 350 million people worldwide are carriers of the virus and it is hyperendemic in parts of the tropics. It is a double stranded DNA hepadnavirus.

Clinical features: the incubation period varies between 1–6 months. The symptoms are the same as in HAV infection, although urticaria and arthralgia are more common with HBV. Severe illness and liver failure may result. Liver damage is mediated by the host cellular immune response to infected hepatocytes. The virus persists in about 10% of infected adults but up to 90% of infants infected at birth. Hepatitis becomes chronic in ~30% of these carriers (particularly if there is super-infection with Hep D virus), with increased risk of cirrhosis and hepatocellular carcinoma (see chronic hepatitis, below). Glomerulonephritis is a rare complication.

Diagnosis: serology/antigen detection. HBV surface antigen (HBsAg) is present from 1 to 6 months after exposure. In some cases, it persists due to viral DNA integration into hepatocyte DNA. The continued presence of HbsAg >6 months after infection defines the carrier state. Carriers may also express the e-antigen (HBeAg) – they have not developed an anti-HBeAg immune response. HBeAg positive carriers are highly infectious. Antibodies to the core antigen (anti-HBc) imply past infection, whilst antibodies against only the surface antigen (anti-HBs) imply previous vaccination. Serum AST is elevated during the period of high infectivity.

Treatment: is supportive. Avoid alcohol during the acute stage (HBsAg positive) and discourage its consumption in the convalescent stage. Ensure adequate nutrition and minimize contacts. Steroids and NSAIDs are not indicated and indeed may *promote* viral replication.

Prevention:

Passive immunization of adults with 3ml hepatitis B immunoglobulin (containing 200IU/ml of anti-HBs) gives encouraging results if given early (preferably within 48hrs and not >7 days) to patients following acute exposure or to their close contacts. A second dose is recommended after 30 days. Half the adult dose given to at-risk babies at birth (or within 12hrs) reduces their chances of developing the carrier state by up to 70%.

Active immunization is required for the at-risk groups mentioned above and would be beneficial for everyone, especially neonates and adolescents. Variations of inactivated HBsAg are used, as a course of 3 doses injected IM in the deltoid or anterolateral thigh (► **not** in the buttock, as resultant antibody titres are much lower[1]). Protective immunity begins ~6 weeks after the 1st dose and wanes after 3–5 years, so consider revaccination. Other vaccine forms are being developed. ► Recent studies in Taiwan have shown that universal vaccination of under-fives reduces the incidence of hepatocellular carcinoma.

1. Shaw FE, 1989, *Vaccine*, 7, 425–30.

Hepatitis D

Only exists in the presence of HBV and is spread by similar routes. An estimated 5% of HBsAg carriers are HDV +ve, with dual infection particularly prevalent in the Mediterranean region, parts of eastern Europe, Africa, the Middle East and S America. Immunofluorescence for the delta antigen (HDAg) signifies infection. The virus is a single stranded circular RNA virus.

Clinical features: coinfection can lead to more severe acute HBV hepatitis or, in the case of chronic HBV infection, it may cause accelerated hepatic failure and cirrhosis. HBV vaccination prevents co-infection. Treatment and prevention is as for HBV.

Serological changes in hepatitis infections

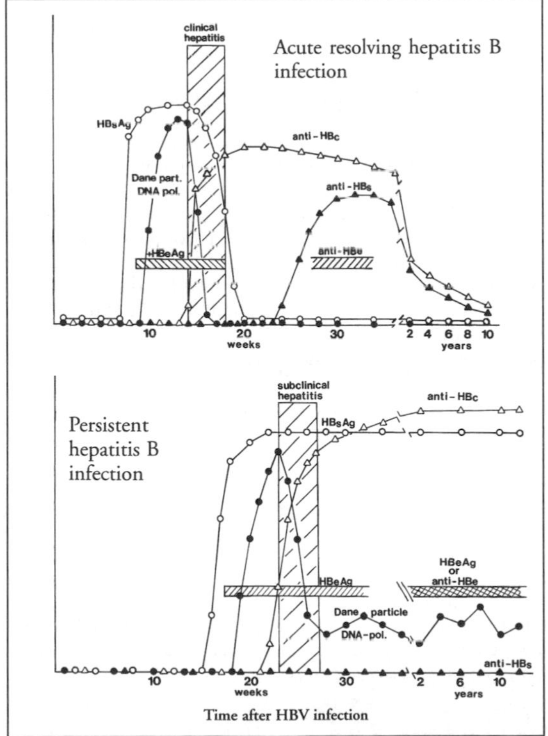

Chronic hepatitis

1. **Chronic passive hepatitis:** is an inflammatory reaction lasting >6 mths which causes portal fibrosis but not necrosis. In the tropics, it is most commonly due to HBV or HCV infection, although alcohol and drugs (notably isoniazid and methyldopa) may play significant roles.
   Clinical features: may follow acute hepatitis. There is hepatomegaly and tenderness, often with no other symptoms. Serum ALT/AST are raised up to 10-fold. Do a liver biopsy to exclude CAH (see below).
   Management: is supportive, since the condition is benign and will remit.

2. **Chronic active hepatitis (CAH):** is a slowly progressive condition which may lead to cirrhosis and hepatocellular carcinoma. It is most commonly caused by infection with HBV (particularly if there is co-infection with HDV) or HCV. (~30% of HBV carriers develop CAH; their mortality may reach 50% from liver failure or hepatocellular carcinoma – see below.) Chronic alcohol excess and lupoid CAH (ANF positive, IgG markedly increased) are other causes.

   Acute hepatitis → CAH → macronodular cirrhosis → hepatoma.

   Histologically there is piecemeal necrosis and fibrosis with plasma cell and lymphocyte infiltration of the hepatic parenchyma +/– the changes of acute hepatitis and cirrhosis.
   Clinical features: jaundice, exhaustion, spider naevi (very difficult to see on dark skin), hepatosplenomegaly.
   Treatment: ► strict alcohol avoidance. Steroids and NSAIDs are contraindicated during the viral replication (HBeAg +ve) stage. Interferon-α is effective in ~40% of patients although up to 50% of those with HCV CAH will relapse when treatment is stopped. Almost all of those who relapse will respond to retreatment. Approximately 20% of patients who respond by clearing HBeAg will also clear HBsAg within a year of treatment (65% will clear it within 6 years). New treatments are currently under trial but are unlikely to be affordable.

Primary biliary cirrhosis

A slowly progressive non-suppurative cholangiohepatitis, with destruction of the small interlobular bile ducts. The aetiology is thought to be autoimmune. 90% of patients are women.
Clinical features: vary widely but include pruritis, hepatosplenomegaly, pale stools, dark urine, clubbing, xanthomata, xanthelasma, arthralgia, fatigue. It is associated with thyroid and pancreatic disease, Sjogrens syndrome and localized cutaneous scleroderma.
Diagnosis: plasma bilirubin usually normal, AlkP raised or normal, AST slightly raised. Biopsy and/or ERCP confirm the diagnosis.
Management: is symptomatic, cholestyramine for pruritis, low-fat diet, vitamin supplementation. Monitor for signs of portal hypertension. Death commonly occurs within 5 years in severe disease.

Haemochromatosis

An autosomal recessive inherited disorder resulting in increased iron absorption from the small bowel. The iron is deposited in cells of the heart, pancreas, liver, pituitary, and joints. If caught early, it is possible to treat and avoid the late complications. Early signs include fatigue, arthralgia, arthritis, gonadal failure, hepatomegaly and bronze-coloured skin. Late complications include chronic liver disease, diabetes, and cardiomyopathy. TIBC is highly saturated (>70%) and ferritin >1mg/ml. Liver biopsy shows the extent of the disease; >2% iron by weight is diagnostic. The patients require regular venesection until they are iron deficient, which may take months.

Wilsons disease

An autosomal recessive inherited disorder of copper metabolism which results in copper deposition in the liver and brain. Clinical features are those of cirrhosis together with signs of basal ganglia damage: tremor, convulsions, and mental disorientation. Check serum copper and caeruloplasmin levels; liver biopsy shows copper and is diagnostic. Treat with penicillamine for life.

Cirrhosis and alcoholic liver disease

Cirrhosis is the *irreversible* destruction of the liver's cytoarchitecture by fibrosis, with nodular regeneration of hepatocytes. The cause is unknown in 30% of cases; otherwise, HBV or HCV infection, alcohol, and CAH are common. Inherited chronic liver diseases such as Wilson's disease, Budd-Chiari syndrome, haemochromatosis, and α_1-antitrypsin deficiency are rare. Although many of these conditions are associated with hepatomegaly, as cirrhosis progresses, fibrotic contraction causes the liver to shrink.

Clinical features: are variable and depend upon the degree of compensation. When present, they are due to hepatocyte failure and portal hypertension. There may be jaundice, pruritus, palmar erythema, spider naevi, leuconychia, Dupuytren's contracture, hepatic fetor, gynaecomastia, small testes, clubbing, liver flap (asterixis; a slow hand tremor made worse by hand extension which is due to encephalopathy), peripheral oedema (owing to hypoalbuminaemia). Portal hypertension may produce haematemesis or melaena (oesophageal varices), splenomegaly, and ascites. Osteomalacia occurs due to altered vitamin D metabolism.

Diagnosis: USS and/or liver biopsy. Do FBC, INR, platelets and LFTs before biopsy – if the INR is prolonged, postpone biopsy until normalized. After biopsy, lie the patient on their right side for 2hrs (bed rest for 24hrs) and carefully monitor vital signs. The following day check for signs of pneumothorax and blood or bile leaks. Tests may show bilirubin ↑, AST ↑, INR ↑, (clotting factors ↓), glucose ↓, albumin ↓.

Treatment: there is none which will reverse the damage.

1. Avoid (or treat) precipitants such as alcohol, dehydration, shock and hepatotoxic drugs.
2. Give nutritional support if the patient is malnourished.
3. Monitor BP if there is risk of bleeding varices.
4. Aspirate the ascites. Send a sample for cytology to exclude other causes (if diagnosis doubtful). A low salt diet and fluid restriction may reduce the ascites, but check U&E, plasma Cr, weight, and urine vol daily.
5. Diuretics (spironolactone or frusemide) may be used in severe ascites – monitor for hypokalaemia and stop if encephalopathy occurs.
6. Treat pruritus with cholestyramine 4–8g daily taken 1hr after other drugs.
7. Watch for signs of liver failure, see p376.

Indian childhood cirrhosis

A disease presenting in children age 1–3yrs from the Indian subcontinent. It may follow a fulminant, acute, or sub-acute course ranging from a viral type acute hepatitis to florid cirrhosis. There is fibrosis with micro- and macronodular degeneration and, although progression to hepatocellular carcinoma is rare, mortality is high. The cause is unknown, although a high copper intake (eg from milk stored in copper vessels), possibly coupled with an inherited defect of copper absorption/metabolism is implicated. There is no specific treatment.

Aetiology and consequences of alcoholic liver disease

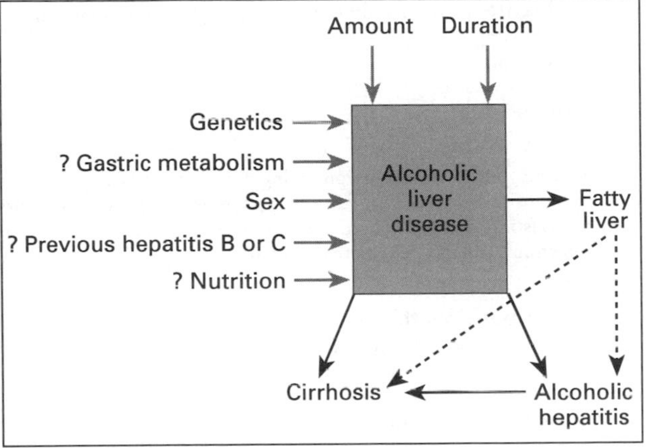

Liver failure

In the tropics, liver failure usually results from viral hepatitis, particularly HBV. Less common causes are other viruses, bacteria, toxins such as alcohol or paracetamol, and acute fatty liver of pregnancy. Beware development of renal failure via the hepato-renal syndrome.

Clinical features: presentation is likely to involve one (or more) of:

- encephalopathy
- hypoglycaemia
- bleeding
- overwhelming infection
- ascites.

The onset may be acute, with no preceding illness or jaundice (fulminant hepatic necrosis). However, liver failure occurs more commonly in patients with pre-existing cirrhosis. These patients have a chronic deterioration with infection, lethargy, GI bleeds, diuretics usage, and/or electrolyte disturbances.

Hepatic encephalopathy

Early signs are: lethargy, delirium, psychiatric symptoms, amnesia, ataxia, tremor, incontinence, ophthalmoplegia, and extra-pyramidal signs. It is due to ammonia, mercaptans and false transmitter excess. Blood ammonium (uncuffed) may be useful in monitoring progress.

Treatment

1. If signs of encephalopathy, manage as for coma (chapter 9).
2. ► Be careful to avoid contamination with blood or secretions.
3. Insert an NG tube, ► unless oesophageal varices are suspected.
4. Monitor TPR, BP, pupils, urine ouput, blood glucose, INR, U&E, LFTs.
5. Consider haemodialysis if there is water overload.
6. Give cimetidine 200mg IV q8h to keep stomach pH >5.
7. If infection is suspected, give gentamicin 2–5mg/kg daily in divided doses *plus* metronidazole 500mg IV q8h *plus* benzylpenicillin 1.2g IV q8h. Otherwise give ampicillin 1.5g IV q6h to sterilize bowel.
8. Watch for convulsions, treating with diazepam (chapter 9).
9. For bleeding, give vitamin K 10mg IV daily for 2–3 days. Platelets and FFP may be needed. Gastric lavage with 100ml cold saline containing 8mg noradrenaline may be useful in gastric bleeding.
10. Give IV glucose if blood glucose level falls below 2mmol/l
11. Beware hypokalaemia.
12. Control pain with normal dose paracetamol or morphine.

► Avoid sedatives, drugs with hepatic metabolism, NSAIDs (risk of GI bleed).

Poor prognosis is associated with grade IV coma, presence of HBsAg, coinfection with HDV, serum bilirubin >20mg/100ml, and sodium <119mmol/l. In one Indian study[1] mortality was ~70%. Liver transplantation before irreversible CNS damage is the only curative treatment.

1. Tandon BN, 1986, *J Clin Gastroenterol*, **8**, 664

Gastroenterology

Hepatic neoplasia

Hepatic secondaries are rare in the tropics compared with the West. They have a characteristic knobbly feeling. Jaundice is relatively uncommon as a presenting feature; unexplained weight loss is more common.

Investigations: USS is the best means of determining the cause of focal liver lesions.

Hepatocellular carcinoma (HCC)

This cancer is the most common 1° cancer of men in sub-Saharan Africa, and is also common in parts of Asia and the western Pacific. Its incidence is as high as 100/100,000 in Mozambique males, with an estimated 1 million deaths/year worldwide. It is strikingly common in the 20–40 age group.

Aetiology

1. **Hepatitis B** and to a lesser extent HCV are thought to cause ~80% of cases world-wide.
2. Non-viral factors which may be involved include:
   - ***Aflatoxin B*** – a toxin produced by the plant mould *Aspergillus flavus*. It grows commonly on groundnuts (peanuts) but is also found on maize, millet, peas and sorghum. Levels of food contamination in Mozambique are the highest in the world and there is good correlation between levels of ingestion and incidence of HCC.[1]
   - ***Cigarette smoking*** – a significant factor in low-risk areas of the world and increasing in importance in the developing world.
   - ***Alcohol*** – HCC is 5-fold more common in males who drink >80mg alcohol per day than in non-drinkers.[2]
   - ***Oral contraceptive pill use*** – some studies suggest a 5-fold increased relative risk for women using the OCP for >5 yrs.

Clinical features: RUQ pain, weakness, and weight loss. Hepatomegaly occurs in 90%, cachexia and ascites in 50%, abdominal venous collaterals in 30%, jaundice in 25%. There may be pathological fractures due to bone metastases and haematemesis from oesophageal varices.

Diagnosis: is clinical. CXR may show a raised R hemidiaphragm. AlkP and α-fetoprotein may be increased. Other Ix: USS, CT scan, biopsy.

Management: is usually palliative. Aim to relieve pain and reduce symptoms – eg with drainage of ascites, anti-pruritic agents, transfusions for anaemia. Chemotherapy, radiotherapy, and transplantation are disappointing. Surgical resection provides the only prospect for cure, although this is only possible in ~2% of cases at presentation. HCC may have a fulminant presentation in the tropics; death occurring within weeks of diagnosis.

Prevention: HBV vaccination.

1. van Rensburg S, 1985, *Br J Cancer*, **51**, 399–405.
2. Yu M, 1991, *J Natl Cancer Inst*, **83**, 1820–6.

Differential diagnosis of the non-smooth liver

Cystic lesions: amoebic (or other pyogenic) abscess, congenital liver cysts, polycystic liver, or hydatid cyst.
Solid lesions: are likely to be malignant. Surgical resection of small, solitary lesions may be attempted. If the patient is terminally ill, omit all investigations and concentrate on palliation.

Primary sites for liver metastases:

male	*female*	*rarer malignancies*
• stomach	• breast	• pancreas
• lung	• colon	• leukaemia
• colon	• stomach	• lymphoma
	• uterus	• carcinoid

Post-hepatic causes of jaundice

Cholestatic jaundice – is caused by blockage of the common bile duct. In the industrialized world, it is normally due to gallstones or pancreatic disease. In the tropics, however, most biliary disease is due to parasitic infection – ascariasis, clonorchiasis, or opisthorchiasis.

Intrahepatic biliary obstruction – may be caused by reaction to numerous drugs (eg chlorpromazine, isoniazid), primary biliary cirrhosis, the cholestatic phase of viral hepatitis (see above), 1° and 2° cancer, lymphoma, or pregnancy. Liver biopsy may be diagnostic. The condition is usually self-limiting, although it sometimes persists for months or years, mimicking primary biliary cirrhosis.

Fascioliasis

Fascioliasis is an animal disease that follows infection with the trematodes *Fasciola hepatica* or *F. gigantica.* Human infection is relatively rare, although epidemics do occur. Human infection occurs after the ingestion of aquatic plants, particularly wild watercress, grown in water contaminated with animal faeces. Transmission is favoured by high humidity, high rainfall, and temperatures between 10–30°C. The trematode's life cycle is similar to the *Clonorchae* (see page 382), using a snail intermediate host and attaching to aquatic plants before they are ingested by ruminants or humans. Cercariae excyst in the gut and migrate to the bile ducts, where they can live for many years.

Clinical features: are due to the host's immune response against the parasite. Although many infections are asymptomatic, there may be bile duct proliferation, dilatation, fibrosis and calcification with stone formation. Symptoms begin ~2 months after ingestion and include diarrhoea, upper abdominal pain, urticaria, malaise, fever, and night sweats. In this acute phase, there is hepatomegaly, anaemia and marked eosinophilia. Obstruction may lead to jaundice, pruritis and fatty food intolerance. In severe cases, there is ascites, profound anaemia, and haemorrhage into the bile ducts. Migration to other tissues causes nodules, granulomata and tracts. Mortality, although rare, is highest in children.

Diagnosis: eggs can be seen in the faeces by 2–4 months after infection; USS, FBC, serology, and antigen ELISA are also useful. In epidemics, ask about dietary history. ► The presence of eggs in the stool may simply indicate that the patient has eaten liver of an infected animal.

Management

1. Bithionol 10–18mg/kg PO tds on alternate days for 10–15 days. [alternative: dehydroementine 1mg/kg IM/SC daily for 10 days may be effective during the acute stage]. Both drugs and multiple courses are often required, sometimes with significant side-effects.
2. Prednisolone is helpful in severe disease
3. Give antibiotics for 2° bacterial cholangitis.

Prevention: improved hygiene, education, and where practicable, treatment of livestock.

Causes of post-hepatic jaundice

- cholestatic jaundice
- *Ascaris lumbricoides*
- *Fasciola hepatica*
- opisthorchiasis/clonorchiasis
- HIV infection
- amoebic liver abscess
- hydatid disease

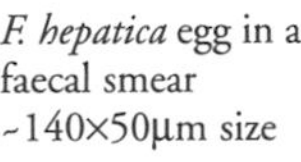

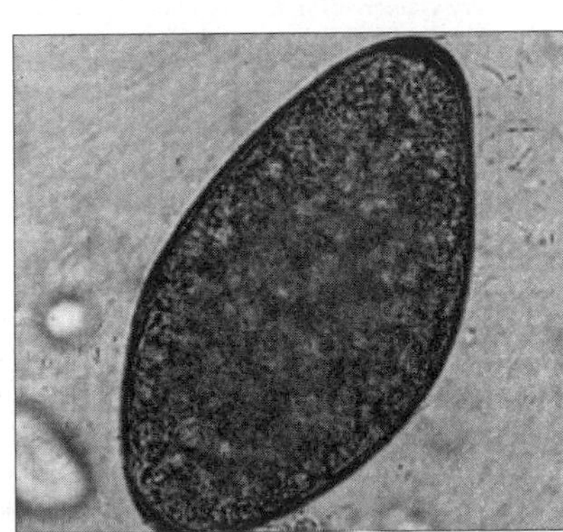

F. hepatica egg in a faecal smear ~140×50µm size

Opisthorchiasis and clonorchiasis

An estimated 200 million people are infected by the human liver flukes: *Clonorchis sinensis* (E Asia), *Opisthorchis felineus* (E Europe, N Asia), *O. viverrini* (Thailand, Laos) and *O. guayaquilensis* (Ecuador). Infection of up to 25% of the population in NE Thailand with *O. viverrini* is believed to be an important factor in their high incidence of cholangiocarcinoma.

Life cycle and transmission: eggs released by adult worms living in the biliary tree pass into the faeces with bile. The excreted parasites pass through snail before developing in fish into metacercaria which are infective to humans. The parasites are ingested by humans in uncooked fish; they then migrate from the bowel to the biliary system where they mature into adults and can live for many years. Pathology results from inflammation around retained eggs.

Clinical features: asymptomatic hepatomegaly is common, although USS often reveals gallbladder enlargement, sludge, gallstones, and poor function in such patients. Symptoms include RUQ pain, diarrhoea, loss of appetite, indigestion and fullness. In more severe cases there may be fever, eosinophilia, obstructive jaundice, weight loss, ascites and oedema. Many patients complain of a feeling of something moving within the liver. Gallstones and intrahepatic stones are common complications of clonorchiasis; the most serious complication is cholangiocarcinoma due to *O. viverrini* infection (5-fold increased risk for mild infection, 15-fold for heavy infection). *O. felineus* can cause acute opisthorchiasis, usually shortly after exposure to a large dose of metacercaria. It is characterized by fever, hepatosplenomegaly, tenderness, and eosinophilia (up to 40% of WCC).

Diagnosis: requires detection of eggs; however, eggs may not be able to pass into the gut in patients with complete obstruction. Percutaneous bile aspiration is dangerous and not recommended due to the high risk of biliary peritonitis and haemorrhage. Others: serology, antigen/DNA assays.

Management

1. Praziquantel 40mg/kg PO as a single dose is often effective.
2. Heavy *Clonorchis* infection may require up to 120mg/kg over 2 days.

Prevention: improved sanitation (preventing eggs from reaching water); education to discourage the consumption of raw fish. Molluscicidal control of snail vectors is not feasible.

Amoebic liver abscess

This is the most common form of extraintestinal amoebiasis. It may present as a complication of acute amoebic dysentery (~10%) or years after exposure with no history of diarrhoea (up to 70%).

Clinical presentation: either acutely with RUQ +/− R shoulder tip pain and hepatomegaly (abscesses may enlarge upwards into the diaphragm) or chronically with dull RUQ ache, weight loss, fatigue, low grade pyrexia and anaemia. The pain of left lobe abscesses often radiates to the left side. There may also be jaundice (usually mild), vomiting, right-sided pleural effusion/collapse, ascites or emphysema.

Life cycle of *O. viverrini*

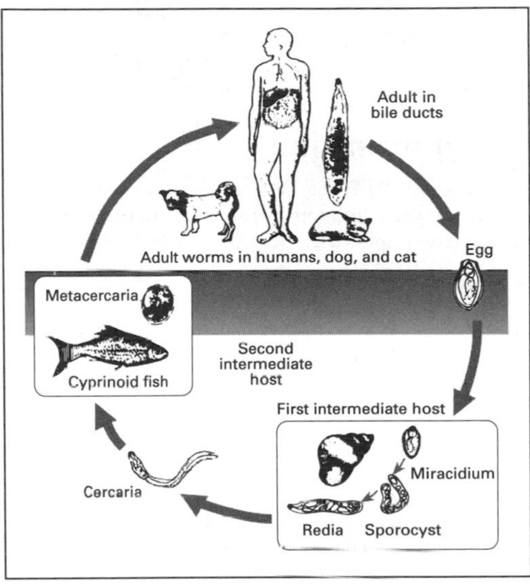

Opisthorchis sinensis egg in faecal smear. 30×15μm size

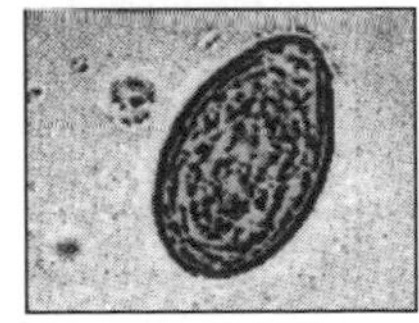

Diagnosis: USS. Stool microscopy is +ve in 50% (culture = 75%). The abscess fluid is odourless and may resemble anchovy paste. Beware misdiagnosis of the acute attack as acute cholecystitis or appendicitis.

Treatment: almost all amoebic abscesses will heal without scarring if treated with drugs +/– drainage (chapter 3D). Drainage is indicated if the abscess cavity is >6cm since there is a risk of perforation and high mortality. ~1% of abscesses, especially those of the left hepatic lobe, involve the pericardium; this requires open drainage (40% mortality).

Hepatomegaly without jaundice

May be due to:

- portal hypertension
- schistosomiasis
- Chagas disease
- sarcoid
- tricuspid incompetence
- trypanosomiasis
- toxocariasis
- beri beri
- hydatid disease
- kwashiorkor
- fascioliasis
- plague
- bartonellosis
- visceral leishmaniasis

Portal hypertension

Portal hypertension (PHT) can be a sequel to any chronic liver disease, although cirrhosis and schistosomiasis are the most common causes in the tropics. It is useful to split causes according to the level of obstruction:

Causes of portal hypertension

Pre-hepatic

- hyperreactive malarial splenomegaly
- portal vein occlusion (lymphoma, pancreatic CA)
- splenic vein occlusion (following umbilical sepsis)
- severe dehydration (cholera, dysentery).

Hepatic (sinusoidal)

- cirrhosis
- schistosomiasis (*S. mansoni* or *S. japonicum*)
- hepatocellular carcinoma
- veno-occlusive disease
- congenital hepatic fibrosis
- drugs (eg dapsone)
- sarcoidosis.

Post-hepatic

- cardiac dysfunction (eg due to RF or TB)
- constrictive pericarditis (endomyocardial fibrosis)
- inferior vena cava obstruction
- hepatic vein thrombosis (Budd-Chiari syndrome eg during pregnancy).

Clinical features: the most serious complication is oesophageal varices which may carry a 70% mortality if they rupture. Signs of PHT include hepatosplenomegaly, *caput medusae*, haemorrhoids, haematemesis or melaena (sign of bleeding oesophageal/gastric varices). See p351.

Management: where possible, treat the cause. Oral β-blockade (propanolol) can lower portal (as well as systemic) pressure and reduce the incidence of bleeding varices. Neither intensive sclerotherapy nor surgical insertion of porto-systemic bypass shunts have shown benefit.

Veno-occlusive disease: caused by ingestion of pyrrolizidine alkaloids contained in certain herbal teas (eg *Helotropium, Crotalaria* and *Senecio*) are an important cause of thrombosis and PHT[1] in Jamaica, S Africa, central Asia and SW USA.

Sites of blockage and veins affected by PHT

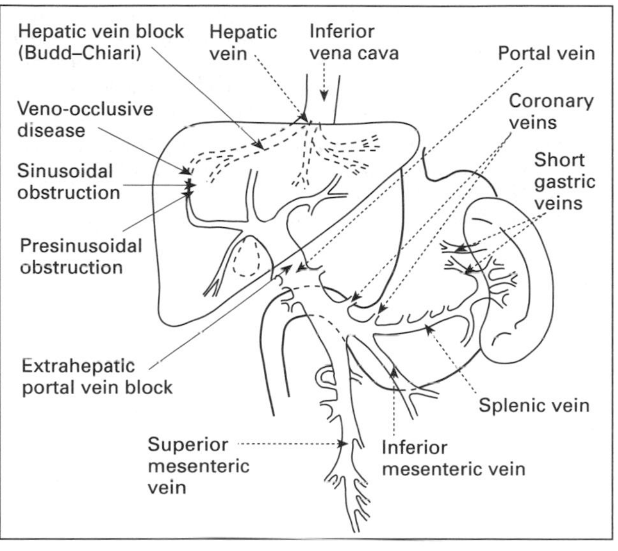

Child's grading of PHT severity

Grade	Serum bilirubin	Serum albumin	Ascites/ encephalopathy	Operative mortality
A	normal	>35g/l	none	2%
B	20–50µmol/l	30–35g/l	mild	10%
C	>50µmol/l	<30g/l	severe	50%

1. *Oxford Textbook of Hepatology*, OUP: Oxford, p1004

Schistosomiasis (bilharzia)

A common, chronically debilitating and potentially lethal disease affecting ~200 million people worldwide. It is second only to malaria in socio-economic importance, with ~600 million people at risk.

It is caused in humans by infection with the mammalian blood flukes or trematodes *Schistosoma mansoni, S. japonicum, S. haematobium* (and occasionally *S. mekongi* and *S. intercalatum*). In the majority of cases, infections are light or moderate; however, *S. haematobium* and *S. mansoni* infections tend to be more serious. It is usually a slow insidious disease but can be lethal and may potentiate other diseases (hepatitis, cirrhosis, bladder CA).

Life cycle: transmission occurs when humans are exposed to water infested with the intermediate snail host while swimming, washing, or collecting water. Schistosome cercariae released from the snails penetrate human skin and enter blood vessels, passing via the lungs to the liver where they mature into adults. The adults mate and start producing eggs, which the female will continue to do for the rest of her life. Some of the eggs pass into the urinary tract (*S. haematobium*) or into the bowel (other species) before being passed in urine or faeces to the outside world. Other eggs embolize in the blood to various sites (eg lungs, liver, CNS) where they stimulate a strong immune response, causing immunopathological disease.

Because adult worms do not multiply in humans, the level of infection and disease is proportional to the extent of exposure. Usually there is a slow rate of accumulation and presentation occurs only after many years. Infection peaks in early adult life with males and females equally affected. However, prevalence and intensity of infection decrease in older age groups due to behavioural changes (↓ water contact) and acquired immunity.

Clinical effects

1. **Early reaction (swimmers' itch):** occurs ~1 day after infection. It is a pruritic papular rash with oedema, erythema, and eosinophilia caused by death of cercariae upon skin penetration. It resolves spontaneously within 10 days and is rare in endemic areas.
2. **Katayama fever (acute toxaemic schistosomiasis):** is a rare, but potentially lethal serum-sickness illness (immune complex mediated) occurring 1–3mths after 1° infection (usually *S. japonicum*). Features include fever, chills, sweating, anorexia, headache, diarrhoea, cough, hepatosplenomegaly, lymphadenopathy, and urticaria. ***Ix*** show eosinophilia, ↑ IgG, IgA, IgM, +/− immune-complex glomerulopathy. The illness is more common in non-immunes and usually subsides after several weeks (although egg output may remain high).
3. **Chronic disease** egg-induced chronic granulomatous inflammation and fibrosis affects many organs. Often asymptomatic, it may present with fatigue, fever, abdominal pain and diarrhoea.

   • ***Pulmonary disease*** – embolizing eggs cause arteritis and pulmonary blood flow obstruction, leading to pulmonary hypertension. There may be fatigue, syncope, chest pain, raised JVP, tricuspid incompetence, and ultimately cor pulmonale.

Distribution of *S. haematobium, S. japonicum and S. mekongi*

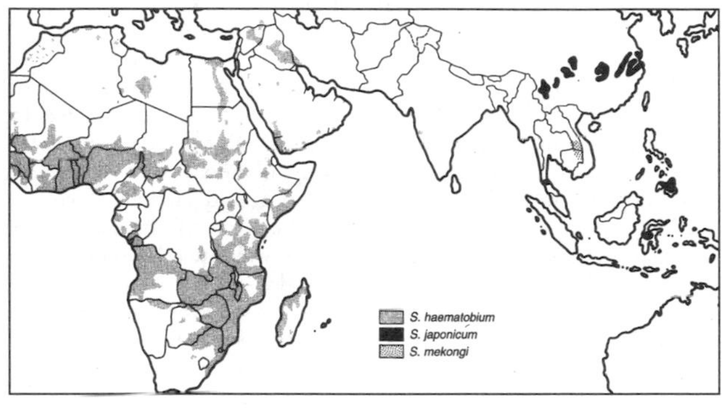

Distribution of *S. mansoni and S. intercalatum*

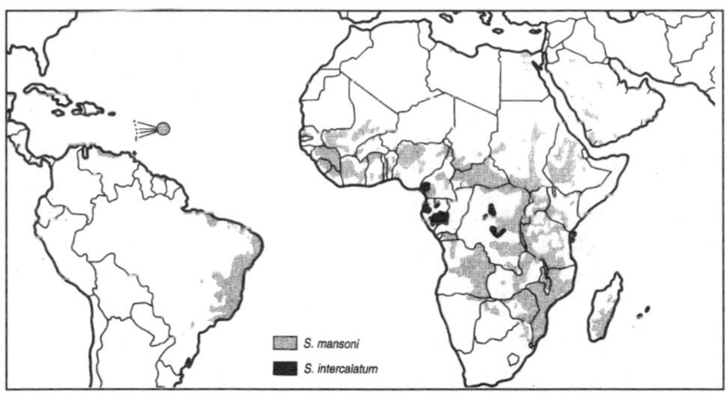

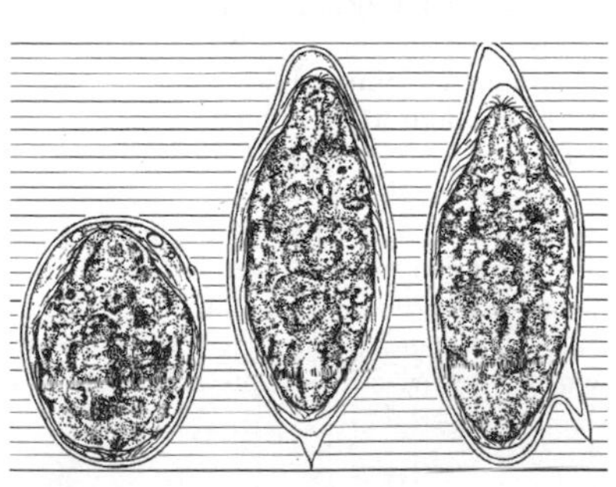

Schematic representation of *S. japonicum, S. haematobium* and *S. mansoni* (from left to right). Total height is 150μm, width 170μm.

- ***Hepatic disease*** – often occurs in the left lobe. Features include portal hypertension and portal-systemic collateral circulation, hepatosplenomegaly (often severe, presenting with RUQ mass), ascites, oesophageal/gastric varices. Liver enzymes are usually normal, with few stigmata of chronic hepatic disease, although in endemic areas hepatosplenic decompensated schistosomiasis may develop in which liver enzymes are abnormal. Hypersplenism may result in pancytopaenia and reduced RBC life-span.
- ***Intestinal disease*** – eggs may reach both the superior and inferior mesenteric venous plexi (and superior haemorrhoidal veins in *S. japonicum* disease) and pass through to the intestinal mucosa to involve both small and large bowel. Chronic inflammation of the large bowel may cause intermittent, bloody diarrhoea with tenesmus, pseudopolyp formation, hypoalbuminaemia, and anaemia, giving a clinical picture similar to that of ulcerative colitis/proctitis. A 'bilharzioma' is a mass of schistosomal eggs, which may be found in the omentum and/or mesenteric lymph nodes. Other features include protein-losing enteropathy, intussusception, and rectal prolapse.
- ***CNS disease*** – is a rare but severe complication of *S. japonicum* and *S. mansoni* disease. Eggs of the former may embolize to the brain to cause meningoencephalitis or focal epilepsy. *S. mansoni* eggs embolize to the spinal cord, causing cauda equina, a transverse myelitis-like syndrome, paraplegia, or bladder dysfunction. Both may present as a space-occupying lesion or encephalitis, although most are asymptomatic.
- ***Other sites*** – very rarely there is placental, genital, arthropathic, or cutaneous schistosomiasis.
- **Salmonella *superinfection*** – *Salmonella* spp may colonize the adult worms, providing a source for bacteraemic episodes.

Diagnosis: rests upon a history of exposure (? itch or fever), clinical signs +/– demonstration of eggs in the urine/faeces or rectal biopsy specimen. Collected eggs may be hatched in fresh water to demonstrate miracidia. Other methods include serology; sigmoidoscopy or Ba enema for intestinal disease; liver biopsy, Ba swallow, oesophagoscopy, USS, and splenoportography for liver disease; CT or myelography for CNS lesions.

Prevention: no repellents, vaccines or prophylactic drugs are yet available. Avoid coming into contact with fresh water (even flowing or deep water), although very fast water with little vegetation (and therefore snails) is likely to be less infective. Beware so-called 'safe lakes' (classically Lake Malawi) or unchlorinated swimming pools. If contact is unavoidable, keep it to a minimum (eg wear boots) and follow with rapid, vigorous drying which may kill cercariae not fully penetrated. Infectivity of cercariae is lost in water left standing for ~20hrs.

At a community level, break the human snail cycle by cleaning and isolating water supplies (however, this is rarely cost-effective). Avoid urination and defaecation near open water. Molluscicides are difficult to implement and ecologically destructive. ► Human treatment and education are the most effective means of prevention.

Management of schistosomiasis

Total cure is reasonable in non-endemic areas but usually unfeasible in endemic areas due to the high risk of re-infection. Egg-count studies have shown that in cases where full cure is not achieved by appropriate treatment, egg production is nevertheless decreased by over 90%.

1. **Early reaction:** antihistamine ointment or tablets may help although they are usually unnecessary.
2. **Katayama fever:** treatment is difficult since most drugs do not affect the early migratory phase of the immature parasites. Give oral prednisolone to suppress the acute reaction, then give praziquantel 75mg/kg PO as a single dose.
3. **Chronic disease:**
   Praziquantel – is effective against all schistosome species (as well as cestodes and other snail-borne trematodes).
   For most species, give 40mg/kg PO as a single dose; for *S. japonicum* give 20mg/kg PO tds for one day only; *S. mekongi* may require repeated doses. In CNS disease give 75mg/kg. Paediatric dosage is the same. Cure rate is ~70%. If possible give the single doses after food.
   Oxamniquine – is cheaper but only effective against *S. mansoni*. Give 15mg/kg PO as a single dose in W Africa and Brazil. In the rest of Africa, give 20mg/kg PO daily for 3 days.
   Metriphonate – is used to treat *S. haematobium* infections. Give 7.5–10mg/kg PO on three days, each 2 weeks apart.
4. Surgical treatment is not recommended – most seemingly irreversible lesions will eventually resolve, especially in the young. Even CNS disease may show resolution after treatment.

Toxocariasis

The canine roundworm – *Toxocara canis* – has a worldwide distribution. Although adult worms do not develop in man, the larvae may persist for >10 years, causing toxocariasis, visceral larva migrans, and ocular disease.

Life cycle: Eggs excreted in dog faeces (particularly from puppies) are ingested by humans. These hatch in the stomach, releasing larvae which penetrate the intestinal mucosa, entering the mesenteric blood vessels. They may remain in the visceral organs or pass through into the general circulation and reach the brain, eye, and other organs.

Clinical features: symptoms depend upon the density of infection.

- ***Visceral larva migrans:*** inflammation and granulomatous reactions in heavy infections of the liver and other organs (eg lungs, brain) results in hepatomegaly, fever, or asthma. Severe cases may have cardiac dysfunction, nephrosis, fits, pareses, and transverse myelitis. The condition usually occurs in children. Most resolve within 2 years, although the disease can be fatal, particularly if the brain is involved.
- ***Ocular toxocariasis:*** subretinal granulomata and choroiditis closely resemble a retinoblastoma in the early stages and tend to occur in the older age groups. Symptoms include strabismus and iridocyclitis with posterior synechiae. The disease is an important cause of decreased visual acuity in the tropics.
- Infected children commonly also harbour *Ascaris* and *Trichrurus* spp; 2° infection with gut bacteria carried by the larvae is also common.

Diagnosis: history of exposure (particularly to puppies), eosinophilia, leukocytosis, reduced albumin:globulin ratio, raised IgG, IgM, anti-A and anti-B isohaemagglutinin titres. CXR may show mottling in lung disease. Larval demonstration is very difficult, though they are sometimes present at the centre of granulomatous lesions at biopsy or post mortem. ELISA tests for antigen are now available.

Treatment

1. Diethylcarbamazine 2–3mg/kg PO tds for 3 weeks
   [alternative: thiabendazole 50mg/kg daily in 3 divided doses for 7–28 days, depending upon tolerance].
2. Steroids may be required for ocular disease.

Prevention: centres around elimination of the infective canine reservoir, with human treatment of symptomatic cases and education regarding child hygiene.

Gastroenterology

Hydatid disease

Echinococcus granulosus and *E. multilocularis* are responsible for causing cystic hydatid disease and alveolar hydatid disease, respectively.

1. Cystic hydatid disease

E. granulosus is a small (3–6mm) cestode tapeworm that lives in the small intestine of dogs and occasionally other carnivores. Eggs passed in canine faeces are infective to humans; following ingestion, they develop into larvae which penetrate the intestinal mucosa and pass to target organs such as the liver (50%), lungs and peritoneal cavity. There the larvae (oncospheres) mature and form an expanding, fluid-filled metacestode vesicle, or hydatid cyst. These may be multiple and reach massive proportions.

Clinical features: are usually due to the expansive growth of cysts and commonly include abdominal pain, hepatomegaly, fever, jaundice, and cholangitis. Rupture can be life-threatening and may be accompanied by anaphylactic shock, although conversely, cysts may disappear or collapse spontaneously.

Diagnosis: USS is usually sufficient. Drainage may show characteristic hydatid sand (protoscolices), ► but because of the high risk of spreading the protoscolices around the body, such aspiration is not recommended. Serological and molecular tests are also available.

Management: cystectomy offers the best chance of cure. However, spillage of cystic contents at surgery causes disease to recur, so great care is needed. Chlorhexidine, hydrogen peroxide, ethanol, and cetrizamide can be used to sterilize the cyst before operation (formalin or hypertonic saline should no longer be used since they may cause tissue damage, hypernatraemia and severe acidosis). Albendazole, mebendazole and praziquantel are believed to be parasitostatic agents, though reliable data are still lacking. Use pre- and post-operatively is thought to give lower recurrence rates, but doses may need to be high (4.5g/day mebendazole or 20mg/kg/day albendazole) and for many months. Life expectancy in successfully operated patients is normal, though those presenting with complications (especially cholangitis) have significant mortality.

2. Alveolar hydatid disease

Alveolar hydatid disease is restricted to the northern hemisphere; it is not a tropical disease. *E.multilocularis* infects humans via their accidental ingestion of faeces from foxes or other canines. After digestion of the eggs, oncospheres penetrate the intestinal mucosa and passes to the liver (a few pass to other sites including the lungs and brain). Maturation produces a characteristic alveolar cyst. Patients present with abdominal pain, hepatomegaly, and sometimes cholangitis. Unlike *E.granulosus*, the cysts expand externally and invade surrounding tissue, resembling a malignant tumour. Metastatic spread occurs in ~10% of patients to CNS, lungs, bone and eyes. Mortality untreated is high, >60% at 10yrs. Surgery requires early presentation to be successful; mebendazole and albendazole may be beneficial but the data is not clear as yet.

Distribution of cystic hydatid disease

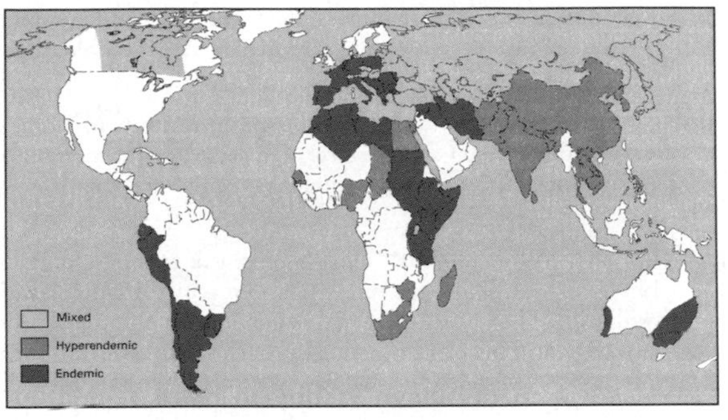

Life cycle of *E. granulosus*

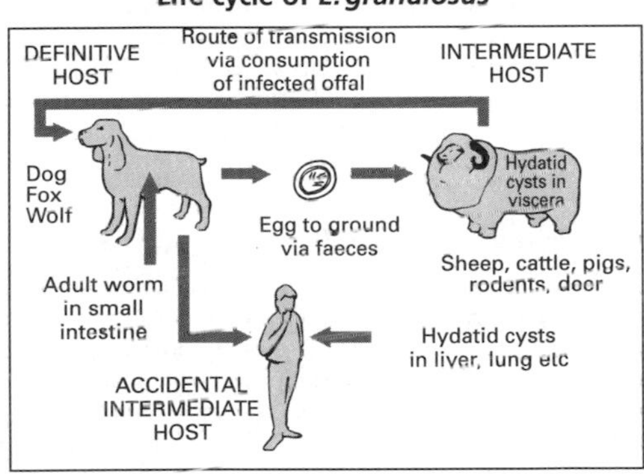

Lower GI bleeding

Lower GI bleeding is seen less frequently than upper GI bleeding in the tropics, but tends to be more difficult to diagnose and manage. Patients present with haematochezia – red, maroon or brownish stools – rather than haematemesis or melaena.

Always perform a thorough abdominal examination and PR examination in any patient with rectal bleeding and exclude other pathology, even if haemorrhoids are present.

Causes: the most frequent causes of lower GI bleeding (without diarrhoea) are typhoid fever, non-specific ulcer, TB, neoplasms, amoebic ulcer, angiodysplasia, others (diverticulosis, ulcerative colitis). Exclude haemorrhoids.

Diagnosis and management: initially consist of resuscitation as for upper GI haemorrhage. Then determine if it is an acute or chronic problem (Hb will help). The history and examination may reveal other features of diseases such as typhoid fever or TB. The colour of the stool is the best indicator of the level at which the causative pathology lies; the darker the stool, the higher the cause. Rectal bleeding leaves bright red streaks of blood on the stool surface. Pass a NG tube if small bowel pathology is suspected; a bile-stained aspirate that is free of blood excludes an upper GI source. Use proctoscopy and sigmoidoscopy to examine the rectum and sigmoid colon. In many cases bleeding will cease with bed rest, IV fluid, and 24hrs nil by mouth. Prolonged bleeding will necessitate further investigation eg with colonoscopy. The patient should be transferred to theatre for exploratory laparotomy if >6 units of blood are needed to replace that lost.

Diverticular disease

A diverticulum is a congenital or acquired outpouching of the gut wall. Most develop when raised intra-luminal pressures force the mucosa to herniate through the muscular layers of the gut wall and present with changed bowel habit, colicky RIF pain (relieved by defaecation), and painless rectal bleeding. Diverticulae can become infected – diverticulitis, giving fever, ↑ WCC and ↑ ESR. Exclude typhoid fever. Treat with bed rest, high fibre diet, and (if infected) antibiotics. Watch for signs of perforation (>40% mortality).

Colorectal carcinoma

Colorectal carcinoma remains uncommon in the tropics. Aetiology includes high fat, low fibre diet, prolonged colonic transit time, polyposis coli and ulcerative colitis. Tumours are annular, polypoid or ulcerous and are staged using Duke's classification. Clinical features are frequently of a change in bowel habit, diarrhoea, blood/mucus PR, and tenesmus. A mass (commonly left-sided) may be felt. Late presentation may be with obstruction or perforation.

Diagnosis and treatment: faecal occult blood, +/– anaemia, pr, procto-colonoscopy with biopsy, where available. The prognosis is poor and surgical resection offers the only hope of cure.

Inflammatory bowel disease (IBD)

Both Crohn's disease and ulcerative colitis are rare in the tropics, although cases have been reported from South Africa and the Indian sub-continent. IBD presents as weight loss, bloody diarrhoea with mucus and associated problems of joint, skin and ocular inflammation, pyoderma gangrenosum, anorectal fissures/fistulae, intestinal obstruction and toxic dilatation of the colon. Diagnosis requires colon-/sigmoidoscopy with biopsy.

Management: of the acute case is with systemic steroids (or topical if disease is localized to the rectum) and life-long sulphasalizine. Complicated cases and those unresponsive to high-dose steroids need surgical treatment.

Haemorrhoids (piles)

Haemorrhoids are prolapsing anal cushions (usually at the 3, 7 & 11 o'clock positions) normally associated with constipation. Haemorrhoids present with bright red bleeding PR, prolapse and discomfort (may be severe if thrombosis occurs) and are classified as follows: •*First degree*: prolapse down the anal canal but not out of it, therefore only recognized at proctoscopy. Treatment is by injection sclerotherapy with 2ml of 5% phenol in oil. Encourage a high fibre diet and avoidance of straining at defaecation. •*Second degree*: prolapse through the anus but reduce spontaneously. Treatment is with sclerotherapy or rubber band ligation. •*Third degree*: As above but require digital reduction. •*Fourth degree*: remain permanently prolapsed.

Management: is with rubber band ligation or haemorrhoidectomy. Thrombosed piles are treated with analgesia and bed rest. The clot may be expressed under local anaesthetic, usually relieving the pain. NB varicocities of the anal canal may occur in severe portal hypertension.

Around the anus

Pruritus ani – may be caused by:

- skin infection or damage such as enterobiasis, tinea cruris, psoriasis, contact dermatitis, lichen planus, lichen sclerosis, leukoplakia, *Corynebacterium minutissimum*;
- surgical conditions such as haemorrhoids, fissure-in-ano, fistula, skin-tags, polyps and carcinoma.

Enterobiasis (threadworm, pinworm)

The soil-transmitted helminth *Enterobius vermicularis* is a common world-wide infection of young children.

Life cycle: infection occurs either by faeco-oral contact (possibly from eggs contaminating dust or bed linen) or by retroinfection in which larvae hatching at the anus migrate back upwards into the bowel. Ingested ova hatch in the stomach and larvae migrate to the appendix and caecum where they invade the crypts and mature in to adult worms (9–12mm long by 2–4mm wide). The female migrates to the anus (usually at night) and lays eggs on the perianal skin and perineum, which are then carried on the faeces or picked up under the finger nails during scratching. There is no multiplication inside the body. The cycle takes about 2–4 weeks.

Clinical features: in the majority of cases, infected individuals are asymptomatic until the female deposits her eggs perianally. This induces intense pruritus. General symptoms include insomnia, restlessness, loss of appetite and weight; children are often irritable and frequently have enuresis. Worms can enter the vulva and cause vulvitis with a mucoid discharge and pruritus. Worms may also be found in the ears and nose. Very rarely the worms gain access to the abdominal cavity and cause chronic peritonitis and granulomata. 2° infection of skin damaged by scratching is a common problem.

Diagnosis: requires detection of eggs in the faeces, on swabs from either the perianal region (use sellotape) or under the fingernails, or the demonstration of adult worms around the anus (usually with an 'element of surprise', at night!).

Management: since reinfection is virtually inevitable in most cases, unless there is simultaneous change in behaviour, treatment is really only beneficial in symptomatic individuals. Where possible, treat the whole family and school members. A single dose of albendazole 400mg (10–14mg/kg in children) or mebendazole 100mg is sufficient.

Prevention: simple measures are the key to preventing reinfection: improving personal hygiene and scrubbing of children's hands before meals and after defaecation, keeping fingernails short, and regular washing of bedclothes.

Life cycle of *E. vermicularis*

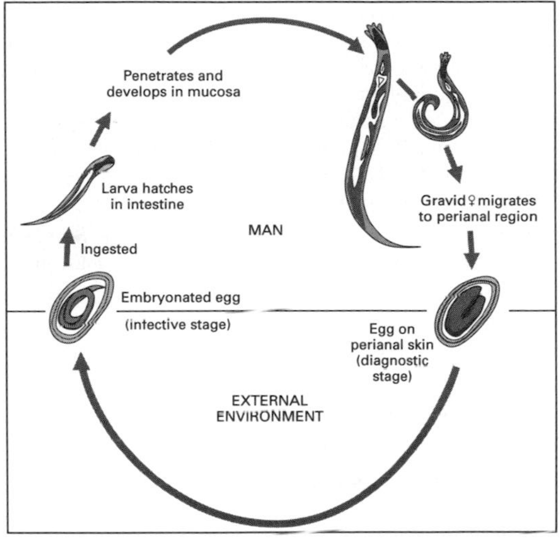

Visible 'worms' in stool

1. Beef tapeworm – *Taenia saginata*

Mature proglottids of the bovine tapeworm *Taenia saginata* are highly motile and conspicuous in the faeces of infected individuals. Occasionally, they may be felt emerging independently from the anus, causing some distress. The adult worm is typically 3–5 metres long (though some reach 10m) and attaches via suckers to the upper small intestine wall. Humans are the only definitive host and usually acquire infection from eating raw or undercooked beef containing a larva-filled cysticercus. Adult worms may shed up to 50,000 eggs per day for 10 years or more. Patients may complain of vague abdominal pain, distension, anorexia and nausea, although infection is often asymptomatic.

Diagnosis: eosinophilia is not usually a feature. Eggs may be seen on faecal microscopy. Intact proglottids (~16×8mm) may sometimes also be speciated.

Treatment
1. Praziquantel 10mg/kg PO as a single dose is highly effective.

Prevention: centres on properly cooking beef (cysts are destroyed by temperatures >48°C) and disposing of human faeces away from areas where cattle (the intermediate hosts) feed.

2. Pork tapeworm – *Taenia solium*

Cysts are eaten in poorly cooked pork (the intermediate host) and mature in the small intestine. The adult worm measures 2–3m (upto 8m) and attaches to the mucosal surface by two encircling rows of hooklets. Unlike *T. saginata*, humans are also readily infected by the larval form of the tapeworm after ingesting eggs excreted by a human carrier (often auto-infection from faecal-oral contamination), causing human cysticercosis (chapter 9). Symptoms of adult worm infection are as for *T. saginata*; the proglottids being smaller (~12×6mm) and less motile.

Treatment
1. Praziquantel 10mg/kg PO as a single dose is highly effective.

3. Dwarf tapeworm – *Hymenolepsis nana*

Measuring 3–4cm, *H. nana* is seldom seen in the stool, but may give rise to abdominal symptoms as for other tapeworms. However, unlike the other tapeworms, *H. nana* has both larval and adult stages in humans and does not require intermediate hosts. Infection with several hundred worms is common. Since encystation occurs within small-intestinal villi, there is immune stimulation resulting in eosinophilia. Characteristic eggs are seen on faecal microscopy.

Treatment
1. Praziquantel 20mg/kg PO as a single dose is highly effective.

Life cycle of *T. saginata*

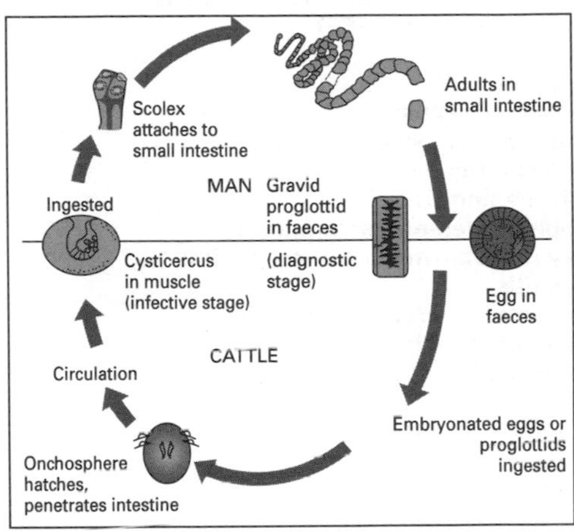

Egg of *H. nana* (30×45μm) and of *T. solium* (30–45μm diameter)

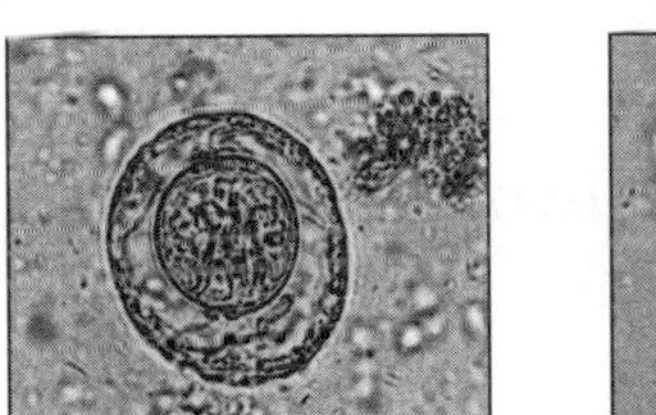

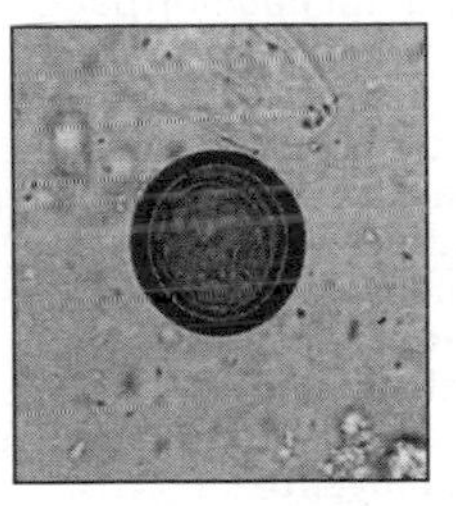

9. Neurology

Acute confusional state 402
Dementia 402
Coma 404
Management of an unconscious patient 406
Glasgow coma score (GCS) 407
Headache 408
Rising intracranial pressure 410
Bacterial meningitis 412
Epidemic meningococcal disease 414
Viral meningitis 414
Chronic meningitis 416
Eosinophilic meningoencephalitis 416
Primary amoebic meningoencephalitis 416
Encephalitis 418
Herpes simplex virus encephalitis 418
Japanese encephalitis 418
Equine encephalitides 419
Rabies 420
Management of rabies infection 422
Tetanus 424
Management of tetanus 426
Stroke 428
Stroke rehabilitation 430
Subarachnoid haemorrhage (SAH) 434
Subdural haemorrhage 434
Extradural haematoma 436
How to do a burr hole 436
Blackouts 438
Space-occupying lesions (SOL) 438
Hydrocephalus 438
Epilepsy 440
Status epilepticus 444
Cysticercosis 446
Weak legs/paraplegia, non-traumatic 448
Poliomyelitis 450
Guillain-Barre syndrome (GBS) 450
Mono/polyneuropathies 452
WHO Differential diagnosis of acute flaccid paralysis 453
Leprosy (Hansen's disease) 454

Neurology

Acute confusional state (ACS)

Clinical features: ►clouding of consciousness is the most important sign. Patients also have a short attention span and are easily distractable. They may be disorientated in time and place. They often appear bewildered and have impaired immediate recall and recent memory.
► Check carefully for signs of reduced consciousness, particularly drowsiness. This may be a warning of impending coma (see page 404). Psychiatric causes of confusion (eg schizophrenia, paranoid state) and early dementia do not present with drowsiness.

Delirium – is more florid than an acute confusional state. It also manifests typically with disorientation, confusion, and reduced attention but, in addition, the patient is often frightened, irritable, and more profoundly disorientated. The patient may have frightening hallucinations and/or delusions, and exhibit aggressive behaviour.

Causes: see box opposite. Most common causes will vary with age.

- Systemic infection
  check chest, urinary tract, surgical wounds, IV cannula sites, CSF.
- Chronic subdural haematoma may present with ACS.

Management

1. Treat cause if one can be recognized.
2. If at night, turn the lights on to decrease the patient's confusion.
3. Give 50ml of 50% dextrose IV if hypoglycaemia is suspected.
4. Treat disturbed behaviour with chlopromazine 25–50mg IM/PO q6h or haloperidol 1.5–5mg IM/PO q6h
5. Avoid benzodiazepines

Nursing is very important in ACS – if possible, use a well lit room with familiar staff. Attempt to reassure the patient.

Dementia

Unlike confusional states and delirium, there is no disturbance of consciousness in dementia. It is a chronic or progressive condition characterized by impairment of higher mental function (eg memory, reasoning, comprehension) and emotional and behavioural changes. Common causes are Alzheimer's disease and multiple strokes (vascular dementia).

Uncommon but treatable causes include communicating hydrocephalus; vitamin B_{12} or B_1 deficiency; hypothyroidism; syphilis; cysticercosis; brain tumour; chronic subdural haematoma. [HIV can cause a dementia which is responsive to antiretroviral therapy.]

Management: ► identify the few patients with treatable causes. Aim to supply others with general support so that they may have the highest quality of life possible. Remember that the family will also need support. Information useful to Alzheimer's disease patients and their carers is available on the web at <www.alz.org>.

Common causes of acute confusion/delirium at presentation (they may all progress to coma)

- CNS infection (cerebral malaria, meningitis, encephalitis, HIV related infections)
- systemic infections
- hypoxia
- metabolic causes eg hypoglycaemia, hyperglycaemia
- alcohol – excess or withdrawal
- drugs
- head injury/concussion
- stroke
- mental illness such as schizophrenia
- raised intracranial pressure
- epilepsy (post-ictal)

Coma

A persistent pathological state of unconsciousness. ► In the comatose patient immediately ensure a clear airway, check that they are breathing, establish haemodynamic stability, and check for life-threatening injuries.

Take a history from relatives or bystanders – did anyone see how the patient became unconscious? Is there any past medical history such as diabetes, alcohol abuse, or drug overdose that might explain the coma?

Examine the patient in an attempt to distinguish metabolic causes of coma from brainstem causes – see below. ► It is particularly important to identify coma due to brainstem compression since surgical relief of the enlarging mass may be urgently required. Use the Glasgow coma score (GCS) – see page 407.

Useful clinical features:

• Fever	→	meningitis or encephalitis
	→	cerebral malaria
	→	metabolic coma of infection
• Hypothermia	→	hypothyroidism; hypothermic coma
• Hypertension	→	coma may be due to stroke
• Hypotension	→	shock
• Pallor, cyanosis	→	metabolic disease
• Bleeding, bruising	→	head trauma.

► Progressive deterioration suggests brainstem compression.
Look for focal CNS signs. Search for asymmetry, for example in response to pain or in the face during expiration. If the response to pain is different, the side with lower response in the GCS is the side with hemiparesis.

Diagnosis – three broad categories

1. *Metabolic*

Normal pupil responses
Normal or absent eye movements depending on the depth of coma
Suppressed Cheyne-Stokes or ketotic respiration
Symmetrical limb signs, usually hypotonic.

2. *Intrinsic brainstem disease* – *from the outset there there may be*

Abnormal pupil responses and eye movements
Abnormal respiratory pattern
Bilateral long tract signs
Cranial nerve signs.

3. Extrinsic brainstem disease due to compression

Papilloedema and hemiparesis *with progressive*
- Loss of pupillary responses
- Loss of eye movements
- Abnormal respiratory pattern
- Long tract signs.

Neurology

Management of an unconscious patient

1. **ABC:** ensure adequate airway, oxygenation, and circulation.

2. **Obtain a reliable history:** check for signs of injury or trauma especially to the head. Record the vital signs: temp, pulse, BP, respiratory rate, oxygen saturations. Do a BM stick to determine blood glucose.

3. **Assess the level of coma:** use the Glasgow coma score (see opposite). Check for meningism, pupillary light reflex, corneal reflexes, fundi, and focal neurological signs in the limbs. Do brain stem reflexes, Doll's eye movements, and caloric tests if brain death is suspected.

4. **Investigate:** do the following – Hb, WCC, urea, electrolytes, glucose, calcium, liver enzymes, and arterial gases. Also do blood cultures if the patient is febrile, a malarial film if the patient is from an area endemic for malaria, a toxicology screen if it is an overdose or poisoning case, or a CSF examination if there is meningism (beware rising intracranial pressure). Do ECG, EEG. X-ray the skull and chest, CT the head if indicated and available.

5. **Determine the cause and treat:**

- ***Coma with focal signs*** – eg subdural or extradural haematoma or space-occupying lesion may require definitive neurosurgical drainage and steroids, mannitol, etc, to lower intracranial pressure.
- ***Coma without focal signs*** – eg hypoglycaemia (give 50% glucose IV); opiate poisoning (give IV naloxone); cerebral malaria (give quinine); overdose (give gastric lavage and/or appropriate antidote).
- ***Coma and meningism*** – eg meningitis or subarachnoid haemorrhage, treat with antibiotics.

6. **Care:** nurse in the ITU or high dependency ward.
    - Monitor the level of consciousness using the Glasgow coma score.
    - Determine pupillary size, equality, and response to light.
    - Check vital signs.

    These should all be done at regular fixed intervals varying from every 15 minutes to every four hours depending on the clinical situation. Pay special attention to respiration, circulation, skin, bladder, and bowels.

7. **Prognosis:** depends mainly on the cause, depth, and duration of the coma. The combination of the absence of the pupillary light reflex and corneal and brain stem reflexes at 24hrs indicates a grave prognosis. The persistence of deep coma for greater than 72hrs also has a poor prognosis.

With thanks to W Howlett.

Glasgow coma score (GCS)

Assess on admission and then at regular intervals to follow progress and predict prognosis.

Best motor response

6 Carries out request (obeys a command)
5 Localizes pain
4 Withdraws limb in response to pain
3 Flexes limb in response to pain
2 Extends limb in response to pain
1 Does not respond to pain.

Best verbal response

5 Oriented in time and place
4 Responds with confused but understandable speech
3 Spontaneous speech but inappropriate and not responsive
2 Speech but incomprehensible
1 No speech.

Eye opening

4 Opens eyes spontaneously
3 Opens eyes in response to speech
2 Opens eyes in reponse to pain
1 Does not open her eyes.

Add together the best response in each group. Roughly

GCS	1 – 8	=	serious injury
GCS	9 – 12	=	moderate injury
GCS	13 – 15	=	minor injury

A simpler version can also be useful:

A Alert
V Responds to vocal stimuli
P Responds to pain
U Unresponsive

Headache

The brain parenchyma is insensitive to pain. Headaches result from distension, traction, or inflammation of the cerebral blood vessels and dura mater. Pain is referred from the anterior and middle cranial fossae to the forehead and eye via the trigeminal nerve and from the posterior fossa and upper cervical spine to the occiput and neck via the upper three cervical nerves. Both infratentorial and supratentorial masses can lead to frontal headaches by causing hydrocephalus.

► The major responsibility of a physician faced with a patient with a headache is to exclude a structural or dynamic cause. Specifically exclude either a space-occupying lesion (SOL) or meningitis. Check for:

• localizing signs • papilloedema • neck stiffness • rash.

Causes of a headache

1. **Acute meningeal irritation** – due to subarachnoid haemorrhage or meningitis caused by bacteria, viruses, fungi, or metastases.
2. **Rising intracranial pressure** – see next page.
3. **Many infectious diseases** cause a headache during the acute phase. Locally important infections need to be determined but examples include malaria, trypanosomiasis, and typhoid, arboviral, typhus fevers.
4. **Giant-cell arteritis** – may rapidly result in blindness. Occurs in elderly people; there may be a tender engorged occipital or temple artery; ESR is markedly raised. Biopsy confirms the diagnosis, but do not delay giving steroids while waiting for the biopsy.
5. **Migraine** – headaches which occur at intervals (not daily) and are associated with N&V, anorexia, photophobia, phonophobia, and in 20% of cases visual, mood, sensory, or motor disturbances. Most individuals have their first attack while young. Identify and avoid precipitating factors; give analgesia (paracetamol, NSAIDs, or codeine) together with metoclopromide 10mg (not in children). Ergotamine is useful in 50% of patients. Chemoprophylaxis may work for regular migraines.
6. **Tension headache** – commonest cause of headache. It is normally a benign symptom due to an identifiable cause: eg overwork, family stress, lack of sleep, or emotional crisis. It is often a daily occurrence unlike migraine headache, getting worse as the day goes on. Visual disturbances, vomiting, and photophobia do not occur. Management involves thorough examination and reassurance of its benign course, analgesia (usually paracetamol 1g qds), and rest. Ask about drugs, caffeine, and alcohol. Amitriphylline starting at 10mg week, increasing by 10mg/week until side effects occur, is also often of benefit.

   ► Tension headaches may be part of a **depressive illness**. Check for other signs or symptoms such as mood change, loss of appetite, weight or libido, or a disturbed sleep pattern.
7. **Others:** •trauma •cluster headaches •hypertension •drugs •indomethacin-sensitive headaches.
8. **Pain may be referred** to the forehead and temple from the orbits, paranasal sinuses, teeth, skull or spine pathology, and venous sinuses.

Neurology

Rising intracranial pressure (↑ICP)

Clinical features: include

- **headache:** often worse in the morning due to CO_2 retention during sleep → cerebrovascular dilatation, possibly waking the patient from sleep; made worse by coughing, straining, standing up; relieved by paracetamol in the early stages
- **alteration in the level of consciousness** (drowsiness)
- **vomiting** (may relieve the headache; sometimes the 1st sign of ↑ ICP)
- hypertension, bradycardia.

  Failing vision and decreasing consciousness are ominous signs.

  Papilloedema is frequently not present.

Pathophysiology: initially, mechanisms such as reducing CSF volume allows the CNS to compensate for ↑ ICP as may occur with a slow-growing tumour. However, if the ICP continues to rise or if the increase is acute and the compensatory mechanisms overwhelmed, the brain often becomes laterally displaced and pushed towards the foramen magnum at the base of the skull. The medial temporal lobe (or uncus) is then forced down through the tentorial hiatus, or a cerebellar tonsil is forced through the foramen magnum, causing the brainstem to become compressed (coning). This produces the following progressive changes:

- level of consciousness decreases, drowsiness → coma
- pupils become dilated and unresponsive, initially on the side of the mass, then bilaterally
- posture becomes decorticate, then decerebrate
- slow deep breaths → Cheyne-Stokes breaths → apnoea.

► Beware ipsilateral hemiparesis and VI nerve palsy as false localizing signs.

Causes: SOL; cerebral oedema; hydrocephalus. The cerebral oedema may surround a tumour or result from infection (cerebral malaria, encephalitis), trauma, or hypoxic cell death.

Management: ► if possible, establish the cause with a scan.

1. Sit the patient up at ~30–40° to increase venous drainage from the brain.
2. Ensure adequate oxygenation – ventilate if necessary.
3. Give mannitol 5ml/kg of a 20% solution over 15 mins IV to reduce cerebral oedema
   - in severe oedema, dexamethasone 12–16mg IV stat by slow IV injection may also be used
   - in less severe oedema, give dexamethasone 4mg IM q6h
   - if the patient has a positive malaria blood film, see chapter 3A for management of cerebral malaria.
4. Control seizures if present.
5. If a SOL is believed to be responsible, refer to a neurosurgeon.

►► If the ↑ ICP progresses rapidly, urgent decompression with burr holes may be lifesaving – see p436.

Neurology

Bacterial meningitis

A multitude of microbes – bacteria, viruses, parasites and fungi – can cause meningitis. However, it is bacterial meningitis which is most important since it has a high fatality rate and is readily treatable. ► All febrile patients with a history of headache should be examined for signs of meningism.

Aetiology: in children and adults, bacterial meningitis is frequently due to:

- *Neisseria meningitidis* (Gram –ve intracellular diplococci)
- *Haemophilus influenzae* B (Hib) (Gram –ve rods)
- *Streptococcus pneumoniae* (Gram +ve capsulated diplococci)

Meningococcus causes epidemics (see page 414), while previous head injury, sinusitis, otitis media, or pneumonia predispose to pneumococcal meningitis. Hib meningitis is most common in children <5 yrs. Other bacteria are less common (eg *S. aureus*, *Pseudomonas* spp) or occur in particular groups (eg Group B streptococcus & *E. coli* in neonates; *Listeria* in pregnant women, immunosuppressed, & neonates).

Clinical features: there is sudden onset of intense headache, fever, N&V, photophobia, and stiff neck. Cardinal signs of meningism are:

- **Neck stiffness:** passively flex the head (chin towards chest), this results in pain and resistance in a patient with meningism.
- **Kernig's sign:** passively straighten the leg with hip flexed (>90°), this causes pain and resistance by stretching inflamed nerve roots.

Neurological signs are not normally focal and include: lethargy, delirium, coma, convulsions. Acute complications include $\uparrow$ ICP, seizures, sepsis, paralysis, syndrome of inappropriate ADH secretion.

► Check the skin (particularly on the back, buttocks, and soles of the feet) and conjunctivae carefully for purpura. This is associated with meningococcal septicaemia which can be rapidly fatal. If present, treat for meningococcal infection without delay.

Diagnosis: blood cultures (1. insert cannula, 2. take out blood for culture, 3. immediately administer antibiotics through cannula if there is clinical suspicion of meningococcal disease); lumbar puncture (if there is no evidence of SOL or $\uparrow$ ICP) for CSF examination. Take blood for FBC, U&E, (+ malarial parasite).

Management:

1. On suspicion, give immediate antibiotics – see opposite.
2. Dexamethasone 0.4mg/kg q12h for 2 days starting just before 1st dose of antibiotics may reduce complications in children in given early.
3. Give supportive measures: fluids, oxygen, maintain normal electrolytes, generous pain relief, and tepid sponging to reduce temperature.

Prognosis: mortality varies with age and organism. Perinatal, neonatal and childhood mortality varies from 50–80%. Similarly mortality is increased in old age. In adults, mortality with pneumococcus is 30–40%, haemophilus 20–30%, and meningococcus 10–15%. The main long-term complications include paralysis, deafness, visual loss, epilepsy, and mental retardation.

Initial empiric antibiotic regimens for presumed bacterial meningitis in adults

Choose one of:

1. **Benzylpenicillin** 2.4g (4 mega units) IV q4h for 10–14 days
   and/or
   Chloramphenicol[1] 12.5–25mg/kg or 1g IV q6h for 10 days.
2. **Ceftriaxone** 2–4g IV daily for 7–10 days.
3. **Ampicillin** 2g IV q6h for 10 days.
4. **Cotrimoxazole** 30mg/kg IV q12h for 10 days.

Local recommendations based on antibiotic sensitivity:

1.
2.
3.

[1] Chloramphenicol

The WHO reaffirms the value of chloramphenicol in infections such as meningitis and severe bacterial infections due to bacteria resistant to other antibiotics. Chloramphenicol has one serious toxicity, aplastic anaemia. Estimates of frequency are one in 10 000 to one in 70 000 courses of therapy (which are similar to estimates of death due to penicillin anaphylaxis: one in 40 000 courses). The WHO's Expert Committee on the Use of Essential Drugs, after due consideration of the risks and benefits of chloramphenicol, concluded that it is essential for modern medical practice in all countries.

Epidemic meningococcal disease[1]

There are at least 9 different serogroups of meningococcus, of which 3 groups A, B and C cause outbreaks of meningitis. Serogroup A meningococcus is the most important. It is responsible for the explosive epidemics that continue to devastate sub-Saharan Africa on an almost annual basis. It is also the main cause of endemic meningitis in this area of Africa with rates that are higher than the epidemic rates in other parts of the world. Types A and C have both been responsible for large outbreaks in the rest of the world.

Some strains of meningococcus appear to be more virulent than others. Large epidemics occur when such strains come into contact with populations of non-immune individuals in areas of poverty during particular climatic conditions (eg dry season, dust storm). In between epidemics, the bacteria survives in the community in the nasopharynx of carriers.

Vaccination: is essential for stopping an epidemic once it has begun. Kits for such campaigns are available from the WHO. Advice on organizing a campaign is also given in a WHO book – see below.

Chemoprophylaxis: only for household contacts of cases: rifampicin 600mg (10mg/kg for a child, 5mg/kg for children <1yr) PO bd for 2 days [alternatives: spiramycin 1g PO bd (child: 25mg/kg) PO bd for five days *or* ciprofloxacin 500mg PO as a single dose].

Viral meningitis

Enteroviruses, such as echo and coxsackie viruses, are important causes of epidemic viral meningitis worldwide while arboviruses cause sporadic disease in endemic regions. Other causes of sporadic viral meningitis include polio, mumps virus, EB virus, HIV, varicella-zoster virus, and CMV.

Clinical features are similar to bacterial meningitis but the headache is less severe and the neck less stiff. It is diagnosed by examination of CSF. The identity of the causative virus during epidemics may already be clear. In sporadic cases, peripheral signs may suggest the aetiology such as genital or rectal lesions (HSV), skin blisters (herpes zoster), orchitis (mumps, lymphocytic choriomeningitis virus), rashes (enterovirus), parotid swelling (mumps). The prognosis is usually good with complete resolution.

Other causes of meningitis

Include
- mycobacteria – *M. tuberculosis* (see chapter 3C and below)
- fungi – *Crypyococcus neoformans, Candida albicans*
- parasites – *Naegleria*

1. For clear details on both setting up a surveillance system and organizing the logistics of a mass vaccination campaign, see the following book from which this information is taken:
Control of Epidemic Meningococcal Disease WHO practical guidelines (Edition Fondation Marcel Merieux, 1995). Available from the WHO.

African meningococcal belt

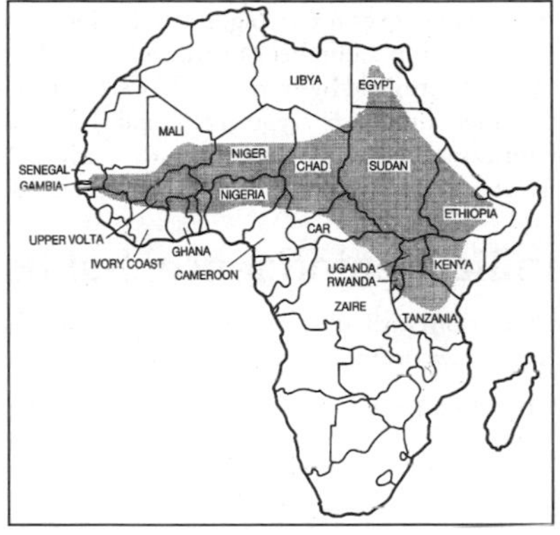

Chronic meningitis

This is commonly caused by TB or *Cryptococcus neoformans* [also: disseminated fungal infections; cysticercosis in children] and presents with chronic headache and low grade fever. Confusion and drowsiness are common and may be due to hydrocephalus. Papilloedema, visual symptoms and cranial nerve lesions may occur. Signs of infection at other sites, eg lungs, will also be found in a number of patients.

The cause can be determined by examination of CSF; subsequently treat for the relevant infection. Both cryptococcal and TB meningitis occur commonly in immunosuppressed patients, particularly AIDS, but they also occur in previously healthy individuals. See chapters 3B and 3C.

Eosinophilic meningoencephalitis

Follows CNS infection with the nematodes *Angiostrongylus cantonensis, Gnathostoma spinigerum* or *Taenia solium.*

- **Angiostrongyliasis** – results from the ingestion of infected snails or contaminated shrimps, fish, and vegetables. The larvae migrate to the brain where they induce an immunoallergic response to dead parasites and then to the eyes and lungs. Initial presentation is of acute, intermittent intense headache without fever; malaise; N&V; cranial nerve palsies; in some, meningism. If severe, there may be fever, decreasing consciousness and spinal cord involvement. The eyes are commonly involved.
  Management: ► do not give antihelminthics since dying parasites elicit a strong immune reaction which can be fatal. It is normally a self-resolving condition – give sedatives, analgesia; the headache responds well to LP every 3–7 days. Eye involvement requires surgery to remove the nematode. Corticosteroids may help in severe disease.
- **Spinocerebral gnathostomiasis** – frequently presents with intensely painful radiculitis followed by ***rapidly advancing*** myelitis → paraplegia with urinary retention or quadraplegia, or as a cerebral haemorrhage in a previously healthy person.
- **Cysticercosis** – see later.

Primary amoebic meningoencephalitis

A rare but commonly fatal infection that follows intranasal infection with *Naegleria fowleri* while swimming in warm fresh water. The amoebae invade the CNS through the cribiform plate and cause extensive tissue necrosis. Headache occurs first, then fever, meningism, coma, convulsions. The patients are seriously ill. The CSF shows neutrophils, red cells, and amoebae on ***wet microscopy***. The prognosis is poor. *Acanthamoeba* cause a similar syndrome, granulomatous amoebic encephalitis (GAE), in immunosuppressed individuals.

Management: amphotericin B 1mg/kg IV daily plus 0.1–1.0mg (TOTAL, NOT /kg) intraventricular (via reservoir) on alternate days.

Cause	***Normal CSF***	***Pyogenic bacteria***	***TB***	***PAM***	***Virus***	***Cryptococcus***
Appearance	Clear and colourless	Cloudy or purulent, contain clots	Clear or slightly cloudy, a fine clot may form	Cloudy	Clear or slightly cloudy	Clear or slightly cloudy
White cells (majority)	<5/mm^3	>200/mm^3 (neutrophils)	>10/mm^3 (lymphocytes +/– RBCs)	>200/mm^3 (neutrophils	>10/mm^3 (lymphocytes)	>10/mm^3 (lymphocytes
Glucose	2.5–4mmol/l (45–72 mg%)	Markedly ↓ or absent	↓	↓	Normal or slightly ↓	↓
Total protein	0.15–0.4g/l (15–40 mg%)	↑	↑	↑	Normal or ↑	↑
Pandy's test	Negative	Positive	Usually positive	Positive	Positive or negative	Positive
[CRP]	Normal	Markedly ↑	Moderately ↑			
Microscopy	None	**Gram:** pus cells and bacteria	**Ziehl/Neelsen:** difficult, requires centrifugation. ? usefulness	**Wet:** motile vacuolated amoebae	None	**Gram:** +ve yeast. **India ink:** double walled yeast

Encephalitis

Virus infection of the brain parenchyma is termed encephalitis. It is characterized by impairment of cerebral function in contrast to meningeal infection which does not affect cerebral function.

Epidemics of encephalitis occur seasonally in many parts of the world and are important causes of death and disability in the young and elderly. The equine encephalitides have recently caused widespread epidemics in South America. ► HSV is the most important cause of sporadic encephalitis worldwide since it is treatable and therefore should be considered in all cases. However, Japanese encephalitis far outstrips HSV in actual numbers.

Clinical features: high fever, headache, N&V, followed by convulsions, confusion and changes in level of consciousness. Some patients also present with meningism, focal neurological signs, abnormal behaviour and/or raised ICP. Severe cases result in prolonged coma, hemiparesis, dystonia, decorticate or decerebrate posturing, and respiratory failure.

Neurological sequelae such as mental retardation, hemiparesis, and behavioural abnormalities are particularly common after Japanese encephalitis, untreated HSV encephalitis, and post-infectious/vaccination encephalomyelitis.

Diagnosis: is via lumbar puncture. ► LP is contraindicated if there is evidence of ↑ ICP or focal signs.

Management: except for HSV encephalitis (see below), management is symptomatic with careful control of seizures (using phenytoin) and pyrexia. Beware respiratory failure, and ↑ ICP (p410). The effectiveness of corticosteroids in preventing cerebral oedema is unclear.

Post-infectious or post-vaccination encephalomyelitis

On rare occasions, infection or vaccination elicits an antiviral immune response which results in CNS immunopathology and an encephalitic picture. It usually occurs after infection with measles, rubella, herpes zoster, mumps, and influenza and after vaccination with the Semple form of the rabies vaccine, but the relative risk is very small compared with the benefits of vaccination.

Herpes simplex virus encephalitis

HSV encephalitis should be considered in the differential diagnosis of any patient presenting with an encephalitic picture. Focal signs relate to the frontal and temporal cortices and limbic system.

It is particularly important since it is the only encephalitis for which there is effective treatment: aciclovir 10mg/kg q8h by slow IV infusion for 10–14 days. Untreated HSV encephalitis has a mortality rate of 40–70% and many survivors have neurological sequelae. Acyiclovir markedly decreases mortality and the incidence of sequelae.

Japanese encephalitis

A common arboviral encephalitis of E, S, and SE Asia. Historically, it has been an infection of young children in wet season epidemics coincident with abundance of its mosquito vector. Widespread childhood vaccination campaigns have shifted the age of most cases from children to adults in a few areas such as north central Sri Lanka. However, in areas where children are still not vaccinated, for example Sarawak, it remains predominantly a disease of young children.

Transmission: is via the bite of the *Culex tritaeniorhynchus* mosquito. The virus's primary hosts are birds such as herons from which it is passed to domestic pigs by mosquitos. It is amplified in these pigs before transmission to humans (a dead-end host). Most infections are subclinical – ~1 in 300 infections results in encephalitis.

Clinical features: after an incubation period of 6–16 days and a non-specific prodrome illness lasting a couple of days, the sudden onset of fever is accompanied by severe headache, meningism, N&V, and hyper-excitability, or decreased consciousness. Seizures are common in children. Neurological signs such as cranial nerve palsies, tremor and ataxia, parkinsonism, and upper limb paralysis develop. Together with a lowered consciousness level, they follow a variable course. Around 25% of patients die; many survivors have serious long term neuropsychiatric disabilities (eg parkinsonism, paralysis, mental retardation). Spontaneous abortion and fetal death may occur in pregnant women. JE virus is now a recognised cause of acute flaccid paralysis.

Equine encephalitides

Three alphaviruses – Western, Eastern and Venezuelan equine encephalitis viruses (EEVs) – cause widespread epizootics of encephalitis in horses in the USA, central America and the northern regions of S America. The virus is amplified during these infections which precede human cases of encephalitis. Rodents and birds are the primary hosts of these viruses; transmission to humans is via *Culex*, *Culiseta* and *Aedes* mosquitos.

The EEVs are not common causes of human encephalitis, but VEEV has recently caused large epidemics in both horses and humans in Colombia and Venezuela. Most infections are subclinical. Some may manifest as a short febrile illness with rigors (in VEE also: sore throat, features of URTI, and diarrhoea). In a few cases, the illness is biphasic: recovery from the febrile illness is followed by encephalitis. Adults do not normally have sequelae; in contrast, many young children and infants are left with some permanent neurological effects after encephalitis. Mortality is high (~10%) in this group.

Rabies

A uniformly fatal infection, still common in many parts of the tropics, that is caused by the rabies virus (or, very rarely, a related lyssavirus). Once clinical symptoms have appeared, the patient will die.

► However, if the infection is caught soon after transmission and before the onset of clinical symptoms, rabies can be prevented by post-exposure vaccination. Increasing the availability and affordability of vaccines and increasing their uptake by rural populations will be pivotal in controlling this disease.

Transmission: is by the bite of an infected mammal in endemic regions most commonly stray dogs (but also wild dogs, wolves, foxes, cats and skunks). The virus does not pass though intact skin; however, infected saliva can infect already damaged skin (eg by dogs' claws) and mucosae. Bites by vampire bats and inhalation of virus in bat-filled caves are methods of transmission in central and south America.

Clinical features: after an incubation period that normally lasts 20–90 days, prodromal symptoms develop itching, pain, or paraesthesia at the site of the bite; followed by fever, chills, malaise, weakness, headache, and neuropsychiatric symptoms. Furious or paralytic rabies develops depending on the major locus of infection.

- ***Furious (brain) rabies*** **–** the pathognomic feature is hydrophobia – inspiratory muscle spasm (arched, extended back with arms thrown up) +/– laryngeal spasm, associated with terror. While initially stimulated by attempts to drink water or wash, it soon becomes provoked by many stimuli. It may end in convulsions with cardiorespiratory arrest. Other features include: hyperaesthesia; generalized arousal (lucid periods alternating with wild, hallucinating, or aggressive periods); cranial nerve defects; meningism; involuntary movements; ANS/hypothalamic changes – hypersalivation, lachriymation, ↑ or ↓ BP and temperature, SIADH, diabetes insipidus.

- ***Paralytic (spine) rabies*** **–** the prodromal symptoms are followed by flaccid paralysis that ascends symmetrically or asymmetrically from the bitten area, with pain, fasciculation, sensory disturbances; paraplegia and loss of sphincter control; ultimately, paralysis of muscles of respiration and swallowing.

Complications include: aspiration and broncho-pneumonia; primary rabies pneumonitis and myocarditis; pneumothorax after inspiratory spasms; cardiac arrhythmias; haematemesis; rarely ↑ ICP.

Diagnosis: history of dog or bat bite plus neurological features; immunofluorescence of viral antigen in base of hair roots in skin biopsy; isolation of virus from body fluids during 1st week.

Prevention: controlling the mammalian reservoir through vaccination; decreasing human exposure to infected mammals; vaccination of persons at high risk and those bitten by mammals post-exposure vaccination. See page 422.

Worldwide distribution of rabies

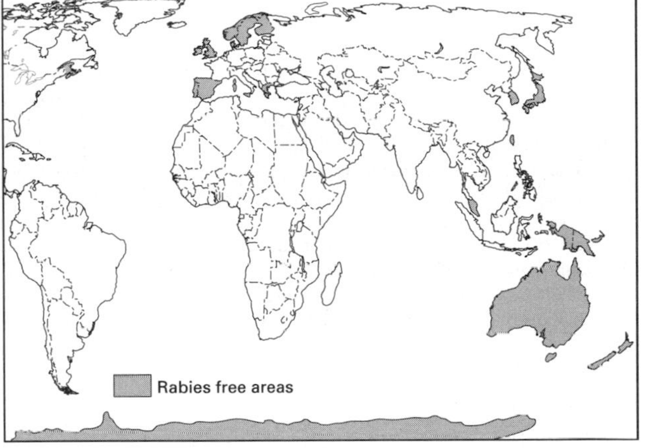

Management of rabies infection

There is currently no effective treatment for a person who is showing signs and symptoms of rabies infection. In this situation, management is purely symptomatic with ► sufficient sedation and analgesia to relieve pain and terror. ITU care will prolong life by preventing or controlling complications.

Post-exposure prophylaxis

Vaccination within days of exposure is 100% effective in preventing the progression of the infection to encephalitis. However, the cheap vaccine which is used most widely in the developing world is itself capable of initiating encephalitis. The Semple vaccine is made by isolating virus from infected sheep's brains. Unfortunately, an immune response to sheep CNS components left in the vaccine can produce severe CNS disease with a 3% mortality.

Recent efforts to make the safer, tissue culture-grown, vaccine more affordable have involved using small doses given intradermally (ID).[1] ► Studies with such regimens have shown that they induce an immune response extremely quickly and that patients require fewer clinic visits. The regimens have been found to be 100% effective and without major side-effects.[1,2]

Procedure: see box opposite

- ***Clean the wound*** – this kills virus in superficial wounds. Scrub wound with soap/detergent and wash under running water >5 mins. Liberally apply virucidal agent: 40–70% alcohol, 0.01% aqueous iodine. Debride as required.
- ***Give antitetanus toxoid***; consider antibiotic cover.
- ***Give vaccine***. The various regimens are:

Sheep brain vaccine (Semple)

Give 2–5mls of vaccine SC into the abdominal wall daily for 14–21 days. Boosters should be given after the course is finished.

Tissue culture vaccines

1. 2-site intradermal method (2-2-2-0-1-1)

Days 0, 3, & 7: 0.1 or 0.2ml ID at each of two sites (deltoids)
Days 28 & 90: 0.1 or 0.2ml ID at one site (deltoid).

2. 8-site intradermal method (8-0-4-0-1-1)

Day 0: 0.1ml intradermally into 8 sites (2× deltoids, suprascapulum, lower quadrant abdominal wall, thighs)
Day 7: 0.1ml intradermally into 4 sites (2× deltoids, thighs)
Day 28: 0.1ml intradermally into 1 site
Day 91: 0.1ml intradermally into 1 site.

ID regimens require the use of Mantoux-like syringes and must cause a raised macule to appear immediately (cf BCG vaccination).

- If possible, give immunoglobulin – either human RIG 20 IU/kg or equine RIG 40 IU/kg. In the latter case, have drugs already drawn up to treat an anaphylactic reaction.

Minor exposure

(including licks of broken skin, scratches, or abrasions without bleeding)

- Start vaccine immediately.
- Stop treatment if the dog remains healthy for 10 days.
- Stop treatment if dog's brain proves negative for rabies by appropriate Ix.

Major exposure

(including licks of mucosa and minor or major bites)

- Immediate rabies IG and vaccine.
- Stop treatment if dog remains healthy for 10 days.
- Stop treatment if dog's brain proves negative for rabies by appropriate Ix.

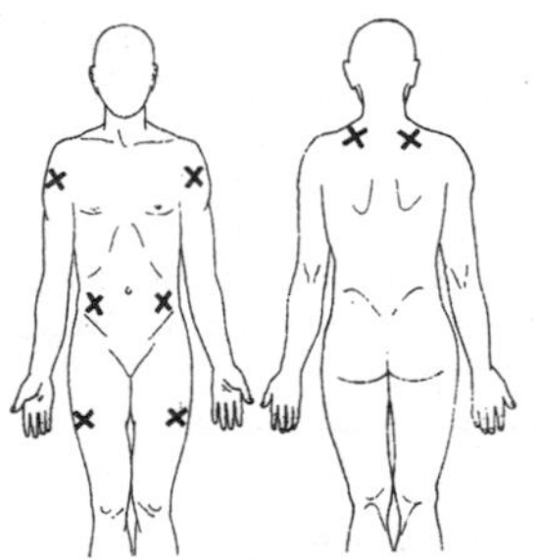

Sites for the 8-site intradermal method of post-exposure vaccination. The use of multiple sites ensures that as many groups of lymph nodes are activated as possible, enhancing the immune response

1. WHO recommendations on rabies post-exposure treatment
2. Warrell MJ, 1985, *Lancet*, i, 1058

Tetanus[1]

Contamination of a wound with the bacterium *Clostridium tetani* results in the production of a powerful exotoxin. This toxin tracks back up the nerves innervating local muscles, entering the CNS. The toxin also enters the blood and passes to other muscles where it is again transported back up peripheral nerves to the CNS. There it blocks the release of inhibitory neurotransmitters, resulting in widespread activation of both motor and autonomic nervous systems. Muscles of the jaw, face and head are involved first because of the shorter axonal paths but all muscle groups become involved in most cases. Activation of opposing groups results in rigidity. Protracted uncontrolled muscular spasms of the chest result in ineffective breathing and hypoxia. Death is due to respiratory complications, circulatory failure, or cardiac arrest.

► Tetanus is easily prevented by vaccination. Its incidence worldwide is directly related to the prevalence of immunization – where immunization rates are high, tetanus is a rare disease. Where immunization is low, it is a common condition of all ages but particularly of neonates who become infected at birth. Immunization of pregnant women prevents neonatal tetanus. Currently ~800,000 babies die each yr.

Transmission: *C. tetani* spores are ubiquitous in the environment and can infect even the most trivial cuts, typically on feet, legs, hands, and feet. Neonatal infection occurs via the cut umbilicus from the use of a dirty knife or the practice of applying dung to the stump.

Clinical features: there is an incubation period of 7–10 days, but this is variable and many patients cannot recall the injury. The **period of onset** is between the first symptom and the onset of spasms; it varies between 1 to 7 days and is a good prognostic indicator – the shorter the interval, the more severe the disease.

The first symptom is often **stiffness** of the masseters producing difficulty in opening the mouth – *trismus*. As the condition progresses, other muscle groups become rigid, including muscles of the • face (producing characteristic look – *risus sardonicus*), • skeleton (→ difficulty in breathing; opisthotonos; rigid limbs) and • swallowing (→ aspiration).

Spasms are an exaggeration of the underlying rigidity, and occur in more severe disease either as a reflex response to stimuli (touch, sounds, sights, emotions) or spontaneously. They may be mild and brief, or prolonged and very painful. Prolonged thoracic spasms may result in respiratory failure, laryngeal spasms in death from anoxia. In severe disease, the patient has a fever, tachycardia and an unstable CVS mostly due to involvement of the autonomic nervous system – see opposite.

Neonatal cases present with inability to suckle; they go on to develop characteristic opisthotonos.

Diagnosis: can be made on clinical features alone.

Prevention: by active vaccination of children and pregnant women (see chapter 15); good wound toilet and passive vaccination following injuries; and provision of clean facilities for childbirth.

1. These pages follow the recommendations of Udwadia FK, *OTM*, p624, 1996.

Grading of tetanus severity

- **Grade I (Mild)** mild to moderate trismus; general spasticity; no respiratory problems; no spasms; little or no dysphagia.
- **Grade II (Moderate)** moderate trismus; well-marked rigidity; mild to moderate but short-lasting spasms; moderate respiratory failure with tachypnoea >30–35/min; mild dysphagia.
- **Grade III (Severe)** severe trismus; generalized spasticity; reflex and often spontaneous prolonged spasms; respiratory failure with tachypnoea >40/min; apnoeic spells; severe dysphagia; tachycardia >120/min.
- **Grade IV (Very severe)** features of grade III plus violent autonomic disturbances involving the CVS. These include: episodes of severe hypertension & tachycardia alternating with relative hypotension and bradycardia; severe persistent hypertension (diastolic >110mmHg); severe persistent hypotension (systolic <90).

Complications

- **Respiratory** collapse; aspiration, lobar, or broncho-pneumonia (often due to Gram –ve organisms: *Klebsiella* spp, *Ps. aeruginosa*, Enterobacter); anoxia due to prolonged laryngeal spasm; severe hypoxia and respiratory failure in severe tetanus if patient is not paralysed and ventilated; unexplained tachypnoea and respiratory distress; ARDS. The complications also include those of tracheostomy and prolonged ventilation.
- **CVS** (mostly mediated by ANS) persistent tachycardia, hypotension or hypertension; labile hypertension; severe peripheral vasoconstriction → shock-like state. Autonomic storms are characterized by sudden sinus tachycardia + severe hypertension followed by sudden bradycardia and hypotension; they may precede cardiac arrest. Increased vagal tone is shown by sudden bradycardia – sucking out of the trachea may lead to an arrest. Arrhythmias include: SVT; junctional rhythms; atrial and ventricular ectopics; short bursts of self-resolving VT. Hyperthermia (hypothermia is very rare).
- **Sudden death** caused by many of the above complications, massive PE, or unidentified event.
- **Sepsis** most commonly iatrogenic
- **Renal insufficiency**
- **Midthoracic vertebral fracture** occurs during severe spasms; there are usually few sequelae and healing occurs without incident.

Management of tetanus

Management of severe tetanus can be extremely difficult, particularly in the open ward where conservative management has an appalling mortality rate. Ideally ALL patients should be treated in an ITU setting.

► However, careful management of the patient with particular attention to critical care and ventilatory support can markedly improve the prognosis where an ITU is not available.

If ventilators are limited, they should be kept for patients with:

- grade IV disease
- grade III disease uncontrolled by sedatives
- serious respiratory complications.

Give immediate care on admission (see box opposite). Subsequent management depends on the severity of the condition.

- **Grade I –** beware complications of septic wound. ***Observe carefully*** since grade I tetanus can progress to more severe disease. For sedation/ muscle relaxation, give diazepam 5mg PO tds (neonatal dose 2mg PO tds). Alternative: chlorpromazine 50mg (adult), 25mg (child), or 12.5mg (neonate) IM qds [phenobarbitone can be added if essential].

- **Grade II –** as for grade I but increase sedation/muscle relaxation. Increase dose of diazepam up to fourfold in adults (do not exceed 80–100mg/day because of respiratory depression). Give by slow IV infusion over 24hrs.

  ► The ideal sedative/muscle-relaxant schedule ensures continuous sedation such that the patient can sleep but also be woken up to obey commands. An objective guide is relaxation of abdominal muscles.

  Perform a tracheostomy (may prevent death due to prolonged laryngeal spasm and anoxia). ► If laryngeal spasm occurs, promptly give chlorpromazine 50mg IV [alternative: diazepam 10–20mg IV].

- **Grade III –** treat as for grade II but also paralyse and ventilate. Reduce diazepam dose to 30–40mg over 24 hrs (↓ risk of CNS depression). Give pancuronium 2–4mg [poorer alternative: gallamine 20–40mg] IV, titrated for each patient to give sufficient neuromuscular blockade for efficient ventilation. Initially give every 0.5–1hr (1st 1–2 weeks) then extend interval as the patient improves. Check with periodic arterial blood analysis, if available. Spasms still occur under paralysis but they need not affect ventilation; pancuronium can be stopped when spasms cease. Continue ventilation until patient can be weaned off.

- **Grade IV –** as above, with addition of drugs that act on the CVS if deemed ***absolutely essential*** for grossly deranged haemodynamics.
  - Hypotension – give volume load; if ineffective or *CI*, use dopamine to keep systolic BP >100mmHg.
  - Hypertension (systolic >200, diastolic >100mmHg) – propranolol 5–10mg PO or nifedipine 5mg sublingual.
  - Bradyarrhythmia or persistent tachyarrhythmias – see peri-arrest protocols in cardiology chapter.

Management on admission. All patients should receive:

- **Antiserum (antitoxin)** preferably human tetanus immunoglobulin 3000–5000 units IV/IM; otherwise equine antiserum 10,000 units by slow IV injection, but ***beware anaphylactic reactions***. Some believe that a sensitivity test should be done first but anaphylactic reactions can occur after a negative sensitivity test. Therefore it may be better to expect anaphylactic reactions in all patients receiving equine antiserum and have treatment ready drawn up in syringes.
- **Antibiotics** – metronidazole 500mg IV q6h or 1g IV q12h, for 7–10 days [poorer alternative: benzylpenicillin 2MU by IM injection or infusion q8h for 8 days].
- **? Local infiltration of antiserum** uncertain efficacy but recommended in some units. 3000 units around obvious wound.
- **Wound toilet** performed after other steps, to remove necrotic tissue. Delay suturing.
- **Vaccination before discharge.**

Critical care and nursing is essential:

- Reduce external stimuli – physical examination must be gentle.
- Keep airway patent – use *gentle* suction to remove saliva and secretions at the back of the throat.
- Take exquisite care of the tracheostomy.
- Gently and frequently change the patient's posture.
- Use physiotherapy to keep lungs patent – ► give a small IV bolus of diazepam before physiotherapy and in the paralysed patient, perform physiotherapy when the action of pancuronium (gallamine) is at its maximum.
- Keep up patient's nutrition – 3500–4000 calories (including >100g protein) by nasogastric tube is required each day.

Overall aims of care:

- Maintain adequate arterial PaO_2 and O_2 saturation.
- Maintain fluid, electrolyte and acid-base balance.
- Maintain circulatory support in grade IV hypotensive patient. A central venous line is very useful if available.
- Prevent, detect and promptly treat any infection.
- Detect early hyperpyrexia – treat with paracetamol and wet cloths.

Stroke

A rapidly developing episode of focal loss of cerebral function which lasts more than 24 hours in a person with no history of recent head injury. In the industrialized world, most are due to cerebral infarction after a thromboembolic event (~80%). The situation may well differ in the developing world – see opposite. Around 20% of stroke patients die within the first month; strokes due to intracranial haemorrhages have a much higher fatality rate than those following cerebral infarction.

Risk factors include: hypertension, ischaemic heart disease, atrial fibrillation, TIAs, peripheral vascular disease, DM, and smoking.
Transient ischaemic attacks (TIAs) – are defined as an acute loss of focal cerebral or monocular function which lasts less than 24 hours. They are believed to be embolic events but ones which are sufficiently transient as to produce ischaemia rather than infarction. They indicate that the person is at increased risk of a stroke (~12% per year) and death due to thromboembolic events such as stroke or MI (~10% per year).

Clinical features: the neurological deficits are varied but commonly come on rapidly. It may be possible to relate the clinical features to the known anatomy of particular cerebral blood vessels but collateral blood supply makes this difficult. Infarcts affecting the cerebral hemisphere may cause contralateral hemiparesis (→ upper motor neurone paralysis after initial spinal shock), sensory loss, homonymous hemianopia, and/or dysphasia. Infarcts affecting subcortical structures such as thalamus and basal ganglia can cause mixed or isolated motor and/or sensory defects or ataxia. Brainstem infarcts can have profound affects: quadraplegia, visual and/or respiratory problems, locked-in syndrome.

There is often a transient hypertension which settles.

Management: ►► it is essential to think about rehabilitation early in the patient's illness. Do not ignore this issue until the patient has developed joint contractures which will prevent physical recovery.

1. Give aspirin 150mg daily if cerebral haemorrhage can be excluded.
2. Take great care of the airway in the unconscious patient. Turn the patient often to avoid bedsores.
3. Ensure adequate nutrition and hydration.
4. Slowly and carefully lower very high BP (>130 diastolic; >240 systolic).
5. If there is an identified source of thromboemboli (other than endocarditis), anticoagulate as for a DVT.
6. Check for treatable causes such as giant cell arteritis.
7. Watch out for causes of neurological deterioration see opposite.
8. If there is evidence of cerebral oedema, consider giving mannitol.

Prevention: since management is unsatisfactory for most patients, prevention is important. Reduce the risk of strokes by controlling the basic risk factors, particularly hypertension and smoking, in both individuals and populations. In patients who have had TIAs or previous strokes, it is especially important to control hypertension and reduce the chance of further thrombotic events by giving aspirin 75mg PO daily. Anticoagulation is required for patients with AF, clotting disorder or recurrent DVTs.

Main causes of stroke in sub-Saharan Africa

- hypertension (haemorrhagic stroke)
- atherosclerosis (thrombotic stroke)
- rheumatic heart disease (embolic)
- others: haemoglobinopathies
HIV
subarachnoid haemorrhage
unexplained (mainly young persons)

Causes of neurological deterioration after stroke:

Local – extension of thrombus; recurrent embolism or haemorrhage; haemorrhagic transformation of the infarct; post-haemorrhage vaso-constriction → further ischaemia; cerebral oedema; brain shift and herniation; hydrocephalus; epileptic seizures.

General – hypoxia (pneumonia, PE, cardiac failure); hypotension; infection; dehydration; hyponatraemia; hypoglycaemia or hyper-glycaemia; drugs; depression.

Stroke rehabilitation

Without rehabilitation and physiotherapy, the patient risks spending the rest of her days in a wheelchair or bed-bound. It is essential to start physiotherapy as soon as the patient is medically stable, to give the best chance of regaining hand and arm function and of walking. In other words, to regain independence.

- Rehabilitation is a 24hr process. Good work during the day can be ruined by a night spent sleeping in a bad position. It may be useful to teach the patient's relatives the basics of physiotherapy so that they can both look out for bad positioning and help the patient perform exercises.
- Initially, encourage the patient to participate in therapy for about 20 mins, three times a day. This can be increased with time.
- The patient needs regular turning to prevent bed sores (q4h).
- Physiotherapy should NEVER be painful. The expression "no pain, no gain" has no place in rehabilitation.

General guidelines

- The stroke patient initially has decreased tone. At the beginning, therefore, rehabilitation attempts to increase power in the limbs. However, over time the tone may increase so much that the patient's limbs become spastic with fixed deformities. A hand left bunched up and curled under the arm is useless. Gentle repetitive exercises should be able to reduce the tone. Work on the opposite movements to those which cause the hand to bunch up – extension at the shoulder, elbow, wrist, and fingers
- Normal movement is easier if the person is completely relaxed This is accomplished by supporting the whole body as in figure 1.
- The aim of stroke rehabilitation is for normal movement. Some patients will neglect one side – ensure that the patient is able to see both arms and hands at all times. Reinforce the message that they are symmetrical. The patient can practice doing actions with her weak limbs (eg picking up a cup, stepping from one foot to the other while sitting) by carefully noting the action with the normal limb, and then copying this with the weak limb.

Repetition of a movement over a period of time reinforces plastic adaption. After a stroke, the brain has to relearn how to do things. It needs to practise. However, repetition can strengthen both bad and good habits, so it is essential to get the practised movements right.

Early stage

1. It is important to support and position the patient carefully, paying particular attention to the hemiplegic shoulder so as to reduce the risk of injury. Figures 1–3 show how to cushion the patient.
2. The relatives or nurses should roll the patient carefully (figure 4). As the patient becomes stronger, teach rolling from side to side, and then how to get up from lying (figures 5, 6). The patient will often need help.
3. Frequent changes in position are good.

1. Supported supine lying

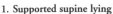

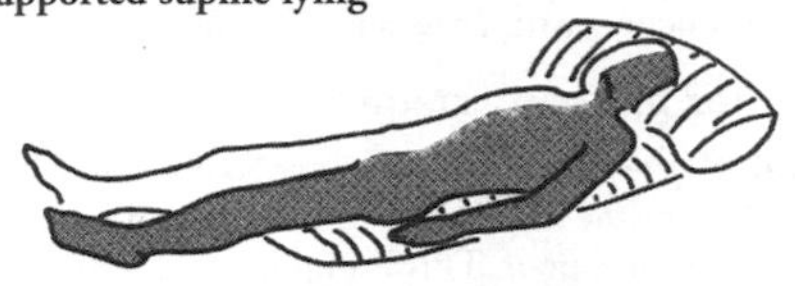

2. Lying on the normal side (coloured white)

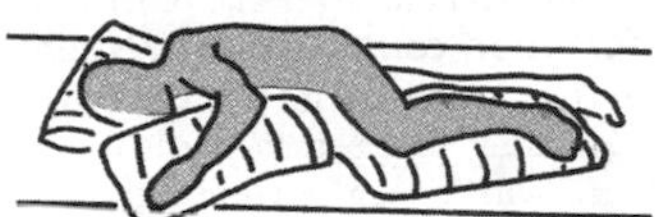

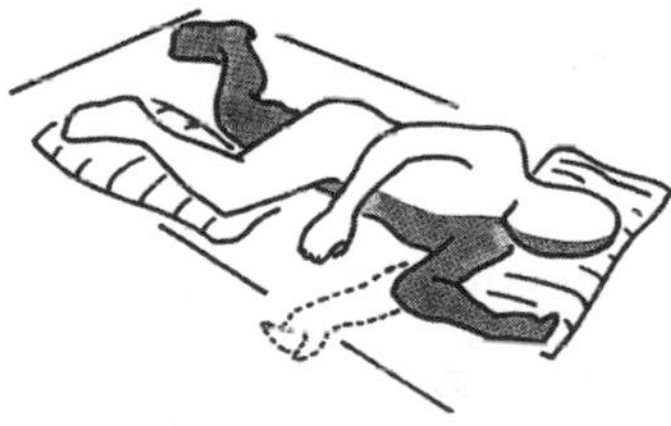

3. Lying on the stroke (hemiplegic) side (coloured black)

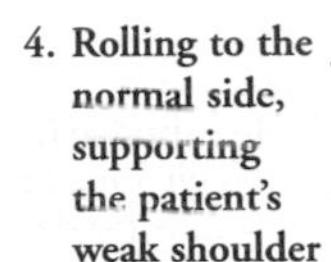
4. Rolling to the normal side, supporting the patient's weak shoulder

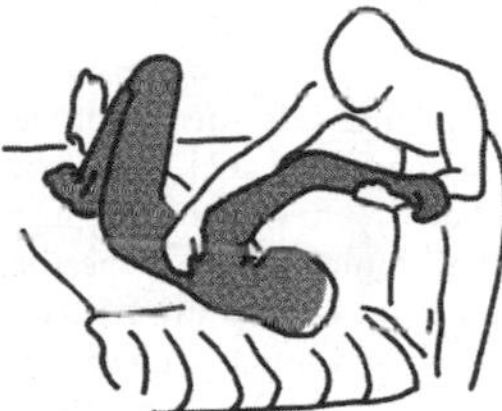

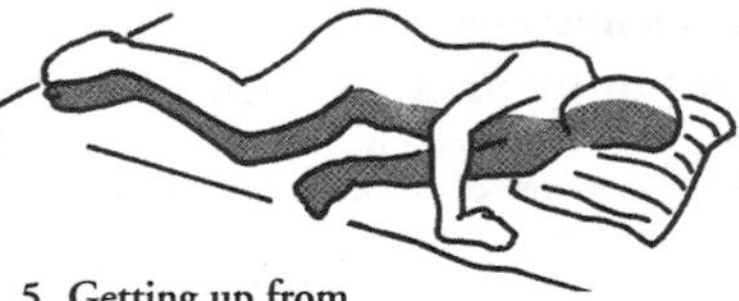

5. Getting up from lying on the stroke side

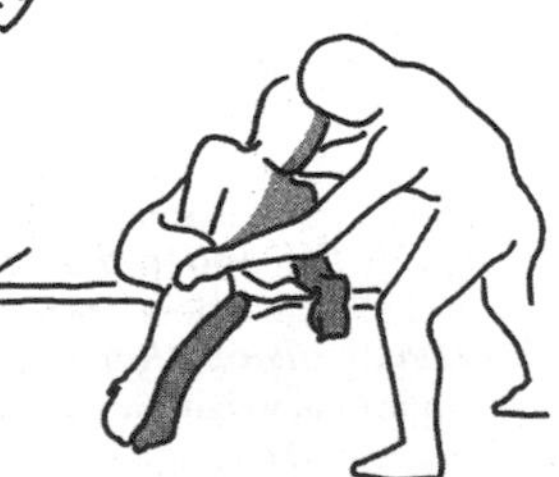

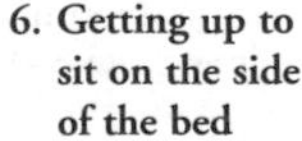
6. Getting up to sit on the side of the bed

4. Aim to maintain muscle length (prevent contractures) with GENTLE passive/active movements into extension, taking particular care over the tendo-Achilles tendon, and the flexors of elbow, wrist, and fingers.
5. Encourage selective and controlled movements. It is better to work slowly to get good control of arm and hand movements than to be able rapidly to regain function with gross abnormal limb movements.

Basic principles for this early stage

- ***Aim for symmetry*** – sit the patient in a good position with adequate support (figure 7). Set the arms forward. Sit the patient out for short periods if trunk control is poor. This is important; practise transferring weight from side to side (figure 11) this will make it easier for her to shift weight from one leg to the other while learning to walk again.
- ***Aim for good control of movement*** – in particular, the patient needs to be able to control the transference of body weight in sitting and in standing. The patient needs to lean forward to get up. This is best learnt with a high seat initially (and something in front to help build confidence; figure 9). With progress, the seat can be lowered and the front support shifted to the side, before trying a chair (figure 12).
- ***Aim for trunk control*** – in sitting before trying to stand, and in particular during the act of moving from sitting to standing.
- ***Aim for balance*** – in standing and stepping before walking.

Walking stage

1. Aim for normal gait – equal stride length and equal time on both sides.
2. The patient may require support on one or both sides.
3. Start off walking with the UNAFFECTED leg. This means that the patient must have already learnt to shift weight from leg to leg.
4. Walkings aids – use a wheeled frame/rollator or a normal walking stick (a quadruped stick should be a last resort.
5. The patient may require help with a 'drop foot' (figure 13).
6. Use mime, gestures, repeating and rephrasing movements, and physical prompts to help the patient. Allow time for slow synapsing.
7. Little and often is a better way to build stamina and sustain carry over from one session to another.

Some "don'ts" for stroke rehabilitation

1. ***Do not ask the patient to try harder*** – AVOID effort as it increases tone and gross patterns of movement.
2. ***Do not ask the patient to squeeze a ball*** – this only encourages the arm flexors which are already too strong.
3. ***Avoid a painful shoulder*** – do not make any arm movements unless the whole shoulder, including the scapula, is relaxed and supple. Support for a weak arm (figure 8) may be useful temporarily, eg while concentrating on walking.
4. ***NEVER lift under the stroke arm or pull it*** – the muscles which hold the shoulder are weak and the joint easily dislocated.
5. ***Prevent dislocation*** – support the forearm and hand forwards with natural weight through the elbow (figure 7).

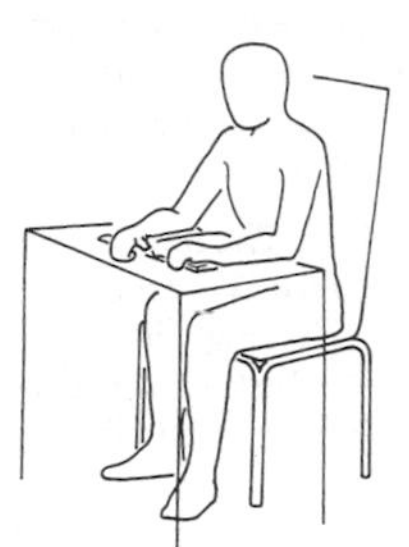

7. A good sitting posture, with the arms out in front

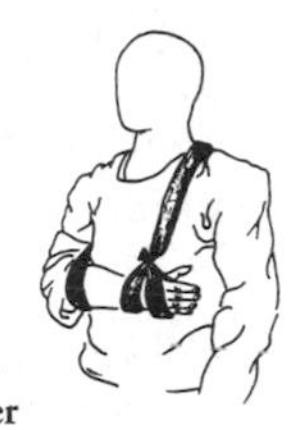

8. Temporary support for a weak shoulder

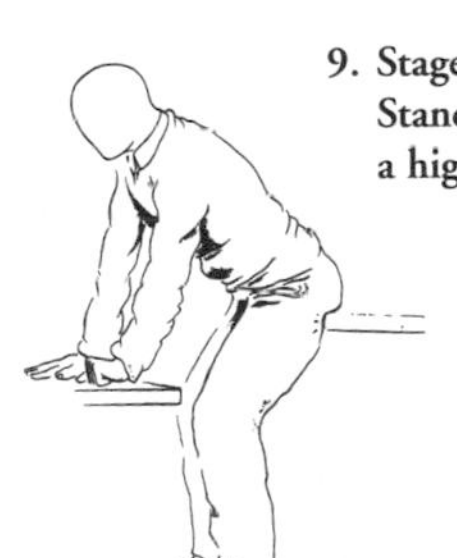

9. Stage 1. Standing up from a high support

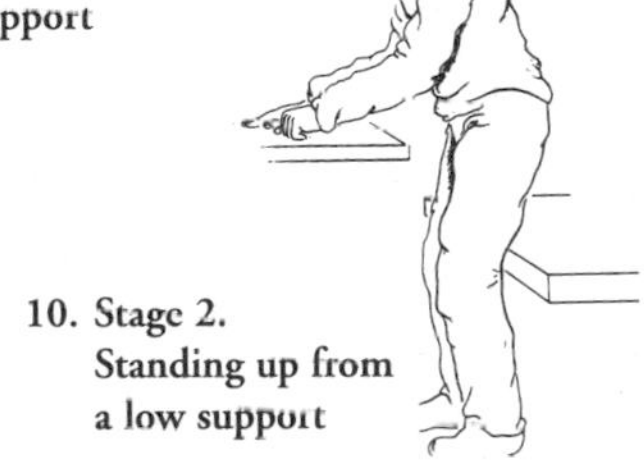

10. Stage 2. Standing up from a low support

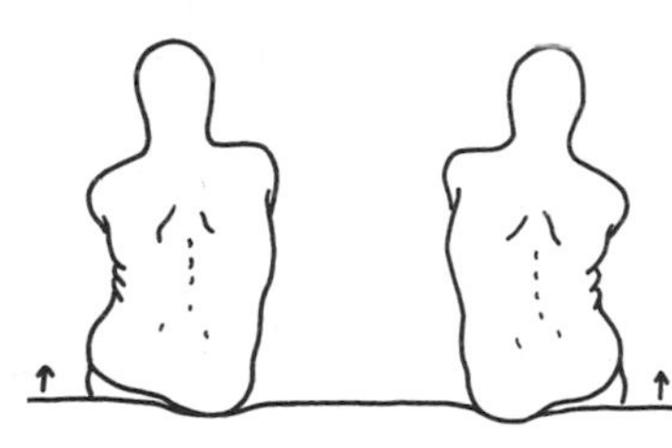

11. Improving trunk control – taking the weight on each side

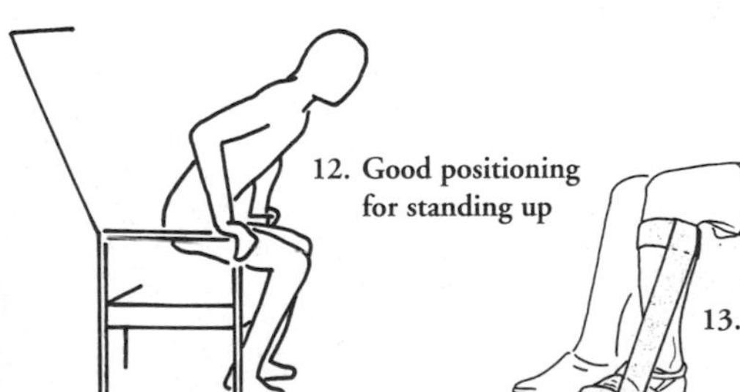

12. Good positioning for standing up

13. Elasticated support for foot drop

Subarachnoid haemorrhage (SAH)

An acute bleed into the subarachnoid space that produces a sudden intense headache, sometimes accompanied by N&V. This is classically described as 'like being hit on the back of the head'. Most cases are caused by ruptured congenital Berry aneurysms. Other causes are rare mycotic aneurysms (due to endocarditis) and arteriovenous malformations (more frequent in young patients). 15% have no identified cause.

Clinical features: the conscious level may be impaired. The more severe the bleed, the lower the conscious level, and the worse the prognosis. Other features include: headache with meningism; vomiting; fits. Focal signs are rare. The patient is often irritable and drowsy; the headache may last for weeks. Complications include vascular spasm which contributes to cerebral ischaemia. ► Beware worsening conscious level, the appearance or worsening of a neurological deficit (eg development of hemiparesis, dilatation of a pupil), or systemic changes such as ↑ BP that may indicate ↑ ICP.

Diagnosis: is by clinical findings with LP (and early CT scan if available). The CSF is uniformly blood stained early on. Xanthochromia (straw coloured supernatant) may be present provided that at least 6 hours have elapsed since the onset of the bleed. It may be present for up to 14 days. ► However, if meningitis is also suspected, the LP should not be delayed.

Management: involves neurosurgery in many cases to evacuate an intracerebral haematoma or clip the aneurysm. Medical treatment involves extended bed rest, analgesia, sedation (beware masking of deterioration in conscious level) and cautious control of hypertension. IV hydration (3L/day) is strongly advised. Nimodipine (60mg PO q4h for 2–3 weeks) decreases the incidence of vascular spasm.

► Many SAHs are preceded by minor herald bleeds which also elicit an intense headache +/– meningism or back pain. If suspected, refer for evaluation since surgical treatment at this time may prevent a later severe bleed. Rebleeding occurs in ~30% of cases; it is a common cause of death.

Subdural haemorrhage

A slow venous bleed that follows damage to veins crossing from the cortex to venous sinuses. It may even occur after a minor accident, such as stepping awkwardly off a bus, in those predisposed: elderly, alcoholics, people with clotting disorders, epileptics. Presentation can occur months after the forgotten accident as chronic bleeding slowly increases the size of the haematoma.

Clinical features: typically there is a lucid interval between the injury and the onset of neurological symptoms. Common acute symptoms include headache, vomiting, fluctuating levels of consciousness; less often: mood changes, irritability, incontinence, drowsiness. Signs may include changes in pupil size, distal limb weakness, and increased reflexes; less commonly fits and dysphasia.

Management of a subdural haematoma

This requires a neurosurgical opinion and if possible a CT scan – evacuation through burr holes is recommended for most cases (see next page). Possibly minor haematomas will resolve by themselves. ► The outcome is good in all ages – ~90% return to normal. Therefore seek the diagnosis in a confused elderly person.

Extradural haematoma[1]

An arterial bleed that normally results from a skull fracture after head injury (eg assault, RTA). The haematoma enlarges rapidly and unless evacuated equally rapidly there is a high risk of brain herniation and the patient's death. ► Suspect when the conscious level declines in a patient with head injury. Unilateral dilation of a pupil, which is sluggish or unresponsive to light, is ipsilateral to the side of the haemorrhage.

Management: do a CT scan if possible to localize the expanding lesion. Further management depends on the distance to a neurosurgeon. If close, give mannitol before transferring the patient. If the neurosurgeon is a long way away, a burrhole will be required to prevent brain herniation.
► In this situation, unless a burr hole is done rapidly, the patient will die or suffer brain damage. You and the patient have nothing to lose and everything to gain. An inelegant burr hole now will do much more good than an elegant operation one hour or more later.

How to do a burr hole

1. Incision
- Shave the scalp if there is time.
- Local anaesthetic is not usually necessary.
- Make a 4 cm incision over the site of fracture or injury. This is usually in the temporal region – just above the zygomatic arch – curved as shown opposite (figure 1) so that it can be enlarged.

2. Incise right down to the bone. Do not stop to control bleeding.

3. Scrape back the pericranium (periosteum) using a periosteal elevator (or similar instrument) to expose the skull.
- Insert a mastoid retractor (figure 2) – this will stop all the bleeding.
- Leave the retractor in.

4. Perforate the bone using a perforator (figure 3)
- Dark blood will ooze out.
- The dura will not be seen as it is stripped away by the blood clot.
- Do no more than ► JUST perforate the skull.
- This will create a conical hole.

5. Enlarge the perforation using a burr (figure 4)
- The burr will enlarge the hole so that it is nearly cylindrical

6. The blood clot will immediately ooze out.
- Suck the blood away by applying a sucker to the burr hole but ► DO NOT INSERT THE SUCKER INTO THE CAVITY. This will cause more bleeding and might damage the brain.

7. It is now safe to transfer the patient to a neurosurgical unit.
- Leave the scalp retractor in. Organize for its return.
- Leave in the endotracheal tube and leave a drip up.

1. With many thanks to Mr C.B.T. Adams, Radcliffe Infirmary, Oxford.

1

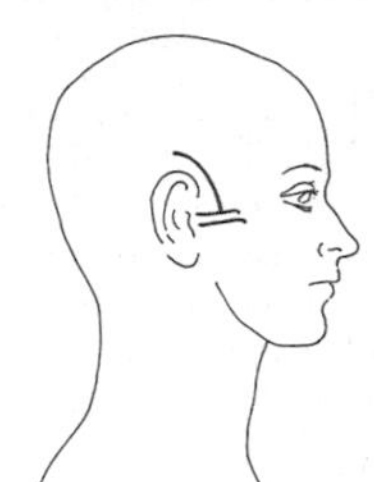

2

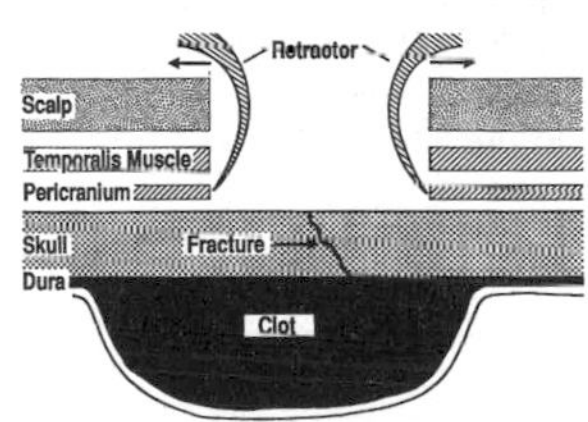
Retractor
Scalp
Temporalis Muscle
Pericranium
Skull
Fracture
Dura
Clot

3

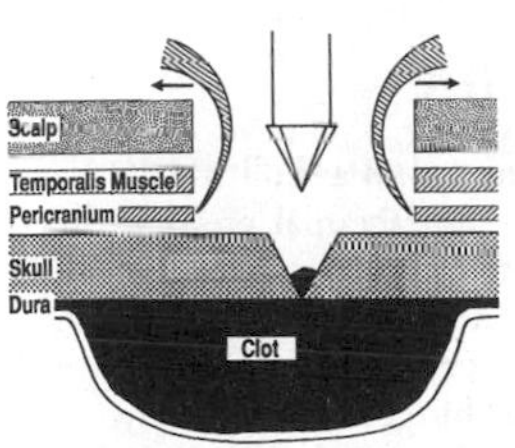
Scalp
Temporalis Muscle
Pericranium
Skull
Dura
Clot

4

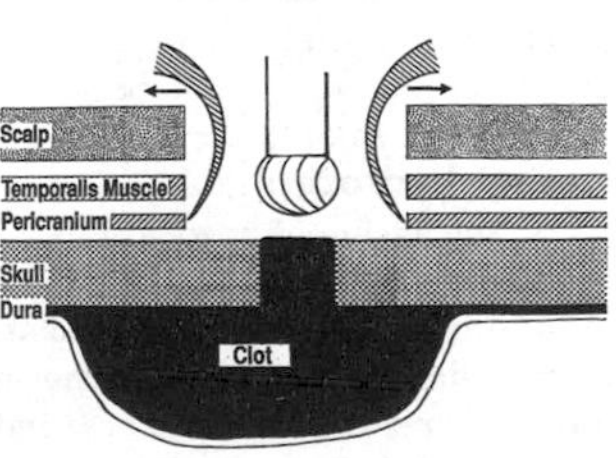
Scalp
Temporalis Muscle
Pericranium
Skull
Dura
Clot

Blackouts

The commonest causes of blackouts are epilepsy (see page 440) and syncope. Causes of blackouts are given opposite. A reliable eyewitness account is helpful.

Syncope is the brief loss of consciousness which results from an acute reduction in cerebral blood flow. It is the commonest cause of recurrent episodes of disturbed consciousness. May be precipitated by anxiety or pain. It is due to reduced venous return to the heart and cardiac output or an inadequate response of the heart when ↑ demand requires ↑ cardiac output. Causes include hypotension, vagal slowing of the heart, neuropathy, arrhythmias, aortic stenosis, vertebrobasilar ischaemia (TIAs), carotid-sinus syndrome.

Space-occupying lesions (SOL)

Classically present with focal neurological signs, ↑ ICP (p410), or seizures. Focal neurological signs can be used to localize the mass but beware false localizing signs from the VIth nerve's long intracranial path.

Causes:

- ***infection*** – tuberculoma, cysticercosis, echinococcosis, bacterial or amoebic brain abscess, paragonomiasis, schistosomiasis, toxoplasmosis, fungal granulomata
- ***tumour*** – glioma, meningioma, metastases, lymphoma, pituitary adenoma, cysts
- ***others*** – aneurysm, haematoma.

Hydrocephalus

The brain is contained within a skull which, in older children and adults, will not expand if the intracranial pressure rises. Blockage of CSF flow through the ventricles or a failure to reabsorb CSF results in a buildup of pressure or hydrocephalus. While producing an increasing head circumference in young children, it results in rising intracranial pressure in older persons which will need urgent management. It exists in two forms:

- **Non-communicating hydrocephalus** – is due to blockage of CSF flow through the ventricles, normally at the foramina or aqueduct between ventricles and/or basal cistern. It is caused by any space-occupying lesion, such as tumour or cyst, or stenosis of the aqueduct. The location of the blockage must be identified and the blockage removed surgically, or a shunt placed.
- **Communicating hydrocephalus** – is due to CSF obstruction in basal cisterns or subarachnoid space (the CSF still flows out of the ventricular system but it cannot be reabsorbed in the arachnoid villi). It may result from intracranial haemorrhage or meningitis (acute pyogenic or chronic); the cause is often unknown. It classically presents with the triad of dementia, incontinence, and gait disturbance (this condition is also called normal pressure hydrocephalus). Repeated lumbar taps with treatment of any underlying cause may be sufficient.

Causes of blackouts

- vasovagal
- postural hypotension
- hyperventilation
- cardiac arrhythmia
- hypoglycaemia
- vertebro-basilar TIAs
- epilepsy
- hypoxia
- hysteria

It is important to measure blood levels of:

- glucose
- Na^+
- K^+
- Ca^{2+}
- Mg^{2+}

Epilepsy

Epilepsy is the continuing tendency to have epileptic seizures – spontaneous paroxysmal discharges of neurons that result in clinical symptoms.

It is a common disease with ~40 million people affected worldwide.[1] Its incidence is higher in the developing world than the industrialized world. Approximately 1% of the population have epilepsy due to the greater incidence of infection and head injury. Unfortunately, at present, only ~15% of cases are treated adequately and many people suffer unnecessarily. As a result, a global campaign is being set up to increase public awareness of both the diseases and its causes.[1] There is also a great need to both reduce its incidence in the developing world (by decreasing the number of head injuries and infections) and find ways of providing adequate supplies of affordable effective antiepileptic drugs to poorer countries.

Causes – 70% unknown, 30% known.

- ***Infection –*** cysticercosis, tuberculoma, schistosomiasis, paragonimiasis, sparganosis, hydatid disease, toxoplasmosis, toxocariasis, cerebral malaria, cerebral amoebiasis, syphilitic gumma, and HIV.
  Epilepsy can also be a late consequence of almost any meningeal or brain parenchyma infection.
- ***Brain injury –*** due to either head injury (such as assault or RTA[2]) or antenatal head injury (may also be due to postnatal injury but this is now believed to be less important).
- ***Unknown*** (many may actually be due to very small areas of focal dysgenesis – hamartomas).
- ***Eclampsia*** during pregnancy is the patient a female of childbearing age? Urgent delivery is required.
- Inherited diseases
- Brain tumour or metastasis
- Degenerative disorders (in elderly)
- Drugs.
- Alcohol
- Metabolic causes
- Vascular disease

Clinical features: will depend on the class of seizure – see below.
- There may be an aura or warning before the attack.
- In grand mal attacks, the person has generalized convulsions usually with tonic clonic movements of all four limbs. The patient loses consciousness and may bite her tongue and be incontinent of urine or rarely faeces.
- Post-ictally there may be a period of confusion, drowsiness, a failure to remember the onset, and a headache with a tendency to sleep.

Seizure classification – important for choice of drug therapy.

1. Origin and spread of the seizure:

- A seizure that remains localized to its area of origin is a ***partial seizure.***
- A seizure that subsequently spreads from this region to involve the whole brain is termed a ***secondarily generalized seizure.***
- A seizure which originates in centrally positioned cells and activates all parts of the brain simultaneously is a ***generalized seizure.***

1. Editorial, 1997, *Lancet*, **349**, 1851 2. Annegers JF, 1998, *NEJM*, **338**, 20

Neurology

2. Clinical features of the seizure:

- **Partial seizures:** have signs and symptoms referrable to a part of one hemisphere.
  Simple (consciousness is not impaired eg in focal motor seizures which may start in a toe, finger, or the angle of mouth).
  Complex (consciousness is impaired with signs of temporal lobe activity eg olfactory aura followed by automatism of facial expression, behaviour; hallucinations).
  Secondarily generalized.
- **Generalized seizures:** do not have any features which are referrable to only one hemisphere.
  Absences (petit mal) brief ~10s pauses (eg stops talking mid-sentence, carries on where left off). Classically, has pathognomic 3Hz activity on EEG.
  Tonic-clonic (grand mal) sudden onset with loss of consciousness, body stiffens for up to 1 minute before jerking, post-ictal drowsiness.
  Myoclonic and ***akinetic*** seizures.

Management: ► if the seizure appears to have a focal onset, look for a treatable underlying cause, particularly infectious (if available, use CT or even better MRI). ► Patients should be warned not to drive.

First-line drugs: ► see a formulary for details of use and side-effects.

- ***Phenobarbital*** – start at 1.5mg/kg PO daily, building up to 3.0 (max. 5.0) mg/kg daily. First choice for partial and generalized tonic-clonic seizures. Its side-effects in children appear to be acceptable.[1]
- ***Carbamazepine*** – start at 100mg PO bd, building up to 600mg bd if tolerated. First choice for tonic-clonic seizures in association with partial seizures; reserve drug for partial seizures alone.
- ***Sodium valproate*** – start at 300mg PO bd, building up to 750mg bd (max = 2.5g/day). First choice for typical absences, myoclonic and akinetic seizures, and tonic-clonic seizures in association with typical absences.
- ***Phenytoin*** – start at 2.5mg/kg PO daily, building up to 5.0 (max ~8.0) mg/kg daily PO. Reserve drug for tonic-clonic and partial seizures (not for absences). It is a toxic drug and plasma levels should ideally be monitored.
- ***Other drugs*** **–** used for epilepsy include clonazepam, ethosuximide, and the newer expensive drugs: vigabatrin, lamotrogine, gabapentin.

Changing drugs: persist with an old drug until it has been used at its maximum dose before considering a change. Introduce the new drug at its starting dose and slowly increase to its mid-range; then start to slowly decrease the dose of the old drug.

Stopping drugs: it is not clear how long any person needs to stay on anti-epileptic drugs once the seizures have been controlled. An MRC trial of stopping medication in people who had not had a seizure for 2 years showed that 59% of those who stopped medication were seizure-free at 2 years compared to 78% who remained on medication. Discuss with the patient what they want: risk of recurrence vs gravity of the side-effects.

Principles of antiepileptic drug therapy

1. Establish a clear clinical diagnosis
2. Get EEG supporting evidence if possible
3. Choose a drug, considering the:
- seizure type(s)
- patient's age
- price
- interaction with other drugs
- possibility of pregnancy

4. Give one drug only
5. Begin with modest dosage building up slowly over 2–3 months.
6. Give full information to the patient concerning
- names and alternative names of the drug supplied
- the main side-effects of the drug
- the need for compliance with instructions
- possible interactions with other medications

7. Monitor progress, seizure frequency and side-effects
8. Ensure adequate supplies

1. Pal DK, 1998, *Lancet*, **351** 19

► Status epilepticus

Status epilepticus has recently been redefined: "generalised, convulsive status epilepticus in adults and older children (>5 years old) refers to at least 5 min of (a) continuous seizures or (b) two or more discrete seizures".[1,2] This definition reflects the current uncertainty about the relationship between the duration of convulsions and CNS damage. It should encourage earlier appropriate treatment of status epilepticus, without waiting 30mins. It can result in death, permanent neurological damage, or the onset of chronic epilepsy – risk factors for such sequelae include aetiology, duration of attack, and systemic complications.

Aetiology: ~40% occur in known epileptics; ***other causes*** include fever or acute CNS infection (particularly in children), head injury, pesticide poisoning, stroke. ► Eclampsia.

Management
1. Stop seizures quickly.
2. Prevent complications.
3. Find and control the underlying causes.

1. Remove patient from potential danger.
2. Secure the airway, preferably with a Guedal airway, and give oxygen.
► Do not attempt to intubate if the jaw is clenched. Wait for sedation to have its effect.
3. Give 50ml 50% dextrose as IV bolus unless hypoglycaemia is excluded.
4. Give thiamine 250mg by slow IV infusion over 20min if the patient is an alcoholic – ensure facilities for managing anaphylaxis is apparent.
5. Give diazepam 10–20mg in 2–4ml IV or PR at a rate of 1ml/min. (For children, give 1mg per year of age.) This should control ~80% of patients. Second (and rarely third) doses may be needed.
► Beware respiratory depression following bolus diazepam.

If convulsions continue after giving diazepam, manage the patient in ICU if at all possible.

1. Give phenytoin 20mg/kg as an IV infusion – at <50mg/min – through a separate giving set. Once seizures are controlled, maintain with phenytoin 100mg IV q6–8h.
2. [Alternatively give phenobarbitone 10–15mg/kg as an IV infusion – at <100mg/min. Do not give more diazepam. Beware respiratory depression and hypotension. Chlormethiazole is an alternative.]
3. Check for and treat raised ICP.

If convulsions continue after phenytoin

1. Exclude pseudostatus.
2. Check drugs have been given correctly.
3. Then give general anaesthetic and ventilate, whilst treating causative condition.

- Give thiopentone 75–125mg (3–5ml of a 2.5% solution) IV over 10–15 secs. Give further doses according to response. ► Beware complicating hypotension. If large amounts are infused over a long period, it will accumulate and delay recovery.

1. Lowenstein DH, 1999, Epilepsia 40 (suppl 1), S3
2. Lowenstein DH, 1999, NEJM 338, 970.

Neurology

Cysticercosis

A condition, caused by the pork tapeworm, *Taenia solium*, which is a common cause of epilepsy worldwide. Humans are the definitive host for this species and normally become infected by eating cysts in undercooked pork meat – see life cycle opposite.

Accidental human ingestion of eggs in faecally-contaminated food results in disease with marked morbidity of the CNS, muscles, skin, and eye. The symptoms are caused by the inflammatory reaction to the living and dying parasites (active disease) and long-term effects of the inflammatory reaction to the cysts – fibrosis, calcification, and granulation (inactive disease).

Transmission: by ingestion of food or water contaminated with pig faeces. Poor personal hygiene, particularly amongst food handlers, and faecal pollution of water and irrigated vegetables predispose to infection.

Clinical features: CNS involvement (neurocysticercosis) normally manifests as epilepsy. However, since the number and localization of cysts varies greatly, neurocysticercosis can manifest in a variety of ways including hydrocephalus, dementia (frontal lobe involvement; often in children); infarcts (due to vasculitis); basal meningitis; cranial nerve defects; spinal symptoms.

Subcutaneous and muscular cysts occur in 25% of cases with CNS involvement, but may also occur in isolation – the calcified cysts appear as small, round, painless, firm nodules. The rare involvement of cardiac muscle can result in conduction defects. ► Ocular cysticercosis often presents with blurring of vision and the sensation of something moving in the eye. If untreated, it may progress to blindness and eye atrophy.

Diagnosis: active CNS lesions can be identified by CT or MRI; calcified inactive lesions can be seen on CT (and sometimes on X-ray). Serology.

Management

► Drugs should not be given to patients with severe active neurocysticercosis because they can elicit a potentially fatal inflammatory reaction. In this situation, manage symptomatically until the disease has settled.

1. Treat inactive or mild CNS disease with praziquantel 10–20mg/kg PO tds for 2–3 weeks or albendazole 7.5–15mg/kg PO bd for 30 days. Albendazole may be more effective but there may also be more SEs.
2. Patients presenting with seizures and a single cyst can be managed with anticonvulsants alone.
3. Surgery is usually reserved for subarachnoid and intraventricular cysts causing compression and resulting in hydrocephalus or cord compression
4. Ocular infection should not be treated with praziquantel. Ocular cysts may need to be treated surgically.

Prevention: health education and public health measures to improve personal hygiene, meat inspection, sanitation on farms, and sewage disposal. Mass treatments in hyperendemic regions and interruption of the parasite's life cycles.

Life cycle of *Taenia solium*

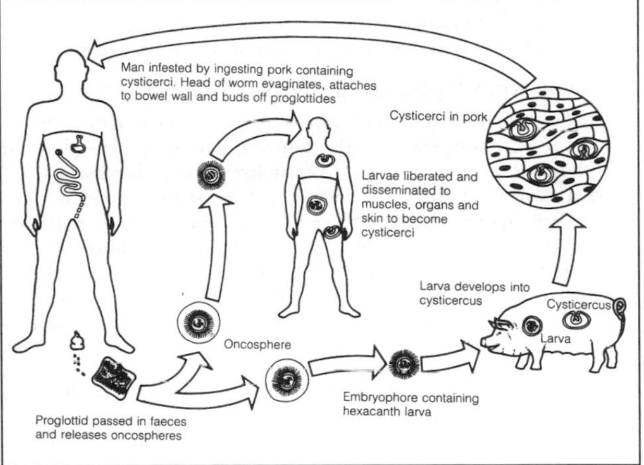
Man infested by ingesting pork containing cysticerci. Head of worm evaginates, attaches to bowel wall and buds off proglottides
Cysticerci in pork
Larvae liberated and disseminated to muscles, organs and skin to become cysticerci
Larva develops into cysticercus
Cysticercus
Larva
Oncosphere
Embryophore containing hexacanth larva
Proglottid passed in faeces and releases oncospheres

Weak legs/paraplegia, non-traumatic

Ask the following questions:

- Was the onset gradual or sudden?
- Is the tone spastic or flaccid?
- Is there sensory loss, in particular a sensory level? – a strong clue to spinal cord disease.
- Is there any loss of sphincter control (bowels or bladder)?
- Is there normal sensation around the sacrum and good anal tone?

1. Sudden weak legs with spasticity

- ***Cord compression*** – spinal or paraspinal infection or abscess due to TB, brucella, pyogenic bacteria; tumours (metastases, Hodgkin's or Burkitt's lymphoma, myeloma); disc prolapse; Paget's disease.

► **Cord compression** is an emergency. It must be considered when there is a rapid progression of leg weakness and/or sphincter failure. Check the perineal area for loss of sensation (saddle anaesthaesia).

- ***Other causes*** – infectious or post-infectious myelitis; cord infarction (due to vasculitis, thrombosis of anterior spinal artery, trauma or compression, dissection of aortic aneurysm, surgery); tetanus; carcinomatous meningitis.

2. Sudden weak legs with flaccidity/acute flaccid paralysis

- ***Cauda equina compression*** – a neurosurgical emergency. Causes: tumour; prolapsed disc; canal stenosis; TB; cysticercosis; schistosomiasis.
- ***Poliomyelitis*** – see page 450.
- ***Other causes*** – acute cord trauma/infarction; myelitis (in early stages with back pain, fever, double incontinence, sensory loss at defined level surmounted by a zone of hyperaestaesia); Guillain-Barre syndrome; rabies; lumbosacral nerve lesion; hypokalaemic periodic paralysis.

3. Chronic spastic paraparesis

- ***Causes*** – cord compression (eg cervical spondylosis); syringomyelia; tropical spastic paraparesis (TSP, due to HTLV-1); MND; subacute combined degeneration of the cord (vit B_{12} deficiency), konzo and lathyrism.

4. Chronic flaccid paraparesis

- ***Causes*** – peripheral neuropathies, myopathies, nerve trauma, and tabes dorsalis.

5. Weak legs + no sensory loss motor neurone disease (MND)

6. Absent knee jerks with extensor plantars

- ***Causes*** – Friederich's ataxia; taboparesis; MND; subacute combined degeneration of the cord.

7. Unilateral foot drop

- ***Causes*** – DM; stroke; prolapsed disc; MND; organophosphate poisoning; common peroneal nerve palsy.

Principles of management of paraplegia

1. Prevention of pressure sores by turning every 2 hours.
2. Attention to bladder and bowels (urinary catheter if incontinent).
3. Adequate hydration and nutrition.
4. Prevent complications, aspiration and pneumonia (ensure adequate swallowing), DVT (support stockings/heparin), contractures (physiotherapy), malaria (mosquito net).
5. Treat the underlying cause.

Tropical pyomyositis – primary *S. aureus* (rarely *Strep. pyogenes*) infection of skeletal muscle that is common throughout the tropics and subtropics, particularly in young men. Presents with localized pain, tenderness, without lymphadenopathy or major skin involvement. Needs to be distinguished from secondary abscesses extending into muscle from skin, bones, or other sites. Management is via surgical drainage and debridement (abscesses are often loculated), and antibiotics – flucloxacillin 0.5–1g IV q6h (unless *Strep. pyogenes* is cultured from pus – benzylpenicillin 2.4g IV q4h).

Clostridial myositis – extensive dirty skeletal muscle injuries are prone to become infected with *Clostridium perfringens*. This Gram +ve rod produces toxins and enzymes that cause necrosis of muscle fibres and interstitial cells, haemorrhage, and vascular congestion. This condition, ***gas gangrene***, must be controlled by removal of dead tissue and antibiotic cover: clindamycin 900mg IV q8h plus benzylpenicillin 2.4g IV q4h [alternatives: ceftriaxone 2g IV bd or erythromycin 1g by infusion q6h].

Poliomyelitis

This disease of young children is caused by the poliovirus, an enterovirus. The virus selectively infects and destroys anterior horn cells in the spinal cord, resulting in the cardinal sign of polio – acute flaccid paralysis (AFP). The clinical disease is relatively uncommon, however: ~99% of infected people show no paralytic manifestations.

A huge worldwide vaccination effort is now under way to eradicate it. While polio has been a major cause of disability worldwide, it may soon be just a disturbing memory, unlike the other major causes – RTAs and mines. Its eradication is revealing other possible causes of AFP eg JE virus.[1]

Transmission: via ingestion of faecally-contaminated food or water, or via droplet spread from the respiratory tract.

Clinical features: the prodromal symptoms are common to many infections and practically indistinguishable: fever, malaise, headache, drowsiness, sore throat.

In a minority, CNS disease (*preparalytic disease*) follows with abrupt onset of fever, headache, body pains, sensory disturbances, and neck stiffness – due to poliovirus meningitis. Flaccid paralysis then occurs in ~65%, developing asymmetrically over a variable time period, particularly affecting the lower limbs. The paralysis rarely progresses after 3 days or after the temperature falls. There is some recovery of function over the following weeks or months, as some damaged anterior horn cells recover. Death is relatively uncommon but results from aspiration or airway obstruction (bulbar paralysis) or respiratory failure (respiratory paralysis). A rare complication is slow deterioration of limb or bulbar function after many years – the *postpolio syndrome*.

Diagnosis: is clinical, with retrospective serological analysis.

Management: is supportive. Bed rest is essential; give analgesia, sedation. Do not give any injections.

Prevention: vaccination and improved public health.

Guillain-Barre syndrome (GBS)

A post-infectious demyelinating peripheral polyneuropathy. Some form of infection, mainly respiratory or diarrhoea, precedes the onset of GBS by 1–2 weeks in as many as 60% of cases. It develops over a few hours (rarely) to several weeks and must be considered a medical emergency.

► Respiratory arrest may occur without notice in severe cases; sudden death may also be caused by ANS disturbance of CVS function. These patients need constant observation, in an ITU setting if possible.

Clinical features: include progressive muscle weakness in the limbs of less than 4wks duration of progress; distal paraesthesia (less often sensory loss). Back and limb pain may be occasionally present. Also cranial nerve palsies (particularly VII); ANS disturbances; ileus. Monitor respiratory function and heart rhythm; plasma exchange or high-dose immunoglobulin if available shortens the hospital stay. Recovery occurs over several weeks or months with remyelination of peripheral nerves.

► The paralytic disease is made worse by IM injections during the preparalytic phase (eg injections of antibiotics) or by the muscles becoming fatigued (eg after exercise), so a high index of suspicion in endemic regions is important to prevent polio being made worse.

► Patients must be carefully observed during the onset of paralysis for signs of life-threatening bulbar and respiratory paralysis. Nurse patients with weak swallowing on their side. Good nursing care including frequent suction and observations may delay the need for a tracheostomy – however, perform a tracheostomy early in serious cases.

Polio rehabilitation

Acute stage

1. Treatment at this stage is based on:
   - rest
   - positioning.
2. Support the wrist and hands in a functional position with a splint or other support (eg pillow).
3. Support the ankle – maintain the ankle at 90° and avoid excessive inversion or eversion.

Subacute stage

1. Progress from passive movements to active assisted movements to active within the normal range.
   The movements will depend on the muscle groups affected
2. Progress to standing and walking with assistance – use walking aids if necessary eg stick, crutches.
   Aim for the best possible function.

Avoid:
- muscle shortening
- malformation due to muscle imbalance.

1. Solomon T, 1998, *Lancet*, 351, 1094

Mono/polyneuropathies

The mononeuropathies are lesions of single nerves, polyneuropathies lesions of multiple nerves normally due to systemic disease. In some conditions such as leprosy, multiple peripheral nerves may be involved simultaneously – this is termed mononeuritis multiplex. Polyneuropathies are symmetrical conditions and often affect the peripheries initially, producing a symetrical glove and stocking distribution.

In the tropics, environmental toxins and nutritional deficiencies are particularly important causes of peripheral neuropathies. They may be seen in epidemic form after toxins are released into the environment by industry or in an endemic form in particular regions. Some toxins are used in local forms of medicine, or they may contaminate food, liquor, etc. They frequently produce an individually recognizable syndrome – as always, there is no replacement for local clinical experience. In these situations, treatment involves removal of the toxin and/or supplementation with the deficient nutrient. ► The effects of many neuropathies are permanent.

Causes

Single nerves can be damaged by: • trauma • compression • DM • leprosy. The latter 2 conditions will often develop into neuropathies affecting multiple nerves, causing a mononeuritis multiplex or widespread peripheral neuropathy.

Polyneuropathies can be caused by:

Deficiencies –

B_1, B_6, B_{12}; a variety of multiple nutrient deficiencies.

Toxins –

- heavy metals: including lead [motor involvement], thallium [found in rodenticides → alopecia], arsenic [nail lines, changes in skin pigmentation]
- drugs: many but particularly isoniazid, ethambutol [affects optic nerve], sulphonamides, chloroquine, clioquinol, metronidazole, phenytoin
- industrial chemicals: solvents eg trio-ortho-cresayl phosphate
- pesticides, particularly organophosphorous (OP) compounds
- excessive consumption of certain foods: eg cassava which contains a cyanogenic glycoside can cause tropical ataxic neuropathy.

Metabolic diseases –

DM, renal or liver failure, alcohol, hypothyroidism.

Infections – leprosy, TB, HIV.

Other causes – genetic diseases, malignancy, connnective tissue disease.

WHO differential diagnosis of acute flaccid paralysis (WHO[ND])

	Polio	*Guillain-Barre syndrome*	*Traumatic neuritis*	*Transverse myelitis*
Installation of paralysis	24–48 hrs, from onset to full paralysis	from hrs to 10 days	from hrs to 4 days	from hrs to 4 days
Flaccid paralysis	usually acute, asymmetrical, principally proximal	usually acute, symmetrical and distal	asymmetrical, acute affecting one limb only	acute, affecting lower limbs, symmetrical
Muscle tone	reduced or absent in the affected limb	global hypotonia	reduced or absent in the affected limb	hypotonia in lower limbs
Deep tendon reflexes	decreased to absent	globally absent	decreased to absent	absent in lower limbs early, hyperreflexia late
Sensation	severe myalgia, backache, no sensory changes	cramps, tingling, hypoanaesthesia of palms/soles	pain in gluteus muscles, hypothermia	anaesthesia of lower limbs, with sensory level
Cranial nerve involvement	only when bulbar involvement is present	often present, affecting nerves VII, IX, X, XI, XII	absent	absent
Respiratory insufficiency	only when bulbar involvement is present	in severe cases; enhanced by bacterial pneumonia	absent	sometimes
CSF findings	inflammatory	albumin-cells dissociation	normal	normal or a few cells
Bladder dysfunction	absent	transient	never	present

Leprosy (Hansen's disease)

Leprosy is a disease that still elicits immense stigma in many communities. It is a chronic inflammatory disease caused by *Mycobacterium leprae* infecting macrophages and peripheral nerve Schwann cells.

Its presentation and progress are determined by the patient's ability to raise a strong cell-mediated immune response to the mycobacterium. Most people (~75%) develop an effective immune response and remove the microbe. The rest are unable to eliminate the bacteria and manifest signs and symptoms of disease – these clinical features fall on a spectrum depending on the strength of their immune response (see table opposite).

- On one extreme, a strong but ineffective immune response keeps mycobacterium numbers at very low levels but also damages microbe-infected peripheral nerves and skin – **TT leprosy.**
- At the other end of the spectrum, a completely ineffective immune response allows the disease to become generalized. There is involvement of multiple organ systems (such as bones, eyes, respiratory tract) in addition to widespread skin and peripheral nerve damage – **LL leprosy.**
- Many patients fall in between these 2 extremes. A number of patients will initially have BB leprosy but then develop an LL form of disease.

Mycobacteria are present in the skin lesions, particularly at the edges where they may be found on biopsy. However, they are very few in TT and BT leprosy because of the immune response and it is difficult to detect them, hence the term ***paucibacillary leprosy*** for these forms. In contrast, the LL forms skin lesions that are absolutely filled with bacteria – ***multibacillary leprosy***.

Transmission: routes are still uncertain but transmission probably occurs via nasal secretions from an LL patient to the upper respiratory tract of a new host. Other routes of entry may be broken skin. The mycobacterium appears to survive for several days in the environment. People in close contact with infected people have a greater chance of becoming infected.

Clinical features: are of skin lesions and peripheral nerve damage.

- ***Skin:*** the first sign of infection is the development of a solitary skin lesion the *indeterminate lesion* (see table). Most of these lesions resolve as the individual's immune response deals with the infection. However, in about 25% of cases, the infection is not controlled and the patient goes on to develop true leprosy and its characteristic lesions. The subsequent skin lesions have been classified into five groups (see opposite).
- ***Nerves:*** characteristic nerves become infiltrated see opposite. Sensory disturbances are often the first symptoms (eg paraesthesia, loss of light touch, temperature, or pain sensation). Muscle wasting can produce claw hands, drop foot, and facial palsy. Nerve dysfunction leads to bone changes secondary to disuse.
- ***Other organs*** may become involved: • eyes (can → blindness) • bones (bone cysts, aseptic necrosis, dactylitis especially phalanges) • lymphadenopathy • mucous membrane ulceration • nails • kidney.

Classification	*Skin lesions*	*Nerve involvement*
Indeterminate	Solitary hypopigmented 2–5cm lesion. Interior may show sensory loss although both Dr and patient are often uncertain about this loss. May become TT-like.	None clinically detectable.
Tuberculoid [TT]	Few lesions (often only 1) with well-defined borders, central flattening and in most cases central sensory loss to heat, pain, soft touch. The patch is not itchy but is often dry (does not sweat) and hairless.	Normally little, with up to 1 nerve involved. Rarely presents with mononeuropathy.
Borderline tuberculoid [BT]	>4 lesions; they tend to be more florid than TT lesions with less clear sensory loss. Satellite lesions occur at the edges.	Asymmetrical peripheral nerve involvement.
Midborderline [BB]	Many lesions with scooped or punched out centres. Satellites are common.	Widespread enlargement of nerves +/− muscle weakness.
Borderline lepromatous [BL]	Many lesions in a bilateral but asymmetrical distribution. The lesions have diffuse borders and there is greater nerve damage.	As above.
Lepromatous [LL]	Numerous nodular skin lesions in a symmetrical distribution. The lesions are not dry or anaesthetic. There are often thickened shiny earlobes, loss of eyebrows, and skin thickening. Early manifestations are always dermal, never neuropathic.	As above.

Diagnosis: is based on the following three findings:

- hypoaesthetic skin patch
- thickened nerves
- skin smear from lesion edge/ear lobe positive for mycobacterium.

Palpate peripheral nerves (both sides at the same time) to assess enlargement, particularly of great auricular nerve, ulnar nerve at the elbow, superficial radial nerve at the wrist, superficial median nerve at the wrist, lateral popliteal nerve at the neck of the fibula, superficial peroneal nerve, and posterior tibial nerve.

Management: if caught early, effective use of antibiotics will eliminate the infection thereby preventing the chronic disabilities that have long been associated with this disease. If there is already a severe peripheral neuropathy, then the patient must be taught how to look after the affected limbs.

Advise the patient to:

- keep her hands under constant observation for swelling or sensory changes
- protect her hands from trauma
- check her feet for ulcers and particularly for any loss of light touch since this is an early indicator of nerve damage
- wear wooden soles and rubber insteps since these help prevent plantar lesions
- soak her feet regularly, removing any callus that builds up.

Antibiotic therapy[1]

LL, BL, and BB patients (plus BT and indeterminate patients with acid-fast bacteria on skin smear, if such tests are performed) are considered multibacillary for determining the choice of antibiotics. The other forms receive paucibacillary regimens. Therapy is safe during pregnancy.

For paucibacillary leprosy, give:

- rifampicin, 600mg monthly (or four-weekly), supervised
- dapsone, 100mg daily.

This is given for 6 months. The patient is considered non-infectious after the first dose of rifampicin.

For multibacillary leprosy, give:

- rifampicin, 600mg monthly (or four-weekly), supervised
- clofazimine, 50mg daily, unsupervised *plus* 300mg monthly (or four-weekly), supervised
- dapsone, 100mg daily.

This is given for at least 12 months and until skin smears are negative. The patient is considered non-infectious after 4–6 doses of rifampicin.

Other regimens: indeterminate leprosy can be treated with a single dose of rifampicin (600mg), ofloxacin (400mg) and minocycline (100mg). Ofloxacin and minocycline can also be used for long term therapy in patients who cannot tolerate rifampicin or clofazimine.

Reactions

These are acute excerbations that normally occur during therapy. ► If not treated promptly and adequately, they often result in crippling deformity. The course of antileprosy chemotherapy must not be stopped during the reaction.

Reversal reaction (type 1 reaction) – 2 forms occur in

- treated BT, BB, BL leprosy groups and non-treated BT patients (upgrading reaction), and
- untreated or inadequately treated BT, BB, or BL patients (downgrading reaction).

The first form occurs a few weeks to months after starting therapy, while the 2nd can occur at any time. The skin lesions become scaly, swollen, erythematous and may ulcerate; new skin lesions develop. Severe reactions have fever, malaise, and/or peripheral oedema. Neuritis (+/– pain) occurs in nerves – without urgent treatment, earlier nerve damage is exacerbated.

Treatment: for severe reactions, is prednisolone 40–60mg PO daily reduced every 1–2wks and stopped at 12wks. A few patients may require maintenance therapy with 15–20mg daily. Splint limbs to rest affected painful nerves. Paracetamol can control mild symptoms.

Erythema nodosum leprosum (type 2 reaction) – occurs in many treated LL (occasionally treated LB and untreated LL) patients some months after starting therapy with the appearance of painful, red nodules. They become purple before resolving after a few days; if severe, some plaques necrose and ulcerate. The skin lesions are accompanied by fever; malaise; bone pain and swollen joints; painful neuritis; lymphadenopathy; iridocyclitis; rarely nephritis. Incurrent infection or increased stress trigger the attack.

Treatment: in severe cases (systemic features or painful nerves), treat in hospital with one of:

- prednisolone 30–40mg PO daily, reduced after 2 weeks by 5–10mg every 2 weeks [best for short episodes]
- thalidomide 200mg bd, reduced to 50–100mg nightly [best drug but ► contraindicated in women of childbearing age]
- clofazimine 300mg daily, reduced after 3 months [preferred drug for premenopausal women; takes 3–4 weeks to have its full effect so should be combined with prednisolone initially].

► Check the patients regularly for iridocyclitis. Treat with steroid and homatropine eye drops. Mild symptoms can be controlled with paracetamol.

1. WHO model prescribing information. Drugs used in leprosy. Geneva 1998

10. Dermatology/skin in systemic disease[1]

Rashes 460
Urticaria 462
Drug eruptions 462
Skin ulcers 464
Dermatitis (eczema) 466
Psoriasis 466
Skin cancers 468
Bacterial skin infections 470
The non-venereal treponematoses 472
Varicella-zoster infection 474
Poxvirus infections 474
Fungal skin infections 476
Cutaneous leishmaniasis 478
Filariasis 480
Onchocerciasis ("river blindness") 480
Dracunculiasis 482
Loiasis 482
Lymphatic filariasis 484
Infestations 488

1. Ryan T, *OTM*, 3rd edn, p3703, Oxford University Press, Oxford.

Dermatology/skin in systemic disease

Rashes

Basis of rashes

- The skin is heterogeneous, varying for example in thickness and quantity of hair or sebaceous glands. Rashes affecting only one component of the skin will have a distribution which reflects this component eg hair follicles in folliculitis or dermatomes in shingles.
- The lesions differ according to the depth of the inflammation. Near the surface it causes vesiculation and scaling while deep dermal or subcutaneous inflammation results in nodule formation.
- The rate of development is determined by the type of inflammatory response. Oedematous weals and blisters are more acute; white cell infiltration, purpura and pustules take longer; while ischaemic necrosis and exfoliation are more chronic responses.
- The distribution of the lesion may be typical – see figure below.
- Endogenous rashes tend to be symmetrical; in contrast, a biting insect knows little of symmetry and may produce groups of bites placed quite indiscriminately. Unlike the rashes of secondary syphilis, the site of the primary chancre is not influenced by host symmetry. Fungus infections tend to be more obvious on one side of the body, whereas psoriasis is usually exactly symmetrical.

Common rashes[2]

Maculopapular rashes

Extensive –
- measles
- chickenpox
- rubella
- dengue
- scabies
- body lice
- typhus
- secondary syphilis.

Sparse –
- gonococcaemia
- typhoid rose spots
- flea bites
- cutaneous myiasis
- Kaposi's sarcoma
- lichen planus
- cutaneous larva migrans
- tungiasis

Hypopigmentation

- postinflammation
- tinea versicolor
- leprosy
- pityriasis alba
- vitiligo
- yaws
- pinta
- post-kala azar dermal leishmaniasis.

Some characteristic rash distributions

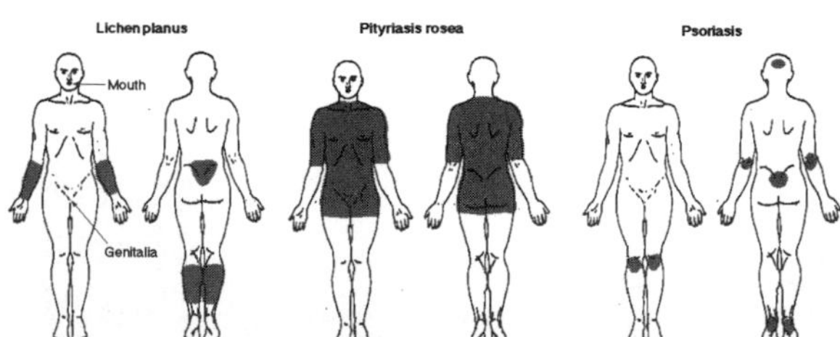

Dermatology/skin in systemic disease

Nodules

- onchocerciasis
- dracunculiasis
- leprosy
- cutaneous myiasis
- fungal infections
- yaws
- Kaposi's sarcoma
- TB abscess
- pyomyositis
- erythema nodosum
- rheumatoid disease
- gout

Plaques/crusts

- fungal infections
- leprosy
- impetigo
- Kaposi's sarcoma
- cutaneous leishmaniasis
- pinta
- any cause of an eschar
- psoriasis

Urticaria

- drugs
- strongyloidiasis
- loiasis
- schistosomiasis
- gnasthostomiasis

Petechiae

- meningococcaemia
- viral haemorrhagic fevers
- typhus
- causes of DIC

Vesicles

- herpes zoster
- herpes simplex
- orf
- papular urticaria
- vasculitis
- monkeypox

Pustules

- bacterial infection
- irritant folliculitis
- psoriasis

Common patterns of dermatitis

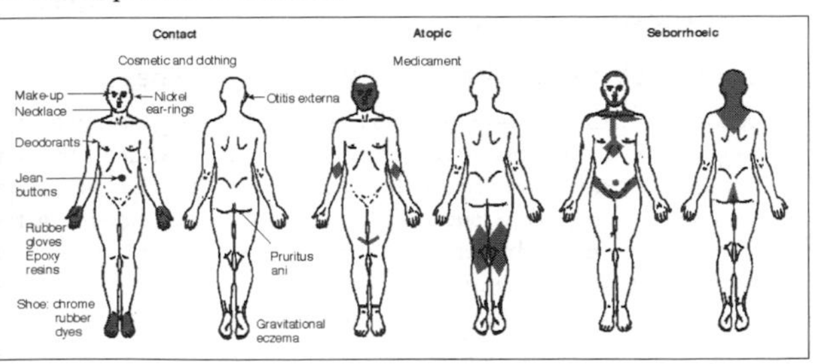

1. Ryan T, 1996, *OTM*, 3rd edn, p3703, Oxford University Press, Oxford.
2. Brook MG, *Manson's Tropical Diseases*, p22

Urticaria

Transient swelling and/or flushing of the skin due to release of inflammatory mediators in the skin. This release is stimulated by allergens (food, drugs) binding to IgE, immune complex disease and complement activation (due eg to antivenom, penicillins, infections), molecules that release histamine directly (eg drugs – morphine, shellfish). The reaction may be accompanied by joint pains, stomach aches, and fever.

►Urticaria is life-threatening when

- it is part of an anaphylactic reaction
- angioedema involves the upper respiratory tract
- it is part of a severe systemic disease (eg septicaemia, SLE).

Papular urticaria: itchy and persistent papules following damage to epidermis, often by an insect bite. They are intensely pruritic, and commonly blister.

Chronic urticaria: urticaria lasting >2–3 months. Most commonly due to parasite infection in the tropics. Check for worm infection (hookworm, tapeworm, roundworm), trichinosis, onchocerciasis, dracunculosis, lymphatic filiariasis, strongyloidiasis. Other causes: drugs, food additives.

Management

Remove the stimulus, treating any infection. Give oral antihistamines eg chlorphineramine 4mg q4–6h or promethazine 10–20mg tds.

Drug eruptions

Adverse drug reactions are a common consequence of the use of both western and altenative therapies. Drug rashes tend to occur in a symmetrical pattern; the rashes are commonly erythematous, urticarial, purpuric or ischaemic. Exfoliation or vesiculation are rare but recognized.

► Ask the patient about previous reactions to drugs. Without this priming, it is unlikely that drugs given for just a few days could have caused the rash. The exception is when an infection primes the body to a medicine (eg cough mixture or antibiotics). In general, most drugs take >5–10 days to initiate a reaction.

Erythema multiforme (Stevens-Johnson syndrome)

A reaction to virus infection (eg HSV, Orf), drugs (eg antimalarials, sulphonamides), neoplasms, or certain systemic diseases, which produces coin-shaped erythematous rashes with central blistering (target lesions) on the hands, feet (to a lesser extent the trunk), and mucosae – mouth, genitalia, eyes. If the mucosal blistering is severe, it is termed Stevens-Johnson syndrome and is often accompanied by fever (+/– anterior uveitis, pneumonia, renal failure, polyarthritis, diarrhoea).

Management of drug eruptions

- stop the use of all drugs likely to have caused the reaction.
- it is possible to restart the drugs one-by-one to identify the causative drug (unless the drug causes anaphylaxis) but there is a high risk of morbidity. Only essential drugs should be restarted.

Cutaneous larva migrans

A cutaneous eruption resulting from exposure of the skin to infective filariform larvae of hookworms (*Ancylostoma* spp) and *Strongyloides* spp for whom humans are not true hosts. They persist under the skin, in which they are visible, but cannot complete their life cycles. ***Treat:*** with thiabendazole (25mg/kg PO bd for 5 days, then 2 days rest before if necessary repeating the 5 day course) or ivermectin. Thiabendazole can also be given topically.

Larva currens – a cutaneous eruption resulting from autoinfection into the skin (often of the buttocks/peri-anal area) by *Strongyloides stercoralis* – see chapter 3D.

Creeping eruptions – can be caused by infection with *S. stercoralis*, *Gnathostoma spinigerum*, cutaneous myiasis (*Hypoderma bovis*, *H. lineatum*), warble fly maggots (*Gasterophilus* spp) and cutaneous *Fasciola hepatica*.

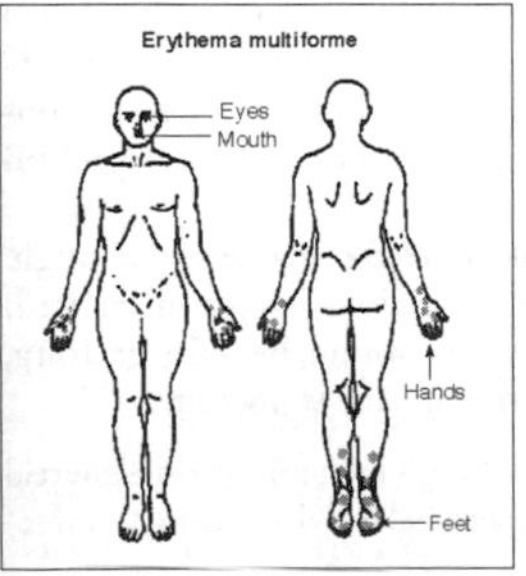

Skin ulcers

- ► The possibility of leprosy should be considered in any patient presenting with a painless burn, injury, or ulcer of one limb.
- ► Trauma is a very common cause of ulceration, particularly in children. Wounds and cuts often become 2° infected → ulceration.

Management of leg ulceration

1. Identify and, if possible, eliminate the cause of the ulcer.
2. Check for arterial disease, particularly absent peripheral pulses.
3. Prevent venous stasis by elevating the legs above the heart (do this during the day by raising the mattress with eg a chair). Elevation should be 45° for most people; if peripheral pulses are absent, do not raise the feet >23cm above the heart. Use compression bandages if difficult to raise legs.
4. Apply clean dressing using short pieces of bandage that do not completely encircle the leg. Dressings wet with saline will encourage healing and soften crusts.

Tropical ulcer

Ulcers due to mixed bacterial infection which predominantly occur on the foot, ankle, or lower leg following minor trauma. A small round painful ulcer forms which then spreads rapidly, exposing the underlying muscles and tendons. The patient is febrile. After a few weeks, the ulcer stops spreading and the pain diminishes. Good treatment in the early stages encourages the ulcer to heal. Neglected ulcers become fibrosed and may be the site of a future squamous cell CA.
Management: if noted early, the ulcers respond well to penicillin and daily dressing. Ulcers >2.5cm require daily dressings and penicillin for one week followed by skin grafting. Chronic ulcers should be excised and skin grafted.

Buruli ulcer

A chronic necrotizing skin disease of tropical forest areas caused by infection with *Mycobacterium ulcerans*. The method of transmission is not known but is presumed to occur through broken skin. The infection starts as a painless nodule which breaks down to form an ulcer that is relatively painless and has edges that may be undermined for 5–15cm. Necrosis is caused by a bacterial exotoxin. There are few systemic signs (although lymphadenopathy occurs). The ulcer may spread rapidly, or become 2° infected. Without treatment, healing is slow and may → scarring, contractures, and deformities. Diagnosis is on typical clinical picture or AFB in the ulcer's base.
Management: completely excise nodule if recognized early enough. Otherwise at the ulcer stage – treat any 2° infection, irrigate ulcer with saline, excise all diseased tissue and cover the wound by skin grafting. Effectiveness of antibiotics (streptomycin, rifampicin) is unclear.

Infective causes of skin ulcers include: bacteria (non-venereal treponematoses anthrax; mycobacteria; superficial or deep fungal infections; parasites such as *Leishmania* spp.

Some causes of skin ulcers

• ulcers on penis or vagina	→ see chapter 3B
• ulcers on breast	→ infection or cancer
• ulcers on foot or leg	→ diabetes → leprosy → venous disease → arterial disease → tropical ulcer → sickle-cell disease → chronic osteomyelitis → guinea worm
• ulcers anywhere	→ cutaneous leishmaniasis → bacterial infection → typhus eschar → trypanosomal chancre → anthrax → buruli ulcer

Dermatitis (eczema)

An inflammatory reaction of the skin that may occur as a normally asymmetrical response to an external injury (irritant or contact allergic) or as a symmetrical endogenous response to a stimulus (atopic).

- **Irritant dermatitis** – the commonest form of dermatitis, generally affecting the hands following contact with industrial irritants at work. The skin is dry and unsupple with deep cracks which may → 2° infected. Previously damaged skin is more susceptible to irritants.
- **Contact allergic dermatitis** – sensitization to an allergen, normally over months or years, results in the onset of dermatitis within hours of subsequent exposure to the allergen eg cosmetics, zips/buttons, food, plants, medicines, and metals. Irritant dermatitis is a risk factor for contact dermatitis. Patch testing identifies the specific allergen.
- **Atopic eczema** – is due to a poorly suppressed humoral immune response to certain foods and environmental agents. The skin is very itchy and dry; it becomes damaged by repeated scratching. Secondary infection produces lymphadenopathy.

Clinical features: the reaction involves both the dermis and the epidermis. Epidermal proliferation results in scaling. Inflammmation in the dermis often produces intense pruritus, pain and swelling. Dermal oedema spreads to include the epidermis, swelling the epidermal cells and producing vesicles (not found in other epidermal proliferation diseases) which burst → exudation. The lesion is papular, confluent in the centre with satellite lesions spreading out on all sides. There is often loss of pigmentation in acute lesions in dark skin, but darkening in chronic lesions.

Psoriasis

A disease of the epidermis in which there is a marked increase in epidermal cell proliferation and migration to the surface. The aetiology is unclear but lesions may occur after skin injury (Koebner phenomenon). Fluctuations in the condition are common, as are spontaneous remissions.

Clinical features: the classic lesion is a sharply demarcated silvery plaque. It is often more active at the edge with a clear centre. At the beginning, or as the plaques resolve, the plaques may be atypical eg scaleless, exudative red lesions. The plaques occur most commonly on knees, elbows, and scalp. Lesions in flexures have decreased scale, and are red, shiny and liable to crack and macerate. Distinct forms occur:

- Guttate psoriasis – small poorly defined lesions (often red with little silvery scale) that occur across the whole body; often in children after streptococcal sore throat or vaccination.
- Palmar/plantar psoriasis – often occurs in isolation; the lesions may develop deep cracks and sterile pustules and the nails become involved. This needs to be differentiated from fungal infection.
- Generalized pustular psoriasis – characterized by presence of fever, arthropathy, bright red erythema followed by the development of multiple pustules. Can occur after removal of steroid therapy. It is self-resolving.
- Polyarthritic psoriasis.

Management of eczema[1]

1. Eliminate or avoid known irritants or allergens.
2. Washing with soap substitutes based on emollients four times a day helps keep the skin moist.
3. Apply steroid creams to affected areas 1–2 times daily. Use the least potent steroid that works for short periods of time only. Avoid strong steroids in children.
4. Severe chronic allergy can be relieved by steroids and other immunosuppressive drugs eg azathioprine.
5. Treat secondary infection vigorously (erythromycin is useful).

Breastfeeding may reduce the risk of atopic eczema. This may be worth emphasizing in infants with a family history of eczema.

Management of psoriasis[1]

The aim is to decrease epidermal cell turnover without causing irreversible tissue damage. Many treatments have been suggested.
Options include:

1. Emollients and reassurance for mild cases.
2. Coal tar applied twice daily to the lesions. Build up from a low concentration intially. Coal tar baths are useful for extensive lesions.
3. Dithranol ointments and creams. Concentrations vary from 0.1–3%. Start with low concentrations – these can be left overnight; higher concentrations should be left on the skin for only 3–60mins. Do not apply to flexures.

   Both coal tar and dithranol can be combined with salicylates which enhance the rate of surface scale loss.
4. Systemic therapy may be required occasionally for generalized illness, particularly in the elderly. Use methotrexate or cyclosporin.
5. Corticosteroids have a limited role. Potent topical steroids should be avoided or given by specialists because they may lead to relapse or vigorous rebound on withdrawal. A weaker steroid (eg hydrocortisone 1%) can be used for short periods (eg 4wks) on the face or in flexures. Systemic steroids should probably be avoided.

1. British National Formulary 13.5.1 and 13.5.2

Skin cancers

Long-term exposure of pale skin to strong sunlight is a risk factor for all these tumours. Therefore Caucasians and pale-skinned Asians should be encouraged always to use sunscreen on sun-exposed parts of their body. Likewise, dark-skinned people with depigmenting disease or who were born with albinism have lost their natural protection and are at high risk of developing skin cancer.

Actinic keratoses: intially dry, wrinkled areas of skin that become pale scaly crusts with a red base. The lesions are caused by chronic exposure of pale skin to intense sunlight and are therefore uncommon in dark-skinned people. They are pre-malignant – while they may disappear in some individuals, in others they develop into one of the malignancies described below. They should be treated before this change takes place.
Treatment: freeze lesions with liquid nitrogen, or daily apply 5% 5-fluorouracil cream directly to the keratoses for 3–4 weeks. The keratoses ulcerate, necrose and become replaced by new skin. The cream may be too strong for the face: cover the neck, face and ears with a 1% solution (5ml 5% cream in 20ml propylene glycol) daily for 3–4 weeks – this treats subclinical lesions as well.

Squamous cell carcinoma: initially a fleshy dry nodule that breaks down to form an ulcerating lesion with hard raised edges. They occur in actinic keratoses, on the lips or inside the mouth of long-term smokers, or at the edges of chronic ulcers and areas of inflammation. They are locally very invasive but do not metastasize systemically.
Treatment: early *wide* local excision is essential; the tumour often infiltrates further into neighbouring tissue than is apparent. If the tumour is removed at its obvious margins, these infiltrations will be left behind and the tumour will recur.

Basal cell carcinoma: initially a slow-growing papule that breaks down in the centre, becoming an ulcer with a rolled 'pearl-coloured' edge. They occur on the face above a line drawn between the chin and ears. If left untreated, they infiltrate slowly causing extensive damage but do not spread from the original site.
Treatment: involves curettage and cauterization of the ulcer's base, or cryotherapy. 5% fluorouracil cream applied to the residual ulcer daily for 2–3 weeks after these procedures may be useful in destroying malignant cells missed by the curretage.

Melanoma: any pigmented lesion that is variably coloured, changes shape or colour, starts to bleed, or ulcerates, should be considered a potential melanoma. Pigmented satellite lesions around a mole also suggest a melanoma. Exposure to direct sunlight is a strong risk factor. They frequently originate in moles; therefore people with many moles should be encouraged to examine them regularly and report changes to a doctor. The tumours are extremely invasive and may only be recognized once they have metastasized to the CNS or other sites. The original lesion may be quite innocuous.
Treatment: is immediate, wide local excision.

Dermatology/skin in systemic disease

Bacterial skin infections

1. **Impetigo:** classically *S. aureus* infection of the epidermis. It often occurs at sites of skin damage – eg cuts, eczema, chickenpox blisters, scabies, insect bites. A blister forms that exudes pus and then scabs over. It is highly infectious by contact, often being spread both to other parts of the same person and to other people. *S. aureus* can be grown from the skin lesions. (*Strep. pyogenes* can also cause impetigo; see below for management.)

   Treatment:
   - if widespread, give cloxacillin 250–500mg qds PO for 5 days.

2. **Erysipelas:** *Strep. pyogenes* infection of the dermis, normally of shin, foot or face. Unlike cellulitis, the area of inflammation *has a distinct edge* as it spreads out from the 1° skin lesion. The skin is tense, swollen, painful and often dark red in colour, with local lymphadenopathy. Severe infection produces skin blistering as the epidermal layers becomes separated. Anaerobic conditions (necrotic tissue) encourages toxin production so the infection becomes worse, with onset of systemic signs, if the infection is not treated.

   Treatment:
   - phenoxymethylpenicillin or erythromycin 500mg PO qds.
   - In severe cases, or where there is no improvement after 24hrs, admit to hospital for benzylpenicillin 2.4g IV q4h for 2–4 weeks, until skin signs have fully resolved.

   ► Bacteraemia may result in erysipelas in unusual sites or the occurrence of lymphangitis or lymphadenitis. This has a high mortality.

3. **Cellulitis:** *S. aureus* or *Strep. pyogenes* infection of the subcutaneous tissues. An erythematous tender swelling *without distinct edge* that often starts in injuries such as small cuts, diabetic ulcers, or skin fissures of the hand, leg, or foot.

   Treatment: differs according to the site of infection:
   - *hand* – cloxacillin 0.25–0.5g PO qds for 5 days
   - *leg/foot* – cloxacillin plus amoxycillin 500mg PO qds (covers *E. coli*)
   - if nidus is *ulceration* (DM; ischaemia) – cloxacillin, ampicillin, plus metronidazole 500mg PO tds.

   ► If cellulitis continues to spread after 24hrs with high fever, admit to hospital for
   - benzylpenicillin 2.4g IV q4h, *plus*
   - flucloxacillin 2g IV q6h *plus if indicated*
   - metronidazole 500mg IV q8h

   ► Take blood cultures.

4. **Necrotizing fasciitis** – an uncommon, severe infection of subcutaneous tissue caused by *Strep. pyogenes*, as a complication of erysipelas or following a simple skin injury. Rapid necrosis of infected tissue leads to intense local pain and high fever; there may be few signs on the skin.

   Treatment:
   - benzylpenicillin 2.4g IV q4h, *plus*
   - metronidazole 500mg IV q8h

   ► Perform an early and wide debridement of involved tissue.

Dermatology/skin in systemic disease

The non-venereal treponematoses

A group of disfiguring and disabling conditions that primarily affect children in communities with poor hygiene. Mass treatment campaigns by the WHO in the 1950–60s effectively controlled their transmission but the last decade has seen a resurgence due to a decreased surveillance. Like syphilis, they have 3 stages with a long period of latency before the manifestation of 3° disease. Unfortunately, unlike syphilis, the 3° lesions are infective which will cause problems for the eradication of these diseases since it is difficult to identify latent carriers.

Transmission: direct person–person through skin contact. The treponemes cannot penetrate intact skin, so abrasions are probably required.

Clinical features: yaws is the commonest and prototypic disease.

1. ***Yaws*** – the primary lesion is a papule which develops into a round/oval 2–5cm painless, pruritic papilloma. It usually occurs on the legs, arms, face, or neck, and normally heals in 3–6 months. Weeks to years after this lesion resolves, multiple 2° lesions occur in crops on any part of the body and last up to 6 months. They are papules or papillomas of various shape; they may ulcerate and form yellow-brown scabs. Other lesions include dermatitis or hyperkeratosis of palms and soles, local lymphadenopathy, dactylitis, long bone swelling, and rarely osteitis of nasal bones, producing swellings on both sides of the nose (*goundou*). After a latent period, the disease reappears with necrotic destruction of skin and bones (gummas). Other clinical features include hyperkeratosis, palatal destruction and 2° infection, goundou, sabre tibia, bursitis.
2. ***Endemic syphilis (bejel)*** – a 1° lesion is rarely seen in this infection. The first lesions are usually painless ulcers of lips and oropharynx (→ sore throat). In addition there is osteoperiostitis of long bones, condylamata lata, angular stomatitis, rarely a 2° syphilis-like rash, and generalized lymphadenopathy. Late lesions include bone destruction (as in yaws), skin ulcers, and palmar and plantar keratosis.
3. ***Pinta*** – an infection that primarily affects the skin. Satellite lesions surround the 1° papule; there is regional painless lymphadenopathy. The 2° stage plaques appear within a few months; these plaques change their colour and occur anywhere on the body. The 3° disease involves depigmentation and atrophy of the skin.

Diagnosis: motile spirochaetes can be seen on dark-field microscopy of lesion exudates. There are no serological or morphological features that differentiate syphilis-causing *T. pallidum* from the other treponemes. The precise diagnosis is clinical.

Management: a single dose of benzathine penicillin G 0.9g IM (½ dose for children) [alternative: erythromicin 500mg (half dose for children) PO qds for 15 days].

Prevention: identification of active cases, followed by treatment of all contacts. If >10% in a community are actively infected, all should receive penicillin.

	Yaws	Bejel	Pinta
Organism	*T. pertenue*	*T. pallidum*	*T. carateum*
Age group	15–40	2–10	10–30
Occurrence	Africa S America Oceania Asia	Africa Middle-East	Latin America
Climate	Warm, Humid	Dry, Arid	Warm

Varicella-zoster infection

This herpesvirus causes two conditions: ***chickenpox*** (or varicella) following 1° infection and ***shingles*** (or zoster) following reactivation of latent virus. The virus is transmitted by inhalation of nasopharyngeal droplets or contact with vesicular fluid. After viraemic spread and 1° disease, the virus becomes latent in sensory ganglia and motor neurones. Reactivation normally occurs in just one sensory ganglia, leading to disease involving neurones of that dermatome only. The stimulus for reactivation is unclear.

1. **Chickenpox** may be severe in neonates and adults but occurs most commonly as a relatively mild infection in children. There is prodromal fever, headache and malaise – minimal in children – followed by the appearance of an itchy rash with *all stages of development* (vesicle → papule → pustule → scab) *present in one area of skin* (cf poxviruses). The scabs fall off on the 10th day without leaving scars, unless the patient has scratched the lesions. ***Complications*** in severe infection include pneumonitis and ARDS; mild encephalitis; thrombocytopenia and purpura fulminans, 2° bacterial infection of pocks (rarely, of respiratory tract). Disseminated disease is common in immunocompromised hosts.
2. **Shingles** is characterized by paraesthesia and shooting pains in the affected dermatome for several days before the appearance of a rash and mild fever. The pocks scab over after 3–7 days; they often become infected with *S. aureus* if left untreated. The rash is typically unilateral and involves only one dermatome; in some cases satellite lesions occur and, very rarely, dermatomes may be involved bilaterally. ***Complications*** occur after involvement of ophthalmic nerve (conjunctivitis; keratitis; periorbital swelling); motor nerves, particularly cranial (palsies); ANS (bladder paralysis; bowel atony). Others include: mild encephalitis; retinal necrosis; purpura fulminans; postherpetic neuralgia (very painful and often difficult to treat; tricyclic antidepressants are beneficial in some patients). Disseminated disease may occur in shingles. While normally mild in immunocompetent patients, it may prove fatal in the immunosuppressed.

Treatment: in severe infections, give aciclovir 10mg/kg IV q8h until 48hrs after the last lesion erupts. Therapy in other patients should shorten and alleviate the symptoms.

Poxvirus infections

Although the eradication of smallpox is one of the success stories of this century, related poxviruses – monkeypox and tanapox – still cause occasional infections across central Africa. The rash (1–2 lesions in tanapox; many covering the whole body in monkeypox) is preceded by a 2–3 day prodromal period with fever and other systemic signs. Lymphadenopathy occurs in monkeypox, characteristically involving both femoral and inguinal nodes ▶ Unlike chickenpox, the lesions are always at the same stage. Both infections tend to resolve without treatment. Human–human transmission has been reported within households with monkeypox.

Dermatology/skin in systemic disease

Fungal skin infections

1. Cutaneous infections

- ***Dermatophytoses (tinea)*** – common skin infections caused by fungi, particularly *Trichophyton* and *Microsporum* spp. They cause scaling or maceration between the toes (tinea pedis); itchy, scaly, red rash with definite edges in the groin area (tinea cruris); annular lesions with raised edges (often itchy) anywhere on the body (tinea corporis); scaling and itching of the scalp with loss of hair (tinea capitis). Treat with local application of Whitfield's ointment (benzoic acid compound) or clotrimazole; for severe cases and nail involvement, use griseofulvin 10mg/kg PO daily for 6–8 weeks or ketaconazole 200mg PO daily for 4 weeks.
- ***Pityriasis versicolor*** – presents as a superficial, hypo- or hyperpigmented, macular rash normally of the upper body. Treat with 2% selenium sulphide shampoo or Whitfield's ointment. Oral antifungals can be used if the rash does not respond to topical therapy.
- ***Superficial candidosis*** – in addition to vaginal and oral infection, *C. albicans* can infect moist skin in folds of skin (groin, under breasts, nappy area of baby) producing a very red rash and skin damage. Treat with topical nystatin or clotrimazole and keep dry.

2. Subcutaneous infections

- ***Mycetoma (Madura foot)*** – a chronic infection of subcutaneous tissue, bone and skin that is caused by actinomycetes (~60%) or fungus species, probably introduced into deep tissue by a thorn. Mycetomas commonly occur on the foot or leg, but may occur anywhere. They start as an area of hard swelling; later sinuses form and discharge fluid. Pain is rarely severe. Underlying bone is eroded and ultimately destroyed and lytic lesions appear in the bone on X-ray. There is some local lymphatic involvement. The cause needs to be determined by microscopy of the sinus discharge. Fungal mycetomas rarely respond to systemic antifungals and frequently require amputation. Actinomycetomas may respond to streptomycin or rifampicin for 2–3 months plus cotrimoxazole for many months until there is clinical improvement.
- ***Sporotrichosis*** – *Sporothrix schenckii* probably enters the subcutaneous tissue through an abrasion. It may present as a single ulcer or nodule. In the lymphangitic form, the fungus spreads down the lymphatics, forming nodules at intervals which may then ulcerate through to the skin. Chronic lesions may look like psoriasis or a granuloma. Systemic disease occurs but is very rare. Treat with saturated aqueous solution of potassium iodide mixed with milk, 0.5–1ml PO tds, increased in small increments to 3–6ml tds, until 1 month after clinical resolution.

3. Skin signs of systemic fungal infection

Systemic mycoses such as histoplasmosis, blastomycosis, coccidioidomycosis, paracoccidioidomycosis, and other fungal infections in immunocompromised individuals, often show skin signs. These include purpura, ulcers, slow spreading verrucose plaques, nodules, papules, pustules, and abscesses.

Dermatology/skin in systemic disease

Cutaneous leishmaniasis

A widespread disease, caused by *Leishmania* parasites, that manifests in different ways depending on the infecting species. After the bite of a sandfly, *Leishmania* multiply in skin macrophages, killing cells and producing the characteristic ulcer. The balance between infection and immune response determines whether the infection remains focused in the skin, healing over many months, or becomes disseminated across the skin and mucosae.

Transmission: occurs via the bite of *Phlebotomus* and *Lutzomyia* sandflies. Reservoirs are rodents or dogs. Transmission is often seasonal.

Clinical features: several days to months after a bite, a nodule develops at the bite site. This grows slowly (up to 5cm) and is covered by a crust. This may drop off to expose a painless ulcer which is dry or exudative, depending on the species. It often heals over months or years, leaving a scar which may be disabling if severe or over a joint. NB the simple lesion may actually vary greatly in shape. Satellite lesions occur; 2° infection is uncommon. *L. mexicana* may cause lesions of the face or pinna – chiclero ulcer (CU) – that take many years to heal, often destroying the pinna.

Two forms of the disease do not resolve spontaneously:

- ***Mucosal leishmaniasis (MC)*** – 2° lesions occur months to years after the 1° lesion has healed. They destroy the mucosa and cartilage of the nasopharynx, larynx, or lips. *L. braziliensis* is the most important cause (although *L. guyanensis* and *L. panamensis* also cause MC)
- ***Disseminated cutaneous leishmaniasis (DCL)*** – the 1° nodule spreads slowly without ulceration while 2° lesions appear symmetrically on limbs and face. Some individuals are not able to mount an immune response to *Leishmania*; their infection (anergic DCL) continues to spread and responds only transiently to chemotherapy.

Diagnosis: identification of Giemsa-stained parasites in skin smears taken from the edge of active ulcers. Species diagnosis is useful for predicting disease course.

Management: depends on the species and manifestation. Simple sores can be left alone to heal spontaneously, unless they are in a disfiguring or potentially disabling position whereupon they will need surgery/curetthage.
► The parasites are killed at 40–42°C, so heating the wound for several days improves healing. The WHO also recommends local infiltration of antimonial compounds into lesions.

Systemic treatment is required for:

- sores potentially caused by agents of MC disease (*L. braziliensis*, *L. guyanensis*, or *L. panamensis*)
- sores too large or badly sited for local therapy
- ulcerated or severly inflamed sores
- disease with lymphatic spread
- lesions with involvement of cartilage
- MC, DCL, or CU disease.

Prevention: efficient case-finding, diagnosis, parasite identification, and systematic treatment; education to decrease vector–human exposure; control of animal reservoirs.

Systemic therapy:

Most infections require:

- 10–20mg antimony/kg IM daily until 4 days after clinical cure *and* negative slit-skin smears.

Except

1. ***L. braziliensis*** cutaneous disease and all **MC** and **DCL** disease require:
   - 20mg antimony/kg IM daily for >4 weeks of therapy *and* negative slit-skin smears.
   - If relapse occurs after a full course, give pentamidine isethionate 3–4mg/kg wkly for >5 weeks, until the lesion is no longer visible.
   - If MC disease does not respond adequately, give 10–15mg antimony/kg IM q12h instead of the daily dose for >4 weeks.
2. **DCL** disease requires:
   - 20mg antimony/kg IM daily for several months after clinical improvement; relapse is common until immunity develops.
3. ***L. aethiopica***, if not self-healing, requires:
   - pentamidine isethionate 3–4mg/kg weekly until the lesion is no longer visible (in cutaneous disease) or for >4 months after negative slit-skin smears (in DCL because relapse is common). Cutaneous ***L. guyanensis*** infection often requires this drug.

Filariasis

One billion people are at risk of infection and 100 million actually infected by this group of parasites. Multiple infections with the different filariae are possible. ► It is important to look for multiple infection and bear this in mind when deciding therapy. In coinfections, such as mixed *O. volvulus* and *L. loa* infections, treatment with diethylcarbamazine (DEC) for loiasis is contraindicated since it may cause a severe Mazzotti reaction due to dying microfilariae. In this situation, ivermectin should be used.

Onchocerciasis (river blindness)

A disease caused by the nematode *Onchocerca volvulus*, which occurs in areas with fast-flowing rivers and biting blackflies of the *Similium* genus, the parasite's vector. In the west African savannah, it is a common cause of blindness; however, successful WHO control work in 11 west African countries has reduced its prevalence in this region. It still causes blindness in other savannah regions while skin and systemic (eg epilepsy) manifestations are more prominent in other parts of its range.

Clinical features: there is considerable variation across the parasite's range, possibly due to differences in the infecting strain of *O. volvulus*.

- Subcutaneous nodules containing adult worms are conspicuous over bony prominences eg iliac crests, ribs, knees, trochanters.
- Microfilariae migrate from nodules into the skin and ocular tissues. The clinical features at these sites are probably related to host inflammatory reactions to dead or dying microfilariae.

The main categories of onchocercal skin disease include:

1. Acute papular onchodermatitis – small scattered itchy papules, +/– vesicles and pustules, +/– skin oedema, often on the trunk and upper limbs.
2. Chronic papular onchodermatitis – larger itchy hyperpigmented, often flat-topped, papules +/– areas of hyperpigmentation.
3. Lichenified onchodermatitis – itchy hyperpigmented papulonodules or plaques which become confluent. The itching is intense initially; the rash is asymmetrical, often affecting one or both legs.
4. Atrophy – loss of elasticity with excessive wrinkles particularly on the buttocks; inelastic folds of inguinal skin form hanging groins, often filled with enlarged lymph nodes.
5. Depigmentation (leopard skin) – patches of decreased pigment or loss contrasted with normally pigmented skin around hair follicles.

Ocular lesions include transient punctate keratitis and potentially blinding conditions such as sclerosing keratitis, iridocyclitis, optic atrophy.

Diagnosis: look for presence of microfliariae in skin snips[1] or in the eye. Ask the patient to put their head between their knees for >2mins before examining the anterior chamber with a slit-lamp. If skin snip and eye examinations are both negative but onchocerciasis is still strongly suspected, perform the Mazzotti test. Give DEC 50mg PO; increased pruritis within 24–48hrs indicates that the patient is infected.

Prevention: long-term ivermectin mass distribution programmes; vector programmes (feasible in small foci); reducing incidence of bites.

Management: a single dose of the microfiliaricide drug, ivermectin (150μg/kg PO), renders an individual essentially amicrofiladermic for about 6–9 months but eventually microfilariae build-up in the skin again and the dose has to be repeated every 6–12 months throughout the lifespan of the adult worms ~15–20yrs). Surgical excision of nodules on the head may decrease the risk of blindness.

1. Murdoch M, 1992, *Tropical doctor*, **22** (suppl 1), 44

Dracunculiasis

A disease of people without a clean water supply that is currently the target of a concerted WHO eradication campaign. It is caused by a nematode, *Dracunculus medinensis*, which infects people after they drink water containing its vector – extremely small copepod crustaceans. Released larvae migrate into body cavities where they mature and mate. Months later, females migrate in the subcutaneous layers of the skin to the extremities where a blister forms. Contact with water, such as when the person walks into a pond to get water, results in the blister bursting and larvae being released.

Clinical features: include a systemic hypersensitivity reaction to infection. Most are identified later when the female worm is seen migrating under the skin or the blister forms or bursts. The tissue around the worm becomes extremely painful and almost always 2° infected with bacteria. Some worms migrate to sites such as brain, joints, or eyes, resulting in cerebral/subdural abscesses, arthritis or blindness. Diagnosis is clinical.

Management: female worms can be removed before they form a blister by making a small incision in the skin at their midpoint and pulling the worm out with careful traction and massage along its track. After a blister has burst, analgesics will be needed before the worm can be pulled out. Metronidazole 25mg/kg PO daily for 10 days relieves symptoms and weakens the anchorage of the worm, making it easier to pull out. Keep the blister clean and covered. **Prevention:** involves improving the water supply or filtering drinking water through cloth to remove the crustaceans.

Loiasis

A condition which is caused by the filarial nematode, *Loa loa*, in the central African rainforests and transmitted by the bite of tabanid flies (genus *Chrysops*). **Clinical features:** bites by infected vectors may cause a painful, itchy swelling. As the injected larvae mature, they migrate away from the site in the subcutaneous layers (producing itching, prickly sensations) or deeper fascial layers (pain, paraesthesia). Transient Calabar swellings occur at intervals, lasting between a few hrs and days and being brought on by local muscle activity. These appear to be an allergic reaction to the worms – the overlying skin is red, painful, hot – and tend to occur on the upper limb, less often the lower limb. Some worms may migrate to the eye producing redness, photophobia, local and periorbital swelling. Diagnosis is clinical; microfilariae *may* be seen in the blood during the day.

Management: diethylcarbamazine 1mg/kg on day 1; 1mg/kg ***bd*** on day 2; 2mg/kg ***bd*** on day 3, and 2–3 mg/kg ***tds*** from day 4–21, all PO. Start persons with heavy microfilaraemia at a low dose of DEC and give steroid cover for the first 2–3 days (due to risk of meningoencephalitis with dying microfiaria). Mazzotti reactions may occur after DEC therapy. Rapid surgery under local anaesthesia is required for worms seen crossing the conjunctivae – you have less than 30 minutes!

Prevention: a weekly dose of DEC 300mg PO may be an effective prophylactic; otherwise, reducing vector contact is important.

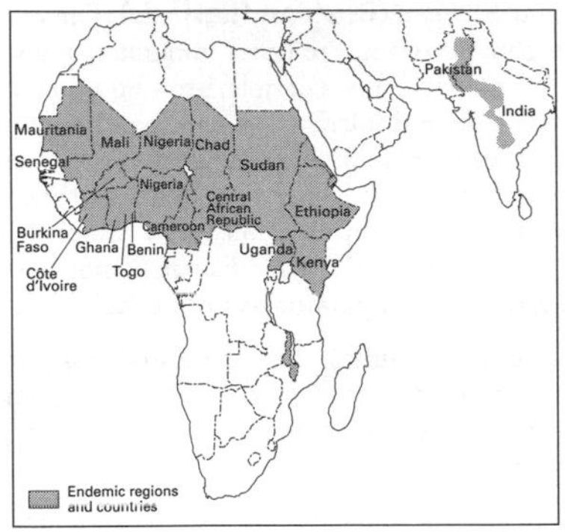

Worldwide distribution of dracunculiasis

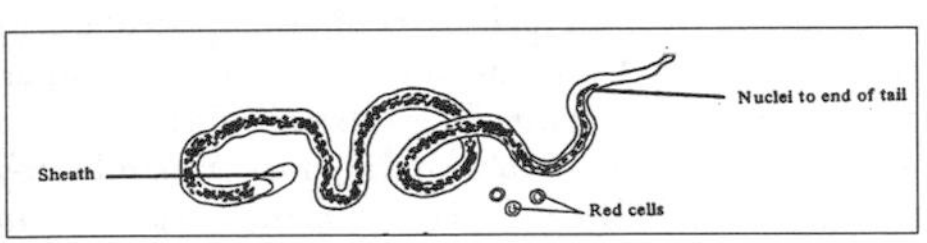

Loa loa as it appears on a blood film

Lymphatic filariasis

A highly variable disease that is caused by infection of the lymphatic system with 1 of 3 species of nematode: *Wuchereria bancrofti* **(Bancroftian filariasis)**, *Brugia malayia*, and *B. timori* **(Brugian filariasis)**. The variation is due to differences in parasite strain, the host's immune response, and the level and incidence of infection. For example, growing up in an endemic region produces immunological tolerance and increased rates of infection but decreased rates of severe immunologically-mediated disease. Immigrants to endemic areas and men have higher rates of severe disease.

The pathology is caused by direct effects of the adults in the lymphatics plus the effects of the host's immune response. Microfilariae do not cause lymphatic pathology but do cause tropical pulmonary eosinophilia.

Transmission: is via the bite of mosquitos. The species of mosquito differs according to the region and particular filiariae, an important point since the anatomical pattern of disease will vary according to the biting habit of the vector (upper vs lower body).

Clinical features: tend to fall into the following spectrum. Features may be locally characteristic – determine what these are.

1. ***Asymptomatic amicrofilaraemia*** in endemic regions where the person is almost certain to have been infected. Probably due to the development of an appropriate immune response and/or the presence of too few parasites to be visible on a blood film.

2. ***Asymptomatic microfilaraemia*** many people have parasites but no apparent disease. ? Due to a hyporesponsive immune system.

3. ***Acute lymphatic filariasis***
   - filarial fever (with chills, rigors, headache, bone & joint pains, malaise, +/– delirium, may be due to 2° infection in some cases. Fever lasts 3–7 days and may recur over many years)
   - limb lymphadenitis and lymphangitis (may → very severe pain; attacks occur at the same time as fever. Commonly affects legs in Brugian disease. Nodes may → abscesses and suppurate → ulcer)
   - funiculitis and epididymo-orchitis (painful swelling of spermatic cord +/– scrotal oedema and redness. Commonest form of acute Bancroftian disease. Often recurs, sometimes repeatedly → chronic disease)
   - abscesses (controversial, but ↓ in number during mass chemotherapy campaigns. Often sterile, occurring in nodes, along vessels, or in muscle [*W. bancrofti*]).

4. ***Chronic lymphatic filiariasis*** a progressive and cumulative disease, probably requiring 10–20yrs of exposure. It may overlap with acute disease. Features include:
   - Hydrocele (normally contains clear, straw-coloured liquid but may become blood- or lymph-stained; repeated tapping of fluid → fibrosis and abscess formation; fluid may contain microfilariae in amicrofilaraemic individuals);
   - Lymphoedema and elephantiasis of the legs is the commonest sequelae of Brugian disease and 2nd only to hydrocele in Bancroftian disease.

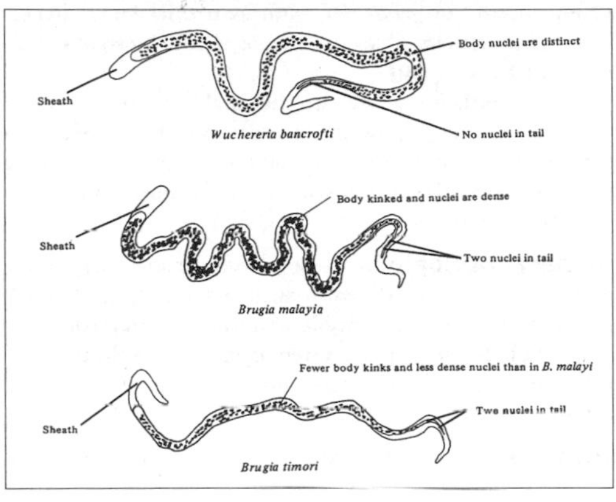

Blood film appearances of the lymphatic filariae

Normally starts at the ankle, spreading onto the foot and up the leg. *Grade I* lymphoedema is transient and pitting, responding well to rest and elevation. With time, ***grading*** → ***II*** (oedema is no longer pitting, becoming brawny).

• Gross swelling occurs in ***grade III***, with skin thickening, hyperkeratosis, and papillomatous changes. Elephantiasis (normally unilateral) develops after a few years;

• Chyluria and lymphuria – rupture into the renal pelvis or bladder of damaged lymphatics draining i) intestines → fat in urine = chyluria or ii) other organs → lymph in the urine. Blood is often present. Chronic chyuria can produce a malabsorption syndrome. Clotting can occur in both cases → urine retention.

Tropical pulmonary eosinophilia: presents with persistent dry cough (often nocturnal); dyspnoea and wheeze (which is typically asthmatic); occasionally crepitations; fever; haemoptysis. If untreated, irreversible airways obstruction and fibrosis leads to persistent dyspnoea, respiratory failure, and cor pulmonale. Eosinophils make up >20% of the peripheral WBCs. Treat early for lymphatic filiariasis.

Other complications: arthritis of the knee joint, endomyocardial fibrosis, skin rashes, thrombophlebitis, and nerve palsies have all been attributed to filarial disease with negative blood films (the microfilaraemia have been destroyed by a hyperresponsive immune response).

Diagnosis: examination of stained films of blood. Microfilariae can be found in the blood during day or night but there is often a peak concentration which the physician must bear in mind when taking blood. In endemic regions, the peak microfilarial density is often between 22.00–02.00 but check locally – in some regions it is during the day. Immuno-diagnosis is being evaluated.

Management: DEC 2mg/kg PO tds for 12 days for *W. bancrofti* infection. Lower doses may be adequate for *B. malayi* or *B. timori* infections: 3–6mg/kg for 6–12 days. ***Mass chemotherapy*** for *W. bancrofti* requires 6mg/kg PO in three divided doses during 24hrs, on 12 occasions, at weekly or monthly intervals. Again lower doses may suffice for the *Brugia* filariae: 3–6mg/kg on 6 occasions. Ivermectin, albendazole, and coumarin have all shown promising results in clinical trials. Further trials need to be carried out to determine their role in the control of filariasis disease.

Surgical management is required for severe hydroceles and lymphoedema, radical surgery may have long-lasting benefits. Conservative treatment can prevent deterioration in lymphoedema and elephantiasis: nocturnal leg elevation, firm pressure bandaging and elastic stockings, careful foot care, control of infections, careful use of diuretics.

Prevention: education to reduce vector–human contact; systematic chemotherapy of individuals and mass chemotherapy of communities with >5% prevalence of infection. Routine addition of DEC to table salt has been used with success in China.

The WHO have recently set up a filariasis eradication programme, aiming to both reduce transmission and control the effects of the disease. The former will be attained by mass community treatment with drugs such as albendazole and ivermectin or through the supplementation of salt with DEC. Community self-help groups are being established to help people reduce the effects of the disease.

The realisation that elephantiasis can be profoundly reduced by simple hygiene and early treatment of infections has stimulated a new approach. Patients are now encouraged to:

- wash the affected part twice daily with soap and water
- raise the affected limb at night
- exercise, to promote lymph flow
- keep nails clean
- wear shoes
- use antiseptic or antibiotic creams to treat small wounds or abrasions, or in severe cases systematic antibiotics.

Such measures help to halt disease progression in those with slight lymphatic damage. People with advanced lymphoedema or elephantiasis can also be helped by these simple methods, as collateral lymphatic channels re-establish lymph flow if kept free from secondary infection.

Examples of simple patient information leaflets are available from the WHO filariasis programme via the WHO website.

Infestations

1. Lice

Six-legged arthropods of the Anoplura order that cause severe pruritis, skin damage due to scratching, and 2° bacterial infection. There are 3 species of medical importance:

- the **head louse** (*Pediculosis capitis*)
- the **body louse** (*P. humanus*)
- the **pubic or crab louse** (*Phthirus pubis*).

The body louse is also important as the vector of epidemic typhus, relapsing fevers, and trench fever. They are transmitted by close personal contact as occurs within families, institutions, or sexual activity. Body louse transmission is increased by poverty, overcrowding, and poor hygiene.

The lice pierce the skin to take a blood meal, injecting saliva and defaecating at the same time. A rash occurs due to a hypersensitivity reaction to the saliva. Blue macules <1cm in diameter occur during pubic louse infection possibly due to injection of an anticoagulant. The body louse lives in the person's clothes, passing onto the skin only to take a blood meal. The other two lice infect the skin directly. Eggs are laid and firmly glued to hairs where they can be seen – the 'nits'.

Management: for head and pubic lice, 0.5% malathion liquid on the affected parts for 8–10 hours (except the eyebrows – thick layer of petrolatum to eyelid margins bd for 8 days). Nits can be removed by soaking hair in 50% vinegar, and combing with 50% vinegar-soaked fine-toothed comb. Treat 2° infection for *S. aureus*.

2. Scabies

An eight-legged mite, *Sarcoptes scabiei*, that is transmitted by close personal contact within families or groups, or through sexual contact. Its prevalence does not seem to be greatly affected by prevailing levels of cleanliness. During the first few weeks following 1° transmission, there are no symptoms as sensitization to mite faeces and saliva occurs. Reinfestation results in almost immediate irritation and in some cases, a generalized urticaria. The infestation is extremely irritating to young children and causes great misery.

Infection causes small polymorphous itchy papules, particularly in the finger webs and on the flexor wrist surface. Other sites commonly include elbows; axillae; genitalia, particularly scrotum; peri-umbilicus; breasts. Head infestation is common in infants. The itching is worse at night. Macules and pustules occur; scratching can be severe in children and result in 2° bacterial infection of the papules. The female burrows into the dermis to lay her eggs – these burrows can be seen as 0.5–1.5cm long irregular tracks. ***Diagnosis*** is either clinical or by finding a female in one of the burrows with a needle.

Management: treat the whole group at the same time since some members may be asymptomatic. Apply malathion 0.5% or permethrin 5% cream to the body below the neck and leave on for 24hrs before washing off. If done properly, a single application is sufficient. Benzylbenzoate 25% can be used but may require repeated applications for 2–3 days. Use 1/2 and 1/4 strength solutions for children 8–12 and 4–7yrs, respectively.

Female *Pediculosis capitis*

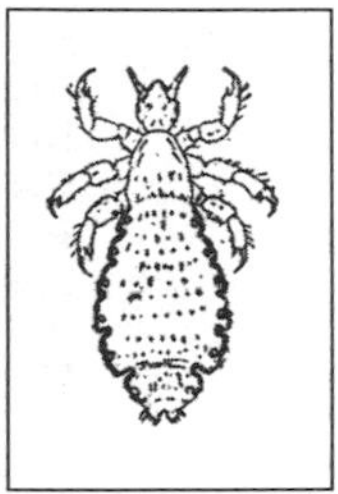

0.3mm length

Female *Pediculosis humanus*

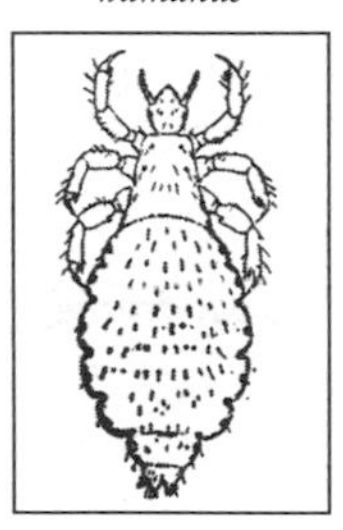

0.4mm length

Female *Phthirus pubis* with ovum within

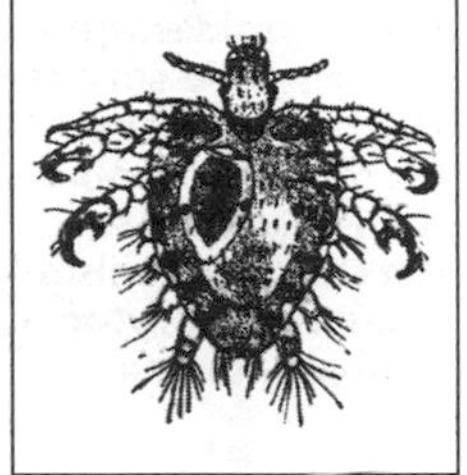

0.3mm length

Female *Sarcoptes scabiei*

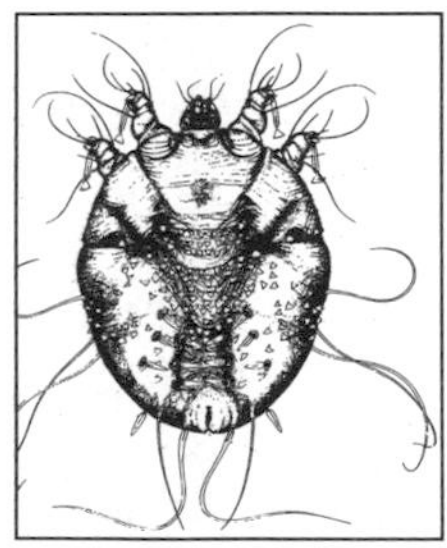

0.4mm length

11. Endocrinology

Diabetes mellitus 492
Treatment of diabetes mellitus 494
Diabetic follow-up 496
Diabetic emergencies 498
The thyroid gland 500
Hypothyroidism (thyrotoxicosis) 500
Hyperthyroidism (myxoedema) 502
Thyroid eye disease 503
Cushing's syndrome 504
Addison's disease 504
Hyperaldosteronism (Conn's syndrome) 506
Phaeochromocytoma 506
Hypopituitarism 506

Endocrinology

Diabetes mellitus

Diabetes mellitus (DM) is a syndrome caused by the lack, or diminished effectiveness of, endogenous insulin and is characterized by hyperglycaemia and deranged metabolism. Several forms of the disease exist and their prevalence throughout the world vary greatly.

Type I DM (insulin-dependent IDDM) is essentially a disease of Caucasians, with highest prevalence occurring in northern Europe. In India there are between 0.06 and 0.7 cases per 1000 population, whilst estimates in tropical Africa suggest 0.03 per 1000. It is usually of juvenile onset and may be associated with other autoimmune disease. Environmental factors may also be important, since a seasonal variation in onset has been noted and also migrants tend to assume the risk of the country they are in. Patients always need some insulin and are prone to ketoacidosis.

Type II DM (non-insulin-dependent NIDDM) is much more common than type I DM and also has marked geographical and ethnic variation in prevalence – 50% of the Pima Indians of the USA and Micronesians of Naura, 10% of Mauritians and 6% of Indian Asians have NIDDM. Asians in S Africa have a prevalence of 20%, whilst Black Africans have the lowest rates. In Caucasians it tends to be a disease of old age, often associated with obesity, whilst in Asians and to a lesser extent Blacks, onset may be earlier. It may progress to IDDM.

Malnutrition-related DM (MRDM) First described in the 50's, the WHO subdivide this disease into 2 classes: ***protein deficient pancreatic diabetes (PDPD)*** and ***fibrocalculous pancreatic diabetes (FCPD).*** Disease prevalence is difficult to assess since there is still argument about precise diagnostic criteria. In both there is an early age of onset in patients of low body weight, in whom high doses of insulin are required, but ketoacidosis is not a feature. In FCPD it is thought that tropical calcific pancreatitis (see gastroenterology chapter) may be a cause. Another theory is that consumption of cyanide-containing foods (eg cassava/manioc/tapioca, ragi in India and kaffir beers in Africa) on a background of protein-calorie malnutrition leads to build-up of toxic hydrocyanic acid, which may directly damage the pancreas. Conversely, some believe that the malnutrition is a result and not a cause of the diabetes.

Other diabetes types Gestational diabetes, slowly progressive IDDM, maturity onset diabetes of the young.

Predisposing factors Drugs (steroids, thiazide diuretics), pancreatic disease (chronic pancreatitis, TCP, post-surgery), endocrine disease (Cushing's acromegaly, phaeochromocytoma, thyrotoxicosis), others (acanthosis nigricans, lipodystrophy and glycogen storage diseases).

Presentation of DM *Acutely*: Ketoacidosis (see below), weight loss polyuria, polydipsia. *Subacutely*: As above, over longer time plus lethargy infection (pruritis vulvae, boils) or may present with complications: infection, cataract, microangiopathy (retinopathy, neuropathy, nephropathy and macroangiopathy (MI, claudication).

Diagnosis[1] requires 2 separate fasting venous plasma glucose levels >7.8mmol/l or a +ve glucose tolerance test (GTT): fast patient overnight, take fasting blood glucose. Give 75g oral bolus of glucose in 300ml water (1.75g/kg in children) and measure blood glucose 2hrs afterwards. DM is diagnosed if the fasting venous plasma glucose is >7.8 and/or the 2hr sample is >11.1mmol/l. If the fasting level is between 6.0mmol/l and 7.8mmol/l, or the 2hr sample is between 7.8mmol/l and 11.1mmol/l then there is impaired glucose tolerance (IGT) and the tests should be repeated at 6 months and the patient monitored. Screening for glyosuria is not a cost-effective way of diagnosis in the general population, especially as *c*.1% have a lowered renal threshold for glucose (normally 10mmol/l). In addition, for PDPD diagnosis, the onset must be below 30yrs of age, the patient must have a BMI (see nutrition chapter) <19kg/m^2, a history of childhood malnutrition and no ketoacidosis. Theses patients will require >60 units of insulin per day. FCPD needs the additional criteria of recurrent abdominal pain and evidence of pancreatic calculi in the absence of alcoholism, gallstones or hyperthyroidism.

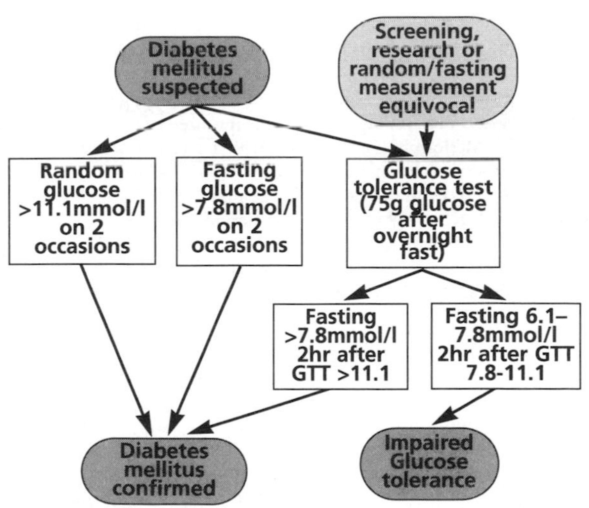

1. DECODE study *BMJ*, 1998; **317**, 371–5

Treatment of diabetes mellitus

Patient education and motivation are the key to success. In the young, compliant person the aim is for normoglycaemia, but if life on the edge of hypoglycaemia is intolerable, this may be modified.

Children are more likely to develop serious ketoacidosis, so the advice of a paediatrician should always be sought on admission. Glycaemic control is especially important during pregnancy, as hyperglycaemia in the first trimester carries a 3-fold ↑ in foetal abnormality and birth complications.

• ***Education*** Emphasize the need for drug and diet compliance. Teach how to monitor blood and urine glucose levels and expose to an insulin-induced hypoglycaemic episode under supervision. Advise the patient to have access to sweets at all times and to alert their family/colleagues to the symptoms of hypoglycaemia. The regular diet, however, should avoid large amounts of rapidly absorbed carbohydrates eg sugar, sweets, fizzy drinks etc. Where possible, arrange for appointments with a dietician and chiropodist and stress the need for regular follow-up.

• ***Conservative*** treatment should always begin with recommending a healthy diet; low in fat, high in starchy carbohydrate, low in sugar, high in fibre with moderate protein, taken at regular times. In most tropical settings this is not a problem. Obese patients should aim to lose weight and other risks of CVS disease should be minimized eg stopping smoking, controlling hypertension, lowering hypercholesterolaemia and taking regular exercise.

• ***Oral drug*** treatment will depend upon the type of diabetes, the options available and the likelihood of patient compliance. Patients with NIDDM are best started on either a biguanide or a sulphonylurea if conservative treatment alone is not able to control glycaemia. Sulphonylureas stimulate insulin secretion and ↑ insulin sensitivity; tolbutamide (0.5–1.0g bd) is short-acting and useful in elderly patients, since hypoglycaemia is less likely. Gliclazide (40–160mg od) and glibenclamide (2.5–15mg od) are longer acting. Metformin is a biguanide, which ↑ insulin sensitivity, ↓ gut glucose absorption, ↓ hepatic gluconeogenesis and ↑ glucose utilization. It may cause anorexia and diarrhoea (may be best for use in obese patients). It does not induce hypoglycaemia, but watch for lactic acidosis. The dose for metformin is 500mg tds with food. If these drugs alone do not control glycaemia, they may be used together. Should this still be insufficient, a sulphonylurea with a slow-acting insulin is recommended.

• ***Insulin*** comes in 1 strength (100units/ml). Soluble is short-acting, peak at 2–4hrs and lasting up to 8hrs. Medium-acting insulins are suspensions and peak at 4–6hrs, lasting up to 16hrs. Long-acting insulins are diverse and may last up to 32hrs.

Treatment regimes are very varied and ultimately will depend upon the will and compliance of the patient. Most will require 20–60 units per day; start with 0.5 units/kg/day, 2/3 given in the morning and 1/3 in the evening and of this, make 1/3 short-acting and 2/3 long-acting. Some patients can cope with 3 daily injections, others with two only. Test glucose before each mealtime initially and adjust the previous insulin dose up or down by 2 units at a time.

Examples of simple insulin regimes

- A single long-acting morning dose, plus 3 short-acting doses pre-meals.
- A mixture of short- and medium-acting insulin before breakfast and before the evening meal.

Diabetic treatment with intercurrent illness

The stress of illness ↑ basal insulin requirements. If calorie intake is ↓ then ↑ long-acting insulin by *c*.20% and ↓ short-acting in proportion to meal size. Check blood sugar regularly. In some cases a sliding scale or GKI regime may be needed.

Sliding scale

Infuse 1l 5% dextrose with 20mmol K⁺ at 100ml/hr. Add 50 units of soluble insulin to 49.5ml of normal saline in a 50ml syringe (ie 1 unit/ml) and infuse this into a separate vein (or IV line) at a rate according to the blood glucose as follows:

<4.5 – 0.5-1 unit/hr
4.5–6.4 – 2
6.5–11 – 3
11.1–17 – 4
>17 – 5 units/hr.

GKI regime

Add 15 units of soluble insulin to 500ml 10% dextrose with 10mmol K^+. Infuse at 100ml/hr and check the blood glucose hourly. Make up new bottles with altered insulin units according to;

Glucose	*Insulin in bottle*
<5	6
5–15	15
>15	25

NB unless the blood glucose is relatively stable, the GKI regime tends to be more wasteful as new bottles need to be made up frequently.

Diabetic follow-up

Careful follow-up is necessary with all diabetic patients, in order to find out any problems which may have been encountered with treatment and to assess the development of long-term complications.

Assess glycaemic control via •home glucose records (aim for 3.5–6.5mmol/l) •history of hypoglycaemic attacks •glycosylated Hb (HbA_1c) indicates mean glucose level over the last 8 weeks and is normally <8%.

Complications of DM

- Infection, lipoatrophy and/or lipohypertrophy at the injection site.
- Vascular disease. MI is 3–5 times more likely in DM, CVA is twice as likely. Treat hypertension vigorously (an ACE inhibitor may also protect against renal disease) and look for and treat any other risk factors for vascular disease.
- Eye disease. Overall 30% of diabetics have some degree of retinopathy. There may also be maculopathy, cataracts and rubeosis iridis (new vessel formation on the iris).
- Neuropathy is usually due to vascular disease of the vasa vasorum and is present in 60% of diabetics overall (20% have a functional deficit). It is usually manifest as a symmetrical, sensory polyneuropathy. The III and IV cranial nerves may be affected by mononeuropathies. Charcot's arthropathy is due to sensory loss at joint surfaces. Autonomic neuropathy is manifest as postural hypotension, gastroparesis, nocturnal diarrhoea, urinary retention and impotence. In all diabetics, particular attention should be paid to the feet, with regular follow-up appointments to assess the extent of any trauma or infection that may be present. Have a low threshold for treating ulcers aggressively.
- Nephropathy. The degree of albuminuria correlates with the risk of death. Check U&Es, Cr clearance and plasma albumin.

The stages of diabetic retinopathy

1 **Background** microaneurysms (dots), microhaemorrhages (blots), and hard exudates.
2 **Pre-proliferative** cotton wool exudates (small infarcts), and extensive blots.
3 **Proliferative** New vessels formed in areas of infarction.
4 **Maculopathy** More common in NIDDM. Acuity is reduced.

Current recommendations for diabetic diet and lifestyle

• *Dietary energy and body weight*	Acheive and/or maintain BMI 19–25. Diet & exercise important.
• *Components of dietary energy*	Saturated fatty acids <10% total energy, polyunsaturated fatty acids <10% total, protein 10–20% total, carbohydrate and other fatty acids making up the rest. Timing of intake essential to IDDM patients.
• *Protein & renal disease*	Total protein intake at lower end of normal range (0.7–0.9g/kg/day) if nephropathy.
• *Vitamins and anti-oxidant nutrients*	↑ foods rich in tochopherols, carotenoids, vit. C, and flavinoids (ie fruit & vegetables).
• *Minerals*	Sodium intake <6g/day, Mg^{2+} supplements may be required in some cases.
• *Alcohol*	1–2 glasses of wine (or equivalent) per day is acceptable. Caution in IDDM, those on sulphonylureas, the obese and hyper-lipidaemia.
• *Special foods*	Low/non-alcohol drinks (if available), no merit in sweeteners or fructose over sucrose.
• *Families*	Most recommendations suitable for the whole family.

Source: Derived from the 1995 recommendations of the American Diabetes Association and the Nutrition Study Group of the European Association for the Study of Diabetes.

Diabetic emergencies

Diabetic ketoacidosis

Since without insulin, glucose is unable to enter into cells, the body is forced to make alternative substrates for metabolism, in the form of ketones produced in the liver. Thus, insulin lack eventually leads to hyperglycaemia and a build-up of acidic ketones. This may be precipitated by infection and often leads to acidosis and coma.

Clinical features Often there is a gradual deterioration over several days – ask a relative if the patient cannot give a proper history. There may be hyperventilation (with sweet, ketotic breath), hyperglycaemia, ketoacidosis, coma. Do: FBC, U&Es, bicarbonate, blood gasses, blood cultures. Test the urine for ketones and bacteruria.

Treatment • Correct dehydration (may be life-threatening) first with 1.5–2 litres/hr of normal saline for 2 hours. • Pass an NGT. • Give IV soluble insulin at 1.5 units/hr (or 6 units/hr IM) until the blood glucose is <14mmol/l. Then either switch to a GKI regime, a sliding scale or (if neither of these are available) simply halve the rate of infusion to 0.75units/hr IV. • Measure K^+ hourly, since hypokalaemia can result as hyperglycaemia is corrected and glucose enters cells, taking K^+ with it. Give 20–60mmol K^+ IV depending upon the measured levels (unless there is oliguria, when K^+ should be withheld). • If unconsciousness is prolonged give 5000IU heparin sc bd. • Monitor vital signs, blood glucose and K^+ every hour. • Look for and treat any infection (check MSU, CXR and blood cultures). Temp may not be elevated. • Be alert to shock, DVT cerebral oedema and DIC. • Some advocate giving 100mmol of bicarbonate IV over 1hr if the pH is <6.9. If there is gross acidosis without ↑ ketones, consider aspirin overdose or lactic acidosis in elderly diabetics.

Hyperglycaemic hyperosmolar non-ketotic coma: There is gradual dehydration and ↑ glucose (>35mmol/l) over *c.*1 week. There is no acidosis since ketones are not made and the plasma osmolality may be >340mmol/kg. (Work out approximate plasma osmolality by: 2[Na^+] + [urea] + [glucose] mmol/l.) Treat as for ketoacidosis, but correct the osmolality slowly (over *c.*3 days) to avoid cerebral oedema after large fluid shifts.

Hypoglycaemia is usually due to excess insulin administration. It presents with altered (aggressive) behaviour, sweating, tachycardia, fits and coma of rapid onset. Treat with 50–100ml of 50% dextrose followed by a saline flush to avoid damaging the vein. Improvement should be rapid. Give dexamethasone 10mg IV stat then 4mg IM q6h in prolonged hypoglycaemia to combat cerebral oedema. If IV access fails, try 0.5–1mg glucagon IM to attempt to prompt conversion of hepatic glycogen to glucose (though in the pre-terminal state, there may be no glycogen left). An infusion of dextrose saline may be needed after recovery from coma to replenish stores.

Endocrinology

The thyroid gland

The thyroid gland is made of two lobes joined by an isthmus and secretes T_4 and T_3 (more active) under the stimulus of TSH from the pituitary. T_3 and T_4 increase cell metabolism, increase catecholamine effects and are vital for normal growth and development. The gland may become enlarged either diffusely (goitre) or in single or multiple nodules and in each case the patient may be euthyroid, hypo-, or hyperthyroid.

Hypothyroidism (myxoedema)

The patient may present with any of: weight gain, lethargy, constipation, dislike of cold, menorrhagia, hoarse voice, depression, dementia, angina, infertility, dry skin, vitiligo.

Signs: coarse features, bradycardia, goitre, CCF, non-pitting oedema, ascites, pleural effusion, delayed reflexes, loss of the outer 1/3 of the eyebrows.

Diagnosis: $\downarrow T_4$ (and T_3). TSH will be ↑ if there is 1° thyroid failure or ↓ if there is pituitary failure. Get an ECG, CXR, FBC (may show anaemia due to iron or folate deficiency), cholesterol and triglycerides may be ↑.

Causes

- ***Iodine deficiency*** (see nutrition chapter). May be endemic (in mountain areas) or sporadic (pregnancy/puberty).
- ***Hashimoto's thyroiditis*** Autoimmune disease usually found in women, leading to goitre from lymphocyte infiltration. Can be euthyroid. 5% → malignancy.
- ***1° atrophic hypothyroidism*** is essentially Hashimoto's with no goitre and is associated with IDDM, Addison's disease and pernicious anaemia.
- ***Dyshormonogenesis*** Autosomal recessive peroxidase deficiency.
- ***Thyroidectomy or radioiodine treatment.***
- ***Drug-induced*** Anti-thyroid drugs, amiodarone, lithium, iodine.

Treatment if healthy and young; life-long thyroxine at 50–150μg/day adjusted according to the clinical state (aim to keep TSH levels <5mU/l). In the elderly begin with 25μg/day and monitor for angina or tachycardia (propanolol may need to be added eg 40mg OD).

Myxoedema coma

Occurs in long-standing hypothyroid patients, often precipitated by infection, MI, CVA or trauma. Look for hypothermia, hyporeflexia, bradycardia and fits.

Treatment Take blood for T_3 & T_4, TSH, FBC, U&Es, cultures and arterial samples. Give O_2 and treat any precipitating cause. If available, give 5–20μg T_3 by slow IV injection, repeated if necessary every 12hrs., with 100mg/8hrs hydrocortisone (especially if pituitary hypothyroidism suspected). Rehydrate with normal saline, avoiding CCF. Correct hypothermia and treat its complications (hypoglycaemia, pancreatitis, arrhythmias). After 3 days, cautiously reintroduce thyroxine orally at the usual dose.

Causes of goitre or thyroid nodules

- Physiological (either endemic or sporadic) colloid goitre
- Nodular goitre
- Hyperplasia (Grave's)
- Goitrogens
- Dyshormonogenesis
- Thyroiditis
- Tumours (benign and malignant).

Complications of goitre

- Tracheal displacement or compression
- Haemorrhage into cyst
- Toxic change
- Malignant change.

Thyroid tumours

- Benign (adenoma)
- 1° malignant (papillary, follicular, medullary, anaplastic, lymphoma)
- 2° (usually local invasion from oesophageal Ca, very rarely blood borne spread).

Hyperthyroidism (thyrotoxicosis)

The patient may present with ↓ weight, diarrhoea, oligomenorrhoea, tremor, emotional lability, heat intolerance, ↑ sweating, itch, fatigue, polyuria/polydipsia, hair-thinning, eye-protrusion.

Signs tachycardia, AF, fine tremor, thyroid eye disease, goitre/nodule(s), thyroid bruit, myopathy.

Diagnosis ↑T_3 & T_4, ECG, FBC, U&Es. Other tests available include the TRH test, thyroid scanning, USS, thyroid auto-antibodies. Test the visual fields and acuity.

Causes

- ***Graves' disease*** Genetic pre-disposition leading to antibodies to TSH receptors and thus a diffuse goitre. There may be pre-tibial myxo-edema (oedematous swellings above the lateral malleoli and shins), normochromic, normocytic anaemia, ↑ESR, ↑Ca^{2+} and abnormal LFTs. It is associated with IDDM and pernicious anaemia.
- ***Toxic adenoma*** is a nodule producing T_3 and T_4.
- ***Subacute thyroiditis*** Often post-partum and possibly triggered by viral illness (mumps, coxsackie), the goitre may be painful.
- ***Others*** Toxic multi-nodular goitre, medication, follicular carcinoma of the thyroid, choriocarcinoma, struma ovarii (ovarian tumour secreting T_3 & T_4).

Treatment Immediate symptomatic control may be achieved with propanolol 40mg qds. Start carbimazole at 15mg tds for 4 weeks, then reduce the dose according to TFTs and maintain on 5mg tds for 12–18 months before stopping. 50% will relapse. NB in the West 0.1% have agranulocytosis on carbimazole, therefore tell the patient to return if she has a sore throat shortly after starting treatment; check the FBC. Other treatments include radioiodine thyroid ablation and partial thyroidectomy.

If there is thyroid eye disease (see opposite), in addition to controlling the hyperthyroidism, it may be necessary to use systemic steroids if there is ophthalmoplegia or gross oedema. Seek specialist referral.

Other complications heart failure, AF, osteoporosis, gynaecomastia.

Thyroid eye disease

This occurs in the presence of specific autoantibodies causing retro-orbital inflammation and lymphocyte infiltration. Where available, a CT scan may be used to do this. In some cases it may precede thyrotoxicosis.

History ↓ acuity, double vision, eye pain and/or protrusion. If there is ↓ acuity it may mean that there is optic nerve compression; seek expert advice.

Signs proptosis, conjunctival oedema, corneal ulceration, papilloedema, optic atrophy, lid lag, lid retraction, ↓ colour vision, ophthalmoplegia.

Treatment does not always respond to treatment and may even develop after the patient has been rendered euthyroid. Try hypromellose eye drops for lubrication. Diuretics +/– steroids may help, but often surgical decompression is needed.

Cushing's syndrome

Cushing's syndrome is due to chronic glucocorticoid (eg cortisol) excess from the adrenal medulla. Cortisol is normally released after stimulus from the hypothalamo-pituitary axis and Cushing's syndrome is classified as either ACTH dependent (ie excess stimulus) or ACTH independent (ie ↑ cortisol without an increased stimulus).

Clinical features wasting of tissues, myopathy, thin skin, purple abdominal striae, bruising, osteoporosis, water retention (hypertension, facial and peripheral oedema), obesity, ↑ infection, poor wound healing, hirsutism, amenorrhoea, hyperglcaemia.

Diagnosis

- 24hr urinary free cortisol (normally <700nmol/24hrs).
- Dexamethasone suppression test; give high-dose dexamethasone (dxm) eg 2mg PO at 11pm. Take blood for plasma cortisol at 9am – normally it will be inhibited to <170nmol/l, but in Cushing's syndrome it will still be high.
- The metyrapone test: metyrapone normally inhibits a step in cortisol synthesis, resulting in an excess of urinary 17-oxogenic steroids (17-OGS). In Cushing's syndrome, as more cortisol is made, there is a greater rise in urinary 17-OGS (>35–135µmol/24hrs). The interpretation of these tests will depend upon the cause of the syndrome (see opposite).

Addison's disease

Adreno-cortical insufficiency, leading to ↓ gluco- and mineralocorticoids.

Clinical features: weakness, apathy, anorexia, weight loss, abdominal pain, oligomenorrhoea. There may be hyperpigmentation, vitiligo, hypotension, sexual dysfunction. Dehydration in crises.

Investigations: synacthen tests (giving an ACTH analogue and looking for the normal rise in plasma cortisol). Contact the lab regarding doses and times of blood collection. Check for hyperkalaemia, hyponatraemia (may be SIADH), uraemia, acidosis, hyercalcaemia, eosinophilia. Get a CXR and AXR (looking for signs of TB).

Causes: idiopathic (probably auto-immune, associated with Grave's disease, Hashimoto's, IDDM, pernicious anaemia), adrenal TB, adrenal metastases.

Treatment: treat cause. Replace steroids with hydrocortisone, 20mg mane, 10mg nocte and adjust the dose according to plasma cortisol (aim for 700–850nmol/l) and clinical symptoms (↑ if postural hypotension, ↓ if patient becomes Cushingoid). Warn the patient about not stopping steroid treatment abruptly and if possible give syringes to give the hydrocortisone IM if vomiting prevents oral therapy. Explain that they need to take more hydrocortisone during intercurrent illnesses. There should be 6-monthly follow-up.

Interpreting test results

Cushing's disease: there is some, but not normal suppression of plasma cortisol with high-dose dxm. Plasma ACTH is ↑, but <250ng/l.
Adrenal tumour: Usually there is no suppression of cortisol with high-dose dxm and there is no change in the metyrapone test. Plasma ACTH is undetectable.
Ectopic ACTH production: ↑ plasma ACTH with no suppression with high-dose dxm or response to the metyrapone test. There may be a hypokalaemic alkalosis.
False positives: Depressive illness, excess alcohol.

Causes and treatment:

- *ACTH-dependent:*
  1. Iatrogenic (ACTH or synacthen treatment) – treat by ↓ dose.
  2. Cushing's disease; ACTH-producing pituitary adenoma – treat either surgically or medically with metyrapone.
  3. Ectopic ACTH (or, rarely CRH) production from tumours, especially small-cell bronchial CA – treat the cause.
- *ACTH-independent:*
  1. Iatrogenic (prednisolone or dexamethasone treatment) – ↓ dose.
  2. Alcohol excess.
  3. Cortisol producing tumours (adrenal adenoma or Ca) – remove tumour.
  4. Carney's syndrome, McCune-Albright syndrome, GIP hypersensitivity.

Addisonian crisis

Look for signs of shock in a known Addisonian or someone on long-term steroids who has omitted their tablets. Often there is preceding infection, trauma or surgery.

Management: •Take bloods for urgent ACTH and cortisol. • Resuscitate with colloid then crystalloids. • Give 100mg hydrocortisone IV, then give same dose IM qds. • Culture blood, urine and sputum. •Give a broad-spectrum antibiotic. • Monitor for hypoglycaemia. • Change to oral hydrocortisone after 72h if stable.

Hyperaldosteronism (Conn's syndrome)

Excessive aldosterone production independent of the renin angiotensin system. Typically there is hypertension, hypokalaemia, alkalosis and mild hypernatraemia. Check plasma K^+, aldosterone, renin, angiotensin. Most cases are due to adrenocortical adenoma (Conn's synd.), but also include adrenal hyperplasia and carcinoma. 2° causes (due to ↑ renin); renal artery stenosis, accelerated HT, diuretics, heart failure, hepatic failure, Bartter's syndrome. **Treatment** is surgical (though dexamethasone may help in hyperplasia) or by treating the cause in 2° disease. Replace K^+.

Phaeochromocytoma

A benign tumour, usually in the renal medulla producing catecholamines. May be inherited as part of the multiple endocrine neoplasia syndrome (MENIIa) and associated with neurofibromatosis and medullary thyroid cancer. There is hypertension, cardiomyopathy, weight loss, hyperglycaemia and crises of fear, palpitations, tremor, and nausea. Test the urine for HMMA or VMA. Cautiously reduce the BP with phenoxybenzamine 10mg daily, increased each day by 10mg, up to 1–2mg/kg in 2 divided doses and propanolol 20mg tds. Add phentolamine 2–5mg IV repeated if necessary during crises. Surgery provids the only cure.

Hypopituitarism

The pituitary produces: ACTH, GH, FSH, LH, TSH and prolactin. ↓ production of one or more of these is termed hypopituitarism and may be due to: cysts, granulomata, abscesses, congenital defects, stroke, basal skull fracture, pituitary adenoma, hypophysectomy, irradiation. There may be atrophy of the breasts, small testes, hair loss, thin skin, hypotension, visual field defects (bilateral hemianopia, initially of upper quadrants). Investigate with: lateral skull XR, assessment of visual fields, U&Es, FBC. Where available: CT head, levels of the above hormones. A specialist centre is needed for treatment, which involves replacement of hydrocortisone, thyroxine and oestrogen/testosterone.

Hyperprolactinaemia presents with amenorrhoea, infertility, galactorrhoea in women and impotence in men. There may be visual field loss due to pressure effects. Causes may be physiological (pregnancy, stress), due to drugs (metoclopramide, haloperidol, methyldopa, oestrogens, TRH) or due to disease: pituitary disease, CRF, hypothyroidism, sarcoid. Treat the cause.

Acromegaly is caused by ↑ secretion of GH from a pituitary tumour (in children, in whom epyphiseal plates have not yet fused this results in giantism). Adults have coarse features, prominent mandibles and hands and feet, large tongues, arthralgia, muscle weakness and paraesthesiae (carpal tunnel synd.). There may be DM, HT and cardiomyopathy. Diagnose by ↑ GH. Treatment is surgical.

Diabetes insipidus results from ↓ ADH secretion from the posterior pituitary, leading to ↓ water resorption by the kidney, polyuria and polydipsia. It may be cranial in cause (head injury, metastases, sarcoid, meningitis, surgery) or nephrogenic (↓K^+, ↑Ca^{2+}, drugs, pyelonephritis, hydronephrosis). Test by early morning urine osmolality (if >800mosmol/l diabetes insipidus is excluded), U&Es, water deprivation test.

12. Haematology[1]

Gayathri Perera

Disorders of red blood cells: anaemia	510
Laboratory findings in anaemia	512
Anaemia in pregnancy	513
Microcytic anaemia	514
Iron-deficiency anaemia	514
Anaemia of chronic disease	516
Sideroblastic anaemia	516
Normocytic anaemia	516
Hookworms	517
Whipworm	517
Macrocytic anaemia	518
Haemolytic anaemias	520
Glucose-6-phosphate dehydrogenase (G6PD) deficiency	522
Sickle-cell anaemia	524
Thalassaemia	528
β thalassaemia major	530
Disorders of white blood cells	532
Lymphomas	532
Leukaemias	536
Myeloproliferative disorders	540
Myeloma	540
Splenomegaly	542
Disorders of haemostasis	544
Coagulation disorders	546
Disseminated intravascular coagulation	548

1. Much of this chapter was based on AF Fleming's chapter *Haematological diseases in the tropics* in *Manson's Tropical Diseases*, 20th ed (G. Cook ed), W. B. Saunders, Philadelphia, 1996.

Haematology

Disorders of red blood cells: anaemia

Clinical features and approach to dealing with anaemia

Anaemia is the most common manifestation and clinical feature of disease in the tropics. Prevalence and morbidity are highest in pre-school children and pregnant women. Although less common amongst other groups, it is still a major health problem.

Anaemia is present when there is a decreased level of haemoglobin (Hb) in the blood – below the reference level for the age, sex, and pregnancy state of the individual. This fall in Hb is often, but not always, accompanied by a fall in the PCV. Alterations in the total circulating plasma volume as well as of the total circulating Hb mass determines the Hb concentration, allowing for altitude effect.

Anaemia can result from:

- haemorrhage or chronic blood loss
- decreased production of red cells
- haemolysis.

These groups are not mutually exclusive and frequently overlap.

Causes of importance in the tropics are:

- nutritional deficiencies (iron, vitamin B_{12}, and folate)
- infections (malaria, hookworm, schistosomiasis, TB, HIV)
- inherited disorders of red cells (G6PD deficiency, thalassaemias, and sickle cell disease).

Classification is useful in terms of management. It is based on the red cell indices: mean cell volume (MCV) and mean cell haemoglobin (MCH). These values indicate the type of anaemia and may suggest an underlying abnormality before there are any clinical features of anaemia.

► The diagnosis of anaemia should always lead to investigation of the underlying problem. The history, examination, and blood film will help determine the aetiology.

Symptoms can occur when the anaemia is chronic, but many patients are asymptomatic. Symptoms which relate to the underlying cause include non-specific complaints such as fatigue, headache, faintness (common in the general population), dyspnoea, palpitations, intermittent claudication, tinnitus, anorexia and bowel disturbance. Susceptibility to infections increases with chronic and severe anaemia, especially in megaloblastic anaemia.

Signs may be divided into general and specific.

***General*:** pallor of mucous membranes; signs of hyperdynamic circulation (tachycardia, bounding pulse, cardiomegaly, and systolic flow murmurs); rarely papilloedema and retinal haemorrhages after an acute bleed (can be accompanied by blindness); heart failure, especially in the elderly.

***Specific*:** koilonychia (spoon-shaped nails) seen in iron deficiency anaemia; jaundice (haemolytic anaemia); bone deformities (thalassaemia major); leg ulcers (sickle-cell disease).

Aetiology of anaemia

1. Blood loss

Acute

Chronic • hookworm • menstruation • childbirth

2. Decreased red cell turnover

Nutritional deficiencies

- iron, folate, vitamin B_{12}
- protein, vitamins A, C & E, riboflavin, pyridoxine, copper

Depressed bone marrow function

- secondary anaemias — infections (eg TB), chronic liver or renal disease, carcinomatosis
- HIV
- aplastic anaemia — drugs/chemicals, infiltration, idiopathic, irradiation, congenital
- thalassaemias α and β

3. Increased red cell destruction

Abnormalities of red cells

- Hb — sickle-cell disease
- enzymes — G6PD deficiency
- membrane — elliptocytosis, ovalocytosis, spherocytosis

Abnormal haemolysis

- immune haemolysis — autoimmune, transfusion, fetomaternal incompatibility
- non-immune haemolysis — infections (eg malaria), hypersplenism, drugs and chemicals, venoms, burns and mechanical injury

Classification of anaemia according to RBC size

Red cell appearance	microcytic	normocytic	macrocytic
Indices	low MCV	normal MCV	high MCV
Bone marrow	normoblastic	normoblastic	megaloblastic
Diagnosis	iron deficiency liver disease thalassaemia chronic disease haemolysis sideroblastic	acute blood loss chronic disease malignancy infection collagen diseases	↓ vit. B_{12} ↓ folate alcohol

Laboratory findings in anaemia

Red cell values: these vary with age, sex, pregnancy state, genetic and environmental factors. The values given are ranges, adjust them according to your local area.

	Hb (g/dl)	***PCV*** (%)	***MCV*** (fl)	***MCH*** (pg)
Birth	13.5–19.5	0.44–0.64	–	–
10–12yrs	11.5–14.5	0.37–0.45	77–91	24–30
Men	13.0–18.0	0.40–0.54	76–96	27–32
Women	11.5–16.5	0.37–0.47	76–96	27–32

Leukocyte and platelet counts: distinguish isolated anaemia from pancytopenia. The counts *increase* in haemolytic anaemia, infections and leukaemias, and there may be abnormal leukocyte or neutrophil precursors.

Reticulocyte count*:* *increases* with the severity of the anaemia, as in chronic haemolysis. A dampened reticulocyte level in the face of anaemia suggests: impaired marrow function (hypoplasia, carcinomatous infiltration, lymphoma, myeloma, acute leukaemia, tuberculosis), deficiency of iron, vit. B_{12} or folate, lack of erythropoietin (renal failure), reduced tissue oxygen consumption (myxoedema, protein deficiency), ineffective erythropoiesis (thalassaemia major, megaloblastic anaemia, myelodysplasia, myelofibrosis, congenital dyserythropoietic anaemia), chronic inflammatory or malignant disease.

Iron binding studies (see table on next page): help distinguish between the different types of microcytic anaemia.

Hb colour scale: a new WHO test gives a good approximation of Hb levels in areas without laboratory facilities.[1]

Blood film: viewed under a simple light microscope, anisocytosis and poikilocytosis point towards specific causes of anaemia. The WCC and its differential, platelet number and morphology as well as the presence or absence of abnormal cells can also be obtained from the film.

Bone marrow: examination when the diagnosis is in doubt can be invaluable. *Aspiration* enables assessment of: the appearance of developing cells, the presence of abnormal cells, and the proportion of cell lineages. Fragments of marrow are needed on the slide in order to assess cellularity. Romanowsky technique and a stain for iron assesses the iron stores in the reticuloendothelial system (macrophages).

Trephine biopsy: may be indicated if the bone marrow aspirate is a dry tap due to fibrosis or increased cellularity (because of leukaemia). A core of bone marrow is taken from the posterior iliac crest with a trephine needle. The bone marrow is fixed in formalin, decalcified and sectioned, and then viewed under a microscope. It provides a panoramic view of the marrow. Although less valuable than an aspirate, since individual cell details cannot be seen, it nevertheless gives a reliable indication of the presence of abnormal infiltrates in the marrow.

Anaemia in pregnancy

Defined by the WHO as a Hb level <11g/dl in a pregnant woman. This means that >20% women will become anaemic. A small fall in Hb is a physiological response to the pregnant state. Those most prone to drop their Hb drastically are those who start pregnancy anaemic eg those with menorrhagia, hookworm, malaria, haemoglobinopathies, poor diet, frequent pregnancies and twin pregnancies.

Anaemia in pregnancy is associated with the increased risk of haemorrhage, puerperal infection and thromboembolic problems. The mother takes longer to recover and there is the increased risk of infection postpartum.

Screening: includes looking for causes of anaemia, especially for haemoglobinopathies, sickle-cell disease, G6PD deficiency and malaria.

Management includes:

1. **Fortification with oral iron** supplements (approx. 750mg extra iron is needed during pregnancy, of which 300mg is required by the baby, mostly after 30 weeks of gestation). 100mg of Fe and 350μg of folate are in 1 tablet of *Pregaday*.
2. **Parenteral iron** may be given to those with iron-deficiency anaemia unable to tolerate oral iron: give 5% iron dextran by slow IV infusion. Dose in ml =

   $[0.0476 \times \text{weight in kg} \times (14.8 - \text{Hb level})] + 16$.

   CI: asthma, renal/liver disease.
3. The rise in Hb takes place over 6 weeks, so **blood transfusions** may be needed for late, severe anaemia (Hb <9g/dl). 1 unit should increase Hb by 0.7g/dl.
4. **Treatment of infections** particularly malaria.

1. Stott GJ, 1995, *Bulletin WHO*, 73, 369

Microcytic anaemia

Four common types: iron-deficiency anaemia, thalassaemia, anaemia of chronic disease, and sideroblastic anaemia.

Iron-deficiency anaemia

The commonest cause of anaemia worldwide, particularly in children and pregnant or breastfeeding women in whom it is a major cause of illness and death. It is the most important cause of microcytic, hypochromic anaemia in which MCV, MCH, and MCHC are all reduced.

Specific clinical features are brittle nails, koilonychia, atrophy of the papillae of the tongue, angular stomatitis, brittle hair, and a syndrome of dysphagia and glossitis (Plummer-Vinson syndrome).

Causes include:

- **Poor diets –** low in animal protein, foods high in factors which inhibit iron absorption. Most iron in food is inorganic which is not readily absorbed.
- **Chronic blood loss –** hookworm, schistosome and whipworm infection; GI losses (oesophageal varices; hiatus hernia; peptic ulcer; CA of stomach, caecum, colon, or rectum; colitis, angiodysplasia; diverticulosis); haematuria; pulmonary haemosiderosis; menorrhagia.
- **Increased demands –** prematurity, growth, pregnancy.
- **Malabsorption –** coeliac disease, gastrectomy.

Diagnosis: take good dietary, menstrual, and medication history; do iron binding studies (see table opposite). Blood film shows microcytic (MCV <80fl) and hypochromic (MCH <27pg) red cells, poikilocytosis (pencil shapes), anisocytosis, and target cells. There is a low reticulocyte count relative to the degree of anaemia. Erythroid hyperplasia is seen along with ragged normoblasts in the bone marrow. Stool examination may show hookworm ova or other parasitic infestation. GI tract investigation may be warranted in some individuals, rectal examination and FOB is required in all.

Management

1. Find and treat the underlying cause.
2. Give iron *replacement* as ferrous sulphate 200mg/8h PO, before food. It takes 6 months to replenish iron stores. Parenteral iron, given as dextran or iron sorbitol, may be indicated in severe malabsorption and in UC and Crohn's disease. Monitor the response to iron with Hb – expect a rise of 1g/dl each week – and reticulocyte count.
3. Correct associated complications.
4. In severe anaemia, blood transfusions may be necessary to prevent sudden death. It is very important to not overload the circulation and precipitate or worsen cardiac failure. The use of exchange transfusion, fast-acting diuretics, and intra-peritoneal transfusion may avoid overload.

Prevention: consider giving i) prophylactic iron to high-risk groups: pregnant women, infants, and pre-school children and ii) antihelminthics to children. It may be possible to locally fortify one or more staple foods.

Iron-binding studies in hypochromic anaemia

	Fe deficiency	*Chronic disease*	*Thalassaemia trait*	*Sideroblastic anaemia*
MCV	reduced	normal	all low	
MCH	reduced	normal	for degree	congenital = low
MCHC	reduced	normal	of anaemia	acquired = high
Serum Fe	reduced	reduced	normal	raised
TIBC	raised	reduced	normal	normal
Serum ferritin	reduced	norm/red	normal	raised
Bone marrow iron stores	absent	present	present	present
Hb electrophoresis	normal	normal	HbA2 raised in β+ form	normal

Anaemia of chronic disease

Anaemia associated with chronic inflammatory or malignant disease.

Causes:

1. ***Chronic inflammatory diseases –***
   - infectious: TB, lung abscess, osteomyelitis, pneumonia, SBE.
   - non-infectious: RA, SLE, other connective tissue disorders, sarcoidosis, Crohn's disease.
2. ***Malignancy –*** carcinoma, lymphoma, sarcoma.

Clinical features of general anaemia and specific features of non-progressive mild microcytic or normocytic and normochromic anaemia. Reduced serum iron and TIBC. Normal or raised serum ferritin levels.

Management is to treat the underlying cause. There is no response to iron supplements. In many cases, it is complicated by the presence of another form of anaemia (such as iron, vitamin B_{12} or folate deficiency), renal failure, bone marrow failure, hypersplenism, or endocrine abnormality.

Sideroblastic anaemia

A refractory anaemia with hypochromic cells in the blood and increased marrow iron. Defined by the presence of pathological ring sideroblasts in the bone marrow. Divided into hereditary and acquired anaemia.

- hereditary form occurs in males; females are carriers and are rarely symptomatic.
- acquired forms are either primary (myelodysplasia FAB type 2) or secondary (other myeloproliferative disorders, drugs such as TB chemotherapy, alcohol, lead, conditions such as haemolytic anaemia, megaloblastic anaemia, and malabsorption).

Management: in secondary disease, treat the underlying cause. The hereditary diseases often respond well to pyridoxine therapy. Give folic acid replacement, especially if megaloblastic anaemia supervenes. In severe cases, repeated blood transfusion is often the only option, bringing with it the dangers of transfusion overload.

Normocytic anaemia

Normocytic, normochromic anaemia is seen in anaemia of chronic disease, in some endocrine disorders (hypopituitarism, hypothyroidism, and hypoadrenalism), and in some haematological disorders (aplastic anaemia and some haemolytic anaemias). It is also seen following acute blood loss before iron stores are reduced. If there is a reduced white cell or platelet count, consider bone marrow failure and perform a bone marrow biopsy.

Management: treat the underlying cause. If the blood loss is severe and shock a possibility, consider blood transfusion to replace and maintain the blood volume.

Hookworms

The soil-transmitted helminths *Ancylostoma duodenale* and *Necator americanus* probably infect more than 900 million people in the tropics and subtropics, flourishing in areas of poverty and malnutrition. They are the commonest cause of anaemia worldwide. Filariform larvae penetrate the skin (usually the feet) and migrate to the small intestinal lumen, maturing to adult worms as they do so. There they attach to the mucosal surface, resulting in chronic, low-grade blood loss. The adult female sheds eggs into the faeces.

This can result in a daily loss of 1mg of iron per 10,000 ova per gram of faeces irrespective of the species. Subacute hookworm anaemia has an element of haemorrhage in its aetiology; acute hookworm anaemia is rare and follows extremely heavy infections. Heavy infections may also lead to hypoproteinaemia and malabsorption.

Whipworm

Trichuris trichiura is one of the most prevalent helminths in the world. Heavy infestations (>800 worms, which = 16,000 ova per gram of faeces) can result in the loss of 4ml blood or 1.5mg iron per day. See diarrhoeal diseases chapter.

Diagnosis and treatment: See p 140 for details Treatment consists of treatment of the anaemia and elimination of the parasites. Albendazole is the drug of choice; 400mg once produces an 80% reduction in egg count, if followed by 200mg daily for 3 days there will be 100% eradication. Mebendazole and levamisole are alternatives.

Prevention: In most areas where hookworm and whipworm are prevalent, reinfection is almost certain. In many instances treatment follows one of two routes; routine drug treatment of a whole target population at set intervals (eg yearly) – especially of children or drug treatment is withheld for only those who are symptomatic. In either case, education about safe disposal of faeces and the wearing of footwear is vital, if the cycle is to be broken.

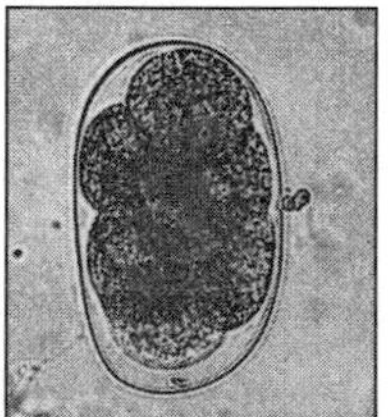

Ancylostoma duodenalis egg. Size ~65×45μm (×40 mag.)

Macrocytic anaemia

Occurs in 2 forms – megaloblastic and non-megaloblastic – which are distinguished by the bone marrow findings at biopsy.

1. Megaloblastic anaemia

Characterized by the presence of megaloblasts (erythroid cells with delayed nuclear maturation) in the bone marrow. There may also be a white cell abnormality (giant metamyelocytes). These changes occur in

- vitamin B_{12} and folic acid deficiency
- abnormalities of red blood cell metabolism, transport and synthesis
- congenital enzyme deficiencies (orotic aciduria)
- acquired enzyme defects (alcohol, chemotherapy).

The aetiology is often multiple.

Clinical features: are general symptoms of anaemia and mild jaundice, glossitis, angular stomatitis, weight loss, purpura due to thrombocytopaenia, macrocytosis of epithelial cell surfaces, neuropathy (subacute combined degeneration of the cord only with lack of vitamin B_{12}), sterility, reversible melanin skin pigmentation, decreased osteoblastic activity, and increased susceptibility to infections. Many remain asymptomatic.

Investigations: show a raised MCV (>95fl) and MCH, normal MCHC, ovalocytes, low reticulocyte count, moderately reduced WCC and platelets in severe cases, and hypersegmented nuclei in neutrophils. Bone marrow is hypercellular with erythroblasts. Metamyelocytes are present. Serum unconjugated bilirubin, hydroxybutyrate and LDH are raised. Serum iron and ferritin are normal or raised.

Management: is with replacement, fortification and dietary modification. Consider prophylactic treatment in patients after partial gastrectomy or ileal resection, pregnancy, severe haemolytic anaemia, on dialysis and in the premature. Folic acid 5mg PO daily for 4 months; maintenance depends on underlying disease. B_{12} replacement is with 6×1mg hydroxycobalamin IM for 1–2 weeks and maintenance with 1mg every 3 months.

2. Non-megaloblastic macrocytic anaemia

Causes: include alcoholism, liver disease, reticulocytosis (after recent bleed), hypothyroidism, myelodysplastic syndromes, sideroblastic and aplastic anaemia.

Investigations: reveal normoblastic, macrocytic anaemia, with round RBCs without hypersegmented neutrophils. Check ESR (malignancy), LFT (including γGT), T4. Exclude vitamin B_{12} and folate deficiency – their levels will be normal. Bone marrow examination for myelodysplasia, aplasia, and myeloma.

Management: diagnose and treat the underlying disease.

Causes of folate and B_{12} deficiencies

	Folate	*Vitamin B_{12}*
Inadequate intake	boiling bottle feeds seasonal shortage prolonged storage of food anorexia famine inappropriate weaning foods prolonged cooking/reheating feeding infants with goats milk alcoholism	breast feeding by B_{12} def. mothers veganism alcoholism
Malabsorption	diarrhoea in infancy acute enteric infections *Giardia lamblia* systemic infections (TB, pneumococcus) *Strongyloides* coeliac disease Crohn's disease	pernicious anaemia gastrectomy chronic *G. lamblia* HIV infection ileocaecal TB *Strongyloides* tropical sprue Crohn's disease
↑ physical demands	growth pregnancy/lactation	pregnancy
↑ pathological demands	haemolysis malignant disease	
Metabolic problems	pyrexia	nitrous oxide chronic cyanide intoxication (cassava)

Haemolytic anaemias

Anaemia due to a reduced red cell life span (normally 120 days) and therefore increased red cell turnover. The bone marrow is able to compensate for a period of time; when it fails, anaemia results.

Causes: the haemolysis is due to genetic or acquired causes. The aetiology is important since it influences therapy.

Genetic

- Membrane defects: hereditary spherocytosis, elliptocytosis, ovalocytosis.
- Haemoglobin defects: thalassaemias, sickle-cell disease.
- Enzyme defects: G6PD and pyruvate kinase deficiency.

Acquired

• Immune:	isoimmune:	haemolytic disease of the newborn, blood transfusion
	autoimmune:	warm or cold antibody mediated, drug-induced.
• Non-immune:	infections:	malaria, septicaemia, parvovirus
	hypersplenism	
	membrane:	paroxysmal nocturnal haemoglobinuria, liver disease
	trauma:	cardiac haemolysis (new valve), microangiopathic anaemia, burns, venoms.

Distinguishing between the different causes involves identifying clinical and laboratory features of increased Hb breakdown and compensatory increase in RBC production. The approach should therefore attempt to identify features of:

- ***extravascular haemolysis:*** jaundice, unconjugated hyperbilirubinaemia, increased urinary urobilinogen, increased faecal urobilinogen;
- ***intravascular haemolysis:*** reduced/absent haptoglobins, reduced haemopexin, haem/methaemoglobin, positive Schumm's test (methaemalbumin), haemosiderinuria, haem/methaemoglobinuria;
- ***increased red cell turnover:*** polychromasia, reticulocytosis, bone marrow erythroid hyperplasia.

Clinical features: are of general anaemia with jaundice; hepatosplenomegaly; leg ulcers due to sickle-cell disease. In the history, check for family history, race, drugs, previous anaemia, jaundice, haematuria.

Investigations: FBC, reticulocytes, bilirubin, LDH, G6PD deficiency, haptoglobin, urinary urobilinogen. Blood films to look for malaria parasite, polychromasia, macrocytosis, spherocytes, elliptocytes, fragmented cells and sickle cells. Direct Coomb's test (DCT), and urinary haemosiderin (stains Prussian Blue).

A. Genetic causes

Hereditary spherocytosis: AD inheritance. Blood films: spherocytes and RBCs show increased fragility. Clinical features: mild anaemia (8–12g/dl) and splenomegaly and gall stones. Diagnosis: osmotic tests. Treatment: splenectomy (delay if in early childhood) and give pneumococcal and haemophilus vaccines.

Hereditary elliptocytosis: AD inheritance. Usually asymptomatic +/– mild haemolysis in homozygotes. There may be episodes of jaundice and moderate splenomegaly following intercurrent infections (malaria may cause severe anaemia). Some elliptocyte variants are said to be resistant to invasion by *P. falciparum*. There is no evidence to confirm this. If treatment is required then splenectomy may help.

South-east Asian hereditary ovalocytosis: AD inheritance. Common in Malaysia, Indonesia, Philippines, PNG, and Solomon Islands. It is not associated with haemolytic anaemia. There appears to be a resistance to malarial parasites, probably due to reduced penetration of merozites.

Pyruvate kinase deficiency: AR inheritance. May present with neonatal jaundice. Later haemolytic anaemia with splenomegaly and jaundice may occur. Diagnosis is by enzyme assay. Treatment is non-specific; splenectomy may improve severe cases.

B. Acquired causes

Drug-induced immune haemolytic anaemia: occurs when drugs cause new RBC membrane antigens (eg high-dose penicillin), immune complexes, or the development of autoantibodies (α-methyldopa, mefenamic acid, L-dopa).

Autoimmune haemolytic anaemia (AHA): can be caused by cold or warm antibodies. They may be primary (idiopathic) or secondary (lymphoma or generalized autoimmune diseases like SLE).

- **Warm AHA** presents as chronic or acute anaemia. Remove underlying cause and treat with steroids (prednisolone 60mg daily, then gradually reduce) +/– splenectomy.
- **Cold AHA** presents as chronic anaemia made worse by a drop in temp, Raynaud's phenomenon, or acrocyanosis. Treatment is to keep warm. Chlorambucil may help; splenectomy does not usually help.
- **Paroxysmal cold haemoglobinuria** is caused by Donnath-Landstiener antibody (mumps, measles, chickenpox, syphilis) sticking to RBCs in the cold, causing a complement-mediated lysis on rewarming.

Glucose-6-phosphate dehydrogenase (G6PD) deficiency

G6PD deficiency has a sex-linked inheritance. It affects over 2 million people in west Africa, Mediterranean, Middle East and south-east Asia. Where *P.falciparum* is or was endemic, G6PD deficiency confers a genetic advantage to female carriers.

Distribution: see map opposite which shows the world distribution of G6PD deficiency. Superimposed are three zones where different G6PD variants reach polymorphic frequencies: zone I ($Gd^{Mediterranean}$), zone II ($Gd^{Mediterranean}$, Gd^{Canton}, Gd^{Union}, $Gd^{Mahidol}$), and zone III (GdA^{-}).

Clinical features:

- Haemolytic anaemia in response to oxidative stress produced by drugs such as primaquine or sulphonamides and food such as fava beans.
- Haemolysis in response to infection (viral or bacterial).

Symptoms arise due to rapidly developing intravascular haemolysis with haemoglobinuria. Many patients remain asymptomatic. Possible precipitants are listed below.

Precipitants of haemolytic anaemia in G6PD deficiency

- antimalarials ► primaquine, chloroquine, fansidar, maloprim
- sulphonamides /sulphones co-trimoxazole, sulphanilamide, dapsone, salazopyrine
- antibiotics nitrofurans, chloramphenicol, nalidixic acid
- analgesics aspirin, phenacetin
- antihelminths β-naphthol, stibophen, nitrodazole
- miscellaneous vitamin K analogues, naphthalene, probenecid, fava beans (possibly other vegetables).

Diagnosis: is by detecting the enzyme deficiency through one of many screening tests. These tests rely on NADPH production and its detection by direct fluorescence or by reduction of a coloured dye (eg methylene blue) to its colourless form. These are sensitive, simple and inexpensive for detecting homozygous males and heterozygous women outside of a crisis.

Following a crisis, blood should be centrifuged and the older cells at the bottom of the column tested, or the dye tests should be delayed for 6 weeks.

During a crisis, the blood film may show contracted and fragmented cells, called “bite” cells and “blister” cells, which have had Heinz bodies removed by the spleen. There are also features of intravascular haemolysis.

Management: withdraw any drug that could have precipitated the crisis and maintain a high urine output (in an attempt to prevent pre-renal failure). Give a blood transfusion if one is warranted. G6PD-deficient babies are prone to neonatal jaundice and in severe cases phototherapy and exchange transfusion are necessary. The jaundice is usually due to the deficiency affecting neonatal liver function.

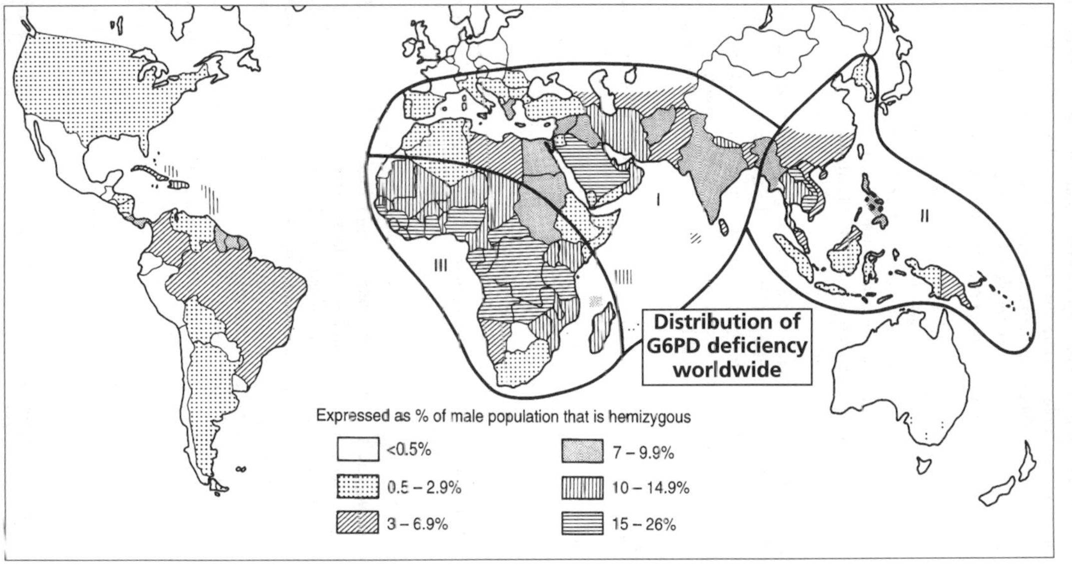

Distribution of G6PD deficiency worldwide

Sickle-cell anaemia

A severe haemolytic anaemia caused by inheritance of a point-mutated β-globin gene. The mutation results in a Glu-Val amino acid substitution in the haemoglobin molecule and the formation of HbS. When deoxygenated, the HbS molecules polymerize into long fibres and cause the RBCs to sickle. Sickled RBCs are fragile and haemolyse easily; they then block the microcirculation in various organs, causing infarcts.

Classification: sickle-cell *disease* arises from the homozygous form, HbSS, while the sickle-cell *trait* is due to heterozygous inheritance, HbAS. The trait is rarely symptomatic, unless crises are precipitated by anoxia or severe infection. Sickle-cell disease is common in Africa and the Indian subcontinent; the trait is common around the Mediterranean and in the mixed populations of Americans.

Clinical features: severe haemolytic anaemia punctuated by crises (see below). Typically, there is anaemia (Hb 6–8g/dl; reticulocytes 10–20%) and jaundice early in life; often with painful swelling of hands and feet (the hand–foot syndrome leading to digits of varying length). Young sicklers alternate periods of good health with periods of acute crises. Later, chronic ill-health supervenes from previous crises.

Complications: include renal failure (papillary necrosis of kidneys due to medullary infarction; failure to concentrate urine leads to dehydration and crisis; nocturnal enuresis is common; glomerulosclerosis is a rare, severe complication); bone necrosis; infections (salmonella osteomyelitis); leg ulcers; splenomegaly in infancy and early childhood which subsequently becomes reduced in size due to infarction (autosplenectomy); proliferative retinopathy; priapism. Micro-infarcts can result in chronic liver damage; bilirubin gallstones are common findings. Survival is strongly linked to socioeconomic conditions.

Crises

- **Painful vascular-occlusive crises** – are frequent and precipitated by infections, acidosis, dehydration, or deoxygenation (altitude, operations, obstetric delivery, stasis of the circulation, exposure to cold, violent exercise). Infarcts may occur in bones (hips, shoulders and vertebrae), the lungs, and spleen. The most serious crises can involve the CNS (in 7% of patients) and spinal cord.

- **Visceral sequestration crises** – are due to sickling within organs and pooling of blood, often with severe exacerbation of anaemia. A severe chest syndrome with pulmonary infiltrates is a common cause of death. Hepatic and girdle sequestration crises and splenic sequestration may lead to severe illness requiring exchange transfusions.
- **Aplastic crises** – may occur due to infection with parvovirus and/or folate deficiency, and are characterized by a sudden fall in Hb and reticulocytes, usually needing transfusion.
- **Haemolytic crises** – are characterized by an increased rate of haemolysis with a fall in Hb but a rise in reticulocytes. They usually accompany a painful crisis.

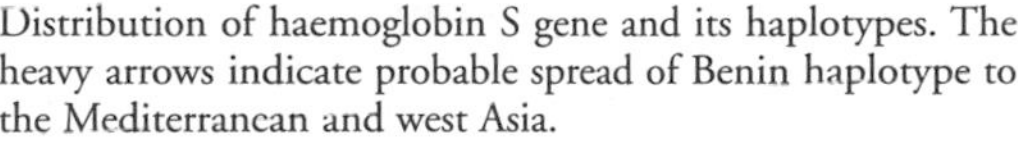

Distribution of haemoglobin S gene and its haplotypes. The heavy arrows indicate probable spread of Benin haplotype to the Mediterranean and west Asia.

Sickle-cell disease and pregnancy

- Sickle-cell disease predisposes to abortion, pre-term labour, still-birth, and sickle-cell crises. To prevent crises, treat with folate supplements, oral bicarbonate, and 3–4 unit blood transfusions every 6 weeks.
- Sickle-cell trait is not a problem, except that pyelonephritis is more common.

Laboratory findings: • Hb 6–8g/dl • sickle cells and target cells in the blood film; features of splenic atrophy (Howell-Jolly bodies) may also be seen • screening tests for sickling in deoxygenated blood (eg with dithionate and Na_2HPO_4) • Hb electrophoresis.

Management: see opposite page, plus

1. **Prophylaxis** – avoid precipitating factors, especially dehydration, anoxia, infections, circulation stasis, and cooling of the skin surface.
2. **Give folic acid and improve general nutrition and hygiene.**
3. **Protect against infection** – vaccinate against pneumococcus and give regular oral penicillin.
4. **Hydroxyurea** – useful for those who present with frequent crises.
5. **Crises** – bedrest, rehydrate with oral fluids and/or IV infusions of normal saline. Give antibiotics if there is infection and bicarbonate if acidotic. Strong analgesics including opiates may be required. Transfuse blood only if there is severe, symptomatic anaemia. Exchange transfusion may be needed for either CNS involvement or a visceral sequestration crisis.
6. **Pregnancy and anaesthesia** – particular care is needed. Routine transfusions are given throughout pregnancy to those with bad obstetric history or a history of frequent crises. Before delivery or operations, patients may be transfused repeatedly with normal blood to reduce the proportion of circulating HbS to less than 30%.

Variants of sickle-cell disease

HbSC disease: occurs in west Africa. The pathophysiology is the same as that for HbSS but the severity is greatly reduced, with most patients being asymptomatic. HbSC is the commonest form of sickle-cell disease to present with complications during pregnancy in west Africa. The Hb value is intermediate between that of HbSS and normal, the MCV is lower than in HbSS, while the reticulocytes are moderately raised. Electrophoresis shows 2 major fractions in the position of HbS and HbC.

HbSβ° thalassaemia: occurs mostly in North Africa, Sicily, and in mixed populations of the Americas. Clinically similar to HbSS; it can be very difficult to distinguish. The definitive diagnosis is made when one parent carries the β^S gene and the other has β° thalassaemia trait.

HbSβ^+ thalassaemia: is the doubly heterozygous condition most commonly seen in Liberia and other parts of west Africa. There is mild anaemia and irreversibly sickled cells are rare. Definitive diagnosis with Hb electrophoresis shows HbA 5–30%, and HbS.

HbSD^{Punjab}: HbD interacts with HbS leading to a disease similar to HbSS. It is seen amongst Sikh and mixed populations. There is moderately severe anaemia; the peripheral blood film resembles HbSS.

Sickle-cell trait: is the inheritance of HbAS and results in a benign condition. Complications occasionally arise due to microinfarcts in the renal medulla and spleen. There is strong evidence, more than with any other inherited abnormality of RBCs, that the trait confers partial protection against *P. falciparum* malaria.

Maintenance of health in sickle-cell disease

1. Early diagnosis

- good laboratory techniques — HbS solubility, Hb electrophoresis
- screening
  - – pregnant women
  - – newborn of mothers with S gene
  - – anaemic children and siblings of patients
- increased clinical awareness.

2. Education

- parents, patients, general public and health professionals.

3. Sickle-cell clinics

- prevent infection
  - – prophylactic antimalarials and penicillin
  - – immunization
- nutrition
  - – folic acid supplements
  - – general nutritional advice
- advice
  - avoid cold, fatigue, dehydration, alcohol
  - – attend clinic regularly
  - – report when ill and pregnant.

4. Hospital

- prompt treatment of crises – rehydration, analgesia, antibiotics +/– hydroxyurea.

5. Obstetrics

- careful supervision of pregnancy, delivery, puerperium
- encourage the woman to have less than 3 pregnancies.

Thalassaemia

The thalassaemias are a heterogeneous group of genetic disorders which result from a reduced rate of synthesis of α or β Hb chains (^{0} indicates total suppression, $^+$ partial suppression). Each individual has two genes for β-globin and four for α-globin. Variation in the normal ratio between these chains leads to globin precipitation; anaemia results from ineffective erythropoiesis and haemolysis. It is possible to correlate clinical severity with genetic deficit.

Distribution is in a band stretching across the Mediterranean, Africa and Asia, and in immigrant populations from these areas.

Thalassaemia intermedia: is less severe than major. It results from the inheritance of one β thalassaemia gene with a HbE gene (in SE Asia) or HbC gene (in west Africa). It also occurs in homozygous β^+ thalassaemia in west Africa, various δβ thalassaemias and Hb Lepore (crossover between δ and β genes) disorders. HbE/β is the commonest form – >40,000 are born each year in SE Asia.

- **Clinical features:** there is a wide range of severity, ranging from mild haemolytic anaemia in HbC/β thalassaemia to severe β major-like disease in HbE/β thalassaemia. Morbidity and mortality are high in the latter condition, especially during childhood, with splenomegaly, recurrent infections, gallstones, skeletal deformities, and chronic leg ulcers.
- **Diagnosis:** hypochromic, microcytic anaemia with target cells. Osmotic fragility is increased. Anaemia is worse in patients with hypersplenism, folate deficiency, intercurrent infection, and in pregnancy.
- **Management:** involves continuous surveillance; folate therapy, active immunization and antimalarial prophylaxis to prevent infections; and prompt treatment of any that do occur. Give blood only during anaemic crises; or when there is a high risk of growth retardation and skeletal abnormality – a high transfusion regime with iron chelation is then indicated. Hypersplenism may increase transfusion requirements; splenectomy should be considered in this situation.

Thalassaemia minor: is of heterozygous inheritance and the carrier is often asymptomatic. Few have palpable splenomegaly.

- **Diagnosis:** Hb is 9–11g/dl; the blood film shows moderate anisocytosis, microcytosis, and hypochromia with a few target cells and cells with punctate basophilia. Marrow biopsy shows mild-moderate erythroid hyperplasia. Electrophoresis shows that the HbA2 is raised to 4–65%; the HbF is also raised to about 3% in approximately half of patients.
- **Management** includes early diagnosis so as to avoid unnecessary treatment of the hypochromic anaemia with iron, offer reassurance that the condition is benign, and allow for genetic counselling.

α thalassaemia: has 4 varieties defined according to the number of defective α-globin genes on chromosome 16. Absence of 1 or 2 genes is very common in the African population and produces a mild anaemia with a low MCV. Epidemiological studies from Melanesia and Papua New Guinea suggest that α^+ thalassaemia has been selected for by malaria.

Clinical classification of thalassaemias	
hydrops fetalis	fatal four-gene deletion α^0 thalassaemia
thalassaemia major (see overpage)	transfusion-dependent, homozygous β^0 thalassaemia (β^0/β^0) or coinheritance of β thalassaemia traits (eg β^0/β^+; most β^+/β^+)
thalassaemia intermedia	homozygous α thalassaemias heterozygous β thalassaemias W African β^+/β^+ thalassaemias coinheritance of β thalassaemia with a β-chain variant (eg HbC/β^0; HbE/β^+) β thalassaemia with hereditary presence of fetal Hb HbH disease
thalassaemia minor	β^0 thalassaemia trait β^+ thalassaemia trait hereditary presence of fetal Hb α^0-thalassaemia trait α^+-thalassaemia trait

HbH disease – the child has β_4 Hb (HbH) due to a lack of α chains. HbH is present at 5–30% throughout life with moderate haemolytic anaemia (Hb 7–10g/dl). Children may have growth retardation and skeletal abnormalities; there is a variable degree of splenomegaly.

Hb Bart's hydrops fetalis – a fatal condition in which the fetus lacks all α genes The infant is stillborn or dies shortly after delivery.

β thalassaemia major

β thalassaemia major is an autosomal recessive disease of children of two heterozygotes or carriers of β thalassaemia trait. Either no β chains (β^0) or small amounts (β^+) are produced. Excess α chains are precipitated in RBCs and in erythroblasts resulting in ineffective erythropoiesis and haemolysis. The greater the α-chain excess, the more severe the anaemia. Over 100 different genetic defects have now been discovered. β thalassaemia major is often due to inheritance of 2 different mutations, each affecting the β-globin synthesis (compound heterozygotes).

Clinical manifestations

- **Failure to thrive –** at 3–6 months of age when the switch from γ to β-chain production should take place.
- **Hepatosplenomegaly –** due to excess haemolysis, extramedullary haemopoiesis, and later in the disease iron overload from transfusions. Splenomegaly increases blood requirements by increasing red cell destruction and pooling and by causing plasma volume expansion.
- **Bone expansion –** as a result of intense marrow hyperplasia → to the characteristic thalassaemic facies: prominent frontal and parietal bones, maxillary enlargement and flattening of the nasal bridge. There is cortical thinning of many bones (→ tendency to fracture) and bossing of the skull with 'hair-on-end' appearance on X-ray.
- **Infections –** are common for a variety of reasons. Anaemic children are prone to bacterial infections. If splenectomy has been carried out without prophylactic penicillin afterwards, pneumococcal and meningococcal infections are likely. Severe gastroenteritis can be caused by *Yersinia enterocolitica* as a result of desferrioxamine treatment of haemochromatosis. Transmission of viral hepatitis is also increased.

Diagnosis: severe hypochromic microcytic anaemia with raised reticulocyte count, normoblasts, target cells, and basophilic stippling in the blood film. Electrophoresis shows absent HbA, raised HbF, and variable HbA2.

Management

1. Aim to keep Hb within 9–14g/dl, suppressing the patient's own abnormal erythropoiesis. This requires 2–3 units every 4–6 weeks. Fresh blood filtered to remove WBCs gives the best red cell survival with the fewest transfusion reactions.
2. Give regular folic acid if there is suspicion of dietary insufficiency.
3. Chelate excess iron with desferrioxamine 1–2g with each unit of blood that is transfused. Give by subcutaneous infusion 20–40mg/kg over 8–12hrs, 3–7 days weekly. It is commenced in infants after 10–15 units of transfusion. ► Excess desferrioxamine in high doses, especially in children, may lead to high tone deafness, retinal damage with night blindness and loss of visual acuity, and growth retardation.
4. Give vitamin C 200mg daily to increase iron excretion.
5. Splenectomy may be needed to reduce the amount of blood required. Delay until after 6 years because there is increased risk of life-threatening infections post-splenectomy before this age.
6. Immunize against hepatitis B.
7. Beware endocrine disorders.

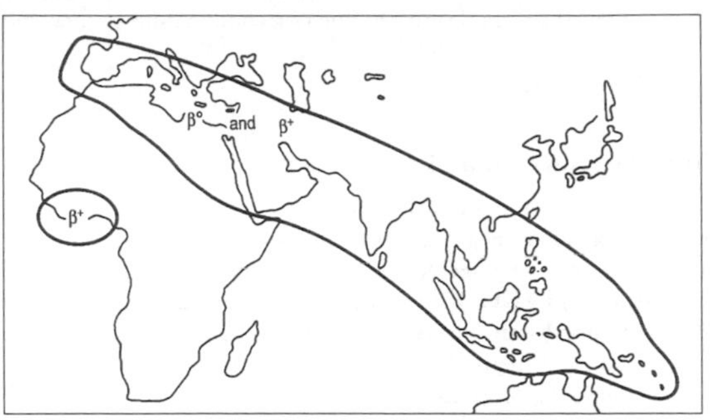

Regions of the world where β thalassaemias reach polymorphic frequencies.

Iron overload due to repeated transfusions: each 500ml unit of blood contains 250mg of iron. Iron accumulation leads to liver damage, endocrine damage (failure of growth, delayed or absent puberty, DM, hypothyroidism, hypoparathyroidism), and myocardial damage. In the absence of intensive iron chelation, death occurs in the second or third decade, usually from CCF or cardiac arrhythmias. Clinically apparent abnormalities usually appear after ~50 units (12g of iron). However, organ damage and skin pigmentation occur before this.

Thalassaemia and pregnancy

In thalassaemia major, the duration of cell survival is reduced. Do not treat with iron as this will overload the already high levels of iron. Transfusions are the mainstay of management. Thalassaemia minor causes a moderate but persistent anaemia during pregnancy. This causes fetal hypoxia, compensatory placental hypertrophy, mild intra-uterine growth retardation, an increased frequency of fetal distress during delivery and a high frequency of low Apgar scores (3 or less at 1 minute) but no significant increase in perinatal mortality. HbF has α chains and the fetus may be anaemic or in severe cases stillborn. β thalassaemia does not affect the fetus.

Disorders of white blood cells

Leukopenia can result from failure of production, inhibition of release from the bone marrow, increased margination in the circulation, and pooling in an enlarged spleen. It is often due to a combination of these factors.

Lymphomas

1. Burkitt's lymphoma (BL)

A lymphoblastic lymphoma which is the commonest childhood cancer in tropical Africa. There is a peak incidence at 5–9 years, with a male predominance. There are three epidemiological patterns: 1) it is endemic in tropical Africa and PNG, with a peak at 4–9 years; 2) it has intermediate incidence in north Africa, western Asia and south America; and 3) it occurs sporadically in the West. Endemicity can be correlated with frequent childhood exposure to and infection with Epstein-Barr virus (EBV) before the age of 1 year, and with a 14q+/8q chromosomal translocation. BL also occurs as a complication of AIDS.

Clinical: often presents with tumours of the jaw and GI involvement. Histology shows a "starry sky" appearance (isolated histiocytes on a background of abnormal lymphocytes).

Management: a single dose of a cytotoxic drug – eg. cyclophosphamide 30mg/kg IV – produces a spectacular remission in some patients.

2. Non-Hodgkin's (non-Burkitt's) lymphoma (NHL)

Heterogeneous group of tumours of B and T cell origin. Low-grade lymphomas run an indolent course but are incurable, while the high-grade ones are more aggressive in nature but long-term cure is achievable. High grade NHLs are more common in Asia and Africa and, in Africa, have a strong association with malarial endemicity.

Clinical features: are rare before 40yrs. Lymphadenopathy is common but extra nodal spread occurs early so first presentation may be in the skin, gut, CNS, or lungs. Although often symptomless; systemic symptoms are as for HL. Marrow involvement may cause pancytopenia; infection is common.

Diagnosis: as for HL. Staging is less important since 70% have spread at presentation. Consider LN biopsy, CXR, (CT), Ba meal.

Management: symptomless low-grade tumours may not need therapy and occasionally show remission. Chlorambucil or cyclophosphamide may control any symptoms which do occur. Splenectomy may help. Radiotherapy can be used for local bulky disease. Optimum treatment for high-grade tumours is 6 weeks of doxorubicin, cyclophosphamide, vincristine, bleomycin, and prednisolone. If it is a lymphoblastic tumour, then treat as for ALL – see below.

Changes in the differential WCC

Neutrophilia >7.5×10⁹/l

acute viral infections
acute bacterial infections (eg *Staphylococcus* spp)
tissue damage; haemorrhage; haemolysis
malignancies; stress states; DKA
drugs, chemicals, steroids, renal failure, pregnancy

Basophilia >0.1×10⁹/l

hypersensitivity; myxoedema; iron deficiency; chronic haemolysis

Lymphocytosis >3.5×10⁹/l

childhood infections, viral infections
protozoan infections (malaria, toxoplasmosis);

Monocytosis >3.5×10⁹/l

protozoan (malaria) and rickettsia infections
chronic bacterial infection: TB, *Brucella*, SBE

Eosinophilia >0.44×10⁹/l

parasitic infections (intra- or extra-GI tract)
asthma, atopy, drugs, lymphoma
connective tissue disease, malignancies
convalescence from viral or other infections

(Values >30% are likely to be due to Katayama fever, infection with *Strongyloides* or *Schistosoma mansoni/japonicum*, or lymphoma).

Leukopenia

Neutropenia <2.0×10⁹/l

- acute malaria
- AIDS
- typhoid
- brucellosis
- hypersplenism
- viral infection in early stages
- megaloblastosis
- overwhelming bacterial infection
- cytotoxic therapy
- idiosyncratic reactions to drugs
- aplastic anaemia
- bone marrow infiltration (eg leukaemia)
- Felty's syndrome
- exposure to chemicals (eg Benzene)
- miscellaneous (racial, familial, cyclic, chronic, idiopathic)

Lymphopenia <1.5×10⁹/l

- viral infections
- AIDS
- corticosteroids
- lymphoma
- acute leukaemias

3. Hodgkin's Lymphoma (HL)

A malignant proliferation of the lymphoid cells which is characterized histologically by Reed-Sternberg cells. HL is not common, with an annual incidence of ~3/100,000 in the West. In the developing world, there are high incidences during childhood in central and south America, north Africa, W Asia and sub-Saharan Africa. There is a predominance of MC and LD forms – see opposite. EBV exposure and infection has been linked to its aetiology, especially in the under 15 and over 50 age ranges.

Clinical features: presentation is with enlarged, painless lymph nodes, usually in the neck or axillae. 25% have general symptoms of malaise, fever, weight loss, night sweats, pruritus, and lethargy. Signs include lymphadenopathy, weight loss, anaemia, hepatosplenomegaly.

Diagnosis: FBC, blood film, ESR, LFTs, uric acid, Ca^{2+}, LN biopsy for definitive diagnosis, CXR, bone marrow biopsy. Staging laparotomy involves splenectomy with liver and LN biopsy. See opposite for staging.

Management: for stages Ia and IIa is radiotherapy, and for stage IIa–IVb chemotherapy: 'MOPP' (Mustine, Oncovin (vincristine), Procarbazine, Prednisolone). SEs: radiation lung fibrosis, hypothyroidism, nausea, alopecia, infertility (men), infection and second malignancies (AML and NHL) and myelosuppression.

4. Adult T-cell leukaemia/lymphoma (ATL)

The type C retrovirus, human T-cell lymphotropic virus type 1 (HTLV-1), causes both ATL and, in a few infected individuals, tropical spastic paresis/HTLV-1 associated myelopathy (TSP/HAM). The virus is endemic in much of the tropics, and becoming more widespread amongst IV drug abusers and homosexuals in N and S. America and western Europe. HTLV-2 is a similar virus which is endemic amongst aboriginal groups in central America. It is now spreading in the USA and Europe via blood transfusions and IV drug abuse.

Transmission: is by sexual intercourse, breastfeeding, and the exchange of blood. Male-to-female transmission is more effective than female-to-male, and enhanced by other STDs. Seroprevalence rises slowly with age, compatible with the slow rate of transmission in endemic areas.

Clinical features: 5 phases are recognized:

1. asymptomatic;
2. acute ATL (2/3 have lymphadenopathy, hepatosplenomegaly and skin lesions: papules, nodules, plaques, tumours, ulcers);
3. chronic ATL (with skin lesions, mild lymphocytosis, and prolonged course);
4. smouldering ATL (skin rashes and low count of ATL cells; remains stable for many years);
5. lymphoma type (clinically like NHL, poor prognosis).

Diagnosis: include LN biopsy, FBC, WCC ($30–130\times10^9$/l), bone marrow biopsy, CXR (pulmonary infiltration and osteolytic lesions).

Management: is supportive; most patients die within 12 months.

Classification of Hodgkin's lymphoma

Classification (in order of incidence)	***Prognosis***
Nodular sclerosing (NS)	Good
Mixed cellularity (MC)	Good
Lymphocyte predominant (LP)	Good
Lymphocyte depleted (LD)	Poor

Staging

I Single LN area
II >2 areas on same side of the diaphragm
III LN on both sides of the diaphragm
IV Spread beyond LNs

A – no systemic symptoms
B – presence of weight loss >10% in last 6 months, unexplained fever >38°C, night sweats.

5-year survival overall 80%; depends on stage and grade.

Leukaemias

The crude incidence of leukaemias is probably the same in tropical and non-tropical areas, but there are distinct differences in the age and gender distribution of the 4 main types. There are relatively few diagnostic problems which are peculiar to the tropics, but there are severe limitations in their management, especially of acute leukaemias.

1. Acute lymphoblastic leukaemia (ALL)

This is a neoplastic proliferation of lymphoblasts.

Clinical features: are due to malignant infiltration (lymphadenopathy, hepatosplenomegaly, bone pain), anaemia, haemorrhage or thrombosis, and infections following immune depression.

Diagnosis: is by blood film (blast cells) and bone marrow biopsy, which shows infiltration by blast cells. The WCC is raised in 2/3 of people.

Management: involves

- **Supportive care** – transfusion for anaemia; platelet transfusion for haemorrhage due to thrombocytopaenia; allopurinol for hyperuricaemia
- **Prevention** – of infection with antibiotics and antimalarials
- **Chemotherapy** – consists of **1.** remission induction with vincristine, prednisolone, L-asparaginase and daunorubicin, followed by **2.** CNS prophylaxis with intrathecal methotrexate and cranial irradiation. **3.** Maintenance chemotherapy – mercaptopurine (daily), methotrexate (weekly), and vincristine and prednisolone (monthly) – is required for 2–3 years. Relapse is common in the blood, CNS, and testes.

2. Acute myeloblastic leukaemia (AML)

This is a neoplastic proliferation of blast cells derived from myeloid elements within the bone marrow.

Clinical features: as for ALL, except that in tropical Africa between 10–25% of all patients and about 1/3 of boys may present with a chloroma – a solid tumour arising from the orbit (may occur at other sites). Gum hypertrophy is seen particularly in M4, M5. DIC is common in M3.

Diagnosis: can be made with the non-specific esterase reaction which is strongly positive with M5 and M4. The myeloperoxidase and Sudan black reaction help distinguish between ALL L2 and AML M1.

Treatment:

- **Supportive** – as for ALL (transfusions, platelets, allopurinol). Survival without treatment is about 2 months.
- **Chemotherapy** – requires specialist centres and improves survival to about 9 months (regimens include daunorubicin, cytosine arabinoside, and thioguanine). Bone marrow transplantation carries a much better prognosis and the possibility of a cure, but it is expensive and needs sophisticated facilities. In AML M3, all-trans-retinoic acid (ATRA) therapy has been shown to be beneficial; it may prove possible in the future to use this to control symptoms in areas with limited resources.

Classification of ALL and AML

Common ALL	75%; defined with a specific antilymphoblast antibody. Phenotypically pre-B. Commonly 2–4 yr olds. M=F.
T-cell ALL	Any age; peak in adolescent males; present eg with a mediastinal mass and high WCC
B-cell ALL	Rare. Very poor prognosis. Surface Igs are present on blast cells.
Null-cell ALL	Undifferentiated, lacking any markers.

Morphological classification of AML

(FAB – French/American/British method)

M1: Undifferentiated blast cells
M2: Myeloblastic
M3: Promyelocytic (associated with DIC)
M4: Myelomonocytic
M5: Monocytic
M6: Erythroleukaemia
M7: Megakaryoblastic

3. Chronic lymphocytic leukaemia (CLL)

Monoclonal proliferation of well-differentiated lymphocytes. 90–95% are B cells; variants include: hairy-cell leukaemia (5–10%; usually of B-cell origin); T-CLL (1%); and B- or T-prolymphocytic leukaemias (<1%).

Clinical features: onset can be insidious with bleeding, weight loss, infection, anorexia. It is asymptomatic in 25%. Signs include hepatosplenomegaly and enlarged rubbery non-tender lymph nodes. The spleen can be enormous in areas of malarial endemicity.

Diagnosis: blood film shows marked lymphocytosis, often with normochromic normocytic anaemia and thrombocytopaenia. Bone marrow biopsy will show infiltration by the malignant clone.

Management:

- **Curative antimalarial therapy** followed by long-term prophylaxis results in partial reduction of spleen size and peripheral WCC.
- **Chemotherapy** is not always needed, but may postpone marrow failure. Chlorambucil (0.1–0.2mg/kg PO daily) is used to decrease lymphocyte count. Prednisolone will help autoimmune haemolysis.
- **Radiotherapy** is used for relief of lymphadenopathy or splenomegaly.
- **Supportive care** involves transfusions and prophylactic antibiotics.

Prognosis: some remain stable for years or even regress. Usually the nodes enlarge. Death is commonly due to infection. Median survival is about 8 years, but it is stage-dependent and shorter in tropical countries.

4. Chronic myeloid leukaemia (CML)

Uncontrolled proliferation of myeloid cells. 90% of cases have the Philadelphia chromosome (22); those without it have a poorer prognosis.

Clinical features: presentation is chronic and insidious with weight loss, lethargy, sweats, fever, haemorrhage, anaemia, bruising, gout, abdominal pain, gross hepatosplenomegaly, generalized lymphadenopathy.

Diagnosis: WCC grossly elevated ($>500\times10^9$/l); ↓ Hb. ↓ leucocyte ALP (on stained film); plasma uric acid and ALP are ↑.

Management:

- chemotherapy following standard regimes of busulphan 2–4mg/24h PO is the mainstay of treatment in the chronic phase. Monitor FBC to avoid pancytopenia. Stop treatment when WCC is 20×10^9/l. Transformation may be signalled by lack of response to previously effective therapy. Treatment of transformed CML is poor.
- autologous bone marrow transplant is another option, starting with chemotherapy and whole body radiotherapy followed by autografting of patient's previously stored haemopoietic stem cells.
- allogenic transplantation, from an HLA matched donor, should be considered during the chronic phase if <55 years. 50–60% of transplanted patients will be cured.

Prognosis: is variable. Typically there are 2 phases: a chronic symptomatic phase, which lasts months or a few years, and then rapid blast transformation with features of acute leukaemia and usually rapid death.

Epidemiology of CLL and CML

Most CLL patients are >40 years; the M:F ratio is 2:1. The lowest incidence rates are in C and S America; the highest in Scandinavia and Canada. In tropical Africa, CLL occurs from 17 years with equal sex distribution. It is rare in India, SE and far-east Asia. B-CLL has been associated with HTLV-1 infection in Jamaica and Nigeria.

CML accounts for 15% of leukaemias. In the West, it occurs most often during middle-age, but in developing countries with younger populations CML can occur in patients <40yrs. There is a slight male predominance.

Staging of CLL

Stage	0	Absolute lymphocytosis $>15\times10^9$/l
	I	Stage 0 + enlarged lymph nodes
	II	Stage I + enlarged liver or spleen
	III	Stage II + anaemia (Hb <11g/dl)
	IV	Stage III + platelets $< 100\times10^9$/l

Myeloproliferative disorders

A group of disorders characterized by proliferation of precursors for myeloid elements: RBC (polycythaemia rubra vera), leukocytes (CML), platelets (essential thrombocythaemia). The proliferating cells retain their ability to differentiate. The disorders share several features such as night sweats, fever, weight loss, itch, and malaise. Each may undergo transformation to acute leukaemia.

- **Polycythaemia:** may be relative (from dehydration due to alcohol, diuretics) or absolute (primary – polycythaemia rubra vera – or secondary due to smoking, chronic lung disease, tumours, or altitude). Radioactive chromium studies help distinguish between the two.
- **Polycythaemia rubra vera (PRV):** is characterised by a high PCV (up to 70%), variably raised WBC and platelets, and splenomegaly (60%). Presentation varies but includes CNS disturbances, angina, bruising, gout. Often found at a routine blood test. An absolute increase in red cell mass makes the diagnosis; the marrow shows active erythropoiesis. WBC, platelets, uric acid, leukocyte ALP are raised (decreased in CML). Treatment is to keep PCV <50% by venesection. Busulphan can be used. Prognosis is variable.
- **Essential thrombocythaemia:** is characterized by very high platelet counts, eg $>800 \times 10^9$/l. Platelet morphology & function is abnormal; presentation may be bleeding or thrombosis. Symptomatic treatment is with busulphan or hydoxyurea. Prognosis is good.
  Differential diagnosis of thrombocythaemia includes bleeding, inflammation, malignancy, post-splenectomy, Kawasaki disease.

Myeloma

Myeloma is a plasma cell neoplasm (IgG: 55%, IgA: 25%, light chain: 20%) which produces diffuse bone marrow infiltration and focal osteolytic deposits. The incidence in the West is 5–10/100,000, with a peak age of 70 yrs and an equal sex distribution. The incidence is higher in the Caribbean and Africa. Young patients are common in Africa: ~65% of patients are 40–60 yrs old; patients in their late 30s are not uncommon.

Clinical features: bone pain and tenderness is common, particularly in spine, ribs, long bones and shoulders. Ca^{2+} increases in 30%. Renal failure results from light chain precipitation, hyperuricaemia, and high Ca^{2+}. Also: anaemia, infection, neuropathy, blurred vision, haemorrhages and exudates in retina, bleeding, and amyloidosis (→ macroglossia).

Diagnosis: abundant plasma cells on bone marrow biopsy; M band or urinary light chains (Bence-Jones protein); osteolytic bone lesions ('pepper-pot' skull). ► Beware rise in Ca^{2+}, urea, creatinine, and uric acid.

Management: supportive analgesia and transfusions for pain, anaemia. Solitary lesions may benefit from radiotherapy. Intermittent melphalan chemotherapy is standard. Consider multiple therapy if there is no response or relapse. Death is commonly due to renal failure, infection or haemorrhage. **Prognosis:** 50% alive at 2yrs. Survival is worse if urea is >10mmol/l or Hb <7.5g/dl.

Haematology

Splenomegaly

The spleen has two major immunological functions: phagocytosis and antibody production. The large number of parasitic, bacterial and viral agents in the tropical world ensures that these functions are stretched to their capacity and induce splenomegaly of varying magnitude. Splenomegaly is therefore a common physical sign in the tropics.

Clinical features: splenomegaly can cause abdominal distension and discomfort. It may also lead to hypersplenism – pancytopenia then occurs as cells become trapped and destroyed in the spleen's reticuloendothelial system, resulting in symptoms of anaemia, infection, and bleeding. The spleen is recognized clinically by its movement with respiration, enlargement towards RIF, +/– presence of a notch, and the fact that one cannot get above it. AXR may help. Check for lymphadenopathy and liver disease.

Investigations: FBC, ESR, LFTs; liver, marrow, or LN biopsy.

Mild splenomegaly (<5 cm below the costal margin):

- **Acute infections** – malaria, septicaemia, viraemias, hepatitis, trypanosomiasis, brucellosis, toxoplasmosis, typhus.
- **Subacute, chronic infections** – TB, brucellosis, syphilis, hydatid disease, meningococcal septicaemia, histoplasmosis, bacterial endocarditis.
- **Miscellaneous** – megaloblastic anaemia, iron deficiency anaemia, immune thrombocytopenia, RA, hyperthyroidism, myeloma, SLE, sarcoidosis, amyloidosis.

Moderate splenomegaly (5–10 cm below the costal margin):

- **chronic haemolysis** – recurrent malaria, haemoglobinopathies, spherocytosis.
- **portal hypertension** – hepatic cirrhosis.
- **haematological malignancies** – CLL, lymphomas, acute leukaemias, PRV.

Massive splenomegaly (>10cm below the costal margin):

- **infections** – hyperreactive malarial splenomegaly (HMS), schistosomiasis, leishmaniasis, tropical splenomegaly syndrome (TSS).
- **blood disorders** – thalassaemia major, CML, myelofibrosis.
- **miscellaneous** – splenic cysts, tumours.

Splenectomies

These operations appear to be going out of fashion. Suitable indications still remain, however, such as trauma, haemolytic anaemias, ITP, and occasionally diagnostic purposes.

Post-operatively there may be a prompt, transient rise in the platelet count. ► All patients, particularly children, are at increased risk of septicaemia (post-splenectomy sepsis), especially pneumococcal. Prophylactic antibiotics, for children, are recommended in the form of penicillin V until age 20yrs. Pneumococcal, meningococcal, and *haemophilius influenzae* B vaccines are recommended.

Haematology

Disorders of haemostasis

Abnormal bleeding results from disorders of:

1. **Initiation of haemostasis** – involving the vascular endothelium and platelets. Manifests as purpura and haemorrhage from or into *superficial* surfaces.
2. **Consolidation of haemostasis** – involving the coagulation and fibrinolytic pathways. Manifests clinically as uncontrolled haemorrhages from or into *deeper* tissues.

Purpura

Disorders of the initiation of haemostasis result from abnormalities of the endothelium (vascular purpura), abnormalities of platelet function, or thrombocytopenia.

1. Vascular purpura – damage to vascular endothelium is a common cause of purpura and haemorrhage in the tropics. Infections are important, causing haemorrhage through either direct toxicity to the endothelium (the haemorrhagic fevers – see chapter 4), or immune damage. In immunocompromised patients, herpesviruses (HSV, VZV) and arboviruses (O'nyong-nyong, African chikungunya) can also cause fatal haemorrhages.

2. Defective platelet function – thrombopathy can complicate the course of some of the haemorrhagic fevers (Lassa, dengue, Marburg, Ebola), alcoholism, hepatic cirrhosis, uraemia, paraproteinaemias, leukaemias, and myeloproliferative disorders. It can also result from ingestion of drugs such as NSAIDS.

3. Thrombocytopenia – an abnormally low platelet count may result from defective production, increased destruction or consumption in the peripheral blood, splenic pooling, or a combination of these. Conditions such as idiopathic thrombocytopenic purpura (ITP) have no epidemiological or clinical features particular to the tropics, except that patients tend to develop splenomegaly and anaemia.

Onyalai – is a profound acquired immune thrombocytopenia of young people in southern Africa which differs from ITP. Clinical features include haemorrhagic bullae on mucous membranes and less frequently the skin (including the soles of the feet), epistaxis, and cerebral haemorrhage. The bleeding normally lasts for ~8 days, but can persist for months and often recurs. Acutely, there is ~3% mortality due to haemorrhagic shock and cerebral haemorrhage. Transfusion is required; splenectomy may be necessary to control bleeding – this is followed by a return to normal platelet counts, but fatal recurrence has occured post-splenectomy.

Causes of haemorrhage due to vascular endothelial damage

Infections

• direct toxicity	viruses (dengue, yellow fever, Lassa fever, other haemorrhagic fevers) bacteria (typhoid, Gram-negative sepsis, meningococcal septicaemia)
• early immune damage	measles, scarlet fever, chickenpox, rubella, TB
• late immune damage	Henoch-Schonlein purpura, purpura fulminans

Drugs

• idiosyncratic reactions	streptomycin, isoniazid, penicillin, aspirin, sulphonamides, quinine, etc.

Others

- uraemia, scurvy, dysproteinaemias (myeloma), fat embolism
- congenital conditions (eg Ehlers-Danlos, Osler-Weber-Rendu)
- senile purpura

Causes of thrombocytopenia

Low production
- infections (eg typhoid, brucellosis)
- megaloblastic anaemia
- alcoholism
- marrow infiltration (eg leukaemia)
- aplastic anaemia
- drugs/chemicals: cytotoxic drugs, idiosyncratic reactions, overdose, occupational exposure (eg benzene)

Increased consumption or destruction
- infections (eg malaria, trypanosomiasis, dengue)
- hypersplenism
- chronic hepatic disease
- DIC
- immune mechanisms:
  ITP, Onyalai, acute viral infection, AIDS
  drugs (quinine, penicillin), lymphomas
  CLL, autoimmune diseases

Coagulation disorders

These conditions occur in two forms:

- congenital – haemophilia A (factor VIII deficiency); haemophilia B (Christmas disease, factor IX deficiency) and Von Willebrand's disease (deficiency or abnormality of factor VIII associated protein) *and*
- acquired – malabsorption (vit. K deficiency), liver disease, disseminated intravascular haemolysis (DIC), and snake envenomation.

1. Congenital forms

Clinical features: bleeding into joints and muscles is a common presentation; it can lead to crippling arthropathy and haematomas with nerve palsies. Boys may also present with haemorrhage post-circumcision. Cerebral haemorrhages may result from the ↑ ICP of persistent coughing.

Diagnosis: is by history, FHx, increased KCCT, and factor VIII assay.

Management: seek expert advice.

- **Haemophilia A –** avoid NSAIDS and IM injections. With minor bleeding, apply pressure and elevate the limb. Desmopressin (0.3–0.4μg/kg /q12–24h IV in 50ml 0.9% saline over 20 mins) raises factor VIII and may be sufficient. Major bleeding requires either factor VIII infusion or cryoprecipitate (rich in factor VIII and can be prepared easily – see box). ► There is a high risk of HIV transmission with cryoprecipitate.
- **Haemophilia B –** is best treated with virus-inactivated factor IX concentrate; cryosupernate or FFP can be given in its absence but there is increased risk of HIV transmission.
- **Von Willebrand's disease –** should be managed with desmopressin although cryoprecipitate may also be required.

Blood products and HIV/hepatitis viruses: ►► HIV, hepatitis B and C, and other microorganisms can be transmitted in blood products that have not been heat inactivated. Such products should only be used when the advantages are judged to outweigh the risks of infection.

2. Acquired hypoprothrombinaemias

- **Vitamin K deficiency:**
  i) Haemorrhagic disease of the newborn is the result of vitamin K deficiency in premature infants and infants of mothers on anti-TB therapy, anticonvulsants or warfarin. Infants may also present later, between 1–3 months of age, with intracranial haemorrhage. It is prevented by prophylactic vitamin K 1mg IM. On the first day of life vitamin K should be given IV. ► Be aware of anaphylaxis.
  ii) Malabsorption – see chapter 8. Diagnosis is via a prolonged PT, which reverts rapidly to normal following treatment with vitamin K 10mg IV; the response will be partial if there is liver disease.
- **Vitamin K antagonism:** is seen with the competitive inhibitor warfarin. Inadvertent overdose, simultaneous administration of other potentiating drugs, and accidental ingestion may all cause haemorrhage. Warfarin's anticoagulant effect remains for a few days after withdrawal; if the bleeding does not resolve, give vitamin K 10mg IV stat.
- **Liver disease:** see opposite.

Haemostatic measurements (for children >2yrs and adults)

blood platelets	150–400 × 10^9/l
prothrombin time (PT)	11–14 seconds
partial thromboplastin time (PTT)	23–35 seconds
blood fibrinogen levels	2–4 g/l
fibrinogen breakdown products (FDP)	<10 mg/l

PT is used for measuring the extrinsic coagulation pathway. Since factor VII has the shortest half-life of the coagulation factors, it is the first factor to become reduced after giving warfarin. Therefore the PT is used to measure anticoagulation due to warfarin.

PTT is used for measuring the intrinsic coagulation pathway. It is therefore used to measure anticoagulation due to heparin.

To prepare a cryoprecipitate and cryosupernatant

Collect donor blood into a multipack plastic blood-collection set. Centrifuge the unit or allow it to sediment; separate the plasma into a second pack and freeze this at -20°C or colder for 24hrs. Thaw the plasma at 4°C and centrifuge; the cryoprecipitate remains in the bag while the cryosupernatant is separated into a third bag. Both should be stored at –20°C until used.

Liver disease and coagulation disorders

Bleeding in liver disease is multifactorial:

1. During acute infectious hepatitis, a mild disorder of haemostasis consisting of reduced levels of factors V, VII and X and a prolonged PT is not unusual.
2. In liver failure, there is severe coagulation factor deficiency, afibrinaemia, and DIC.
3. Patients with chronic hepatic disease or cirrhosis show impairment of synthesis of all vitamin K-dependent factors and fibrinogen and reduced platelet function. The PT is prolonged and vitamin K has little or no effect.

Bleeding with liver disease should be treated by transfusion of cryosupernatant, FFP, or factor concentrates.

Disseminated intravascular coagulation (DIC)

DIC is the widespread or uncontrolled deposition of fibrin in the circulation. It may be triggered by a large number of conditions.

Mechanisms:

1. Damage to the endothelium with activation of the intrinsic pathway of the coagulation cascade.
2. Release of thromboplastin-like materials from tissues with the activation of the extrinsic pathway.
3. Injection of procoagulants in snake venom.
4. During pregnancy, there is normally a potential hypercoagulable and hyperfibrinolytic state. A wide range of obstetric disorders can trigger severe DIC – see opposite.

The dominant feature of DIC is haemorrhage, which is multifactorial. The end state is one of depleted platelets, coagulation factors, and fibrinogen. DIC is therefore also known as 'consumption coagulopathy'. Fibrinogen degradation products (FDPs) are released into the circulation where they have an antithrombin activity. Their incorporation into clots makes the clots friable.

Clinical features: presentation is usually with the underlying condition. DIC can range from a minor derangement of coagulation without bleeding to a severe haemorrhagic state. It is a dynamic condition which can progress rapidly. The common manifestations of bleeding include haemorrhage in mucous membranes, skin, venepuncture sites, or from the uterus.

Microangiopathic haemolytic anaemia: results from subacute and chronic DIC. Obstruction of small blood vessels may cause ischaemia, tissue necrosis, and renal failure; pituitary failure and adrenal failure are rare complications.

Diagnosis: the platelet count is reduced, PTT, PT and thrombin times are prolonged, and the plasma FDPs are raised. In severe DIC, the simple clotting time is prolonged. Microangiopathic haemolytic anaemia shows features of intravascular haemolysis: there are many small, fragmented RBCs with bizarre shapes (schizocytes) in the peripheral blood.

Management:

1. Treat the underlying condition; if this has a rapid response, the DIC will correct spontaneously.
2. Restore and maintain blood volume via transfusion of whole blood (if unavailable, use concentrated RBCs plus saline, or saline and colloids).
3. If haemorrhage cannot be controlled, give platelets, FFP, and/or cryoprecipitate to restore the missing coagulation factors.
4. In subacute or chronic conditions, in which the primary cause cannot be cured, the patient may be heparinized in order to break the cycle. Aim to keep the simple clotting time just above 15mins.

Main causes of DIC in the tropics

Acute

• infections	viraemia, liver disease, sepsis, renal disease, protozoan infections
• obstetric	septic abortions, abruptio placentae, ruptured uterus, amniotic fluid embolus
• shock	accidental trauma – birth anoxia, head injury, fractured femur, surgical trauma, burns, heat stroke
• envenomation	snake bites, *Lonomia achelous* caterpillars
• others	acute hepatic necrosis, cytotoxic therapy, incompatible blood transfusion

Subacute

• obstetric	pre-eclampsia, eclampsia, retention of dead fetus hydatidiform mole
• malignancy	AML M3
• others	purpura fulminans

Chronic

• metabolic	
• malignacy	cg prostatic carcinoma

13. Nutrition

Weight loss and malnutrition 552
Malnutrition and infection 552
Defining and assessing weight loss and malnutrition 554
Oedematous malnutrition/kwashiorkor 558
Severe wasting/marasmus 560
General principles of treatment 560
Specific problems 562
Rehabilitation 568
Failure to respond to treatment 572
Disasters and refugee camps 578
Malnutrition in adults and adolescents 580
Goitre 582
Scurvy 584
Tooth decay and gum disease 584
Rickets and osteomalacia 586
Vitamin B_2 deficiency (ariboflavinosis) 586
Beriberi 588
Pellagra 590
Vitamin A deficiency 592
Vitamin B_{12} deficiency 594
Vitamin E deficiency 594
Vitamin K deficiency 594
Obesity 596

The following two sources have been used extensively for this section:
Savage King F and Burgess A, 1993, *Nutrition for developing countries*, 2nd Ed, OUP, Oxford; and
Cook GC, 1996, Nutrition – associated disease, in *Manson's Tropical disease*, 20th Ed, Cook GC, WB Saunders, London

Nutrition

Weight loss and malnutrition

The syndrome of malnutrition and weight loss is common throughout the tropics, occurring as a primary complaint or secondary to some other illness, and in varying degrees of severity. It is both a medical and social disorder, in that the medical problems of the child result from the social problems of the home in which he or she lives. The disease is the end result of chronic nutritional and, frequently, emotional deprivation by caretakers who, because of poor understanding, poverty, or family disintegration, are unable to provide the child with the nutrition and care he or she requires. Successful treatment of the severely malnourished requires that both the medical and the social problems are recognized and corrected. Failure to do so will often mean that the child is likely to relapse once medical treatment is stopped.

It is estimated that around 100 million children worldwide suffer from moderate malnutrition and that 10 million are severely malnourished and at risk of death.[1]

The daily energy requirement of a 25-year-old male working for 8hrs is estimated at 3200 calories (13,000kJ). Breast-feeding mothers and growing children require proportionally more and are therefore the groups at greatest risk of developing malnutrition. Since bacterial and parasitic infections are also prevalent (again, particularly in children) and since the daily diet is not well balanced in many instances, it is easy to see how a chronic calorie deficit develops.

► The presentation of one child with malnutrition is likely to mean that other children of the same family (and usually others in the community) are also malnourished and warrant further investigation.

Malnutrition and infection

Malnutrition may be both a cause and a consequence of infection. Not only is immunocompetence reduced in the malnourished, but certain infections may also predispose to or worsen malnutrition.

- Intestinal infections cause decreased absorption of nitrates from the GI tract, an increase in urinary excretion of nitrogen, and a decrease in dietary intake owing to anorexia.
- Viral illnesses also exert an adverse effect on nitrogen balance. In addition, measles infection is believed to be an important factor in the development of kwashiorkor by W African children.
- Very heavy parasite infestations (eg *Ascaris*) can consume a significant proportion of the dietary intake.
- Hookworm infection is the commonest cause of iron-deficiency anaemia worldwide (due to chronic GI haemorrhage).
- Heavy infections with *Giardia lamblia* or *Strongyloides stercoralis* may interfere with intestinal absorption.

► We use length and height interchangeably. Length is used when infants or children are too ill to stand. Such children are measured lying down.

1 1993, *Bull World Health Org*, 71, 703

Points in the history and physical examination

History:

- Usual diet before current illness
- Breast-feeding history
- Food and fluids taken in past few days
- Recent sinking of eyes
- Duration, frequency, and nature of any vomiting or diarrhoea
- Time when urine was last passed
- Contact with measles or tuberculosis
- Any deaths of siblings
- Birthweight
- Milestones reached (eg sitting, standing etc)
- Immunizations

Physical examination:

- Weight and length/height
- Oedema
- Enlarged or tender liver, jaundice
- Abdominal distension, bowel sounds
- Severe pallor
- Signs of shock – cold hands or feet, weak pulse, decreased consciousness, thirst
- Temperature – hypothermia/fever
- Corneal lesions suggestive of vitamin A deficiency
- Evidence of ear, mouth, or throat infection
- Infection or purpura of skin
- Respiratory rate and type
- Facial appearance

Non-nutritional causes of weight loss

Malignancy (virtually any), TB (pulmonary or extra-pulmonary), AIDS, visceral leishmaniasis, brucellosis, giardiasis, hydatid disease, anaemia, chronic diarrhoea, malabsorption, depression.

… and assessing weight loss and …rition

…ute (weeks or months) or chronic? What was the pre-morbid or …rmal weight? Indirect assessment, such as loosening of clothes, might be the only clues. The **body mass index** (BMI) takes into account the size (height) of the patient when assessing weight and is found by:

$$\text{Weight (kg)} \div \text{Height}^2 \text{ (m)}$$

It normally lies between 21 and 26. A patient with BMI <17 needs urgent nutritional help. Body fat stores can be quickly estimated by the thickness (in mm) of a single skinfold over the triceps muscle. Biochemical markers such as plasma albumin concentration do not give an accurate index of protein status, since it varies according to the patient's level of hydration and also whether fluid is sequestered in the extravascular space, eg during sepsis.

Other methods for determining nutritional status

1. Using growth charts

A commonly used alternative to the weight-for-height and height-for-age reference levels is the weight-for-age or growth chart (see opposite). This chart has three solid reference curves on it –

- the upper one is *97th centile* curve, below which 97% of a healthy population of children will lie
- the middle one is the *median* curve, or *50th centile,* below which 50% of a healthy population of children will lie
- the lower one is the *3rd centile* curve, below which only 3% of a healthy population will lie.

► The dotted curve represents 60% of the median curve; no healthy child's weight is below this line.

Although there is some variation between boys and girls (and separate charts for each sex do exist), for practical purposes healthy children of either sex will have their weights between the 97th and 3rd centile curves. The slope of the curve shows the *rate* at which the child gains (or loses) weight and should be roughly the same as that of the reference curve.

Weighing a child once will only give you an estimate of the child's growth and nutritional status since children of the same age vary greatly in weight. However, if a single measurement falls below the 3rd centile, the child is *probably* malnourished. If it falls below the 60% line, it is almost certainly malnourished.

Weighing a child at regular intervals and recording the results on a growth chart gives much more information. For example, a child's weight may fall just below the 3rd centile, but remain parallel to it as the child grows and eats a healthy diet – indicating that the child is simply one of the 3% of small, well-nourished children. ► The clinician should be alerted when weight plots cross the reference lines or deviate abnormally. This may indicate that a child is becoming malnourished and not growing as fast as he should, or even losing weight.

Common mistakes with growth charts

- writing January in the first box instead of the child's birth month
- writing the month in which the child was first weighed instead of her birth month in the first box
- missing out months
- writing the months as numbers and confusing them with ages
- forgetting to miss out blank boxes if the child has not been weighed for several months
- not using the calendar and estimating the child's age each time
- recording a child's weight in the wrong year
- putting the weight dot the wrong side of the kilogram line.

Standard growth chart showing centiles

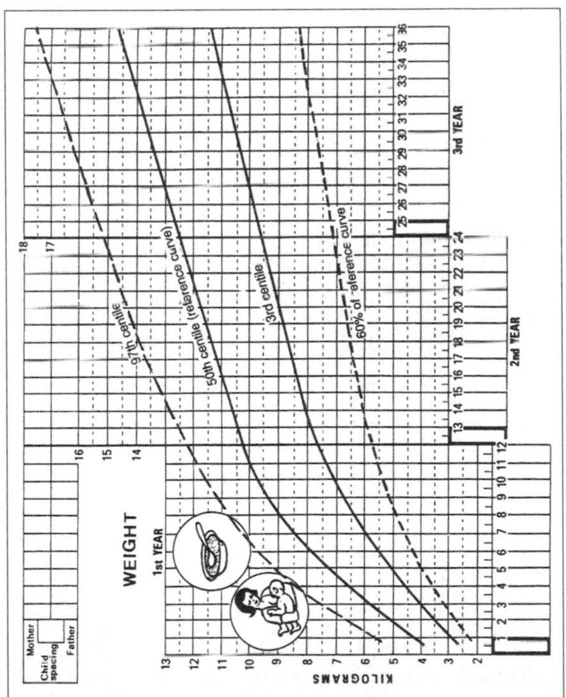

2. Measuring the mid-upper arm circumference (MUAC) – The figure opposite shows an *arm circumference for age chart.* The reference line on the chart rises very steeply in the first year and is thus not very useful for children below 1yr of age. From the age of 1yr, however, it rises only slowly and may be used to assess nutritional status, since there is little variation between ages. In this case:

- A 1–5yr old child with a MUAC <12.5cm is severely malnourished.
- A 1–5yr old child with a MUAC of 12.5–13.5cm is moderately malnourished.
- In different countries, or in different populations, there may be different cut-off points, but the general principle is the same.

3. Using a Shakir strip – Relies on the same principle as the MUAC but uses a purpose-made strip for nutritional assessment. Cut a strip 25cm long and 1–2cm wide from material which does not stretch or tear easily (eg an old X-ray film, a strip cut from a plastic bottle, strong card, etc). Measure and mark: a point 5cm from one end; a point 12.5cm from the first mark (ie 17.5cm from the end) and a point 1cm from the second mark (ie 18.5cm from the end). Colour the strip to the left of the second mark red, between the second and third marks yellow, and to the right of the third mark green.

4. If you don't know the child's date of birth

If the baby is very small: with the aid of the mother, estimate in which month the child was born. Stick to this month for all future references on the growth chart – the *exact* position of the growth line is less important than its overall shape.

If the child is older: estimate the age of a child <3yrs old to within 3 months, which for most purposes will make little difference to the growth line. With the aid of the mother, try to determine the season in which the child was born.

5. Using the child's development

6–8 weeks	the baby begins to smile
3 months	he can control his head
6 months	she can sit up with help
9 months	she can sit up without help
12 months	he can pull himself up to stand
15 months	he can walk.

Problems: some children walk early; some (especially if undernourished) will not walk until they are 18 months old. A child who becomes malnourished may stop walking, even though it was once able to walk.

► Always ask the mother how her child has developed in relation to others.

6. Using the child's teeth – From the age of about 6 months until 2yrs, a child grows approximately one tooth per month. Therefore, estimate the child's age in months by counting the teeth and adding six. However, some perfectly healthy children do not begin to develop teeth until they are over 1yr old, while others start at 3 months. If the child has been chronically malnourished teeth may erupt later. Nevertheless, if a child has 20 or more teeth, he or she is almost certainly at least 2yrs old.

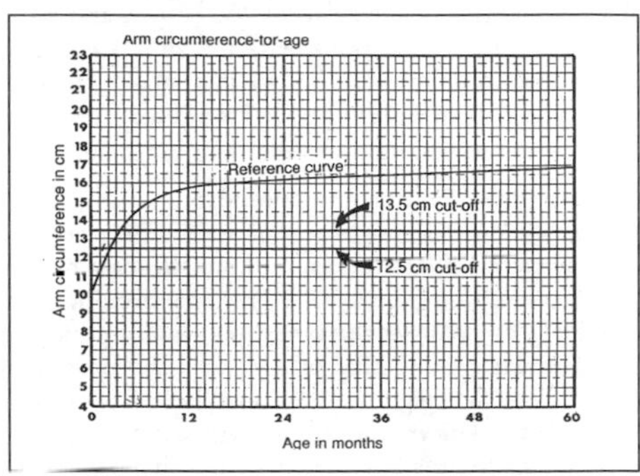

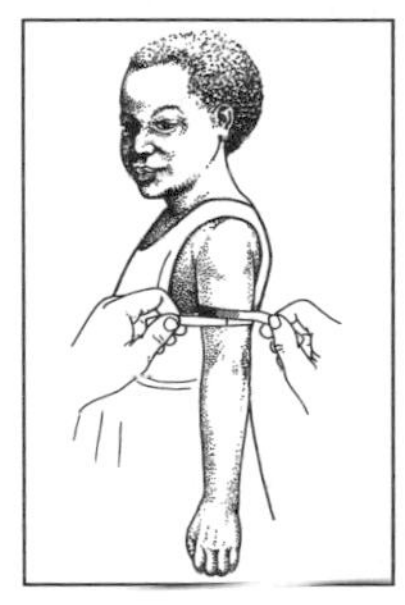

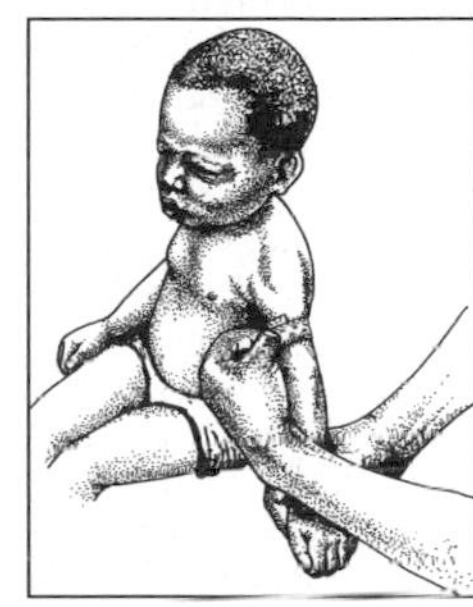

The Shakir strip

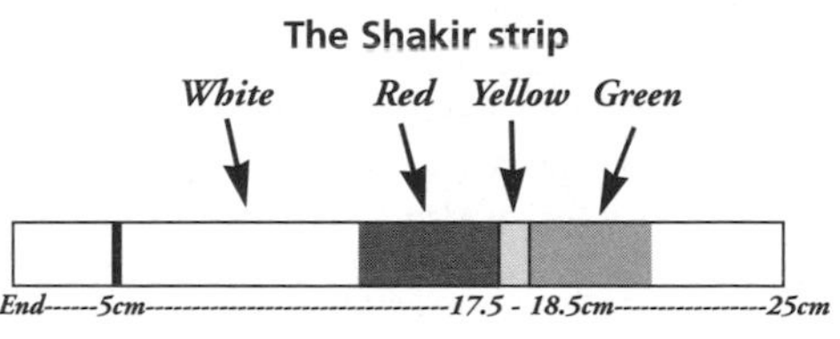

To use: wrap the tape around the upper arm of the child with the colours showing, so that it is tight but comfortable. If the first mark meets the green coloured part of the strip, the child is well nourished. If the first mark meets the yellow coloured part of the strip, the child is moderately malnourished. If the first mark meets the red coloured part of the strip, the child is severely malnourished.

Oedematous malnutrition/kwashiorkor

From the Ghanaian for deprived child, kwashiorkor results primarily from an inadequacy of dietary protein in growing children. It usually occurs when breastfeeding is only partial, or has ceased, and passive immunity declines. Deficiency of micronutrients (eg zinc, selenium) may further decrease natural immunity leading to increased infections, which may themselves exacerbate the malnutrition via direct effects or anorexia. There may be an association between kwashiorkor and aflatoxin ingestion.[1]

Clinical features (see diagram opposite)

- *Failure to grow:* check weight records or growth chart if available. The onset may coincide with cessation of breastfeeding or an infection.
- *Oedema* (pitting): may be localized or extensive, including the eyelids. It may make an onlooker think that the child is plump and well.
- *Skin lesions*: atrophy, patches of erythema and/or hyperpigmentation, desquamation, hypopigmentation, usually beginning around the perineum. Skin breakdown leads to ulceration and gangrene.
- *Hair changes*: the hair becomes dry, thin. It may also become depigmented (achromotrichia), appearing brown, yellowy-red, or even white.
- *Diarrhoea* is non-specific: in chronic malnutrition, it may be 2° to malabsorption owing to GI damage. Hepatomegaly is common.
- *Vomiting*: is common; with diarrhoea, it may result in hypovolaemia, even in an oedematous child.
- *Mental changes*: the child is lethargic and miserable, with reduced expression and comprehension. An encephalitis-like syndrome may occur – coarse tremors, postural abnormalities, ↑ reflexes, and clonus.
- *Cardiovascular changes:* cardiomyopathy results in a small heart with low output. Anaemia and fluid retention may precipitate failure. Hypokalaemia and hypomagnesaemia may cause dysrhythmias.
- *Associated deficiencies*: notably of vitamin A leading to eye lesions.
- *Increased infections*: especially URTIs which may progress rapidly to pneumonia and death.

Famine oedema is the same condition in adults. It is characterized by a reduced total serum protein concentration (<40g/l).

Management: consists of giving a protein-rich diet to the child and correcting fluid or electrolyte imbalances. Eggs, beans, lentils, and nuts are all good sources of protein and usually more easily obtained than meat or fish. During treatment, there may be ECG changes and, paradoxically, other infections may flare up (eg malaria) due to the improved nutritional state of the child. Regaining the normal weight for height may take several months and in a few cases there is a permanent defect (nutritional dwarfism) or sequelae of deficiencies eg bow-legs owing to rickets.

► **For full treatment details, see the following pages.**

Prevention: a complex matter centring on economic and cultural factors. The mothers can be counselled about the dangers of artificial feeding and encouraged to use readily available foodstuffs with high protein content at the time of weaning.

1. Leading article: *Lancet*, 1984, **ii**, 1133

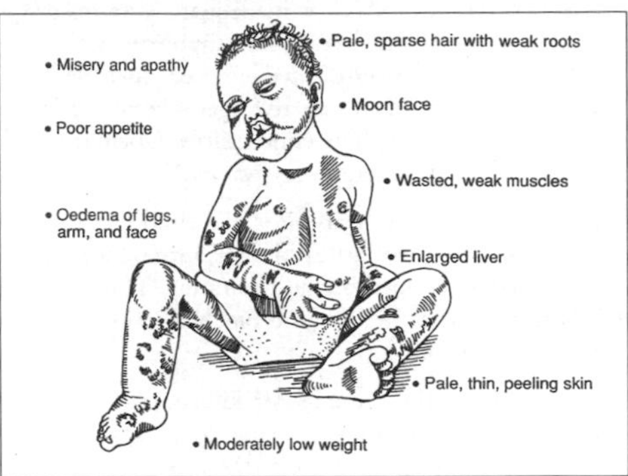

Typical signs and symptoms in Kwashiorkor

Classification of malnutrition (MN)[a]

	Well-nourished	Malnutrition Mild	Moderate	Severe
Symmetrical oedema?	NO	NO	NO	YES = *oedematous MN*[b]
Weight-for-height	90–120%[c] (+2 to −1 SD)	80–89% (−1 to −2 SD)	70–79% (−2 to −3 SD)	<70% = *severe wasting*[d]
Height-for-age	95–110% (+2 to −1 SD)	90–94% (−1 to −2 SD)	85–89% (−2 to −3 SD)	<85% = *severe stunting*

Notes:

a The diagnoses are not mutually exclusive. A child can have severe wasting and oedematous malnutrition, or severe wasting and severe stunting, etc.

b This corresponds to the definitions of "kwashiorkor" and "marasmic kwashiorkor" in other classifications. To avoid confusion with the clinical syndrome of kwashiorkor (which includes other features), the term "oedematous malnutrition" is preferred.

c Percentage of the median WHO standard and standard deviation (SD). For weight-for-age and weight-for-height, one SD unit is about 10% of the median, except in children less than 6 months old. For height-for-age, one SD unit is about 5% of the median.

d This corresponds to "marasmus" (without oedema) or "grade III malnutrition". To avoid confusion, the term "severe wasting" is preferred.

Severe wasting/marasmus

Marasmus most often results from inadequate energy provision in the diet of growing children. The disease develops in infants either fed on milk from a malnourished mother (which is inadequate in terms of quantity), by prolonged breastfeeding with inadequate supplementation, or inadequate artificial feeding with over-diluted cow or powdered milk. The latter may also expose the child to infective agents resulting in diarrhoea, thus compounding the situation. The child utilizes subcutaneous fat, then muscular tissue, as alternative energy sources.

Clinical features (see diagram opposite)**:** the child is extremely emaciated with thin, flaccid skin – the 'little old man' appearance. There may be dehydration associated with diarrhoea and vomiting. The child is alert and irritable. Hair is normal and there are no biochemical or haematological changes diagnostic of the condition.

Treatment: is essentially the same as for kwashiorkor. If caught early, almost all cases will recover with a diet higher in energy than is normally required by a child. Prognosis is worse if there is concurrent infection, dehydration, and/or electrolyte imbalance. Failure of an adequate diet to promote weight gain usually signifies some underlying condition, commonly TB, kala azar or AIDS. **For full treatment details see below.**

General principles of treatment

When first seen, a child with malnutrition often presents as a medical emergency.

1. Admit the child to a special area of the hospital, under constant monitoring.
2. Keep the child warm and dry.
3. Keep handling to a minimum.
4. Avoid giving intravenous infusions unless they are essential (eg in severe shock or dehydration) since the child is at increased risk of infection.
5. IM injections, when required, should be given in the buttock using a small gauge needle and the smallest possible volume.

Initial treatment

This lasts until the child is stable and can eat, usually 2–7 days. If it takes longer than this, the child is considered to be "failing to respond".

Priorities are to:

1. Treat or prevent hypoglycaemia and hypothermia.
2. Treat and prevent dehydration and restore electrolyte balance.
3. Treat incipient or developed septic shock, if present.
4. Start to feed the child.
5. Treat infection.
6. Identify and treat other problems (eg vitamin deficiency, anaemia, heart failure).

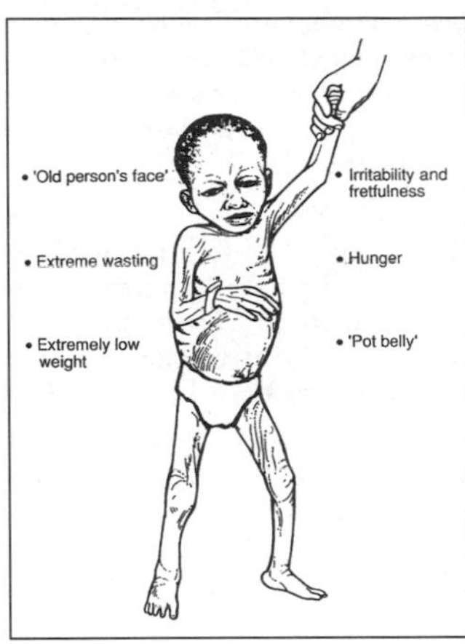

Typical signs and symptoms in marasmus.

Biochemical changes in kwashiorkor and marasmus

Substance	*kwashiorkor*	*marasmus*
Plasma albumin	very low	usually normal
Plasma amino acids	low tyrosine	normal
Serum amylase	very low	normal or low
Plasma (total) cholesterol	very low	normal or low
Plasma free fatty acids	increased	increased
Plasma growth hormone	raised	not as high
Fasting blood glucose	normal or low	low
Plasma urea	low	not as low
Plasma urate	low	raised
Plasma zinc	low	not as low

Specific problems

1. **Hypoglycaemia:** (blood glucose <3mmol/l or <54mg/dl) leads to ↑ risk of infection, hypothermia, lethargy, and confusion. Often confusion is the only sign before death. Give 1ml/kg of 50% glucose IV upon admission, followed by 50ml of 10% glucose (or sucrose) by NG tube to prevent recurrence. As consciousness recovers, begin feeding with the **F-75 diet** (see page 564) or 60g/l glucose in sterile water. Give prophylactic antibiotics as outlined below.

2. **Hypothermia:** (rectal temp <35.5°C) the child will need warming – wrap her in a blanket and place under (but not touching) a non-fluorescent lamp. Alternatively, adopt the 'kangaroo' technique: the mother lies supine with her child on her chest, covered by her clothes and blankets. Avoid hyperthermia by over-heating. All hypothermic children with malnutrition should be treated for hypoglycaemia and infection.

3. **Dehydration and septic shock:** for signs of dehydration, see chapter 3D. The table opposite may help differentiate septic shock from dehydration. With incipient septic shock, the child is usually limp, apathetic and profoundly anorexic, but is neither thirsty nor restless. With developed septic shock, superficial veins are dilated rather than constricted. Pulmonary vessels may also dilate, resulting in dyspnoea.

   ► ***In dehydrated, malnourished children,*** use oral fluids whenever possible, since IV infusion can lead to overhydration and heart failure. ►► Full strength ORS should not be used, since total body sodium is high and potassium low in malnourished children. In the absence of pre-packaged sachets of oral rehydration solution for severely malnourished children (ReSoMal), dilute one standard sachet of ORS in **2 litres of water** instead of 1 litre and add: 50g sucrose (25g/l) and 2 packets of mineral mix powder *or* 40ml (20ml/l) of mineral mix solution (see section on dietary treatment, below).

   ReSoMal should be given as 70–100 ml per kg body weight over 12hrs to restore normal hydration, starting at 10ml/kg/hr for the first 2hrs and reducing to 5ml/kg/hr for the remainder. Use an NG tube at first and switch to oral administration as the child's condition improves. Assess the child frequently, in particular the presence of thirst, diarrhoea, urine output, and level of consciousness. Stop giving ReSoMal if the respiratory rate increases, the jugular veins become distended, or there is increasing abdominal distension.

   ► Only give fluids IV if the child is severely dehydrated or in septic shock. Use:
   - half-strength Darrow's solution with 5% dextrose, or
   - Ringer's lactate with 5% dextrose, or
   - 0.45% (half strength) normal saline with 5% dextrose (+ 20mmol/l of KCl if available).

   ► Continue breastfeeding and start the F-75 diet as soon as possible, beginning by NG tube and changing to oral administration as soon as the child can tolerate it.

Comparison of features of dehydration and septic shock in the severely malnourished child

	Some dehydration	Severe dehydration	Incipient septic shock	Developed septic shock
Diarrhoea	yes	yes	yes/no[a]	yes/no[a]
Mental state	restless/irritable	lethargy/coma	apathetic[a]	lethargy
Sunken eyes	yes[b,c]	yes[b,c]	no[a]	no[a]
Thirsty	drinks eagerly	drinks poorly	no[a]	drinks poorly
Cool hands or feet	no[b]	yes	yes	yes
Weak/absent radial pulse	no[b]	yes	yes	yes
Urine flow	good	poor	good	poor
Hypothermia	no	no	yes/no	yes/no[a]

a Signs that may be useful in diagnosing septic shock.
b Signs that may be useful in diagnosing dehydration.
c If confirmed as being of recent onset by the mother.

Consequences of malnutrition

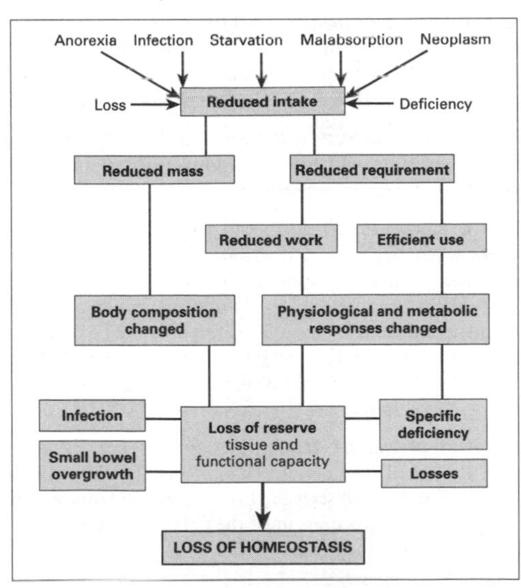

4. **Septic shock:** should be treated with broad-spectrum antibiotics. Keep the child warm and avoid excessive handling. Feed with the F-75 diet by NG tube. Septic shock should be corrected with one of the fluids listed in the dehydration section (previous page). Give 15ml/kg/hr; watch for signs of overhydration and heart failure. As soon as the radial pulse becomes strong, continue rehydration orally, as above.

   ► ***If there are no signs of improvement within 2hrs,*** or there are signs of heart failure, give a blood transfusion of 10ml/kg slowly over 3hrs, with a diuretic. If blood is unavailable, give plasma. If there are signs of liver failure (purpura, jaundice, tender hepatomegaly) give a single dose of vitamin K 1mg IM. During the blood transfusion, nothing else should be given either PO or IV. Steroids should not be used. After the transfusion, give the F-75 diet by NG tube as outlined below.

5. **Dietary treatment:** a formula diet should be started immediately in all children not requiring emergency treatment. Breastfeeding should be continued normally. Record the type of feed, the amount taken, and whether the child vomits. If she does vomit, the quantity of vomit should be estimated and deducted from the daily intake total.

   Severely malnourished children do not tolerate the usual amounts of dietary protein, fat, and sodium, and therefore require a diet low in these ingredients and high in carbohydrate. Two formula diets are used for severely malnourished children: **F-75** (75kcal/100ml) in the initial treatment phase and **F-100** (100kcal/ml) during the rehabilitation stage, when the appetite has returned. These formulas can be purchased as ready-mixed powder, or made from basic ingredients (see opposite) and the mineral and vitamin mixes.

   Give the food frequently and in small amounts throughout the day and night: this avoids overloading the small intestine, liver, and kidneys. The food can be given from every hour to q3h. Children too weak to eat can be fed by continuous NG drip. Do not feed by IV.

   Give the child between 80 and 100kcal/kg per day: if less is given, malnutrition will continue. Quantities greater than this may cause serious metabolic imbalances.

   Patience is required: nearly all malnourished children have poor appetites when first admitted to hospital. At each feed, however, the food should be offered by mouth, after which the remainder is given by NG tube. When the child takes 3/4 of the daily diet orally, or takes two consecutive feeds fully by mouth, the tube should be removed. It should be reinserted, however, if the child fails to take at least 80kcal/kg/day. If the child develops abdominal distension during NG feeding, give 2ml of magnesium sulphate IM.

   The initial phase of treatment ends when the child becomes hungry; this usually occurs after 2–7 days. The child is now ready to begin rehabilitation and start the F-100 diet. Food intake should remain at 100kcal/kg/day, however, until the child has achieved good appetite and readily finishes each meal offered to her.

The composition of liquid diets

Ingredient	*F-75 diet*	*F-100 diet*
Dried skimmed milk	25g	80g
Cane sugar	60g	50g
Oil	25g	60g
Rice/other cereal flour	50g	nil
Mineral mix	20ml (1 packet/*l*)	20ml (1 packet/*l*)
Vitamin mix	see below	see below
Water	to make 1 litre	to make 1 litre

To make 1 litre of mineral mix

Ingredient	*Amount*	*Ingredient*	*Amount*
Potassium chloride	89.5g	Tripotassium citrate	32.4g
Magnesium chloride	30.5g	Zinc acetate	3.3g
Copper sulphate	0.56g	Sodium selenate	0.001g
Potassium iodide	0.005g		

Add water to make 1 litre

To make 1 litre of vitamin mix

Vitamin	*Amount*		
Thiamine	0.7mg	Riboflavine	2.0mg
Niacin	10mg	Pyridoxine	0.7mg
Cobalamin	1mg	Folic acid	0.35mg
Ascorbic acid	100mg	Panthothenic acid	3mg
Biotin	100mg	Retinol	1.5mg
Calciferol	30mg	Tocopherol	22mg
Vitamin K	40mg		

Add to 1 litre of liquid diet

► All children on the F-100 diet should be offered additional water between feeds. Milk intolerance may develop at this stage, although it is rare and should be diagnosed only if:

- copious, watery diarrhoea occurs promptly after milk feeds are begun
- and it improves when milk is reduced or stopped.

In such cases, milk should be substituted (totally or partially) by another liquid, but milk feeding should be attempted again before discharge, to determine whether the intolerance has resolved.

6. Infection

Bacterial: nearly all severely malnourished children have bacterial infections when first admitted to hospital. These may be multiple and, unlike the situation in well nourished children, signs of infection such as fever and inflammation may be absent. Early treatment with effective antimicrobials improves the nutritional response to feeding, prevents shock, and reduces mortality. ► Antibiotics should thus be given to all children with severe malnutrition upon admission:

- first choice treatment is co-trimoxazole for children without signs of infection;
- children with septic shock, oedematous malnutrition, hypothermia, hypoglycaemia, or suspected infection should receive penicillin (2 days IM, then oral) *and* gentamicin IM;
- if second line treatment is needed (the child fails to improve or a specific diagnosis is made), *add* chloramphenicol PO or cefotaxime IM;
- *add* nalidixic acid PO for children with dysentery.

Antimicrobials should be continued for at least 5 days and only stopped once the child has gained weight for 3 consecutive days. Treat any specific infections (eg malaria, schistosomiasis) appropriately.

Measles vaccine should be given to *every* malnourished child admitted to hospital to protect from the associated high mortality of measles infection. Give a second dose before discharge.

7. Vitamin A and other deficiencies: severely malnourished children are at risk of developing blindness owing to vitamin A deficiency. Therefore, give vitamin A to *all* severely malnourished children on admission. See section on vitamin A deficiency for further details.

All malnourished children should also receive folic acid 5mg PO on admission. Many children are also deficient in riboflavin, ascorbic acid, pyridoxine, thiamine, and the fat-soluble vitamins (D, E, K). These are replaced by giving vitamin mix in the diet.

8. Very severe anaemia: is Hb <40g/l (<4g/dl), packed cell volume/haematocrit <12%. Children with this level of anaemia need a blood transfusion. Give 10ml of packed cells (or whole blood) per kg body weight *slowly* over 3hrs. If there are signs of heart failure, withdraw 2.5ml/kg of blood before starting the transfusion and at hourly intervals during it, so that the total volume transfused = that removed. Where testing for HIV and HBV is not possible, only transfuse if the haemoglobin falls below 3g/dl (haematocrit <10%) or there are signs of life-threatening heart failure. Do not give iron during the initial treatment, as it can have toxic effects and can reduce resistance to infection.

9. Heart failure: is usually a result of overhydration (especially with IV infusion) but may also be due to severe anaemia, blood plasma transfusion, or giving a diet with a high sodium content. Signs of heart failure are: respiratory rate >40/min in infants under 2yrs (>30/min in older children), rapid pulse, ↑ JVP, cold peripheries, and cyanosis of the finger tips and beneath the tongue. Heart failure must be differentiated from respiratory infection and septic shock – both of which tend to occur within 48hrs of admission.

If heart failure is caused by fluid overload:

- Stop ***all*** oral and IV fluids; the treatment of heart failure takes precedence over feeding the child, even if it takes 24hrs.
- Give frusemide 0.5–1.5mg/kg IV (max 20mg/day in children; *never* use diuretics to reduce oedema in oedematous malnutrition).
- Only give digitalis if the diagnosis of heart failure is definite *and* the plasma potassium concentration is not low. A single dose of 5μg/kg should be given IV (PO if IV route is not possible).

10. Dermatosis of kwashiorkor: this is characterized by areas of hyperpigmentation and hypopigmentation and other skin lesions which may easily become infected. These usually resolve as the child's nutritional status improves, but in the intervening period should be left dry and exposed. If, however, the skin is very painful or infected, apply zinc and castor oil ointment, petroleum jelly, or paraffin gauze dressings. Use nystatin cream/ointment *and* oral nystatin if the skin becomes infected with *Candida*.

Affected areas may be bathed with 0.01% potassium permanganate solution for 10–15mins daily, helping to dry the lesions, prevent loss of serum, and inhibit infection. 10% betadine may also be used (sparingly for large lesions, since it has significant systemic absorption). ► All children with this condition must receive systemic antibiotics.

Rehabilitation

► A child enters the rehabilitation phase when a good appetite returns. A child who is being fed by NG tube is not yet in the rehabilitation phase.

The aims of this phase of treatment are to:

- encourage the child to eat as much as possible;
- stimulate emotional and physical development;
- prepare the mother to continue to care for the child after discharge.

During this stage, feeding with the F-100 diet should continue q3–4h, night and day. Increase the amount given by 10ml at each feed until the child cannot finish the feed. If the total intake is <130kcal/kg per day, the child is failing to respond (see below).

Never reuse food for the next feed. Be patient and encourage the child. Continue to give the F-100 diet until the child achieves at least 90% of the standard weight for height (the target weight for discharge), but remember that oedematous children may *lose* weight initially, as oedema decreases. If the child is not gaining weight or losing oedema, or there is increasing oedema, then there is a failure to respond.

In all cases, the diet should be supplemented with water, especially in children <6mths. This is especially important if she has diarrhoea or fever.

For older children: it is appropriate to introduce solid food. Most mixed diets, however, have a lower energy density and higher water content than liquid diets and are more likely to be mineral and vitamin deficient. For this reason, they should be fortified (eg with vitamin and mineral mixes and vegetable oil to increase energy density) and given *between* feeds with the F-100 diet. Additional water should always be offered. Prior to discharge, there should be a supervised transition to less frequent feeds throughout the day. The F-100 diet is gradually reduced and the mixed diet increased until the child is eating what he or she will do at home.

Iron and folic acid: should be added to the feeds during the rehabilitation phase, and continued for 2–3 months. A child with moderate or severe anaemia should be given 3mg/kg of elemental iron per day as a single oral dose (divided in to 2 doses for children <1yr old) and 5mg of folic acid (500μg/kg for children <1yr) per day. Tablets of combined 30mg iron and 100μg folic acid are available and may be given daily, ground up and dissolved, or mixed with food if necessary.

► All children should be weighed daily and the weight plotted on a graph. The usual weight gain is 10–15g/kg per day. A child who does not gain at least 5g/kg per day is failing to respond. With high-energy feeding, most children reach the target weight of 90% weigh-for-height within 2–4 weeks.

How to help a mother to relactate

Explain why it would help her baby to breastfeed exclusively and what she needs to do to increase her breastmilk supply. Explain that it takes patience and perseverance.

- Build up her confidence. Help her to feel that she can produce enough breastmilk for her baby. Try to see her at least twice a day.
- Make sure that she has enough to eat and drink.
- Encourage her to rest more and to try to relax when she breastfeeds.
- Explain that she should keep her baby near her, give him plenty of skin-to-skin contact and let him do as much as possible for himself. Grandmothers can help if they take over other responsibilities, but they should not care for the baby at this time. Later they may do so again.
- Explain that the most important thing is to let her baby suckle more, at least 10 times in 24hrs, more if it wants
  - she can offer the breast every 2hrs;
  - she should let baby suckle whenever he seems interested;
  - she should let baby suckle longer than before at each breast;
  - she should keep baby with her and let him breastfeed at night;
  - sometimes it is easier to get a baby to suckle when it is sleepy.
- Discuss how to give other milk feeds, while she waits for her breast-milk to flow and how to reduce these milk feeds as her own milk increases.
- Show her how to give the other feeds from a cup, not from a bottle.
- She should not use a pacifier.
- If her baby refuses to suckle on an empty breast, help her to find ways to give the baby milk whilst it is suckling, for example with a dropper or syringe.
- For the first day or two, she should give the full amount of artificial feed for a baby of his weight or the same amount that he has been having before. As soon as her breastmilk begins to flow, she can start to reduce the daily total by 30–60ml each day.
- Check the baby's weight gain and urine output, to make sure that he is getting enough milk. If he is not getting enough, do not reduce the artificial feed for a few days – if necessary, increase the amount of artificial milk for a day or two.
- If a baby is still breastfeeding sometimes, the breastmilk supply increases in a few days. If a baby has stopped breastfeeding, it may take 1–2 weeks or more before much breastmilk comes.

Emotional and physical stimulation

Severely malnourished children have delayed mental and behavioural development, which, if not treated, can be the most serious long-term result of malnutrition. It is essential that stimulation through play programs, at which the mother is present as often as possible, be started during rehabilitation and continued after discharge. It is vitally important that the mother be with her child as much as possible during the stay in hospital and that she be encouraged to feed, hold, comfort and play with her child as much as possible, as well as helping the nursing staff to prepare meals. The number of other people interacting with the child should be kept to a minimum and any potentially painful procedures should be done by the most skilled person available, away from other children and the child be held and comforted immediately afterwards. Anything that gives the environment a relaxed, happy, and welcoming atmosphere is to be encouraged.

Training the parents

Before discharging the child, ensure that you have taken the time to explain to the parents the causes of malnutrition and how to prevent it recurring. This should include methods of correct feeding and continuing to stimulate the child's mental and emotional development. The parents should be able to detect the early signs of dehydration and infection and know how to obtain treatment.

- ► The parents should never be blamed for the child's problems or made to feel unwelcome or humiliated. Only if the child is abandoned or the conditions at home hopeless (perhaps due to the death or absence of a parent/guardian) should a foster home be sought.

Discharge

- ► The child should remain in hospital until *all* the criteria opposite are fulfilled.

The home diet should provide at least 110kcal/kg body weight, per day, as well as sufficient vitamins and minerals to support continued growth. Breast feeding should continue and be supplemented with animal milk, where available. Solid foods should contain a well cooked staple cereal, to which 5–20ml of vegetable oil should be added to enrich its energy content. If possible include fresh vegetables, fruit, eggs, milk, fish and meat.

Follow-up

As the risk of relapse is greatest immediately after discharge, the child should be seen at 1 week, 2 weeks, 1 month and 6 months after discharge, with at least one home visit if possible in the first weeks. Further visits should be planned for every 6mths until the child has reached 3yrs, as long as the weight remains above the 90% weight-for-height line. Children with frequent problems should remain under supervision for a longer period. Ask about the child's recent health, feeding practices, and play. The child should be examined, weighed, measured, and the results charted. Take the opportunity to give outstanding vaccinations.

Criteria for discharge

The child:
- eating well
- mental state has improved – smiles, responds to stimuli, interested in surroundings
- sits, crawls, stands or walks
- normal temperature
- no vomiting or diarrhoea
- no oedema
- gaining weight >5g/kg body weight per day for 3 successive days
- middle of the night feed no longer needed
- no medical problem requiring hospital stay
- immunization (eg measles) is complete

The mother:
- knows how to prepare appropriate foods and to feed the child
- knows how to make toys and stimulate healthy play
- knows how to give home treatment for diarrhoea, fever, and when to get help

The home
- there is a willing and able caretaker for the child
- follow-up for the child and mother has been planned

Failure to respond to treatment

Normally, if the guidelines are followed, a severely malnourished child without complications should show signs of improvement within a few days and continue to improve thereafter. A child who meets any of the criteria in the table opposite should be diagnosed as having *failed to respond.* In such cases, it is essential that practices in the treatment unit are carefully reviewed and the child is thoroughly re-evaluated in an attempt to identify the cause. Treatment should never be altered blindly as this is likely to be harmful to the child.

The most frequent causes of failure to respond are given opposite.

Problems with the treatment facility

1. **Poor environment:** a severely malnourished child is less likely to respond to treatment when treated on a general medical ward. The risk of cross-infection is increased, it is harder to provide special feeding and attentive care, and staff are less likely to have the necessary skills and attitudes for such specialized management. Whenever possible, malnourished children should be managed on a paediatric ward, or better still, a unit specialized in the treatment of malnourished children.

2. **Staff:** an effective management system should ensure careful monitoring of the child, effective training of nursing and auxiliary staff, use of the most experienced staff as supervisors, and ensure a reliable supply of necessary drugs and food, as well as reliable record-keeping. Where possible, try to avoid rotating staff frequently as this disrupts the child's routines. Staff attitudes towards a particular child can also determine whether treatment succeeds or fails. If it is thought that the child is beyond hope they may give it less attention, so there is failure to respond, seeming to confirm the staff's opinion.

   ► It is essential to remind the staff frequently that the child's wellbeing depends upon their efforts and that every child deserves full attention.

3. **Weighing machines:** (both for the children and the food being prepared for them) should be checked and adjusted *daily* following a standard procedure.

4. **Food:** the preparation, storage, and handling of food should be under strict hygiene control. Cooked food which is going to be stored should be refrigerated. Reheated food should be heated thoroughly and allowed to cool slightly before serving. Persons with hand infections should not handle food. Observe the diets being prepared and check that staff are weighing, measuring, mixing, and storing food correctly.

   Ensure that sufficient time is taken with the feeding of each child. Assuming that an average of 15 mins is needed to feed one child and assuming that food is given every 3hrs, one person will be needed day and night to feed 12 children. When food is given every two hours, or hourly, even more staff will be needed – the mother's assistance may help relieve the situation.

Criteria for failure to respond

1. Primary failure to respond	*Time after admission*
• Fails to regain appetite	By day 4
• Fails to start to lose oedema	By day 4
• Oedema still present	By day 10
• Fails to gain weight at >5g/kg/day	By day 10
2. Secondary failure to respond	
• Fails to gain >5g/kg/day for 3 successive days	During rehabilitation

Usual causes of failure to respond

Problems with the treatment facility

- poor environment for malnourished children
- insufficient or poorly trained staff
- inaccurate weighing machines
- food prepared or given incorrectly

Problems with individual children

- insufficient food given
- vitamin or mineral deficiency
- malabsorption
- rumination
- infection
- serious underlying disease

Problems of the individual child

1. Feeding:

- *Is enough food being given?* Recalculate the food and energy requirements of the child and ensure that the correct amount is offered at the right times and that the amount taken by the child is measured and recorded accurately.
- *Is feeding during the night taking place?*
- *Are the family able to feed the child properly during the rehabilitation phase or at home?*
- *Is the child absorbing the food?* There may be pancreatic insufficiency, gastroenteritis with diarrhoea, or another cause of malabsorption. Check for fat in the stool and if necessary carry out pancreatic and other gut function tests.
- *Is the child receiving enough vitamins and minerals?* Ensure that the mineral and vitamin mixes are being added properly to the food.
- *Is the child ruminating?* Rumination is a form of self-stimulation that may occur in up to 10% of severely malnourished, emotionally deprived children. A ruminating child regurgitates food from the stomach into the mouth, chews it and spits much of it out, usually when not observed. The child may have vomit-stained clothes/bedding or smell of vomit. Distinguish rumination from normal vomiting (the child is not distressed by vomiting after ruminating). The problem should be treated by experienced staff giving the child more frequent attention. They need to show disapproval when the child begins to ruminate, without being intimidating, and encourage play and other forms of emotional stimulation.

2. Infection: is a frequent cause of failure to respond. The infections most often overlooked are: pneumonia, UTI, otitis media and TB. Other common causes are hepatitis B, malaria, HIV, and dengue. Examine the child carefully, measuring temperature, pulse rate, BP, and RR every 3hrs. Infection in a malnourished child may cause hypothermia. Further *Ix* may include: CXR, microscopy and culture of blood, urine, sputum and stool, and CSF examination.

- ***Diarrhoea:*** give ReSoMal to prevent dehydration (see above and chapter 3D). If the stool contains blood, treat for *Shigella*. Other common causes include *Giardia* and *E. histolytica*. Blind antimicrobial treatment should be discouraged; antidiarrhoeal drugs should never be given.
- ***Otitis media:*** occurs frequently and is often associated with a hospital-acquired URTI. Signs are non-specific (fever, restlessness), although the child may pull on her ears due to the pain. If the tympanic membrane ruptures, there may be a purulent discharge. Examine the ear with an otoscope and treat with co-trimoxazole, ampicillin, or amoxycillin for 5 days. A cotton wick will help to dry any discharge.
- ***Pneumonia:*** look for a RR >40/min in a child <1yr (>50/min in an older child), tracheal tugging, and indrawing of the chest. The common signs of pneumonia are frequently absent in the malnourished. The CXR may appear normal. Treat as for otitis media, but add benzyl penicillin IM for at least 3 days (or until there is improvement) if there is indrawing of the chest. Give oxygen if the RR is >70/min.

Growth chart showing a child failing to respond

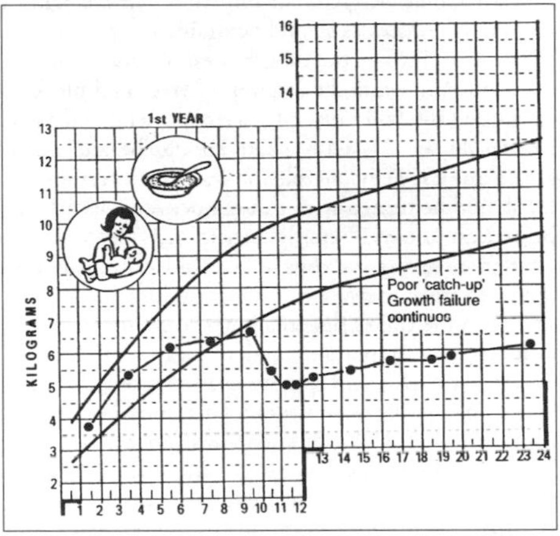

- ***UTI:*** occur frequently and are usually asymptomatic. Diagnose by urine microscopy or 'dip-stick' methods. Co-trimoxazole for 5 days is usually effective [alternative: ampicillin].
- ***Bacterial infections:*** including pustules, impetigo, infected fissures, and indolent ulcers. Treatment involves careful cleansing with soap and water and applying betadine ointment or chlorhexidine lotion to the area. Penicillin should be given for impetigo, lymphangitis, cellulitis, or infected bullae. Abscesses should be drained.
- ***Candidiasis:*** can involve the mouth, oesophagus, stomach, rectum, moist skin, and if systemic the respiratory tract and blood. Oral nystatin suspension (100,000 units qds) is recommended for oesophageal, oral, or rectal disease. Nystatin cream should be applied to affected areas of the skin. Use ketoconazole for systemic infections.
- ***Scabies:*** should be treated with gamma benzene hexachloride cream (1%) for at least 2 days. Benzylbenzoate (12.5%) is an alternative, though is more irritating and thus to be avoided in malnourished children where possible. Beware 2° infection of the lesions through scratching. Trim the child's fingernails and treat the family.
- ***Tuberculosis:*** is an important cause of treatment failure. Diagnosis should be made by CXR and sputum examination. The Mantoux test may be negative in severe malnutrition, becoming positive as the nutritional status improves. HIV^+ children are at greater risk of developing TB. Since the recommended drugs are hepatotoxic, they should be used with caution in a child with a tender or enlarged liver.
- ***Helminthiasis:*** infection with roundworm, hookworm, *Strongloides*, or whipworm is common in older children who play outside. See chapter 8.
- ***Malaria:*** often appears during the rehabilitation phase, as the nutritional status improves. Treat the child with a full course of antimalarial therapy, with the dosage based on body weight. See chapter 3A.
- ***HIV and AIDS:*** in some countries, up to half the children presenting with severe malnutrition are HIV^+. Such children are particularly prone to interstitial lymphocytic pneumonia (ILP). This should be looked for on CXR, treated with systemic steroids. An HIV test is only necessary if ILP is suspected.

3. **Serious underlying disease:** malnutrition can result from unrecognized serious congenital abnormalities, inborn errors of metabolism, malignancies, immunological disease, and other diseases of major organs. Any examination of a severely malnourished child should include a search for such diseases. Whether the underlying disease is treatable or not, the malnutrition should be treated as outlined above.

Learning from failure

Accurate records should be kept of all children who fail to respond and of all deaths due to malnutrition. Periodic review of these records can help to identify areas where management practices should be carefully examined and improved. The objective should be to achieve a case fatality of <5%.

Nutrition

Disasters and refugee camps

Health workers in disaster areas or refugee camps may have to manage a large number of severely malnourished children. Although the principals of treatment are the same as in non-disaster situations, treatment must follow a routine rather than an individual approach and a therapeutic feeding centre may have to be set up. This is usually necessary when a survey shows that >10% of children, aged 6 months to 5yrs, are <80% weight-for-height.

Therapeutic feeding centre (TFC)

In the ideal situation, the TFC should be within or near a hospital and could serve up to 100 children. The minimum staffing requirement will be: 1 part-time doctor, 3 nurses, 10 nursing aides, and the mothers/carers of the children admitted. It should include a *special care unit* to provide 24hr care during the initial treatment and a *day care unit* for care during rehabilitation. There must be a supply of clean water (at least 10 litres/child/day) and a latrine and bathing area for every 20 people served. Secure storage is needed for food and supplies and there should be an area for food preparation and cooking.

Admission and discharge criteria are as for non-disaster situations, though they may be modified according to national guidelines or the TFC's resources, but should always be clearly defined. Principles of treatment are as for hospital management, but are applied uniformly to all children, rather than to individuals. The doctor should evaluate each child daily. Multivitamins, minerals, antihelminthics and antimicrobials should be given with the initial treatment.

Evaluation of the TFC

A medical team should monitor the health and nutrition status of the *entire* population by:

- calculating mean daily mortality rates at weekly intervals
- monitoring food availability, including its macronutrient and micronutrient content at monthly intervals
- conducting anthropometric (weight and height) surveys every 3mths.

Using these data, the coverage, success and mortality rates of the TFC should be regularly evaluated by the following criteria:

- *Coverage rate:* the number of severely malnourished children admitted, divided by the total number of severely malnourished children in the population (ie refugee camp), based on the latest survey.
- *Success rate:* the number of children reaching criteria for discharge, divided by the number of children admitted within a given period.
- *Mortality rate:* the number of deaths in the centre, divided by the number of children admitted at the centre within a given period.

The results of these assessments depend upon local conditions, resources, and agreed health priorities. Most TFCs can cover >80% of severely malnourished children in a population, with >50% success rates and mortality rates <15%.

Nutrition

Malnutrition in adults and adolescents

Severe malnutrition occurs as a primary condition in adults and adolescents in conditions of extreme privation and famine. It also occurs in situations of dependency, such as in elderly people, the mentally or physically handicapped, or prisoners.

It is commonly associated with other illnesses such as chronic infection, malabsorption, alcoholism and drug dependency, liver disease, endocrine and autoimmune diseases, cancer, and AIDS. In such cases, both the malnutrition and the underlying disease need to be treated.

The physiological changes and principles of management for adults and adolescents with severe malnutrition are in general the same as those for children, although there are differences in the classification of malnutrition, the amount of food required, and the dosage of drugs. Adults are often reluctant to associate their diet with wasting or oedema, and may be reluctant to eat anything except traditional foods, even in famine conditions. Moreover, they may be restricted from eating some foods for cultural or religious reasons and in such cases will need to be persuaded that the formula feeds are actually medicine. These problems should not be underestimated when faced with treating severely malnourished adults; patience, understanding and explanation are needed.

Management

1. Take a careful dietary history.
2. Take blood to measure glucose level (to exclude diabetes mellitus).
3. Begin giving the same formula feeds as used in children, although the amount needed per kilo body weight actually *decreases* with increasing age, see opposite.
4. Adults and adolescents are also susceptible to hypothermia and hypoglycaemia and should be treated as for children.
5. Give systemic antimicrobials.
6. Give a single dose of retinyl palmitate, ► except pregnant women.

Rehabilitation: an improving appetite indicates the beginning of rehabilitation and is often accompanied by requests for large amounts of solid food. Traditional food may be given, with the addition of vegetable oil, mineral mix, and vitamin mix. Continue to give the formula feed if possible, perhaps presenting it as medicine.

Discharge: adolescents and adults may be discharged once they have begun to steadily gain weight and are free from other associated problems. Make sure that time is taken to discuss the nature of the problem with the patient and, if necessary, with his or her spouse and family in an attempt to educate them to prevent recurrence. Supplementary feeding at home should continue until the BMI is >18.5 or the weight-for-height is >90% in adolescents.

Treatment failure: is usually a result of:

- unrecognized infection or illness
- a nutrient deficiency
- refusal to follow the regime.

Classification of malnutrition in adults and adolescents

1. Adults (>18 yrs):

Assess by calculating the body mass index (BMI):

[weight in kg divided by the square of the height in metres – ie kg/m^2]

BMI	***Nutritional status***
>20	Normal
18.5–20	Marginal
17–18.4	Mild malnutrition
16–16.9	Moderate malnutrition
<16	Severe malnutrition

When an adult is too ill to stand, or has a spinal deformity, the ***demi-span*** should be measured. This is the distance from the middle of the sternal notch to the tip of the middle finger in metres, with the arm held out horizontally to the side. Height then equals:

$$[0.73 \times (2 \times \text{demi-span})] + 0.43$$

The BMI can then be calculated as before.

► Examine the peripheries for pitting oedema. If present, non-nutritional causes such as pre-eclampsia, nephrotic syndrome, nephritis, filariasis, heart failure and wet beriberi should be excluded.

2. Adolescents (12–18 yrs)

The BMI is normally lower in adolescents than in adults and therefore this system should not be used for them. Use the weight-for-height charts as for children. Severe malnutrition is diagnosed if the weight-for-height is <70% or there is nutritional oedema.

Amount of diet for malnourished adolescents and adults

Age (years)	*Total kcal (kcal/kg/day)*	*F-75 (ml/kg/hr)*	*F-100 (ml/kg/hr)*
7–10	75	4.2	3.0
11–14	60	3.5	3.5
15–18	50	2.8	2.0
19–75	40	2.2	1.7
>75	35	2.0	1.5

Goitre

Endemic goitre is found worldwide in areas where dietary iodine is deficient – usually for geographical reasons (eg mountainous regions with poor soil and high rainfall). It also occurs where goitrogen-containing foods such as cassava (manioc) and cabbage are regularly consumed. These vegetables contain compounds that impose an abnormally high demand upon the thyroid or interfere with iodine metabolism within the gland. It is estimated that 1 billion people are at risk of iodine deficiency.

Clinical features: follicular thyroid enlargement occurs due to pituitary thyroid-stimulating hormone (TSH) release. Eventually nodular formation occurs, with the risk of calcification and haemorrhage. Tracheal pressure may compress the recurrent laryngeal nerve resulting in dysphagia and hoarseness. The patient is usually euthyroid. There is no evidence that malignancy is a complication of chronic goitre.

Pregnancy: severe iodine depletion (urinary iodine excretion <20μg daily) during pregnancy interferes with neuronal dendrite formation in the foetus leading to cretinism, of which there are two forms:

- ***neurological cretinism***, characterized by mental retardation, deaf mutism, spastic diplegia, and strabismus
- ***myxoedematous cretinism***, in which there are signs of hypothyroidism.

Management:

1. Make up a 0.15% solution of potassium iodide (30mg of potassium iodide in 20ml of boiled water).
2. Give 4–6 drops daily for as long as dietary insufficiency persists.
3. Lugol's iodine (often kept for sterilization) may also be given as 1 drop every 30 days, or 1 daily teaspoon of a solution containing 1 drop of Lugol's iodine in 30ml of water.
4. Massive goitres may need surgical treatment.
5. Iodine should be given to women in endemic regions before conception to prevent cretinism.

Prevention: is best achieved by a single 5ml IM injection of iodized oil containing 400mg iodine/ml; this is effective for several years. Iodized salt is also available. Iodine replacement can also be carried out by treating children at school with potassium iodide solutions or by adding iodine to public water supplies.

Iodine deficiency surveys: are best done using urine collection in schoolchildren aged 6–12yrs in poor or remote villages. School age children are easy to reach and show well how much iodine deficiency there is in a population.

If a survey cannot be carried out, a severe iodine deficiency problem exists in an area if >10% of people have a *visible* goitre.

Worldwide distribution of iodine deficiency

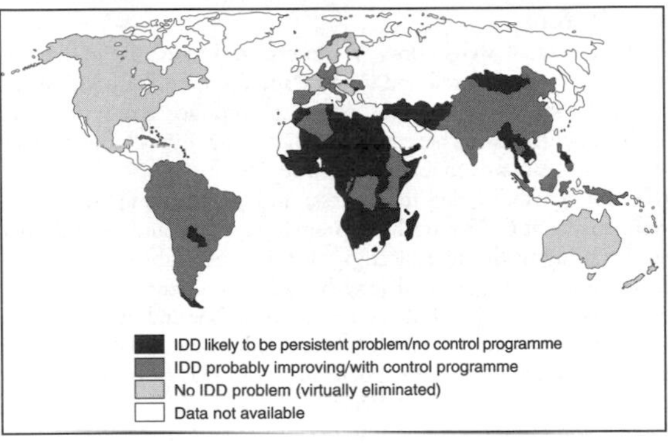

Scurvy

Vitamin C (ascorbic acid) is essential for metabolic oxidation and the formation of collagen. Its deficiency, scurvy, results from dietary insufficiency and is found worldwide in areas where fruit and vegetables are sparse. Children require 30–50mg/day of ascorbic acid, adults 70mg/day.

Clinical features

- ***Adults:*** gradual weight loss, weakness, and muscular stiffness with bruising. The gums swell and become spongy, eventually with bleeding and tooth loss. Subcutaneous petechiae produce scorbutic purpura. Wounds fail to heal. There may be microcytic, hypochromic anaemia, which only responds to ascorbic acid replacement.
- ***Infants:*** irritability, leg tenderness, and pseudoparalysis, commonly commencing at 6–12 months in premature babies and those artificially fed. Erupting teeth cause bleeding of the gums; subperiosteal haemorrhage causes limb pain and may be palpable at the distal end of the femur and proximal end of the tibia. Costochondral beading may also be palpated (scorbutic rosary). Occasionally there is bloody diarrhoea. Anaemia is microcytic and hypochromic, but may be megaloblastic due to accompanying folate deficiency. Bone X-rays show epiphyseal changes and ground glass appearance of the shafts.

Diagnosis: differentiate from rickets (which may coexist) using the Hess test – petechiae appear upon occlusion of venous return in the arm with a sphygmomanometer. Measure urinary vitamin C excretion following a saturating dose of ascorbic acid; if it is decreased, the patient has scurvy.

Management: ascorbic acid 250mg qds until all signs have disappeared. In infants give 50mg qds for 1 week, followed by 50mg bd for 1 month. A glass of fresh orange juice daily will do equally well.

Prevention: avoid overcooking vegetables (vitamin C is destroyed by prolonged heat), consume fresh fruit (especially oranges, guava, limes) and if necessary (eg in refugee camps) give tablet supplementation.

Tooth decay and gum disease

The increasing consumption of sugary food without accompanying increase in dental hygiene is increasing the incidence of tooth and gum disease in the developing world. Such problems should be referred to a dentist but, since this is not always possible, the health worker is often faced with having to do the best she can.

Tooth decay results from bacterial infection gradually eroding holes in teeth. It can be extremely painful, preventing a person from eating, and progress to abscess formation. Yellow plaque initially coats the teeth; this accumulates and hardens to form tartar which needs to be removed by a dentist.

Gum disease (*periodontal disease*) is usually due to bacterial infection affecting the tissues surrounding and supporting the teeth. There may be bleeding (gingivorrhoea), an unpleasant taste in the mouth, and bad breath. Gum disease is often not painful so the person may be unaware of it until teeth become loose and fall out.

Prevention of tooth/gum disease

This is difficult, since patients will rarely stop eating sweet foods and toothbrushes are often scarce. Brushing teeth at least once per day is the best way to prevent disease (even without toothpaste, it is of great benefit; a chewing stick can substitute for the toothbrush). Other good practices include flossing between the teeth before brushing (to break up plaque) and rinsing the mouth with water after meals (to remove small pieces of food). Hot salty water helps to sterilize the mouth if there are caries or an abscess. Educate the patient about eating less refined sugar and eating more naturally sweet foods, such as fruit (these contain fibre which helps prevent sugar sticking to teeth).

Rickets and osteomalacia

Rickets and osteomalacia are infantile and adult diseases, respectively, of abnormal bone calcification, resulting from vitamin D deficiency. Vitamin D_2 is produced in human skin by the action of sunlight on a cholesterol metabolite and the disease therefore tends to affect children and/or women deprived of sunlight due to social or religious reasons. There is also evidence of an 'anti-calcifying' factor present in the flour used to make chupatties in Asia.[1] The diseases may also result from renal failure, anticonvulsant use, and cirrhosis – all of which alter vitamin D metabolism.

Clinical features

- ***Rickets***: onset is within the first 2yrs of life. The child is pale, irritable, and mentally and physically retarded. There may be delayed closure of the fontanelles, and deformities of the spine, chest (pigeon chest, rachitic 'rosary' – due to swollen costochondral junctions), pelvis and limbs (bow-legs, knocked-knees), and bossing of the skull (craniotabes). Hypocalcaemia may cause tetany and laryngeal stridor.
- ***Osteomalacia***: usually occurs in women, often during the first pregnancy, and presents with softened, painful bones (pelvis, ribs, femora) and fractures. Hypocalcaemia produces tetany and there may be spontaneous fractures and anaemia.

Diagnosis

- ***Rickets:*** the line of osteochondral calcification is broadened and rarefied leading to cupped, ragged metaphyseal surfaces.
- ***Osteomalacia:*** uncalcified osteoid tissue at the growing ends of bone results in enlargement. Loosers zones are partial fractures without bony displacement (often of lateral scapular border, inferior femoral neck, or medial femoral shaft). Hypocalcaemia is common (6–7mg/dl).

Management: provide calcium (500ml of milk) and vitamin D (2000–5000 IU) daily. Give advice regarding sunlight exposure (and ? chupatty consumption). Look for causes of renal/liver disease, or alter anticonvulsant therapy if this is a possible cause.

► Vitamin D therapy can cause dangerous hypercalcaemia.

Vitamin B_2 deficiency (ariboflavinosis)

Found world-wide, often in association with other syndromes of malnutrition and dietary deficiencies, ariboflavinosis is due to vitamin B_2 (riboflavin) deficiency. An ideal daily intake of riboflavin is 2mg, the main sources being meat, vegetables, milk, and wholemeal flour. The vitamin is essential for normal oxidative metabolism.

Clinical features: sore red lips, increased vertical fissuring of the lips (perleche), angular stomatitis, and a purplish raw tongue with enlarged papillae. There may be facial dyssebacea (plugging of sebaceous glands with sebum, giving a roughened appearance) and scrotal dermatitis.

Management: is with 2–5mg of riboflavin daily and advice regarding diet. The condition is rapidly cured.

1 Dunnigan MG, 1976, *Lancet*, **i**, 1346

Nutrition

Beriberi

Vitamin B_1 (thiamine) is vital for carbohydrate metabolism, acetylcholine synthesis and neuronal transmission. Its deficiency results in beriberi. Thiamine is present in most raw foodstuffs, but notably is absent from white rice which has been 'polished' to remove the pericarp layer. The vitamin is not denatured by normal cooking. The minimum daily requirement in a 70kg adult is 300IU (1mg), rising during pregnancy, lactation and childhood. 2° beriberi may result from alcoholism (beriberi heart) and nitrofurazone treatment of trypanosomiasis.

Alterations in carbohydrate metabolism primarily affect central and peripheral nervous tissue (*dry* or *paraplegic beriberi*) and cardiac muscle (*wet* or *cardiac beriberi*). A mixture of the two forms is common.

Clinical features

- ***Dry beriberi:*** is essentially a peripheral neuropathy with mixed sensory and motor defects. There is a gradual onset of weakness and wasting, commencing in the lower limbs, often with foot drop and wasted calves. Weakness spreads proximally, eventually involving the upper limb muscles. The knee and ankle jerks and upper limb reflexes are lost; affected muscles show myoedema and painful contraction when hit. Anaesthesia spreads simultaneously in a 'stocking and glove' fashion (distinguishing beriberi from motor neurone disease) and there is a loss of postural sensation. A severe ataxia develops, with a characteristic high-stepping, broad-based gait requiring the use of a stick. The vagus may be involved and sphincter dysfunction occurs in the terminal stages. Death is from generalized and diaphragmatic paralysis.
- ***Wet beriberi:*** is high output right heart failure (RHF) with generalized oedema and oliguria. The extremities are initially well-perfused; the JVP raised, with marked pulsation due to tricuspid incompetence, and the BP low, with a high pulse pressure. The heart sounds become evenly spaced, giving a 'tick-tack' rhythm and there is a loud pansystolic murmur heard over the whole praecordium. Tender pulsatile hepatomegaly may occur. Frequently, there is unilateral or bilateral hydrothorax and ascites. Death occurs due to RHF (may be sudden), pulmonary oedema, hydrothorax, or hydropericardium.
- ***Infantile beriberi:*** normally occurs in infants who are breastfeeding from a B_1-deficient mother. Onset is typically during the 2nd or 3rd month after birth. Their irritability and slight oedema may initially be confused with kwashiorkor, but cardiopulmonary signs (similar to adults) occur rapidly and death may follow in as little as 36hrs (it is thought that breakdown products from incomplete carbohydrate metabolism are toxic to neonates). Slightly older children may progress to a chronic form of disease similar to that in adults.

Diagnosis: ECG and CXR shows signs of right heart failure in cardiac beriberi. There is increased plasma pyruvate (up to 2mg/dl in the acute stage) and increased lactate. In Volhard's diuresis test, the patient is kept nil-by-mouth for 12hrs overnight, then given 1 litre of water to drink. Normally 1l of urine will be passed within 4hrs. In beriberi, there is water retention which disappears following thiamine administration.

Management

1. *Wet beriberi*

- Give 50–100mg thiamine IV tds during the acute phase, until serial CXRs shows regression of cardiomegaly.
- Give the injection into the jugular vein in moribund adult patients.
- In severe cases, venesect 300ml of blood from the arm – this may be life-saving.
- Non-urgent cases require bed rest, fluid restriction, and a high protein low salt diet, supplemented with regular thiamine IM injections or tablets.

2. *Dry beriberi*

- Give thiamine injections.
- Pain is relieved rapidly; signs of peripheral neuropathy take months or years to resolve.

3. *Infantile beriberi*

- Give 25mg thiamine IV immediately followed by thiamine 25mg IM once or twice daily until symptoms have subsided. Then switch to oral treatment: thiamine 10mg PO daily for 3–4 weeks.
- Treat the mother of breast-feeding symptomatic infants. Stop breastfeeding for 24hrs while the mother is being treated. Express and discard the milk during this time; after 24hrs the mother can start breastfeeding again.

Prevention: rests upon dietary education, principally in the avoidance of white rice. Yeast is an excellent source of vitamin B_1.

Pellagra

Primary pellagra now occurs primarily in south and east Africa (although it is also found in Brazil, Cuba, and India). It is due to metabolic imbalance of nicotinic acid (niacin) and its precursors or analogues. The daily requirement of niacin is 10–15mg, although a diet high in tryptophan (a precursor) will substitute. Nicotinic acid deficiency leads to metabolic disturbances in many tissues; especially the nervous system. It occurs equally in both sexes, usually during the 2nd–4th decades, and is common in prisons and mental institutions. It is often complicated by arabiflavinosis.

Aetiology: pellagra is common in communities where maize is the staple food, since nicotinic acid in maize is in a bound form which is unavailable even after digestion. Sorghum is also important since it is rich in leucine which affects nicotinic acid and tryptophan metabolism. 2° pellagra also occurs due to reduced intestinal absorption; prolonged treatment for TB with isoniazid (>300mg daily); GI surgery; alcoholic gastritis.

Clinical features: are classically diarrhoea, dermatitis, and dementia. The patient may initially have vague abdominal symptoms, giddiness, and joint pain (termed the pre-pellagrous state). The sclerae may appear bluish and the patient's character may change, becoming irritable and morose. With time, other signs develop.

- ***GI:*** there is gingival swelling and/or bleeding; the tongue becomes scarlet, raw, and fissured, and may atrophy. Dysphagia occurs due to pyrosis (a burning sensation in the oesophagus) as well as abdominal tenderness, diarrhoea (often steatorrheic), although constipation can occur.
- ***Skin:*** lesions appear at sites exposed to sunlight or subject to pressure. An erythematous eruption appears on the back of the hands and feet, spreading to the rest of the body in irregular patches. Classically there is a symmetrical lesion behind the mastoid process, or a collar-like ring around the neck (Casal's necklace). Lesions are swollen, itch or burn, commonly have petechiae and are worse on exposure to sunlight. The eruption usually lasts 10–14 days and is followed by hyperkeratosis and desquamation. Atrophic patches of skin remain in the interdigital clefts and the nails become brittle and atrophied.
- ***CNS:*** signs may be present from the start or occur during convalescence. They include insomnia, anxiety, depression, photophobia; acute mania or psychosis (which may be permanent), with cogwheel rigidity of the extremities and primitive reflexes. Often there is profound melancholia and suicidal tendencies. Confusion may precede death.

- ***PNS:*** disease is variable in onset in relation to other symptoms. Signs include: neuropathy and/or paraplegia (spastic or ataxic), tremors, rigidity, paraesthesiae, exaggerated reflexes, upgoing plantar reflex. The cranial nerves are sometimes involved.
- ***Eye disease:*** features include conjunctival oedema, corneal dystrophy and lens opacities extending from the periphery to the centre.

Symptoms may regress and remit according to seasonal and dietary changes, but usually progress over a period of years.

Prevention: requires alteration of dietary habit through education and careful attention to institutional catering.

Diagnosis: a plasma nicotinic acid <0.31mg/dl in acute disease. One needs to distinguish the neurological symptoms from those occurring in hysteria, syphilis, ergotism, lathyrism (acute spastic paralysis in *Lathyrus* pea eaters), and other neuropathies.

Management:

1. Provide a high energy balanced diet which is rich in the various B vitamins eg 25–30g yeast daily.
2. Give 50mg nicotinic acid PO tds for 10–14 days.
3. The dose may be doubled in severe disease, or given as 300mg tds IV in acute mania or encephalopathy. Chronic psychiatric and spinal symptoms are usually resistant to treatment.
4. Sorghum-eating pellagrins have been successfully treated with isoleucine (which counteracts the metabolic effects of leucine) at 5g/day for 15 days.

Vitamin A deficiency[1]

Xerophthalmia causes blindness in about 250 000 children each year, particularly in south and SE Asia. It is due to vitamin A (retinol) deficiency and is usually a consequence of malnutrition associated with measles infection. WHO reports that ~40 million pre-school children are vitamin A deficient world-wide and that ~1/3 of these have some ocular damage.

Vitamin A is required for rhodopsin production in the retina and also for an effective immune response. Its deficiency makes the child night-blind and susceptible to systemic infections, particularly measles. The cornea is also particularly dry which makes it even more prone to damage during measles infection.

Clinical features: eye signs correlate approximately to severity (and duration) of retinol deficiency and are classified XN, X1, X2, X3 and XS:

- ***Night blindness (XN):*** occurs due to rhodopsin-deficiency in retinal cone cells. It is difficult to assess in infants – ask the mother whether the child bumps into objects in poor lighting.
- ***Conjunctival xerosis (X1a):*** dryness of the conjunctival epithelia results in increased susceptibility to infection and trauma.
- ***Bitot's spots (X1b):*** are foamy, white spots found on the surface of the conjunctiva, commonly at the corneoscleral junction on the temporal side. As the cornea is not involved, vision is normal. They may be bilateral and/or pigmented and may persist in older children beyond the period of vitamin A deficiency.
- ***Corneal xerosis (X2):*** similar to X1a, but the cornea is now involved. It is most common in children aged 2–4yrs and may herald the onset of visual impairment and, thus, severe disease.
- ***Corneal ulceration (X3a):*** may be superficial or deep. If it is central, it will profoundly affect the vision.
- ***Keratomalacia (X3b):*** in severe vitamin A deficiency, the cornea may suddenly melt (keratomalacia). It occurs most commonly in children aged 1–3yrs, and may be bilateral.

  Many children at this severe, acute stage of xerophthalmia will not survive many months longer, since they have greatly increased susceptibility to intercurrent infection and tolerate systemic disease poorly.
- ***Corneal scarring (XS):*** the permanent result of healing (after vitamin A supplementation) of stages X2–3. The severity of visual impairment depends upon the extent of scarring.

Prevention: centres around dietary education in communities where the disease is prevalent. Instruct mothers and health workers as to which foods are rich in vitamin A: spinach, carrots, sweet potatoes, mangos, papaya, milk, eggs, red palm oil, liver, fish liver oils. In the short-term, vitamin A capsules, 200,000IU may be given every 3–6 months to children aged 1–6yrs (half this dose if <1yr old). Any child with measles should be given one 200,000IU dose of vitamin A (give the full 3 doses if the child has ocular signs or is from a community known to be at risk). Better, long-term measures include immunisation against measles and encouraging families and farmers to cultivate vitamin-rich crops, particularly oils which are very rich in vitamin A.

Management – especially in the advanced stages – is not merely to save vision, ► but also to save the child's life.

1. For adults and children >1yr old, give 3 doses of vitamin A:
- immediately give vitamin A 200,000IU PO (66mg retinyl acetate, or 110mg retinyl palmitate equivalent).
- on the next day, give vitamin A 200,000IU PO.
- between day 7 and day 28, give vitamin A 200,000IU PO.

2. ► For children <1yr old, or <8kg, use half these dosages.

3. With the first vitamin dose, give topical antibiotic eye ointment (eg tetracycline 1% or chloramphenicol 1%) to be applied tds for 10 days.

4. If the cornea is involved, the eye should be closed and gently covered with an eye pad and the patient referred to a specialist.

► High doses of vitamin A are contraindicated during pregnancy. If a pregnant woman presents with signs of xerophthalmia, she should be given 10,000IU vitamin A PO daily for 2 weeks. At birth, this should be followed by the standard regime, above, which will ensure an adequate supply for both mother and breastfed baby.

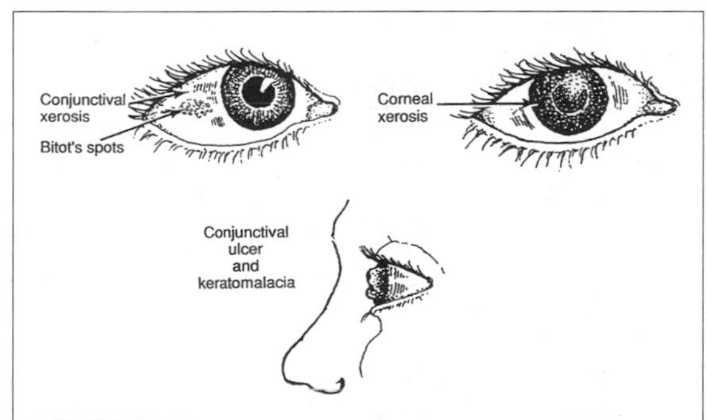

1. McGavin M, 1996, *Manson's Tropical Diseases*, 20th Ed, WB Saunders, London.

Vitamin B_{12} deficiency

Vitamin B_{12} (cobalamin) and folate are essential for the synthesis of DNA; deficiency of either produces megaloblastic anaemia. Total body cobalamin is ~1–10g (most of which is in the liver). Since an adult's daily requirement is ~2mg, normal stores are adequate for 3–4yrs in the absence of dietary intake. Deficiency may result from inadequate intake; pernicious anaemia; malabsorption due to ileal disease, and disturbed metabolism following nitrous oxide or cyanide poisoning.

Clinical features: usually seen in infants/neonates born to, and breast-fed by, women deficient in vitamin B_{12} (commonly due to tropical sprue or pernicious anaemia; more rarely in strict vegans). The child may show developmental retardation, involuntary movements, reduced muscle tone, peripheral neuropathy, optic atrophy, psychiatric disturbances, and subacute combined degeneration of the cord. Commonly, there is hyperpigmentation of the palmar and plantar skin and mucous membranes.

Diagnosis: low plasma B_{12}; megaloblastic anaemia with hypersegmented neutrophils and macro-ovalocytes on blood film. There may also be anisocytosis, poikilocytosis, leukopaenia, and thrombocytopaenia. The Schilling test diagnoses malabsorption and pernicious anaemia.

Prevention: give advice about eating foods rich in vitamin B_{12}; such foods include liver, kidney, bivalve molluscs, eggs, and milk products. Fruit and vegetables are *low* in vitamin B_{12}.

Vitamin E deficiency

Vitamin E is an antioxidant, required for cellular protection against oxidative stresses. Normal plasma concentration is 0.5–1.2mg/dl. The best dietary source is unsaturated mineral oil, but the vitamin is destroyed by prolonged storage, heat, or exposure to oxidants. Deficiency commonly affects neonates fed with milk rich in polyunsaturated fatty acids and supplemented with iron, causing haemolytic anaemia and retrolental fibroplasia. In adults deficiency may cause myopathy and sensory neuropathy. Treatment is with 300mg (400IU) up to twice daily.

Vitamin K deficiency

Essential for the formation of several clotting factors (II, VII, IX & X) and coagulation inhibitors (proteins C & S), deficiency of vitamin K results in a haemorrhagic syndrome. The vitamin is found in leafy green vegetables and is also produced by normal intestinal flora. Deficiency affects poorly fed neonates, adults with malabsorption, or adults who have had their intestinal microflora reduced by antibiotic treatment or occasionally vitamin K antagonist anticoagulant therapy. The PT is ↑ and plasma levels of the above clotting factors are reduced. Treatment is with phyloquinone (up to 10mg IV as a single dose) in cases of haemorrhage. Dietary advice suffices in most non-bleeding cases.

Management of vitamin B_{12} deficiency

1. Give 6 doses of hydroxycobalamin 1000µg IM over 1–2 weeks to replenish body stores.
2. For patients with malabsorption, continue to give 100µg every 3 months (if necessary, for life).
3. Neonates may be given 0.1µg per day PO, whilst also treating the deficient mother.

Obesity

In practice the terms overweight and obese are interchangeable and imply that a person is too heavy for their height compared with standard references. A few very muscular people are overweight due to muscle bulk, but this is usually obvious. Obesity is not yet a problem in most of the tropics; however, in certain areas, usually where relative wealth has appeared at a rapid rate, obesity is a significant problem.

People become obese because they take in more calories in food and drink than they use up in essential metabolic processes and energetic work. The extra calories are stored as fat. There is a high calorific intake when people eat large amounts of food at each meal; when they eat foods containing many calories (fatty foods and sugary foods); when they eat energy-rich snacks between meals; when they drink a lot of beer. People burn few calories when they have a low *basal metabolic rate* or when they do little physical activity. Thus, obesity tends to be a disease of the better-off, those who live in cities and those who have sedentary jobs.

It is important because it increases the risk of:
- coronary heart disease
- stroke
- hypertension
- type II diabetes
- gallstones and other digestive disorders
- back problems
- arthritis of the knees and hips
- accidents, fractures, and fatigue.

Diagnosis: obesity can be assessed using the BMI (see p554) in adults (excluding pregnant women). A BMI >25 indicates probable obesity, >30 definite obesity. Children are overweight if they are greater than the 97th centile on either the weight-for-height curve or the weight-for-age curve (growth chart). Be careful not to confuse the oedema of oedematous malnutrition with obesity.

Management: of obesity is notoriously difficult, particularly in those cultures where being fat is seen as a symbol of wealth.

1. Advise the patient to eat foods containing more fibre and less fat or sugar. For snacks, they can eat fruit or maize cobs, while avoiding sweets, chips, crisps, and cakes.
2. Cut down on their alcohol intake, especially beer.
3. Exercise for a minimum of 20 mins per day at a level just enough to raise the heart and respiratory rates, eg walking to work, using stairs instead of lifts. It is pointless setting your patient an exercise regime more suited to athletes in training – be realistic and always offer encouragement not scorn.
4. It is also wise to advise about the benefits of stopping smoking as a means of reducing the risk of coronary heart disease.

Goals of obesity therapy

- Weight loss – set realistic goals, in stages
- Increased mobility
- Control of associated disorders: diabetes, hypertension, sleep apnoea, arthritis
- Reduction in medications
- Change in body shape
- Improved cardiovascular fitness
- Psychological and social factors
- Individual goals: firring into clothes, ability to have surgery, reduction in pain

Treatment algorithm for obesity

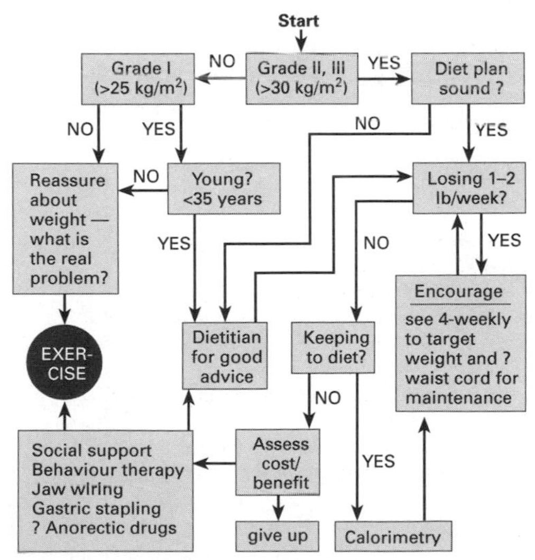

14. Injuries/poisoning

Pre-hospital care 599
Burns 600
Trauma and penetrating injuries 601
Acute poisoning 602
Attempted suicide 603
Acute poisoning – specific treatment 604
Snake bite 608

Pre-hospital care[1]

Some guidelines:

- Know your area. This means knowing not only its geography, and possible points of weakness in transport and communications, but also knowing the pattern of diseases within it.
- Learn about seasonal variations in disease incidence and prepare for them.
- Know you own equipment. It is pointless having expensive equipment and not knowing how to operate it, worse still know how to operate it, but find that it is broken when most needed.
- Know your limitations; if you are about to perform a potentially dangerous procedure but don't feel confident about it, there is no shame in asking for help.
- Cultivate good relations with other regional (and national) medical units - you may need to transfer patients urgently at times, so be prepared for this.
- Thus, know your local means of transport, from 'piggy-back' carrying to helicopter evacuation. How quickly (and at what cost ?) can it be summoned?

It has been shown in Ghana[2] that no changes in hospital practice which were inexpensive enough to implement, could improve outcomes in traumatic injuries resulting in death. Improving pre-hospital care and reducing transport time to hospital may be the only means of reducing deaths from trauma in the developing world.

Patience, tenacity, good communication with the right people and opportunism are all necessary when attempting to improve medical resources. Initiative and improvization are often the order of the day.

Many thanks to Dr. Bob Mark.

1. Adapted from a chapter by RC Mark and TM Tomlins in *Pre-Hospital Medicine – the Principles and Practice of Immediate Care*. Ian Greaves, and Keith M Porter. Edward Arnold Publishing, with kind permission (in press).
2. Mock CN *et al.* 1993, *Journal of Trauma* 35, 518–23

Burns

Burns are common in the tropics, where in many instances open fires are used for cooking and heating.

Major burns • Ask the nature of the burn; whether there was a blast; if fumes (?noxious) were inhaled; if there was pre-existing cardio-pulmonary disease; if the patient is tetanus immune.

- Look for signs of a respiratory burn (burnt nasal hairs or soot in the mouth, hoarseness/stridor, headache or confusion suggesting CO poisoning).
- Check for associated injuries and circulatory collapse. Get necessary X-rays and ECG (especially for electrical burns).
- Determine the extent of the burn using Wallace's 'rule of nines' (adults): Head (whole) = 9%; Torso (front) = 18%; Torso (back) = 18%; Each arm (whole) = 9%; Each leg (whole) = 18%; Genital area = 1%. Thus express any burn as an estimate (%) of total body area (in children head and legs = 14%).
- Assess the depth of the burn; *full thickness burns* are browny/white, painless and do not blanch to pressure. They require skin grafting. *Partial thickness burns* are red, blistered and very painful. They heal in 10–14 days.

  Management: resuscitation ('A, B & C') • Consider intubation if the airway is compromised; • give 100% oxygen (hyperbaric if CO poisoning is suspected – COHb >20%. Give 20ml 1.5% dicobalt edetate IV if cyanide poisoning from plastics burn);
- Stop any major bleeding and replace fluids (for burns >15% in adults or >10% in children); *[% area burn × weight (kg)] ÷ 2* = ml of colloid to give over each unit of time since the burn (not since time of presentation). Time units; 4hr, 4hr, 4hr, 6hr, 12hr. Thus, if there has been a delay in reaching hospital, rapid replacement may be necessary. In addition, give 1.5–2.0ml/kg/hr of 5% dextrose. NB: adjust all volumes and rates of infusion according to clinical response.
- Give morphine analgesia; • ensure tetanus immunity; • dress the burn with Vaseline gauze/silver sulphadiazine/saline-soaked gauze and cover. Do not burst blisters.
- Refer all burns >15% area (10% in children) or burns affecting face, hands or genitals to a burns unit or plastic surgeon if possible.

Minor burns: The assessment is essentially the same as above; cause/associated injuries/area/thickness. Bathe the burn in cold water, clean it and apply a non-adherent dressing. Give oral analgesia, tetanus prophylaxis and see the patient in OPD at 2–5 days for review and dressing change.

Trauma and penetrating injuries

Most penetrating wounds will need exploration under GA to repair and exclude damage to deep structures. Even small superficial injuries may hide much internal damage, depending on the mechanism of injury or weapon used (eg high velocity bullet). Cardiorespiratory depression often signifies very severe damage, as patients are often young and have greater reserves. NB do not remove weapons or large foreign bodies from the wound until in theatre as there is increased risk of exsanguination.

Management consists of the time-honoured 'A, B & C' for resuscitation with Airway, Breathing and Circulatory assessment, with further 'D' for Disability, followed by 'E' for Exposure/Environmental control. This is best coordinated by adopting a standardized routine for assessment as used in the ATLS (Advanced Trauma and Life Support) course. This involves;

- a rapid *primary survey* to identify life-threatening conditions which need immediate correction.
- resuscitation of vital functions along the A, B & C pathway, not progressing to further stages until each problem is identified and corrected. At all stages the C-spine is protected until injury is ruled out.
- a *secondary survey* with more detailed head to toe examination of the patient, proceeding to X-rays (usually C-spine, CXR – erect if possible – and pelvic XR as a minimum) and other diagnostic tests such as bloods, peritoneal lavage etc. Do a rectal examination and, if the pelvis is not involved, insert a urinary catheter.
- Assess disability by careful neurological survey and checking for facial injuries.
- Expose the patient fully and check for evidence of penetrating or blunt trauma. Cover any exposed viscera with saline-soaked gauze.
- definitive care is the management of all injuries identified in order of priority, including surgery, fracture stabilization, hospital admission or transfer if necessary.

Expect serious injuries in the following high-risk patients:

High speed impact, ejection or death of another vehicle occupant.
Entrapment within wreckage.
Fall greater than 5m (15ft).
Motorcyclist, or pedestrian struck.
Abnormal vital signs eg systolic BP <90, GCS <12, resp. rate <10 or >30 breaths/min.

Chest wounds: may damage pleura, lung, great vessels, heart, mediastinum, diaphragm or abdominal contents. Haemopneumothorax requires a chest drain – if drainage is initially >1500 (or 300ml/hr) thoracotomy may be needed. Close sucking wounds with an air-tight dressing. Be highly suspicious of pneumothorax and cardiac tamponade development.

Abdominal injuries: All but the most superficial will need admission for exploration and observation.

Limb injuries: Damage may be to nerves, tendons, vessels, muscle and bone. Always check peripheral pulses and sensation distal to the wound and watch for developing ischaemia and compartment syndrome. Never use a torniquet.

Acute poisoning

The tens of thousands of deaths caused by pesticides throughout the developing world every year are both personal tragedies and huge strains on limited medical resources. The scale of this problem stands in stark contrast to the very limited amount of attention it attracts in terms of research and national health policy.[1]

Management:

Get a history. What has been taken? How much and when? Have a handbook available that lists pesticides by both their chemical class and trade name since many people will only know the latter.

- Clear airway and check respiration. If required, give oxygen.
- If secretions are building up (eg after organophosphates), suck them out to keep the airway clear.
- Check consciousness level. If she has impaired consciousness, is having seizures, or has taken a corrosive or petroleum-based compound, insert a cuffed endotracheal tube to prevent aspiration.
- Place the patient on her side or semi-prone.
- ► Watch out for and control convulsions – see chapter 9.
- Give IV antibiotics if there is risk of aspiration pneumonia.

► **Gastric lavage and induced emesis are now no longer recommended for most poisonings.** While theoretically useful if given within 1–2hrs of poison ingestion, clinical trials (although all flawed in design to some degree) have failed to show any benefit for either. Gastric lavage in particular is associated with increased admissions to intensive care and incidence of aspiration pneumonia. (They may be useful for removing large pieces of vegetable matter eg oleander seeds – trials are required to determine local guidelines.)

► **Instead oral adminstration of activated charcoal is currently believed to be the most beneficial intervention.** Activated charcoal offers a large surface area for the poison to interact with, decreasing the absorption through the GI tract into the body. Give 50mg (15–30mg for children) dissolved in 240ml water q4h for 24hrs until it is seen in the faeces.

► **Multiple doses of activated charcoal** – some poisons such as cardiac glycosides are excreted in the bile and then reabsorbed from the terminal ileum – the enterohepatic circulation. This can be blocked by regular administration of activated charcoal q4h – this should be continued as long as clinically required. 30% of plasma digoxin can be removed daily in this way. Its value for many other poisons is unknown but it may be worth doing for all poisons.

Osmotic cathartics may further decrease absorption by causing diarrhoea and removing the poison from the bowel; however, their clinical value in practice is unclear. Give 150–250ml of a 10% solution of $MgSO_4$ or $NaSO_4$ (1–2ml/kg for a child). $MgSO_4$ is contraindicated if renal failure is present or predicted. $NaSO_4$ is contraindicated by severe hypertension, heart or renal failure. Both are contraindicated in ileus.

The attempted suicide[2,3]

Proper management of these patients requires you to:
- assess and manage medical harm
- assess future suicide risk (ie over next few weeks)
- determine whether the patient has a mental illness
- clarify the main problems which can then become the focus of help and a management plan.

Psychiatric assessment: be sympathetic, despite the hour. Interview relatives and friends if possible. Aim to establish:

1. Intentions at the time: was the act planned? What precautions against being found were made? Did he seek help afterwards? Does he think the method was dangerous? Was there a final act (eg suicide note)?
2. Present intentions.
3. What problems led to the act; do they still exist?
4. Was the act aimed at someone?
5. Is there a psychiatric disorder present (depression, alcoholism, personality disorder, schizophrenia, dementia)?
6. What are his resources (family, friends, work, personality)?

Assessment of future suicide risk: nearly all the research on attempted suicide has been carried out in the West. This has shown that the features which indicate someone is at increased risk of future suicide include:
- original or present intention is to die
- previous suicide attempts
- psychiatric disorder
- poor resources/social isolation
- male sex.

► Relatively little is known about this problem in many parts of the developing world.

1. Eddleston M, 1998, *BMJ*, 317, 133
2. Tony Hope, and *OHCM* p744, OUP, Oxford
3. Hawton K, Catalan J, *Attempted Suicide, a Practical Guide to its Nature and Management* 2nd Ed, OUP, Oxford

Acute poisoning – specific treatment

Relatively few poisons commonly used in the tropics have specific antidotes – the main aim of management of most patients will be to reduce absorption of the poison and then control symptoms.

Anticoagulants – determine prothrombin time if possible. If time is prolonged, or not available, vitamin K administration should be considered. Treat life-threatening haemorrhage with vitamin K 5mg by slow IV injection plus fresh frozen plasma and blood; less severe haemorrhage warrants 0.5–2mg vitamin K by slow IV injection.

Barbiturates – overdose may cause decreased consciousness, respiratory depression, signs of shock, hypoglycaemia, and hypothermia. Give 50mls of 50% dextrose IV to counter hypoglycaemia. If a long-acting (eg phenobarbitone) or intermediate-acting (eg amylobarbitone) barbiturate, perform a forced alkaline diuresis until she is conscious. Dialysis may be necessary in severe poisoning.

Benzodiazepines – presents with drowsiness, slurred speech, ataxia, rarely coma (small pupils/hyporeflexia), or respiratory arrest, due to the drugs' inhibitory effect on the CNS. Most patients can simply be observed. In case of respiratory arrest (often with newer, short-acting drugs) give ventilation. [Severe poisoning can be reversed with flumazenil 0.2mg IV over 15secs repeated with doses of 100µg at 60sec intervals if required, up to a maximum of 1mg. This drug must not be used if there are signs of tricyclic antidepressant toxicity.]

Cardiac glycosides – can be due to overdose of digoxin medication or ingestion of a source of natural glycoside (eg oleander seeds). Main effects are on the heart – arrhythmias and conduction block. Give atropine 0.5mg IV for bradycardia; repeat if necessary. Temporary cardiac pacing can tide the patient through 3rd degree heart block, but only antidigoxin antibodies can reverse DC-shock resistant VF or cardiogenic shock which occurs with severe poisoning.

Corrosives – these compounds cause necrotic ulceration of oropharynx, oesophagus, stomach, and rarely duodenum, with subsequent risk of perforation and mediastinitis, peritonitis, and shock. ► Do not induce vomiting or perform gastric lavage. Beware life-threatening laryngeal oedema. Give milk or water but not so much as to cause vomiting. Anticipate shock, infection, or perforation; in case of latter, get urgent surgical opinion. Sequelae include scarring and stenosis.

Cyanide – late presentations include dyspnoea, cyanosis, or unconsciousness. Altered mental status, tachypnoea (in absence of cyanosis), unexplained anion gap metabolic acidosis, and bright red blood are earlier signs. Adminster O_2; correct acidosis; give amyl nitrite by inhalation over 30sec each minute until other drugs are prepared. Then give: dicobalt edetate 300mg IV over 1 min followed by 50mls of 50% dextrose. Repeated ×2 if required. [Alternative: sodium nitrite 300mg by IV infusion over 3 min followed by sodium thiosulphate 12.5g IV over 10 min.]

Isoniazid – may cause decreased consciousness, convulsions, coma, respiratory arrest, metabolic acidosis. If severe, give pyridoxine IV (quantity equal to the quantity of isoniazid taken. If quantity is not known, give 5g by slow IV injection) and repeat at 5–20 min intervals if there is no response.

Kerosene – if aspirated, leads to chemical pneumonitis (if severe, can lead to fatal haemorrhage). ► Give gastric lavage if: poisoning is severe, kerosene contains other toxic substances, or you suspect >1ml/kg has been ingested. Give supportive care.

Lithium carbonate – has effects on CNS, heart, and kidney. Haemodialysis is the best method to remove lithium in severe poisoning. Check serum electrolytes often; if hypernatraemia is present, give 5% dextrose until plasma Na^+ returns to normal.

Metal ions (eg gold, mercury, zinc, lead, copper) – acute poisoning can cause coma, convulsions, and death, or affect multiple organ systems. Anticipate and treat shock, renal or hepatic failure. Give penicillamine 1–2g PO daily in 4 divided doses (2 hrs before meals, if possible) for 2–4 weeks – get senior opinion. An alternative option (preferred in mercury poisoning) is dimercaprol (BAL) 2.5–3mg/kg q4h for 2 days; then q6h on the 3rd day and bd for days 4–10 or until recovery.

Opiates – are found in analgesics and recreational drugs. Features include pinpoint pupils, decreased consciousness and respiratory depression. Give naloxone 0.8–2mg IV; if no response, repeat as necessary every 3 mins up to 10mg. If no response to 10mg, review diagnosis. An infusion may be needed after improvement to sustain it – 0.4–0.8mg/hr.

Paracetamol – give N-acetylcysteine IV unless paracetamol blood levels can be measured and shown to be safe (NB charcoal may delay its effect). Dose = 150mg/kg in 200ml of 5% dextrose over 15mins followed by 50mg/kg in 500ml of 5% dextrose over 4hrs and 100mg/kg in 1litre over 16hrs. Continue even if liver failure develops since it may decrease morbidity/mortality. If unavailable, give methionine 2.5g PO repeated 3× q4h. Check liver and kidney function. ► Closely monitor blood glucose levels, watching for hypoglycaemia.

Salicylates – severe poisoning may present with CNS depression; haematemesis; hyperthermia. However, lethal doses may not affect consciousness. Lesser poisoning produces GI pain, N&V, tinnitus. Metabolic acidosis occurs in young children; respiratory alkalosis more commonly in older patients. Give charcoal and correct electrolyte imbalances. If there are neurological signs, give 50mls of 50% dextrose IV; repeat if necessary. Give forced alkaline diuresis to increase salicylate excretion.

Tricyclic antidepressants – may present with signs of CNS toxicity (convulsions; ophthalmoplegia; muscle twitching; delirium; coma; respiratory depression), anticholinergic effects (dry mouth; blurred vision; dilated pupils); cardiotoxicity, hypothermia, pyrexia. Give charcoal, control convulsions; monitor heart and correct arrhythmias; control acidosis. Physostigmine salicylate 2–4mg IV over 2 min followed by 6mg/hr can be used for prolonged coma but beware bradycardia, hypotension and convulsions.

Pesticides

Bipyridylium (eg paraquat): severe poisoning produces multisystem failure and death within a few days. The lungs are selectively damaged in moderate poisoning and the patient dies from lung fibrosis several days to weeks after ingestion. Give charcoal and magnesium cathartic. For most patients, supportive measures are all that is available.

Carbamates: treat as for organophosphates but do not use pralidoxime since it is of no value. For poisoning with both classes of pesticide, give pralidoxime 1g in 250ml 5% dextrose by slow infusion. ► Stop the infusion if the patient's condition worsens.

Organochlorides: severe poisoning may present with status epilepticus or coma and multisystem damage. Phenobarbitone 100–200mg PO can be given as prophylaxis for convulsions. Treat status epilepticus as per chapter 9. General anaesthesia and ventilation may be required. Beware respiratory depression. ► Do not give adrenaline since it may initiate fatal cardiac arrhythmias.

Organophosphates: have three main effects on the:

- muscarinic receptors (N&V; sweating; salivation; defaecation; small/pinpoint pupils; pulmonary oedema; cardiac arrhythmias)
- nicotinic receptors (muscle twitching; weakness; paralysis; fascicultions)
- CNS (decreased consciousness; fits; respiratory depression).

► Sudden respiratory depression may occur after apparent recovery. Other effects include hyperglycaemia and pancreatitis.

Management – the best treatment for organophosphate poisoning is not yet clear. Atropine reverses the muscarinic effects of the pesticide while pralidoxime is reported to reverse its nicotinic effects. Recent studies from south Asia have questioned the role of pralidoxime and whether atropine should be given as an infusion or as boluses. The current recommendations are to:

1. Give atropine 2–10mg IV depending on severity of muscarinic effects, repeating 2mg IV every 10mins (or set up an infusion). Keep the heart rate between 120 and 140 beats/min. The pupil should not be small during atropine therapy. Maximum atropine is 100mg in 24hrs. ► Withdraw atropine slowly so that a rebound effect does not occur.
2. Give pralidoxine (2-PAM) 30mg/kg by slow IV injection in any severe or progressive intoxication, followed by an infusion of 8–10mg/kg/hr until there is clear clinical improvement.
3. Temporary cardiac pacing may be required for arrhythmias.

Thallium: presents with multisystem effects; death may occur due to respiratory arrest or shock. Give potassium ferric hexacyanoferrate (Prussian blue) 5–10g PO stat then 1g PO tds or by duodenal tube. Anticipate renal failure. Give additional KCl in IV fluids. Forced alkaline diuresis may increase thallium excretion.

Injuries/poisoning

Valuable information on many of these poisons is available from the National Poison Centre, Malaysia on the internet at <http://prn.usm.my>.
An excellent practical handbook is: Fernando *Management of Acute Poisoning*, Colombo, National Poisons Information Centre.

Snake bite

Untreated, less than 10% of people bitten by venomous snakes will die. With treatment, the outcome is even more favourable. Therefore, the first thing to do with a bitten patient is to calm and reassure them. Then attempt to find out the identity of the snake since this may affect which antivenom should be given.

Signs of envenoming: will vary according to the species of snake. However, the effects of most seriously venomous snakes fall into 2 categories – neurotoxic and haemorrhagic. In the former, the patient may die from respiratory arrest; in the latter, the patient may die from haemorrhagic shock. Some venoms will affect both systems. Other systems affected include muscles and kidneys.

► **Examine the patient regularly for signs of systemic envenoming**. Local symptoms support the idea that the person has been envenomed but are frequently not in themselves an indication for specific antivenom.

- **Local –** pain; swelling; blistering; regional lymphadenopathy.
- **Bleeding –** in gingival sulci; from venepuncture sites, skin wounds, or fang marks; haematuria; if severe, haematemesis or haemochezia may occur. Beware the patient going into shock – raise the foot of the bed and give plasma expanders. Subclinical bleeding that requires antivenom can be detected with a 20min clotting assay.
- **Neurological –** initial symptoms: blurred vision; heaviness of eyelids; drowsiness; signs: contraction of frontalis muscle; ptosis; ophthalmoplegia; limb weakness. ► Look for signs of respiratory muscle paralysis – dyspnoea, exaggerated abdominal respiration and intercostal muscle contraction, cyanosis.
- **Other systems –** • trismus and generalized muscle tenderness indicates rhabdomyolysis; • decreased urine output indicates acute renal failure (due to haemolysis and/or direct renal effect of venom); • dark urine may indicate either haemolysis or rhabdomyolysis.

If there are no signs of systemic envenoming, keep patient under observation for at least 24hrs.

Management: give antivenom if there are • systemic signs, • local swelling involving >half a limb, or • other signs recommended locally as an indication for antivenom.

- There is no point giving a test dose since it poorly predicts the individuals who will have an anaphylactoid response to the antivenom. Instead have already drawn up adrenalin, chlorpheniramine and hydrocortisone for use if anaphylaxis does occur.
- Give the recommended dose of antivenom by slow IV push over 10–20 minutes. (IV infusion in normal saline over 1 hour is another method but the equipment is more expensive and it takes longer to set up.)
- Give tetanus toxoid, and penicillin to prevent infection. If the wound has been tampered with give gentamicin. Necrotic tissue must be rapidly excised.

Locally recommended indications for antivenom therapy:

-
-
-
-
-
-

Rehabilitation

Following bites to hands or feet it is essential to think about rehabilitation early. Careful positioning and physiotherapy will reduce complications of the bite and improve the chance of normal function returning.

15. Immunization[1]

Immunization 612
Basic immunization strategies and schedules 614
Tetanus immunization of women of childbearing age 616
Adverse reactions 616
Contraindications 618
EPI vaccines 620
Other vaccines 622
New vaccines – under development and required 625

1. The information for this chapter is taken from two recent publications produced by the Global Programme for Vaccines and Immunization (GPV), Expanded Programme on Immunization (EPI), of the WHO, Geneva.
Immunization Policy, EPI/GPV, WHO 1995
State of the World's Vaccines and Immunization, WHO/GPV and UNICEF 1996.

The Expanded Programme on Immunization (EPI)

In 1974 when the Expanded Programme on Immunization was launched by the WHO, less than 5% of the world's children were immunized during their first year against the targeted 6 diseases. Now almost 80% of the 130 million children born each year are vaccinated before their first birthday. The EPI is preventing the deaths of at least 3 million children each year. In addition, every year, 750,000 fewer children become blind, crippled, mentally retarded, or otherwise disabled.

Immunization is the only medical breakthrough that has been made available to the vast majority of the world's population, not just 10 or 20%. Immunization contacts have opened up opportunities for other health care interventions – health education for mothers, vitamin and mineral supplements for children, and routine health checks. In recognition of this, the World Bank Report of 1993 stated that an EPI "package" also incorporating vaccines against hepatitis B and yellow fever together with supplements of vitamin A and iodine (the 'EPI plus') offered the highest cost-effectiveness of any health care measure in the world today.

Yet neither hepatitis B nor yellow fever vaccines are currently available in many of the countries in greatest need, illustrating one of the basic problems facing immunization programmes – some countries are simply unable to afford these extra vaccines, and donor countries show little interest in funding them. As a consequence, children are dying despite the availability of low cost effective vaccines

Many others are dying with diseases against which no vaccine currently exists. But here research is making progress – scientists are now studying a range of potential vaccines against >60 diseases. We are now at the threshold of a major scientific development that could change the face of preventative health care for children. But will it be affordable for the majority? The new vaccines will be much more expensive than the old.

The WHO and UNICEF are taking a 2-pronged approach to transforming imunization – boosting coverage through improving existing vaccines and adding a range of new vaccine against diseases that are not yet preventable. Strong advocacy will be required to ensure that vaccine research and development is not only driven by commercial interests but by public health goals as well.

The Children's Vaccine Initiative has been set up in collaboration with other interested organizations to further these aims. Its role is to improve the global supply of vaccines by working with the manufacturers to create a multi-tiered pricing system to ensure that vaccines will be priced at levels suitable for poor countries. The CVI will also work to advocate the value of disease prevention using vaccines. Changing attitudes to vaccines will save both money and needless suffering for children and their families by saving lives, reducing expensive treatment of unvaccinated children, and preventing disabilities.

Although excellent new vaccines already exist to save children from cholera, typhoid, and Hib disease, they are currently only affordable in industrialized countries. It is surely neither just nor equitable to allow life-saving vaccines to filter down slowly over many years to children in the developing world when they are so desperately needed now.

Immunization

Although the number of children fully vaccinated by the age of 1 year has increased from 5% in 1974, when the Expanded Programme on Immunization was set up, to ~80% in the 1990s, 12 million children under the age of 5 yrs are still dying each year.

Many of these deaths are due to diseases that could be prevented by vaccination in principle but for which vaccines have not yet been developed. However, two million deaths are due to diseases that can be prevented by the vaccines already on offer through the EPI. In 1994, over one million children died from measles, almost 500,000 from neonatal tetanus, and 400,000 from whooping cough.

These deaths occur for two reasons – because not all existing vaccines are 100% effective and because each year ~20% of the world's children are not fully immunized in their first year of life with the EPI vaccines.

Research work around the world is working to improve the effectiveness of vaccines to work on the first problem. In response to the second problem, the WHO is also working on ways of increasing coverage, setting a target of improving the immunization coverage globally for all EPI vaccines from 80% to over 90% by the year 2000. They have noted that many opportunities to give vaccines are not taken – the so-called 'missed opportunities'. Reduction in these missed opportunities would likely markedly improve global coverage.

Increasing immunization coverage – the importance of missed opportunities

Various studies have identified the following as the most important reasons for a child or woman of childbearing age coming to a health facility and not receiving the vaccines for which she is eligible:

- the failure to administer simultaneously all the vaccines for which a child was eligible
- false contraindications for vaccination – see p618
- health worker practices, including not opening a multi-dose vial for a small number of persons to avoid vaccine wastage
- logistical problems such as vaccine shortage, poor clinic organization, and inefficient clinic scheduling.

Missed opportunities can be reduced by health centres that see women and children by:

- offering immunizations as often as possible
- routinely screening the immunization status of all women and children that the centre serves
- teaching health workers which are true and which are false contra-indications
- ensuring that good practice procedures are followed.

The following section follows the guidelines of the Expanded Programme on Immunization for childhood vaccination. However, the epidemiology of the diseases which the EPI aims to combat will differ in each and every country. As a result, the vaccinations that are suitable for a particular country will likely differ between countries. For example, since yellow fever is endemic only in Africa and S. America, vaccination against this disease will be of little benefit in Asian countries. In addition, earlier immunization campaigns have greatly altered the epidemiology of a number of diseases, such as polio, thereby altering the importance of vaccination against these diseases.

To reflect this variation in circumstances, policy needs to be made at the national level to decide which vaccines should be included in the country's infant and childhood immunization schedules. ► These national policies will take precedence over the EPI guidelines presented here. Space has been left on page 615 for national guidelines to be written into this handbook.

Abbreviations for particular vaccines:

BCG	Bacille Calmette Guerin
DT	Double vaccine consisting of diphtheria toxoid and tetanus toxoid for use in children less than 10yrs old
DTP	Triple vaccine consisting of diphtheria toxoid, pertussis, and tetanus toxoid
MMR	Triple vaccine consisting of vaccines for measles, mumps, and rubella
MR	Double vaccine consisting of measles and rubella vaccines
IPV	Injected polio vaccine (Salk vaccine)
OPV	Oral polio vaccine (Sabin vaccine)
Td	Double vaccine consisting of tetanus toxoid and low-dose diphtheria toxoid for use in children older than 10yrs old and adults.
TT	Tetanus toxoid vaccine

Basic immunization strategies and schedules

The decision to immunize at a particular age is, for the most part, a compromise between

- the desire to immunize as early as possible, thereby protecting the child before she becomes exposed to the infectious agent, *and*
- the requirement to wait both for the infant's immune response to mature, and for the maternally-derived antibodies that crossed the placenta prenatally to disappear, so that the immunization will be effective.

In general, vaccines are recommended for *the youngest age group at risk* for developing the disease whose members are *known to develop an adequate antibody response* to immunization *without adverse effects* from the vaccine.

The basic schedule calls for all children to receive one dose of BCG vaccine, 3 doses of DTP vaccine, 4 doses of OPV, and one dose of measles vaccine before their first birthday – see opposite. In countries where HBsAg carriage rates are >2%, universal infant vaccination with Hep B vaccine is recommended. Where HBsAg carriage rates are lower, adolescent immunization can be considered as an alternative or addition. For the rationale behind this schedule, please see the WHO/GPV document *Immunization Policy*, cited at the beginning of this chapter.

Some vaccines require the administration of >1 dose for development of an adequate immune response. The doses *should not be given less than 4wks apart* since it may lessen the antibody response. Although increasing the interval will increase the antibody response, the child is then susceptible to infection for a longer time.

► It is important to complete the primary series quickly and therefore offer protective immunity to the infant as soon as possible.

Other points:

- As many vaccines as possible should be given in one visit to reduce the number of contacts required.
- If a child has missed the EPI schedule, she can receive the first dose of all the vaccines that a child of her age should have already received simultaneously.
- All the EPI vaccines can be safely given at the same time but they should be injected into different sites.
- Different vaccines should not be mixed and administered in one syringe.
- If vaccines cannot be given on the same day, then live vaccines should be spaced at least four weeks apart. A shorter interval may result in interference between the vaccines and a reduction in the immune response.

WHO-recommended infant immunization schedule

Age[1]	Vaccines	Hepatitis B[2] Scheme A	Hepatitis B[2] Scheme B
Birth	BCG, OPV 0	HB-1	
6 weeks	DTP-1, OPV-1	HB-2	HB-1
10 weeks	DTP-2, OPV-2		HB-2
14 weeks	DTP-3, OPV-3	HB-3	HB-3
9 months	Measles[3] and/or Yellow fever		

1. Babies born prematurely should be vaccinated at exactly the same times after birth as babies born at term.
2. Scheme A is recommended where perinatal transmission of Hep B is common (eg SE Asia). Scheme B may be used in countries where perinatal transmission is less common (eg sub-Saharan Africa).
3. Where there is a high risk of mortality from measles among children under 9 months (such as hospitalized or HIV-infected infants, or refugee camps) measles vaccination should be carried out at both 6 & 9 months.

National recommendations

Age	Vaccines
Birth	
6 weeks	
10 weeks	
14 weeks	
6 months	
9 months	

Tetanus immunization of women of childbearing age

The immunization of pregnant women with tetanus toxoid vaccine is a highly effective means of protecting the newborn child from neonatal tetanus. The optimal schedule for this vaccination depends on the immunization history of the woman.

- **Schedule A.** Regions in which women were not vaccinated during infancy and childhood, or where there is insufficient documentation for previously vaccinated women to be identified, should administer a full TT five-dose schedule for all women of childbearing age. The details of these schedules are presented on the opposite page. The regions concerned need to determine the age group to be included in the schedule eg 15–35 or 15–44.
- **Schedule B.** Regions in which women have documentation of previous vaccination with TT-containing vaccines during infancy or childhood can apply more selective schedules for tetanus vaccination – see opposite. (It is likely that more and more countries will start to fall into this group with the recent worldwide increase in tetanus vaccination during infancy. The EPI recommends that countries start to use schedule B when DTP vaccination during infancy has reached 80%.)

Adverse reactions

Although modern vaccines are extremely safe, some vaccines may lead to adverse reactions. It is difficult to prove that a vaccination causes a specific event. Instead, population studies must be carried out to look for an association between the vaccination and the adverse event – eg clustering of cases in vaccines or a higher incidence in vaccinees compared to unvaccinated groups. Adverse reactions tend to be caused by:

- **Faults of administration** (programmatic errors) – eg abscesses after poor mixing of vaccines or use of non-sterile needles or syringes; or disseminated disease in immunosuppressed patients after administration of BCG or measles vaccines.
- **Properties of the vaccines** – the reactions may be caused by the immunizing antigen itself or by other components such as antibiotics (used in growth of the virus), preservatives, or adjuvant.

Mild adverse events are common – eg 20–50% of DTP recipients experience mild local reactions while some measles vaccine recipients get a rash and fever. Booster doses of toxoids may induce hypersensitivity reactions in some people.

► Severe reactions such as encephalitis after mumps or measles vaccines are extremely rare. DTP vaccination has been reported to be associated with many adverse affects but comprehensive studies have failed to link this vaccination to many of these adverse effects. Vaccine-associated severe events are much less common than the severe complications caused by the disease itself.

► It is essential to detect serious adverse events and to identify the underlying cause since such reactions will influence community acceptance of the vaccinations, lowering immunization rates.

Schedule A. TT immunization schedule for women of childbearing age

Dose	*When to give*	*Expected duration of protection*
TT-1	At first contact or as early as possible in pregnancy	None
TT-2	At least four weeks after TT-1	1–3 yrs
TT-3	At least six months after TT-2	5 yrs
TT-4	At least one year after TT-3 or during subsequent pregnancy	10 yrs
TT-5	At least one year after TT-4 or during subsequent pregnancy	All childbearing years

Schedule B. Guidelines for TT immunization of women who were immunized in the past

Age at last TT immunization	*Previous TT immunizations*	*Recommended immunizations* At present contact	later (at interval of >1 year)
Infancy	3 DTP	2 TT	1 TT
Childhood	4 DTP	1 TT	1 TT
School age	3 DTP + 1 DT/Td	1 TT	1 TT
School age	4 DTP + 1 DT/Td	1 TT	none
Adolescence	4 DTP + 1 DT at 4–6 yrs and 1 TT (or Td) at 14-16 yrs	none	none

Contraindications

► There are relatively few absolute contraindications to vaccination.

► Every opportunity to vaccinate a child or woman of childbearing age should be taken, particularly in outpatient clinics – see 'missed opportunities' on p612. There is a high risk that delaying vaccination until the child is better will result in that child not getting her full complement of vaccinations because she did not return again and was lost to follow-up. Many programmes have contraindications which are inappropriate. Such false contraindications are listed opposite.

True contraindications to vaccination include:

- Illnesses severe enough for the child to be hospitalized – if the child is vaccinated but then dies from the pre-existing illness, the vaccine may be thought to have killed the child. ► However, immunize as soon as the child's general condition improves. Give measles vaccine on hospital admission if possible because of the risk of nosocomial transmission.
- For **LIVE** vaccines, immunodeficiency diseases or immunosuppression due to malignant disease, therapy with immunosuppressive drugs, or irradiation. HIV/AIDS is a special case – see below.
- A severe adverse event (anaphylaxis, collapse or shock, encephalitis, encephalopathy, or non-febrile convulsion) after a previous dose of vaccine. If the adverse reaction occurs with a dose of DTP vaccine, omit the pertussis component and complete the vaccination with the DT vaccine.
- For vaccines prepared in egg (yellow fever, influenza) a history of anaphylaxis following egg ingestion. Vaccines prepared in chicken fibroblast cells (measles or MMR) can usually be given to such people.
- Live vaccines should not be routinely administered to pregnant women except where there is a high risk of exposure and the need for vaccination outweighs any possible risk to the fetus. In adult women, pregnancy should be avoided for >1 month after vaccination with a live vaccine.

Live vaccines include

- BCG
- measles
- mumps
- yellow fever
- typhoid
- rubella
- oral polio vaccine (OPV).

Immunization of HIV-infected persons

There has been concern that HIV-induced immune system impairment might make HIV-infected people more susceptible to severe vaccine-associated diseases. There has so far been no evidence to support this concern. Instead, since both measles and TB are associated with higher mortality in HIV^+ patients, there is clearly a great need for these persons to be vaccinated. Most HIV^+ infants and adults are able to mount a good immune response to vaccination and should receive all EPI vaccines as early as possible.

The WHO/UNICEF guidelines for immunization of HIV-infected individuals are presented opposite.

Conditions which ARE NOT contraindications to immunization and which MUST NOT prevent a child from being vaccinated

- Minor illnesses such as URTI or diarrhoea, with fever <38.5°C
- Allergy, asthma, other atopic manifestations, hay fever, or snuffles.
- Prematurity, small-for-date infants
- Malnutrition
- Child being breastfed
- Family history of convulsions. (▶ However, if there is a *Hx* of febrile convulsions, offer advice on the treatment of fever before giving vaccine – for a 2–3 month infant, give 60mg paracetamol followed by a 2nd dose 4–6 hrs later if required. Advise parents to see a doctor if the fever persists after a 2nd dose of paracetamol)
- Treatment with antibiotics, low-dose corticosteroids or locally acting (eg topical or inhaled) steroids
- Dermatoses, eczema or localized skin infection
- Chronic diseases of the heart, lung, kidney and liver
- Stable neurological conditions, such as cerebral palsy and Down's syndrome
- History of jaundice after birth

WHO/UNICEF recommendations for the immunization of HIV-infected children and women of childbearing age

Vaccine	Asymptomatic HIV infection	Symptomatic HIV infection	Optimal timing of immunization
BCG	Yes[1]	No	Birth
DTP	Yes	Yes	6, 10, 14 weeks
OPV[2]	Yes	Yes	0, 6, 10, 14 weeks
Measles	Yes	Yes	6, 9 months[3]
Hepatitis B	Yes	Yes	As for uninfected children
Yellow fever	Yes	No[4]	
TT	Yes	Yes	5 doses – see above

1. If the local risk of TB infection is low, then BCG should be withheld from individuals known or suspected to be HIV infected.
2. IPV can be used as an alternative in symptomatic HIV⁺ children.
3. Because of the risk of severe early measles infection, HIV⁺ infants should receive measles vaccine at 6 months and as soon after 9 months as possible.
4. Pending further studies.

EPI vaccines

► Always consult the manufacturer's data sheet before using a vaccine.
► See previous page for general contraindications.

Some vaccines produce very few reactions while others such as measles and rubella may produce a mild form of disease, with a very small risk of serious complications – see page on adverse reactions. Some vaccines produce discomfort at the site of injection, mild fever, and malaise.

► Anaphylactic reactions are extremely rare but may be fatal.

BCG – is a freeze-dried preparation of a live attenuated strain of *Mycobacterium bovis* that is given in a single intradermal injection. The vaccine appears to be most effective in preventing TB meningitis and miliary TB in infants, hence its early administration. Its long-term protective effects are unclear as are the stability of the protective immunity induced and the value of booster doses. There is also good evidence that BCG vaccination protects against leprosy. ***Cautions:*** apart from neonates, any person being considered for BCG vaccination should be given a skin test for hypersensitivity to tuberculoprotein. Except in infants, >3 weeks should be left between administration of any live vaccine and BCG. ***Contraindications:*** BCG should not be given to subjects with generalized septic skin conditions. ***Side-effects:*** a small swelling forms 2–6wks post-vaccination that may progress to a benign ulcer. Healing occurs in 6–12wks.

Diphtheria toxoid vaccine – is a formaldehyde-inactivated preparation of diphtheria toxin, absorbed onto aluminium salts to increase immunogenicity. It is normally given in the form of a triple vaccine with tetanus and pertussis vaccines (DTP), but can be given with tetanus alone when pertussis vaccine is contraindicated. The vaccine does not prevent infection but rather inhibits the toxin's effects, preventing systemic illness. ► A low dose vaccine (combined with tetanus, Td) should be used in children >10 yrs old and adults requiring immunization to decrease the risk of serious reactions to the vaccine.

Hepatitis B vaccine – is a suspension of inactivated hepatitis B surface antigen (HBsAg) absorbed onto aluminium salts. It is given by IM injection in 3 doses – the 2nd and 3rd doses are given at one month and six months (the deltoid muscle is the preferred site in adults, the anterolateral thigh in infants/children; the buttock should not be used as it may decrease vaccine efficacy). It is available as a recombinant vaccine and as a plasma-derived vaccine; both are safe and highly efficacious. If available, one dose of Hep B immunoglobulin should be given immediately to infants newly born to mothers who became infected during the pregnancy or are Hep e-antigen positive.

Measles vaccine – is a freeze-dried preparation of live attenutated virus that is given by single SC injection. It is normally given at around 9 months but an additional dose can be given at 6 months in those at high risk – see schedules. In industrialized countries, it has now been replaced by a triple vaccine that combines measles, mumps and rubella vaccines (MMR). This vaccine is given after 12–15 months and then again at age 3–5 before school entry.

The vaccine can be used to control outbreaks of measles. It should be offered to susceptible children within 3 days of exposure to infection. The measles vaccine normally contains >1000 units of infectious virus. ***Side-effects:*** may be associated with a mild measles-like illness with rash and fever 1wk after vaccination. Convulsions and encephalitis are rare complications.

Pertussis vaccine – is available in 2 forms: whole-cell vaccine (pertussis bacteria killed by chemicals or heat) or the recently introduced, expensive acellular vaccine. They are normally given by IM injection in a triple vaccine with diphtheria and tetanus vaccines (DTP). The whole-cell vaccine is effective at preventing serious disease but not infection. The induced immunity decreases with time. However, the importance of this vaccine has been shown by a resurgence in disease in the UK and Sweden after vaccine uptake rates fell. Since the vaccine requires 3 doses to elicit a strong immune response, it cannot be used to control an epidemic. The acellular vaccine contains purified immunogenic components of the bacteria – normally the toxoid and 2–4 other components. Side-effects appear to be much less common. Researchers are still looking at the efficacy of these vaccines. ***Side-effects:*** convulsions and encephalopathy have been reported as very rare complications but it is not certain that they were caused by the vaccine.

Poliomyelitis vaccine – is available in 2 forms – a live attenuated virus vaccine given by mouth (OPV, Sabin vaccine) and an injectable killed virus vaccine given by IM injection (IPV, Salk vaccine). Each vaccine contains strains of three different types of poliovirus (types 1, 2 and 3), offering wide protection.

The EPI recommends the OPV because of its low cost, ease of administration, superiority in conferring intestinal immunity, and potential for infecting household and community contacts, thereby providing secondary immunity. OPV has been shown to be the vaccine of choice for eradication due to its ease of administration in campaigns and the dramatic impact gained by breaking chains of transmission. ***Cautions:*** patients with D&V require a further dose after recovery. ***Contraindications:*** living with an immunodeficient person – the IPV should be used for these cases. ***Side-effects:*** vaccine-associated poliomyelitis in vaccine recipients and contacts is rare – about 1 case per 2 million vaccinations each year in the UK. However, very strict personal hygiene needs to be emphasized, particularly for the contacts of a recently vaccinated baby.

Tetanus toxoid vaccine – is a formaldehyde-inactivated preparation of tetanus toxin absorbed onto aluminium salts that is given by IM or deep SC injection. It is normally given to infants in the form of a triple vaccine with diphtheria and pertussis vaccines (DTP), but can be given with diphtheria alone (DT) when pertussis vaccine is contraindicated. The administration of tetanus toxoid (TT) to a pregnant woman induces antitoxin antibodies which pass across the placenta and prevent neonatal tetanus. Some countries recommend booster doses of TT for all persons at school entry, at school leaving, and then at 10yr intervals. A full primary course of immunization can be given to adults who did not receive a childhood course. For serious potentially contaminated wounds, anti-tetanus immunoglobulin is valuable in addition to wound toilet, vaccination (at a different site), and antibiotic cover. ***Cautions:*** TT should not be given at <10 yr intervals because of the risk of hypersensitivity reactions.

Yellow fever vaccine – consists of freeze-dried preparation of live attenuated virus (17D strain) that is grown in egg embryos and given by SC injection. It is highly immunogenic and offers at least 10 years of immunity. ***Contraindications:*** do not give to infants under the age of 6 months, unless infection with yellow fever is unavoidable, since there is a small likelihood of encephalitis in this age group.

Other vaccines

► Always consult the manufacturer's data sheet before using a vaccine.

Cholera vaccine – is currently a preparation of heat-killed Inaba and Ogawa subtypes of *V. cholera*. Unfortunately this vaccine is poorly antigenic and provides only partial protection of limited duration. Its use is no longer recommended. Oral one-dose candidate vaccines against the El Tor biotype and 01 and 0139 serotypes are currently under development and field trials.

Haemophilus influenzae* type b (Hib) vaccines** – consist of Hib polysaccharides conjugated to either diphtheria or tetanus toxoids or the meningococcus outer-membrane protein complex. The vaccine is given by IM injection in a schedule of 3 doses during infancy (normally with DTP and OPV), in some countries followed by a booster dose at age 12–18 months. Since the risk of serious Hib infection falls sharply after the age of four, it is only recommended for individuals at high risk of infection in this age group (sickle-cell disease, during treatment of malignant disease, following splenectomy). ***Contraindications: see p618 for general contraindications. ***Side-effects:*** include fever, headache, malaise, N&V, prolonged crying, anorexia, diarrhoea, rash. Rarer side-effects include convulsions, erythema multiforme, transient lower limb cyanosis.

Hepatitis A vaccine – is a formaldehyde-inactivated preparation of hepatitis A virus grown in human diploid cells that has been absorbed onto aluminium salts. It is given by IM injection, preferably into the deltoid muscle. A booster is recommended at 12 months. ***Contraindications:*** see p618 for general contraindications. ***Side-effects:*** include transient soreness, erythema and induration at the injection site. A mild flu-like illness, and generalized rashes have been reported.

Influenza vaccine – consists of inactivated influenza virus that has been grown in eggs. Since the virus is continually altering its haemagglutinin (H) and neuraminidase (N) surface proteins, different strains that express the H and N proteins of the prevalent strain must be used each year. The WHO recommends which strains should be incorporated into the vaccine each year after surveying the virus across the world. The vaccine can be given by deep SC or IM injection annually to those at risk – people, particularly the elderly, with the following conditions: chronic respiratory (including asthma), renal and CVS disease, diabetes mellitus, other endocrine disorders, immunosuppression. It may also be of benefit to those living in nursing homes or other long-stay facilities.

Japanese encephalitis vaccine – a formalin-inactivated preparation of virus grown in either mouse brain or cultured hamster cells. The mouse brain preparation has had brain proteins removed and is not associated with CNS damage. This vaccine has been widely used in Asia and shown to be both effective and safe. Two doses are given by SC injection 1–2wks apart. An additional dose is given at 4 wks and boosters recommended every 1–4 yrs. The hamster cell vaccine has been developed and used extensively in China since 1967. Because of the severity of the disease, the EPI recommend that every country where JE is epidemic consider incorporating this vaccine into their immunization schedules. ► Research is required to ascertain the earliest age at which this vaccine can be given, the necessity of booster doses, and whether it can be given simultaneously with other EPI vaccines.

Meningococcal vaccines – currently consist of capsular polysaccharides purified from various serogroups of *N. meningitidis*. At present, monovalent vaccines exist for groups A and C, bivalent vaccines for both A and C, and a quadrivalent vaccine for serogroups A, C, W-135 and Y. A single dose of the monovalent A group vaccine given by deep SC or IM injection elicits protective immunity for 1–3 years in persons >2 yrs. The response is poorer in children <2 yrs – 2 doses are required 3 months apart to achieve protective immunity. Group C vaccines are effective in adults but not children. The current vaccines are not recommended for infant vaccination programmes but may be used together with antibiotics to protect household contacts. They also play an important role in controlling meningococcal A/C epidemics.

Mumps vaccine – consists of a live attenuated strain of virus grown in chick embryo cells in tissue culture. It is normally given by IM injection with measles and rubella vaccines in the MMR triple vaccine at age 12–15 months and again at 3–5 yrs. See ***Measles vaccine*** for side-effects and contraindications.

Pigbel vaccine – is an inactivated preparation of toxin from *Clostridium perfringens* type C that is given by IM injection. It is effective in infants and children and has been given routinely to children in Papua New Guinea at ages 2, 4 and 6 months, simultaneously with their DTP vaccination, since 1980. Protection lasts for 2–4 yrs.

Pneumococcal vaccines – consist of capsular polysaccharide antigens from 7, 9, 14 or 23 different serotypes of *S. pneumoniae*. Unfortunately these antigens do not induce a protective immune response in children <2 yrs old, one of the age groups with highest attack rate. Alternative strategies are being developed to produce a vaccine that is effective in infants, using protein components of the bacteria. The vaccine is recommended for persons >2yrs old who are at high risk for severe infection: sickle-cell disease, CRF, immunosuppression, CSF leaks, HIV infection, asplenia, chronic liver, heart or lung disease, DM. If possible, give the vaccine at least 2 wks before either splenectomy or chemotherapy. ***Contraindications:*** pregnancy, breastfeeding, during infection. ***Side-effects:*** hypersensitivity reactions may occur. They are more frequent with revaccination therefore routine revaccination is not recommended. ▶ However, revaccination should be offered where the risk of fatal infection is judged to be high (>4 yrs after 14 serotype vaccine and >6 yrs after 23 serotype vaccine). Children at high risk can be revaccinated after 3–5 yrs if they are still <10 yrs old.

Rabies vaccine – is available as a freeze-dried inactivated preparation of virus grown in either sheep brain or cultured human diploid cells. The former vaccine is still used in some parts of the world but it is associated with an unacceptably high rate of post-vaccination severe neurological complications (~1:1000). This is due to immune responses to sheep brain antigens that contaminate the virus preparation. The cultured vaccine is far safer but much more expensive. Its use around the world is increasing, however, particularly as novel cheaper ways of administering the vaccine are developed. See chapter 9 for prophylactic and post-exposure vaccination schedules.

Rubella vaccine – is a preparation of the live Wistar strain of the virus. It is given by deep SC or IM injection in industrialized countries either to • infants as part of the triple measles, mumps, and rubella (MMR) vaccine or • as a monovalent vaccine to prepubertal girls between their 10th and 14th birthdays. The purpose is to reduce the incidence of primary infection in pregnant women and therefore reduce the incidence of congenital rubella syndrome in their offspring. Universal immunization is not recommended at present by the EPI because incomplete coverage would just increase the age at which most infections occur, increasing the likelihood of infection in childbearing women. ***Contraindications:*** avoid immunizing women during early pregnancy. Advise women not to become pregnant for >1 month after immunization. However, there is no evidence at present that the vaccination is teratogenic.

Typhoid vaccine – occurs in three forms – • a killed whole-cell suspension, • a purified form of the capsular polysaccharide Vi (both given by deep SC or IM injection), and • an oral live attenuated preparation of the bacteria. *None are substitutes for good personal hygiene*. All elicit protective immunity in adults and children >2yrs but not in children <2yrs. They are therefore not recommended for immunization during infancy. • The whole-cell vaccine is given in 2 doses 4–6wks apart but requires boosters every 3yrs and it is associated with a high incidence of adverse reactions – see below. • The capsular antigen vaccine is given as a single dose with boosters every 3 years. • The oral vaccine is given in 3 doses on alternate days. Residents of endemic regions who are frequently exposed to *S. typhi* require boosters every 3yrs; visitors to these regions who will be less exposed require boosters every year. ***Cautions:*** the second dose of the whole-cell vaccine and subsequent boosters should be given by intradermal injection to reduce adverse reactions. The oral vaccine is inactivated by concomitant administration of antibiotics or sulphonamides. Mefloquine must not be taken for 12hrs either side of giving the oral vaccine, and preferably should only be started >3 days after vaccine administration. ***Side-effects:*** local reactions including pain, swelling and erythema may appear 2–3 hrs after administration of the whole-cell vaccine and 48–72hrs after administration of the capsular antigen vaccine. Systemic reactions such as fever, malaise and headache may also occur after administration of the whole-cell vaccine.

New vaccines – under development and required

New and better vaccines are continually required. Important vaccines currently under development include vaccines for:

- enterotoxigenic *E. coli*
- meningococcus B
- para-influenza viruses
- respiratory syncitial virus
- HIV
- dengue
- rotaviruses
- schistosomiasis.
- malaria
- rotaviruses
- shigellae

16. Laboratory investigations

Due to space considerations, we have been unable to include a section on laboratory investigations as we had first hoped. In its place, we therefore recommend the following book for information on standard laboratory techniques in the developing world:

District Laboratory Practice in Tropical Countries
Monica Cheesbrough, Tropical Health Technology: March, England 1998

Contents:

- Importance and integration of the laboratory in district health care
- Training of district laboratory personnel
- Total quality management and SOPs
- Health and safety in district laboratories
- Equiping district laboratories and equipment maintenance
- Parasitology tests (Major colour section of the book)
- Clinical chemistry tests
- Appendices: preparation of reagents, tables, figures, useful addresses

Available from: Tropical Health Technology – see opposite, for £10.90 in developing countries and £33.30 in other countries (includes P&P).

A useful approach to screening

(courtesy of Tony Moody, London School of Hygiene and Tropical Medicine)

1. Blood film	• anaemia	Giemsa stain
	• differential WCC	Giemsa stain
	• parasites	Giemsa stain – thick/thin
	• bacteria	culture
2. Sputum	• TB	Ziehl-Nielsen stain
	• paragonomiasis	wet film
	• schistosomes	wet film
	• pneumocystis	Giemsa (silver stain)
	• cryptosporidiasis	Ziehl-Nielsen stain
3. Stool	• ova	
	• cysts	
	• other – blood, mucus, trophozoites	
4. Others: CSF	• cells	Giemsa stain
	• parasites	concentrate, then stain
	• cysts	
pus	• bacteria	Gram stain
exudate	• cells	Giemsa stain
urine	• schistosomes	
lymph node	• parasites	Giemsa stain

Giemsa stain can be replaced with the more rapid Field's stain.

17. Contact addresses

The World Health Organization, 1211 Geneva 27, Switzerland [http://www.who.int/; *Weekly Epidemiological Record*: www.who.int/wer/]

British National Formulary, c/o Royal Pharmaceutical Society of Great Britain, 1 Lambeth High Street, London SE1 7JN.

International Association for Medical Assistance to Travellers, 40 Regal Rd, Guelph, Ontario, N1K 1B5, Canada.

Liverpool School of Tropical Medicine, Pembroke Place, Liverpool L3 5QA. United Kingdom (tel 0044 151708 9393).

London School of Hygiene and Tropical Medicine, Keppel Street, London, United Kingdom [http://www.lshtm.ac.uk].

The Centres for Disease Control and Prevention (CDC), 1600 Clifton Road, NE Atlanta, GA 30333, USA [http://www.cdc.gov/].

The Wellcome Trust, 210 Euston Rd, London NW1 2BE, UK [http://www.wellcome.ac.uk; tel 0044 171 611 8888).

Tropical Health Technology, 14 Bevills Close, Doddington, March, Cambs PE15 0PT, UK (tel 0044 1345 740825).

WHO Collaborating Centre for Research, Training and Control in Diarrhoeal Diseases, International Centre for Diarrhoeal Disease Research, Bangladesh (ICDDR, B), GPO Box 128, Dhaka 100, Bangladesh.

Index

A

abdominal pain 354–5
abetalipoproteinaemia 156
abortions, septic 200, 201
abscesses, lung 304, 305
accelerated hypertension 275
ACE inhibitors 271
acid-alcohol-fast bacilli 111
acquired immunodeficiency syndrome, *see* human immunodeficiency virus (HIV)/AIDS
acromegaly 506
actinic keratoses 468
acute abdomen 354–5
acute bronchitis 180
acute cholecystitis 364
acute confusional state 402, 403
acute flaccid paralysis 448, 450, 453
acute lymphoblastic leukaemia 536, 537
acute myeloblastic leukaemia 536–7
acute myocarditis 281
acute necrotizing ulcerative gingivitis 347
acute nephritic syndrome 326
acute pancreatitis 360–1
acute paracoccidioidomycosis 308
acute pericarditis 251, 282
acute poisoning 602–6
acute post-infectious measles encephalitis 234
acute progressive encephalitis 234
acute renal failure 332–5
acute respiratory infections 180–1
acute severe asthma 296–7
acute toxic schistosomiasis 386
acute tubular necrosis 334
Addisonian crisis 505
Addison's disease 504–5
adenitis
  mesenteric 357
  tuberculosis 118
adenocarcinoma 302
adult T-cell leukaemia/lymphoma 534
advanced life support (ALS) protocols 262–5
Aedes aegypti 238
Aedes albopictus 236, 238
African histoplasmosis 308
African trypanosomiasis 222–5
AIDS, *see* human immunodeficiency virus (HIV)/AIDS
airways disease 298
alcoholic liver disease 374, 375
algid malaria 28
allergic alveolitis, extrinsic 312
allergic bronchopulmonary aspergillosis 306
α thalassaemia 528
alveolar disease 298
  hydatid 392
American tick typhus 208
American trypanosomiasis 226–7
amodiaquine 41
amoebiasis 136
amoebic colitis 358
amoebic dysentery 136–7
amoebic liver abscess 382–3
amoebic meningoencephalitis 416
amopyroquin 41
amplifier hosts 236
amyloidosis 340
anaemia 510–12, 566
  cancer 202
  of chronic disease 516
  haemolytic 520–1, 548
  iron-deficiency 514–15
  macrocytic 518–19
  malaria 24, 26
  normocytic 516
  in pregnancy 513
  sickle-cell 342, 524–7
  sideroblastic 516
anaphylactic shock 273
Ancylostoma duodenale 517
angina 254–5
  post-infarct 260
angiostrongyliasis 416
anorexia 58
anthrax 220, 221
antibiotic-associated colitis 140–1
antibiotics
  bacterial meningitis 413
  leprosy 456
  melioidosis 221
  resistance and rational use 6–7
antidiarrhoeal drugs 175
antiepileptic drugs 443
anticoagulant poisoning 604
antimicrobial drugs 131, 190
anuria 322
aortic incompetence 250
aortic stenosis 250
aphthous ulcers 346
aplastic crises 524
appendicitis 356–7
arboviruses 236–7

arenavirus haemorrhagic fever 244, 245
Argentinian haemorrhagic fever 244, 245
ariboflavinosis 586
arrhythmias, cardiac 252, 260, 264–7
artemether 40
artemisinins 40
artesunate 40
arthritis 276, 342
ascariasis 362
Ascaris lumbricoides 140, 362, 363
aspergilloma 306
aspergillosis 306–7
Aspergillus flavus 306
Aspergillus fumigatus 306
Aspergillus niger 306
aspiration pneumonia 188
asthma 294–7
asymptomatic HIV infection 52, 78–9
atopic eczema 466
atovaquone 41
atrial fibrillation 266, 267
atrial flutter 267
atrial septal defect 251
atypical mycobacteria 112, 114
atypical pneumonia 184–5
autoimmune haemolytic anaemia 521

B

bacillary dysentery 132
Bacille Calmette Guerin (BCG) vaccination 115, 124, 620
Bacillus anthracis 220
bacteraemia 305
bacteria, staining for 111
bacterial meningitis 412–13
bacterial prostatitis 331
bacterial skin infections 470
bacterial vaginosis 106
bacteriuria in pregnancy 331
Balantidium coli 134
Balantidium enterocolitis 134
Bancroftian filariasis 484
barbiturate poisoning 604
Bartonella bacilliformis 210
Bartonella henselae 210
Bartonella quintana 210
bartonellosis 210, 211
basal cell carcinoma 468
basic life support 262
BCG vaccination 115, 124, 620
beef tapeworm 398, 399
behaviour changes 72
bejel 472, 473
benign malaria 20, 25, 38
benzodiazepine poisoning 604
Berger's disease 327
beriberi 588–99
β thalassaemia major 530–1
bilharzia 386–9
biliary cirrhosis 372
biliary colic 364
biliary obstruction, intrahepatic 380
bipyridylium 606
Bitot's spots 592, 593
blackouts 438, 439
blackwater fever 28
bladder cancer 321
bladder pain 322
Blantyre Coma Scale 27
Blastomyces dermatitidis 308
blastomycosis 308
blood donations 80
blood films 30, 31, 32–5, 195
body louse 488, 489
body mass index 554
Bolivian haemorrhagic fever 244, 245
bone disease in chronic renal failure 337
Borrelia duttoni 212
Borrelia recurrentis 212
Borrelia 213
bradycardia 260, 264, 266
brain rabies 420
breastfeeding
  dehydration 167, 168
  HIV infection 80
  persistent diarrhoea 172
  relactation 569
  TB 123
breathlessness 288
British National Formulary (BNF) 7
bronchial obstruction 305
bronchiectasis 300
bronchiolitis obliterans 312
bronchitis 180, 298
Brucella melitensis 216
brucellosis 216–17
Brugia malayia 484, 485, 486
Brugian filariasis 484
Brugia timori 484, 485, 486
bubonic plague 218
buccal mass 347
Burkholderia mallei 220
Burkholderia pseudomallei 220
Burkitt's lymphoma 347, 532
burns 600
burr holes 436–7
buruli ulcers 464

C

calcific pancreatitis 156
calculi, renal 338–9

Calymmatobacterium granulomatis 104
Campylobacter coli 134
Campylobacter enterocolitis 134
Campylobacter jejuni 134
Campylobacter laridis 134
cancer 202–5
  bladder 321
  buccal 347
  colorectal 394
  gastric 353
  hepatocellular 378–9
  lung 302–3
  oesophageal 348
  prostatic 323
  renal 324
  skin 468
  tongue 346
Candida albicans 108
candida vaginitis 108
candidiasis 66, 346, 577
candidosis, superficial 476
carbamate poisoning 606
carbamazepine 442
carcinoid tumours 302
cardiac arrest 262–3
cardiac failure 268–71
cardiac glycoside poisoning 604
cardiac rupture 261
cardiogenic shock 260, 272
cardiology 248
  advanced life support protocols 262–5
  angina 254–5
  arrhythmias and conduction 266
  atrial fibrillation 266, 267
  bradycardia 266
  cardiomyopathies 280–1
  chest pain 248–9
  ECG abnormalities 252–3
  heart failure 268–71
  hypertension 274–5
  infective endocarditis 278–9
  myocardial infarct 256–61
  pericardial disease 282–3
  praecordial signs in common heart conditions 250–1
  rheumatic fever 276–7
  shock 272–3
cardiomyopathies 280–1
carditis 276
cat scratch disease 210, 211
ceftazidime resistance 6
cellulitis 470
Central Drug Research Institute, India 2
cerebral malaria 24, 26, 30, 37
cervicitis 88
Chagas disease 226–7
chancroid 104, 105
chemoprophylaxis
  cholera 149
  HIV infection/AIDS 51
  malaria 42–3
  TB 124
chemotherapy
  HIV infection/AIDS 51
  malaria 36, 38–41
  TB 122
chest medicine
  aspergillosis 308–9
  asthma 294–7
  bronchiectasis 300
  chronic obstructive pulmonary disease 298–9
  cough 286
  diffuse parenchymal lung disease 312–13
  dyspnoea/breathlessness 288
  fungal pulmonary infections 306, 308–9
  haemoptysis 286
  lung abscess 304, 305
  lung cancer 302–3
  paragonimiasis 310–11
  pleural effusion 292–3
  pneumothorax 290–1
  pulmonary embolism 304
  wheezing/stridor 288
chest pain 248–9
chest X-rays
  heart failure 269
  pneumonia 190
chickenpox 474
chikungunya 238
childbirth 13
children
  brucellosis 217
  cholera 149
  diabetes mellitus 494
  diarrhoea 172, 173, 174, 175
    dehydration, *see* dehydration
  equine encephalitides 419
  immunization, *see* immunization
  Integrated Management of Childhood Illness 16–17
  intestinal flukes 160
  malaria 24, 26, 28, 36, 42
  measles 232, 234
  nutrition, *see* nutrition
  portal hypertension 385
  rheumatic fever 277
  TB 119
Children's Vaccine Initiative 611
chlamydial infections 102
Chlamydia trachomatis 82, 102
chloramphenicol 413
chloroquine 39, 42, 44
cholangitis, sclerosing 364
cholecystitis 364

cholera 131, 146–9
  vaccine 622
cholera sicca 146
cholestatic jaundice 380
chorea 276
chronic bronchitis 298
chronic calcific pancreatitis 156
chronic cholecystitis 364
chronic constrictive pericarditis 251
chronic disease, anaemia of 516
chronic flaccid paraparesis 448
chronic hepatitis 372
chronic lymphocytic leukaemia 538, 539
chronic malaria 25
chronic meningitis 416
chronic myeloid leukaemia 538–9
chronic obstructive pulmonary disease 298–9
chronic pancreatitis 361
chronic paracoccidioidomycosis 308
chronic renal failure 336–7
chronic spastic paraparesis 448
chronic urticaria 462
chylothorax 292, 293
chyluria 318
cirrhosis 374
  Indian childhood 374
  primary biliary 372
clindamycin 141
clonorchiasis 382
Clonorchis sinensis 382
clostridial myositis 449
Clostridium difficile 140
Clostridium difficile colitis, *see* antibiotic-associated colitis
Clostridium perfringens 150, 449
Clostridium tetani 424
clothing, protective 12, 13, 14, 15
coagulation disorders 546–7
Coccidioides immitis 308
coccidioidomycosis 68, 308
cold autoimmune haemolytic anaemia 521
colic
  biliary 364
  renal 338–9
colitis
  amoebic 358
  antibiotic-associated 140–1
  HIV infection 66
collagen-vascular disease 312
colorectal carcinoma 394
coma 404, 406, 498, 500
  Blantyre Coma Scale 27
  Glasgow coma score 407
communicating hydrocephalus 438
community-acquired pneumonia 183, 184
conception 38
conduction disturbances 252, 260, 266–7
confusion 402, 403
congestive cardiomyopathy 280
conjunctival xerosis 592, 593
conjunctivitis, gonococcal 100
Conn's syndrome 506
constrictive pericarditis 283
contact allergic dermatitis 466
continuous ambulatory peritoneal dialysis 333
contraception 94, 123
convulsions 174
copper poisoning 605
corneal scarring 592
corneal ulceration 592
corneal xerosis 592, 593
corrosives, poisoning with 604
coryza 180
cough 286
counselling, HIV infection 57, 78
Coxiella burnetti 210
crab lice 488, 489
creatinine clearance 315
creeping eruptions 463
crescentic glomerulonephritis 327
Crigler-Nagar syndrome 366
Crimean-Congo haemorrhagic fever 242, 245
crusts, skin 461
cryoprecipitate preparation 547
cryosupernatant preparation 547
cryptococcosis 76
cryptogenic fibrosing alveolitis 312
cryptosporidiosis 150
Cryptosporidium parvum 150
Cushing's syndrome 504
cutaneous larva migrans 463
cutaneous leishmaniasis 478–9
cutaneous manifestations, HIV infection 64–5
cyanide 604
cysticercosis 416, 446–7
cystic hydatid disease 392, 393
cytomegalovirus 62

D

dapsone 42
Darrow's solution 171
dehydration 162, 562, 563
  assessment 163
  fluid defect, estimation of 164
  oral rehydration solution 164–5
  treatment plan A 166
  treatment plan B 167–9
  treatment plan C 170–1
  types 162
delirium 402, 403
dementia 72, 402

dengue fever 236, 238, 239
haemorrhagic 242, 243
dengue shock syndrome 242
dental procedures, prophylaxis before 279
dermatitis 466, 467
dermatology, *see* skin
dermatophytoses 476
dermatosis of kwashiorkor 567
diabetes insipidus 506
diabetic ketoacidosis 498
diabetes mellitus 492–8
diabetic nephropathy 340, 496
dialysis 333
diarrhoeal diseases 130
acute diarrhoea with blood 132, 133
acute diarrhoea without blood 142, 143
amoebic dysentery 136–7
antidiarrhoeal drugs 175
antimicrobial drugs 131
bacillary dysentery 132
Balantidium enterocolitis 134
Campylobacter enterocolitis 134
cholera 146–9
chronic diarrhoea 152, 156–7
classification 130
Clostridium perfringens 150
complications 174
cryptosporidiosis 150
dehydration 162–71
enterohaemorrhagic *E. coli* 132
enterotoxigenic *E. coli* 142
enterotoxin-producing *S. aureus* 142
faecal smear 129
food poisoning 151
giardiasis 144–5
HIV infection 66
home therapy, difficulties 177
intestinal flukes 160–1
malabsorption and steatorrhoea 152–3, 156, 157
malnutrition 574
persistent, management 172–3
post-infective malabsorption 154–5
prevention 176
rotavirus 142
Salmonella enterocolitis 138
strongyloidiasis 158–9
traveller's disease 142, 143
trichuriasis 140, 141
Yersinia enterocolitis 134
diffuse parenchymal lung disease 312–13
digoxin effect 253
dilated cardiomyopathy 280
diphtheria toxoid vaccine 620
directly observed treatment strategy, TB 113, 124
disasters 578
disinfectants 14, 15
disposal of infected wastes 14
disseminated cutaneous leishmaniasis 478
disseminated intravascular coagulation 28, 548–9
diverticular disease 394
donovanosis 104
doxycycline 40, 42
dracunculiasis 482, 483
Dracunculus medinensis 482
Dressler's syndrome 261
drug eruptions 462–3
drug-induced immune haemolytic anaemia 521
dry beriberi 588, 589
dwarf tapeworm 398, 399
dysentery
amoebic 136–7
antimicrobial drugs 131
bacillary 132
dyspepsia 352
dysphagia 66, 348, 349
dyspnoea 288
dysuria 322

E

Ebola virus 241, 244
Echinococcus granulosus 392, 393
Echinococcus multilocularis 392
Echinostoma spp 160
echinostomiasis 160
eczema 466, 467
education 5
see also health education and promotion
Ehrlichia spp 210
ehrlichiosis, human 210
elderly people, urinary tract infection 331
electrocardiogram 251–3, 256, 257
electrolyte disturbances, diarrhoeal diseases 174
elliptocytosis, hereditary 521
emphysema 298
empyema 292
encephalitides, equine 419
encephalitis 418
herpes simplex 418
Japanese 419
measles 234
encephalopathy
hepatic 376
HIV 52
endemic syphilis 472, 473
endocarditis, infective 278–9

endocervicitis 102
endometriosis 92
endocrinology
Addison's disease 504–5
Cushing's syndrome 504
diabetes mellitus 492–8
hyperaldosteronism 506
hyperthyroidism 502
hypopituitarism 506
phaeochromocytoma 506
thyroid eye disease 503
thyroid gland 500–1
Entamoeba histolytica 136, 137
enterobiasis 396
Enterobius vermicularis 396, 397
enterocolitis
Balantidium 134
Campylobacter 134
necrotic 150
Salmonella 138
Yersinia 134
enterohaemorrhagic *E. coli* 132
enteropathogenic *E. coli* 156
enterotoxigenic *E. coli* 142
enterotoxin-producing *Staphylococcus aureus* 142
enuresis, nocturnal 322
eosinophilia, pulmonary 312, 486
eosinophilic meningoencephalitis 416
epidemic meningococcal disease 414, 415
epidemics 8–11
cholera 148–9
epididymo-orchitis 86
epilepsy 440–4
equine encephalitides 419
eruptions, drug 462–3
erysipelas 470
erythema multiforme 462
Escherichia coli
enterohaemorrhagic 132
enteropathogenic 156
enterotoxigenic 142
Essential Drugs Programme 6–7
essential thrombocythaemia 540
ethambutol 123
Expanded Programme on Immunization 611, 620–2
extradural haematoma 436
extravascular haemolysis 520
extrinsic allergic alveolitis 312
exudates 292, 293

F

faecal smears 129
falciparum malaria 20, 24–5
chemotherapy 38, 39, 40, 41
diagnosis 30
management 36
multidrug-resistant 44
severe malaria 26
famine oedema 558
Fansidar (pyrimethamine) 40, 42
fasciitis, necrotizing 470
Fasciola gigantica 380
Fasciola hepatica 380, 381
fascioliasis 380
fasciolopsiasis 160
Fasciolopsis buski 160, 161
febrile convulsions 174
fetus, HIV infection 74
see also pregnancy
fevers
arbovirus haemorrhagic 242–5
arenavirus haemorrhagic 244, 245
Argentinian haemorrhagic 244, 245
Bolivian haemorrhagic 244, 245
cancer 202
Crimean-Congo haemorrhagic 242, 245
dengue 236, 238, 239
dengue haemorrhagic 242, 243
diarrhoea 174
differential diagnosis 194–7
filovirus haemorrhagic 244
HIV infection 58
Lassa 244, 245
paratyphoid 206–7
Q 210
relapsing 212–13
rheumatic 276–7
Rift Valley 242, 245
trench 210
typhoid 206–7
typhus 208–9
viral haemorrhagic 15, 240–1
yellow 242, 243
F-100 564, 565, 568
fibrocalculous pancreatic diabetes 492
filariasis 480
lymphatic 484–6
filovirus haemorrhagic fever 244
flaccid paralysis 448, 450, 453
flaccid paraparesis 448
fluid defect, estimation of 164
fluid overload 268
flukes
intestinal 160–1
lung 310–11
focal neurological signs, HIV infection 72
focal segmental glomerulonephritis 327
focal segmental glomerulosclerosis 327

focal *Toxoplasma* encephalitis 74
folate deficiency 519
food poisoning 150, 151
fourth heart sound 250
F-75 564, 565
fungal pulmonary infections 306–9
fungal skin infections 476
furious rabies 420

G

gallstones 365
Gambian sleeping sickness 222, 223, 224
Gardnerella vaginalis 106
gastric cancer 353
gastritis 352
gastroenterology
  acute abdomen 354–5
  alcoholic liver disease 374, 375
  amoebic liver abscess 382–3
  appendicitis 356–7
  ascariasis 362–3
  cirrhosis 372, 374
  clonorchiasis 382
  dyspepsia 352
  dysphagia 348, 349
  enterobiasis 396–7
  episthorchiasis 382, 383
  fascioliasis 380, 381
  gastric cancer 353
  gastritis 352
  haemochromatosis 373
  hepatic neoplasia 378
  hepatitis 368–72
  hepatocellular carcinoma 378–9
  hepatomegaly 366, 384
  hydatid disease 392–3
  jaundice 366–7, 369, 380, 381
  liver disease 366
  liver failure 376
  lower GI bleeding 394–5
  mouth and pharynx 346–7
  oesophageal carcinoma 348
  oesophageal varices 351
  pancreatitis 360–1
  peptic ulcer 352
  peritonitis 358–9
  portal hypertension 384–5
  pruritus ani 396
  reflux oesophagitis 348
  right upper quadrant pain 364–5
  schistosomiasis 386–9
  toxocariasis 390
  upper GI bleeding 350
  visible "worms" in stool 398–9
  Wilson's disease 373
gastrointestinal symptoms
  HIV infection 66–7
  malaria 29
  TB 118
genetic drift 231
genetic shift 231
genital herpes 108
genital ulcers 84, 85
genitourinary hydatid disease 325
genitourinary pain 322–3
genitourinary TB 118
gentamicin 190
giant-cell arteritis 408
Giardia agilis 145
Giardia intestinalis 131, 144, 145
Giardia muris 145
giardiasis 144
Gilbert's syndrome 366
gingivitis 346–7
gingivorrhoea 346, 584
gingivostomatitis 346
girls, education 5
glanders 220
Glasgow coma score 407
Global Programme on AIDS 60
glomerular disease 326, 327, 328
glossitis 346
gloves, protective 12, 13, 14
glucose-6-phosphate dehydrogenase deficiency 522–3
goitre 501, 582–3
gold poisoning 605
gonococcal conjunctivitis 100
gonorrhoea 82, 100–1
government health care provision 4–5
granuloma inguinale 104
granulomatous amoebic encephalitis 416
granulomatous vasculitides 312
growth charts 554–5
Guillain-Barre syndrome 450–1, 453
gum disease 584, 585
gunshot wounds 601
guttate psoriasis 466

H

haematology
  anaemia, *see* anaemia
  coagulation disorders 546–7
  disseminated intravascular coagulation 548–9
  glucose-6-phosphate dehydrogenase deficiency 522–3
  haemostatic disorders 544–5
  hookworms 517
  leukaemias 536–9
  lymphomas 532–5
  myeloma 540

myeloproliferative disorders 540
splenomegaly 542
thalassaemia 528–31
whipworms 517
haematuria 318, 319
haemochromatosis 373
haemoglobinuria 318
haemolytic anaemias 520–3, 548
haemolytic crises 524
haemolytic-uraemic syndrome 334
haemophilia A 546
haemophilia B 546
Haemophilus ducreyi 104
Haemophilus influenzae type B 184
vaccine 622
haemoptysis 286
haemorrhagic fever 197
arbovirus 242–5
viral 240–1
haemorrhoids 395
haemostatic disorders 544–5
haemothorax 293
halofantrine 40
hand washing 12, 13, 14
Hansen's disease (leprosy) 454–7
HbSC disease 526
HbSβ° thalassaemia 526
HbSβ^{+} thalassaemia 526
HbSD^{Punjab} 526
Hb Bart's hydrops fetalis 529
HbH disease 529
headache 72, 408
head lice 488, 489
Heaf test 115, 120, 121
health education and promotion
cholera 148
diabetes mellitus 494
malaria 44
TB 124
heart failure 268–71, 566–7
Helicobacter pylori 352
helminthiasis 576
hepatic disease 66
hepatic encephalopathy 376
hepatic neoplasia 378
hepatocellular carcinoma 378–9
hepatomegaly 366, 384
hepato-renal syndrome 334
hepatosplenomegaly 530
hepatitis 371, 372
hepatitis A 368
vaccine 622
hepatitis B 370
vaccine 620
hepatitis C 369
hepatitis D 371
hepatitis E 368
hepatitis F 368
hepatitis G 368
herbal medicines 2
hereditary elliptocytosis 521
hereditary ovalocytosis 521
hereditary spherocytosis 521
hernia, hiatus 352
herpes, genital 108
herpes simplex virus encephalitis 418
heterophyasis 160
Heterophyes heterophyes 161
Heterophyes spp 160
hiatus hernia 352
histoplasmosis 68, 308
Hodgkin's lymphoma 534, 535
hookworm 140, 362, 363, 517
human ehrlichiosis 210
human immunodeficiency virus (HIV)/AIDS 50–1
clinical features 52–3
clinical presentation and management 58–77
diagnosis 54–7
encephalopathy 52
and genital herpes 108
and genital ulcers 84
immunization 618
and malaria 24
malnutrition 24, 576
management of asymptomatic patients 78–9
prevention and control 80
and TB 58, 126–7
universal precautions 12, 13
wasting syndrome 52
human sleeping sickness 222–5
hydatid disease 392–3
hydrocephalus 438
Hymendepsis nana 398, 399
hyperaldosteronism 506
hypercalcaemia 202, 204, 253
hyperglycaemia hyperosmolar non-ketotic coma 498
hyperkalaemia 253
hypernatraemic dehydration 162
hypernephroma 324
hyperparasitaemia 29
hyperprolactinaemia 506
hyperpyrexia 28
hyperreactive malarial splenomegaly 25
hypersensitivity vasculitides 312
hypertension 274–5
portal 384–5
hyperthyroidism 502
hypertonic dehydration 162
hypertrophic cardiomyopathy 281
hypocalcaemia 253
hypoglycaemia 28, 174, 498, 563
hypokalaemia 253
hyponatraemic dehydration 162
hypopigmentation 460
hypopituitarism 506

ypoprothrombinaemias, acquired 546
hypothyroidism 500–1
hypotonic dehydration 162
hypovolaemic shock 272
hypothermia 562

I

iatrogenic pneumothorax 290
immunization 612–13, 622–5
  adverse reactions 616
  contraindications 618–19
  Expanded Programme on Immunization 611, 620–2
  new vaccinations 625
  strategies and schedules 614–15
  tetanus 616, 617
immunoglobulin A nephropathy 327
impetigo 470
incontinence 322
Indian childhood cirrhosis 374
infantile beriberi 588, 589
infected wastes, disposal of 14
infection control 12
infectious mononucleosis 230
infective endocarditis 278–9
inflammatory bowel disease 395
influenza 230, 231
  vaccine 622–3
inguinal bubo 84
injections, universal precautions 13
injuries 599–601
insulin-dependent diabetes mellitus 492
Integrated Management of Childhood Illness 16–17
intermittent peritoneal dialysis 333
interstitial lung disease 312–13
interstitial nephritis 326
intestinal flukes 160–1
intestinal lymphoma 157
intracranial pressure, rising 410
intrahepatic biliary obstruction 380
intra-uterine contraceptive device, removal 94
intravascular haemolysis 520
intravenous urography 317
invasive aspergillosis 306
invasive procedures, universal precautions 13
invasive salmonellosis 138
Investing in Health 4–5
iodine deficiency surveys 582–3
Ippy virus 245
iron-deficiency anaemia 54
iron overload 531
irritant dermatitis 466
ischaemic heart disease 255
isolation precautions 15
isoniazid 132, 604–5
isotonic dehydration 162

J

Japanese encephalitis 419
  vaccine 623
jaundice 366
  hepatocellular causes 369
  investigations 367
  malaria 26
  post-hepatic causes 380, 381
  pre-hepatic causes 366–7
Junin virus 244, 245

K

kala-azar 228–9
Kaposi sarcoma 64–5
Kaposi sarcoma associated virus 64
katayama fever 386, 389
keratomalacia 592, 593
kerosene poisoning 605
ketoacidosis, diabetic 498
kidney lumps 324
kidney tumours 324–5
Koebner phenomenon 466
kwashiorkor 558–9, 561
  dermatosis of 567
Kyasanur Forest disease 242

L

laboratory investigations 626
laboratory specimens 14
lactic acidosis 28
large-cell carcinoma 302
larva currens 463
larva migrans 463
Lassa fever 244, 245
laundry 14
lead poisoning 605
left atrial myxoma 281
left ventricular aneurysm 261
left ventricular failure 260, 268
Legionella pneumophila 185
legionnaires' disease 185
Leishmania aethiopica 479
Leishmania braziliensis 479
Leishmania chagasi 228, 229
Leishmania donovani 228, 229
Leishmania guyanensis 479
Leishmania infantum 228, 229
leishmaniasis
  cutaneous 478–9
  visceral 228–9
lepromatous leprosy 454, 455
leprosy 454–7
Leptospira interrogans 214
leptospirosis 214

leukaemias 536–9
lice 488, 489
life support 262–5
linen 14
lipoid pneumonia 312
lithium carbonate poisoning 605
liver
amoebic abscess 382–3
metastases 379
non-smooth 379
liver disease 366
alcoholic 374, 375
coagulation disorders 547
liver failure 376
Loa loa 482, 483
loiasis 482
louse-borne relapsing fever 212
louse-borne typhus 208, 209
lower abdominal pain 92–4
lower GI bleeding 394–5
lung abscesses 304, 305
lung cancer 302–3
lung disease, diffuse parenchymal 312–13
lung fluke disease 310–11
lymphadenopathy 60–1
lymphangiectasia 156
lymphatic filariasis 484–6
lymphoblastic leukaemia 536, 537
lymphocytic leukaemia 538, 539
lymphocytic pulmonary infiltration 312
lymphogranuloma venereum 102
lymphomas 532–5
intestinal 157

M

Machupo virus 244, 245
macrocytic anaemia 518–19
maculopapular rashes 460
Madura foot 476
maintenance hosts 236
malabsorption 152–6
malaria 20
benign 20, 25
chemoprophylaxis 42–3
chemotherapy 38–41
diagnosis 30–1
epidemiology 22–3
falciparum 20, 24–5
fever 195
future 44
identification of parasites on blood films 32–5
life cycle and transmission 20–1
malnutrition 576
management 36–7
multidrug-resistant 44, 45
severe 20, 26–9
treatment failure 44
uncomplicated 20
malarone (proguanil) 41, 42
malignant disease, renal manifestations 342
malnutrition 580–1
defining and assessing 554–7
and diarrhoea 173
infection 552–3
and malaria 24
measles 232
oedematous 558–9
malnutrition-related diabetes mellitus 492
Maloprim 42
Mantoux test 115, 120
marasmus 560, 561
Marburg virus 245
massive myoglobulinuria 334
measles 232–5
vaccination 566, 620–1
Medline 2
mefloquine 38, 40, 42
megaloblastic anaemia 518
melanoma 468
melioidosis 220, 221
membranoproliferative glomerulonephritis 327
membranous glomerulonephritis 327
meningism 72, 406
meningitis
bacterial 412–13
chronic 416
diarrhoeal diseases 174
headache 408
tuberculosis 118
viral 414
meningococcal disease 414, 415
meningococcal vaccine 623
meningoencephalitis
amoebic 416
eosinophilic 416
mercury poisoning 605
mesenteric adenitis 357
metabolic acidosis 174
metastases 302
metal ion poisoning 605
metriphonate 389
microangiopathic haemolytic anaemia 548
microcytic anaemia 514–16
micturating cysturethrogram 317
micturition dysfunction 322
mid-upper arm circumference 556, 557
migraine 408
miliary TB 116
mineral mix 565
minimal change glomerulonephritis 327

mite typhus 208
mitral incompetence 250
mitral stenosis 250
mononeuropathies 452
mononucleosis, infectious 230
Mopeia virus 245
morphine 204
mouth-to-mouth resuscitation 12
mucosal leishmaniasis 478
multibacillary leprosy 454, 456
multidrug resistance
  malaria 44, 45
  TB 124
multiple myeloma 342
mumps vaccine 623
mural thrombus 261
murine typhus 208
mycobacterial infection 62, 112, 114
Mycobacterium 112
Mycobacterium bovis 112, 114, 115
Mycobacterium leprae 454
Mycobacterium tuberculosis 112, 114, 126, 127
Mycobacterium ulcerans 464
myelitis, transverse 453
myeloblastic leukaemia 536–7
myeloid leukaemia 538–9
myeloma 540
  multiple 342
myeloproliferative disorders 540
myetoma 476
myocardial dysfunction 260
myocardial infarct 256–61
myocarditis, acute 281
myoglobinuria 318, 334
myositis, clostridial 449
myxoedema 500–1

N

NAPRALERT 2
Necator americanus 517
necrotic enterocolitis 150
necrotizing fasciitis 470
necrotizing ulcerative gingivitis 347
needlestick injuries 12, 13, 80
Neisseria gonorrhoeae 82, 100
neonates
  BCG vaccination 124
  malaria 24, 42
  syphilis 99
  tetanus 424
nephritic syndrome 326
nephritis 340
  interstitial 326
  SLE 327
nephroblastoma 324
nephropathy, diabetic 340, 496
nephrotic syndrome 328–9
nephrotoxins 334
neuritis, traumatic 453
neurology
  acute confusional state 402, 403
  acute flaccid paralysis 453
  bacterial meningitis 412–13
  burr holes 436–7
  blackouts 438, 439
  chronic meningitis 416
  coma 404, 407
  cysticercosis 446–7
  dementia 402
  encephalitis 418–19
  eosinophilic meningoencephalitis 416
  epidemic meningococcal disease 414
  epilepsy 440–4
  extradural haematoma 436
  Guillain-Barre syndrome 450–1
  headache 408
  HIV infection 72–7
  hydrocephalus 438
  intracranial pressure, rising 410
  leprosy 454–7
  mono/polyneuropathies 452
  poliomyelitis 450, 451
  primary amoebic meningoencephalitis 416–17
  rabies 420–3
  space-occupying lesions 438
  stroke 428–33
  subarachnoid haemorrhage 434
  subdural haemorrhage 434–5
  tetanus 424–7
  unconscious patients, management 406
  viral meningitis 414–15
  weak legs/paraplegia 448–9
neurosyphilis 98, 99
neutropenia 204
nicotinic acid 590
night blindness 592
nocturnal enuresis 322
nodal rhythms 260
nodules
  skin 461
  thyroid 501
non-Burkitt's lymphoma 532
non-communicating hydrocephalus 438
non-Hodgkin's lymphoma 532
non-insulin-dependent diabetes mellitus 492
non-megaloblastic macrocytic anaemia 518
non-venereal treponematoses 472–3
normal saline 171
normocytic anaemia 516

nosocomial pneumonia 188
notifiable diseases 9
nutrition
  assessment of acutely sick infants 550–1
  beriberi 588–9
  disasters and refugee camps 578
  failure to respond to treatment 572–6
  goitre 582–3
  malnutrition, *see* malnutrition
  obesity 596–7
  osteomalacia 586
  pellagra 590–1
  rehabilitation 568–71
  rickets 586
  scurvy 584
  severe wasting/marasmus 560–1
  specific problems 562–7
  tooth decay and gum disease 584–5
  vitamin A deficiency 592–3
  vitamin B^2 deficiency 586
  vitamin B^{12} deficiency 594, 595
  vitamin E deficiency 594
  vitamin K deficiency 594

O

oat-cell carcinomas 302
obesity 596–7
obstructive cardiomyopathy 281
occupational exposure to HIV infection 80
ocular toxocariasis 390
oedematous malnutrition 558–9, 561
oesophageal candidiasis 66
oesophageal carcinoma 348
oesophageal varices 351
oesophagitis, reflux 348
Old World tick typhus 208
oliguria 322
Onchocerca volvulus 480
onchocerciasis 480–1
onyalai 544
opiate poisoning 605
opisthorchiasis 382
Opisthorchis felineus 382
Opisthorchis guayaquilensis 382
Opisthorchis sinensis 382
Opisthorchis spp 160
Opisthorchis viverrini 382, 383
opportunistic infections 50, 52
oral candidiasis 346
oral rehydration solution 164–5, 166, 167, 168–9, 170
organochloride poisoning 606
organophosphate poisoning 606
Ornithodoros spp 212
oropharyngeal pathology 346–7
Oroya fever 210
osteodystrophy, renal 337
osteomalacia 586
otitis media 574
outbreaks 8–11
  cholera 148–9
ovalocytosis, south-east Asian hereditary 521
overcrowding 232
overflow incontinence 322
oxamniquine 389
oxygen therapy 299

P

pain and cancer 202, 204–5
palmar psoriasis 466
pancreatic calcification 156
pancreatic dysfunction 156
pancreatitis 360–1
Panstrongylus megistus 227
papular urticaria 462
paracetamol poisoning 605
Paracoccidioides brasiliensis 308
paracoccidioidomycosis 308
paragonimiasis 310–11
paralysis, acute flaccid 448, 450, 453
paralytic rabies 420
paraneoplastic syndromes 202
paraparesis 448
paraplegia 448–9
paratyphoid fever 206–7
parenchymal disease 312–13
paroxysmal cold haemoglobinuria 521
paraquat 606
patent ductus arteriosus 250
paucibacillary leprosy 454, 456
Pediculosis capitis 488, 489
Pediculosis humanus 488, 489
Pediculus humanus 212
pellagra 590–1
pelvic inflammatory disease 92, 94
penetrating wounds 601
penicilliosis marneffei 62
peptic ulcer 352
perianal discomfort 66
pericardial effusion 282
pericardial TB 118
pericarditis 251, 261, 282, 283
peripartum cardiac failure 269
periodontal disease 584
peripheral neuropathy 72
peritonitis 354, 358–9
persistent generalized lymphadenopathy 60
pertussis vaccine 621
pesticide poisoning 606
petechiae 461

phaeochromocytoma 506
pharyngitis 347
pharynx 346–7
phenobarbital 442
phenytoin 442
Phthirus pubis 488, 489
physiological saline 171
piercing, skin 13
pigbel 150
  vaccine 623
pigmented buccal lesions 347
piles 395
pinta 472, 473
pinworm 396–7
pityriasis versicolor 476
plague 218–19
plantar psoriasis 466
plaques, skin 461
Plasmodium falciparum 20, 24, 30, 36
  chemotherapy 38, 39, 40, 41
  identification on blood films 33–5
  multidrug resistance 44
  severe malaria 26
Plasmodium malariae 20, 24, 25, 33–5
Plasmodium ovale 20, 25, 33–5, 39
Plasmodium vivax 20, 24, 25
  chemoprophylaxis 42
  chemotherapy 39
  identification on blood films 33–5
  multidrug resistance 44
platelet disorders 544
pleural effusion 292–3
pleurodesis 290, 291
pneumaturia 322
pneumococcal pneumonia 186–7
pneumococcal vaccines 624
pneumoconioses 312
Pneumocystis carinii 70
Pneumocystis carinii pneumonia 70
pneumocystosis 70–1
pneumonia 182
  aspiration 188
  atypical 184–5
  classification 183
  clinical features 182
  community-acquired 183, 184
  legionnaires' disease 185
  lipoid 312
  malnutrition 574
  management 189–90
  nosocomial 188
  pneumococcal 186–7
  recurrent 188
pneumonic plague 218
pneumothorax 290–1
poisoning 602–9
poliomyelitis 450, 451, 453
  vaccine 621
polyarthritic psoriasis 466
polycystic kidney disease 324
polycythaemia 540
polycythaemia rubra vera 540
polyneuropathies 452
pork tapeworm 398, 399, 446, 447
portal hypertension 384–5
post-infective malabsorption 154–5
post-kalar dermal leishmania 228
post-mortem procedures 13
post-primary TB 114, 116–18
Pott's disease 118
poverty 4
poxvirus skin infections 474
praecordial signs in common heart conditions 250–1
praziquantel 389
pre-eclampsia 334
pregnancy
  acute renal failure 332, 334
  anaemia 513
  asymptomatic bacteriuria 331
  brucellosis 217
  cardiac failure 269
  goitre 582
  gonorrhoea 100
  hypertension 274
  immunization 616, 617
  lower abdominal pain 94
  malaria 24, 38, 39, 42
  sepsis 200–1
  sickle-cell disease 525, 526
  syphilis 99
  thalassaemia 531
  tuberculosis 123
  see also fetus
primaquine 39
primary amoebic meningoencephalitis 416
primary biliary cirrhosis 372
primary pneumothorax 290
primary TB 114, 116
proctitis 102
progressive multifocal leukoencephalopathy 76
proguanil 41, 42
proliferative glomerulonephritis 327
prostatic carcinoma 323
prostatic pain 322
prostatitis, bacterial 331
protective clothing 12, 13, 14, 15
protein-deficient pancreatic diabetes 492
proteinuria 329
pruritus ani 396
pseudomembranous colitis 140–1
psoriasis 466, 467
psychogenic headache 408
pubic lice 488, 489
puerperal sepsis 200, 201

pulmonary aspiration 305
pulmonary embolism 253, 304
pulmonary eosinophilia 312, 486
pulmonary haemorrhagic disorders 312
pulmonary infections, fungal 306–9
pulmonary oedema 28
pulmonary TB 116, 117, 120, 126
purpura 544
pustular psoriasis 466
pustules 461
pyogenic pericarditis 282
pyomyositis, tropical 449
pyrazinamide 123
pyridoxine 123
pyrimethamine 40, 42
pyruvate kinase deficiency 521
pyuria, sterile 331

Q

Q fever 210
quinidine 40
quinine 38, 39, 40

R

rabies 420–3
  vaccine 624
rashes 197, 460–1
recurrent pneumonia 188
red blood cells disorders
  anaemia, *see* anaemia
  glucose-6-phosphate dehydrogenase deficiency 522–3
  hookworms 517
  thalassaemia 528–31
  whipworms 517
reflux oesophagitis 348
refugee camps 578
relactation 569
relapsing fever 212
renal calculi 338–9
renal carcinoma 324
renal colic 338–9
renal disease
  chyluria 318
  creatinine clearance 315
  genitourinary pain 322–3
  glomerular disease 326, 327
  haematuria 318, 319
  interstitial nephritis 326
  kidney lumps 324
  kidney tumours 324–5
  micturition dysfunction 322
  nephrotic syndrome 326, 328–9
  prostatic carcinoma 323
  renal calculi and renal colic 338–9
  renal failure 332–7
  renal manifestations of systemic diseases 340–2
  urinary schistosomiasis 320–1
  urinary tract infection 330–1
  urine 316–17
renal failure 332–7
renal impairment, malaria 26
renal osteodystrophy 337
renal pain 322
renal parenchymal disease 334
renal syndrome 244
renal vein thrombosis 328
reserve antibiotics 7
resistance
  antibiotics 6–7
  malaria 44, 45
  TB 124
ReSoMal 562
respiratory infections 180–1
  see also pneumonia
respiratory manifestations, HIV infection 68-71
restrictive cardiomyopathy 280
resuscitation, mouth-to-mouth 12
rhabdomyolosis 334
rheumatic fever 276–7
rheumatoid arthritis 342
Rhodesian sleeping sickness 222, 223, 224
rickets 586
rickettsial infections 210–11
rickettsial pox 208
Rickettsia spp 208
rifampicin 2, 123
Rift Valley fever 242, 245
right upper quadrant pain 364–5
right ventricular failure 268
right ventricular infarct 261
Ringer's Lactate solution 170, 171
rotavirus 142
rubella vaccine 624
rumination 574

S

salicylate poisoning 605
Salmonella enteritidis 138
Salmonella enterocolitis 138
Salmonella spp 388
Salmonella typhimurium 138
salpingitis (pelvic inflammatory disease) 92, 94
sarcoidosis 312, 342
Sarcoptes scabiei 488, 489
scabies 488, 576
Schilling test 152
Schistosoma haematobium 320, 321, 386, 387, 389

Schistosoma intercalatum 320, 386, 387
Schistosoma japonicum 386, 387, 388
Schistosoma mansoni 386, 387, 388
Schistosoma mekongi 386, 387
schistosomiasis 386–9
  urinary 320–1
scleroderma 342
sclerosing cholangitis 364
scrotal swelling 86–7
scrub typhus 208
scurvy 584
secondary pneumothorax 290
seizures 72
Semple vaccine 422
sepsis 198–9
  female genital tract 358
  during pregnancy 200–1
septal defect
  atrial 251
  ventricular 250
septic abortions 200, 201
septicaemia 305
septic shock 198, 562, 563, 564
severe asthma 296–7
severe malaria 20, 24, 26–9
severe wasting 560, 561
sexual behaviour 80
sexually transmitted diseases 48–9
  bacterial vaginosis 106
  candida vaginitis 108
  chancroid 104, 105
  chlamydial infections 102
  genital herpes 108
  gonorrhoea 100–1
  granuloma inguinale 104
  symptomatic management
    genital ulcers 84, 85
    inguinal bubo 84
    lower abdominal pain 92–4
    scrotal swelling 86–7
    urethral discharge 82–3
    vaginal discharge 88–91
  syphilis 96–9
  trichomoniasis 106
  see also human immunodeficiency virus (HIV)/AIDS
Shakir strips 556, 557
sharp injuries 12, 13
Shigella boydii 132
Shigella dysenteriae 132
Shigella flexneri 132
Shigella sonneii 132
shigellosis 132
shingles 474
shock 272
  anaphylactic 273
  cardiogenic 260, 272
  malaria 28
  septic 198, 562, 563, 564
short-course chemotherapy 122
sickle-cell anaemia 342, 524–7
sickle-cell trait 526
sideroblastic anaemia 516
sinus bradycardia 260
skeletal TB 118
skin
  bacterial infections 470
  cancers 468
  cutaneous leishmaniasis 478–9
  dermatitis 466, 467
  dracunculiasis 482, 483
  drug eruptions 462–3
  filariasis 480
  fungal infections 476
  infestations 488–9
  loiasis 482, 483
  lymphatic filariasis 484–6
  non-venereal treponematoses 472–3
  onchocerciasis 480–1
  poxvirus infections 474
  psoriasis 466, 467
  rashes 197, 460–1
  ulcers 464–5
  urticaria 462
  varicella-zoster infection 474
skin-piercing 13
sleeping sickness 222–5
small-cell carcinoma 302
small-form histoplasmosis 308
smear-negative pulmonary TB 117
smear-positive pulmonary TB 117
snake bite 608–9
socioeconomic factors, TB 124
sodium valproate 442
sore throat 181
south-east Asian hereditary ovalocytosis 521
space-occupying lesions 438
spastic paraparesis, chronic 448
spherocytosis, hereditary 521
spinal cord compression 204
spine rabies 420
spinocerebral gnathostomiasis 416
splenomegaly 542
splenectomies 542
sporotrichosis 476
Sporothrix shenckii 476
spotted fever 208
squamous cell carcinoma 302, 468
stable malaria 22
staining 111
Staphylococcus aureus 142, 184, 198, 431
status epilepticus 444
steatorrhoea 152, 157
sterile pyuria 331
Stevens-Johnson syndrome 462
stranguary 322

Streptococcus pneumoniae 182, 184, 186
Streptococcus pyogenes 198, 470
streptokinase 259
streptomycin 123
stress incontinence 322
stridor 288
stroke 428–33
Strongyloides stercoralis 158, 159
strongyloidiasis 158
subacute sclerosing panencephalitis 234
subarachnoid haemorrhage 434
subdural haemorrhage 434–5
suicide, attempted 603
sulfadoxine-pyrimethamine 40
superficial candidosis 476
supraventricular arrhythmias 252, 260
swimmer's itch 386
Sydenham's chorea 276
symptomatic HIV infection 52, 54
syncope 438
syphilis 96–9
  endemic 472, 473
systemic collagen-vascular diseases 312
systemic lupus erythematosus (SLE) 342
  nephritis 327
systemic manifestations, HIV infection 58–62
systemic sclerosis 342

T

tachycardia 260, 264–5
Taenia saginata 398, 399
Taenia solium 398, 399, 446, 447
tapeworms 398–9
tension headache 408
tension pneumothorax 290
testicular pain 322
testicular torsion 86, 87
tetanus 424–7
  immunization 616, 617, 621–2
tetracycline 40, 41
thalassaemia 526, 528–31
thallium poisoning 606
therapeutic feeding centres 578
thiacetazone 123
third heart sound 250
threadworm 396–7
throat soreness 181
thrombocythaemia, essential 540
thrombocytopenia 544, 545
thrombosis, renal vein 328
thyroid eye disease 503
thyroid gland 500
thyroid nodules 501
thyroid tumours 501
thyrotoxicosis 502
tick bites 197
tick-borne relapsing fever 212
tick typhus 208
tinea 476
tongue 346
tooth decay 584
torsion of the testis 86, 87
toxic shock syndrome 198
Toxocara canis 390
toxocariasis 390
Toxoplasma gonii 74
toxoplasmosis 74
traditional health care systems 2
transudates 292, 293
transverse myelitis 453
traumatic neuritis 453
traumatic pneumothorax 290
traveller's diarrhoea 142, 143
treatment plan A 166
treatment plan B 167–9
treatment plan C 170–1
trench fever 210
Treponema pallidum 96
Trichomonas vaginalis 82, 106
trichomoniasis 106
trichuriasis 140
Trichuris trichiura 140, 141, 517
tricyclic antidepressant poisoning 605
Tropheryma whippei 156
Tropical Medicine Resource 3
tropical pulmonary eosinophilia 486
tropical pyomyositis 449
tropical splenomegaly syndrome 25
tropical sprue 154–55
tropical ulcers 464
true incontinence 322
Trypanosoma brucei spp 222, 223, 225
Trypanosoma cruzi 226, 227
Trypanosoma rangeli 226
trypanosomiasis
  African 222–5
  American 226–7
tuberculin test 115, 120
tuberculoid leprosy 454, 455
tuberculosis 112
  clinical features 116–19
  diagnosis 120–1
  directly observed treatment strategy 113
  disease and pathogenesis 114–15
  global burden 113
  and HIV 58, 126–7
  malnutrition 576
  microbiology 112
  staining 111
  transmission 112

treatment 122–5
tuberculosis adenitis 118
tuberculosis meningitis 118
tuberculous pericarditis 282
tubular necrosis, acute 334
typhoid 206–7
vaccine 624–5
typhus fevers 208–9

U

ulcerative gingivitis, acute necrotizing 347
ulcers
aphthous 346
corneal 592
genital 84, 85
peptic 352
skin 464–5
ultrasound 317
uncomplicated malaria 20, 36
chemotherapy 38, 39, 40, 41
United Nations
UNAIDS 56
UNICEF 16–17, 611
universal precautions 12–14
unstable angina 254
unstable malaria 22
upper GI bleeding 350
upper respiratory tract infections 180
uraemia 355
ureteric pain 322
urethral discharge 82–3
urethral syndrome 331
urethritis 102
urge incontinence 322
urinary catheters 331
urinary schistosomiasis 320–1
urinary tract 317
infection 330–1, 576
urine 316
urothelial tumours 324
urticaria 461, 462

V

vaginal discharge 88–91
vaginitis 88
candida 108
vaginosis, bacterial 106
varicella-zoster infection 474
varices, oesophageal 351
vascular-occlusive crises 524
vascular purpura 544
Venezuelan haemorrhagic fever 245
ventricular arrhythmias 252, 260
ventricular septal defect 250
Vibrio cholerae 146, 147
viral haemorrhagic fever 15, 240–1
viral hepatitis 368–71
viral meningitis 414
viral respiratory infections 180–1
visceral leishmaniasis 228–9
visceral sequestration crises 524
visual impairment, HIV infection 72
vitamin A deficiency 174, 566, 592–3
vitamin B^2 deficiency 586
vitamin B^{12} deficiency 519, 586, 594, 595
vitamin C deficiency 584
vitamin D deficiency 586
vitamin E deficiency 594
vitamin K antagonism 546, 594
vitamin K deficiency 546
vitamin mix 564, 565
von Willebrand's disease 546

W

warm autoimmune haemolytic anaemia 521
waste disposal 14
wasting, severe 560, 561
weak legs 448–9
weakness, HIV infection 58
weight loss 552, 553, 554–7
cancer 202
HIV infection 58
Weil's disease 214
Wellcome Trust, Tropical Medicine Resource 3
west beriberi 588, 589
wheezing 288
Whipple's disease 156
whipworm 140, 141, 517
white blood cells
leukaemias 536–9
lymphomas 532–5
white cell counts 195–6
Wilm's tumour 324
Wilson's disease 373
women
conception 38
empowerment 5
HIV infection 80
pregnant, *see* pregnancy
tetanus immunization 616, 617
urinary tract infection 331
World Bank, World Development Report 4–5
World Health Organization
cancer 203
cholera 148
Essential Drugs Programme 6–7
Expanded Programme on Immunization 611
HIV infection and disease 52, 54, 56, 60

  Integrated Management of
      Childhood Illness 16–17
  malaria, severe 27
  tuberculosis 113
Wuchereria bancrofti 484, 485, 486

xerophthalmia 592–3
xerosis
  conjunctival 592, 593
  corneal 592, 593
xylose absorption test 152

yaws 572, 573
yellow fever 242, 243
  vaccine 622

Z

Ziehl-Neelsen test 112
zinc poisoning 605